I0634252

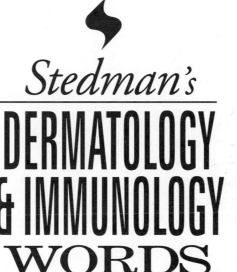

Stedman's

DERMATOLOGY & IMMUNOLOGY WORDS

WORDS

INCLUDES RHEUMATOLOGY, ALLERGY, & TRANSPLANTATION

THIRD EDITION

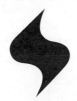

Stedman's

DERMATOLOGY & IMMUNOLOGY

WORDS

INCLUDES
RHEUMATOLOGY, ALLERGY, & TRANSPLANTATION

THIRD EDITION

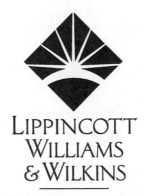

LIPPINCOTT
WILLIAMS
& WILKINS

Publisher: Julie K. Stegman
Senior Product Manager: Eric Branger
Associate Managing Editor: Steve Lichtenstein
Production Coordinator: Jason Delaney
Typesetter: Josephine Bergin
Printer & Binder: RR Donnelley

Copyright © 2005 Lippincott Williams & Wilkins
351 West Camden Street
Baltimore, Maryland 21201-2436

All rights reserved. This book is protected by copyright. No part of this book may be re-produced in any form or by any means, including photocopying, or utilized by any information storage and retrieval system without written permission from the copyright owner.

Printed in the United States of America

Third Edition, 2005

Library of Congress Cataloging-in-Publication Data

Stedman's dermatology & immunology words : includes rheumatology, allergy & transplantation.— 3rd ed.
    p. ; cm.— (Stedman's word books)
Includes bibliographical references.
    ISBN 0–7817-5530–1
    1. Dermatology—Terminology. 2. Immunology—Terminology.3. Allergy—Terminology. 4. Rheumatology—Terminology. 5. Transplantation of organs, tissues, etc.—Terminology. I. Title: Dermatology & immunology words. II. Title: Stedman's dermatology and immunology words. III. Series.
    [DNLM: 1. Dermatology—Terminology—English. 2. Rheumatology—Terminology—English. 3. Transplantation—Terminology—English. WR 15 S8121 2005]
RL41.S74 2005
616.5'001'4--dc22
                                                                                2004021176
                                                                                04 05 06
                                                                3 4 5 6 7 8 9 10

Contents

Acknowledgments

An important part of our editorial process is the involvement of medical transcriptionists—as advisors, reviewers, and editors.

We extend special thanks to Sandy Kovacs, CMT, and Carrie Donathan, CMT, FAAMT, for editing the manuscript, helping to resolve many difficult content questions, and reviewing material for the appendix sections. We also extend special thanks to Helen Littrell, CMT, for performing the final prepublication review.

We are also grateful to our MT Editorial Advisory Board members, including Marty Cantu, CMT; Patricia Gibson; Robin Koza; and Peg Nelson, CMT. These medical transcriptionists and medical language specialists served as important editors and advisors.

Other important contributors include Jeanne Bock, CSR, MT, who composed the appendix sections, as well as Susan Bartolucci, CMT, Cheri Bruno, Susan Caldwell, Heather Little, and Beverly S. Oberline, CMT, who were crucial in developing and revising content.

Lisa Fahnestock played an integral role in the process by reviewing the files for format, updating the content, and providing a final quality check.

As with all our Stedman's word references, this resource incorporates the suggestions and expertise of our many contacts in the medical transcriptionist community. Thanks to all of our advisory board participants, reviewers, and editors; AAMT meeting attendees; and others who have written us with requests and comments—keep talking, and we'll keep listening.

Editor's Preface

How many of you have gone to a symposium or AAMT convention and wished you had an extra suitcase? I have thought about taking an almost empty suitcase with me, but I haven't remembered to do that yet. What good is an empty suitcase, you ask? To fill it with all the new reference books you will buy at the meeting, of course. In my 26 years as a medical transcriptionist, I have never gone to a meeting and not bought at least one book and usually I buy quite a few. I guess you could call me a "reference book junkie."

In today's trend of increased patient information documentation, many of the medical specialists are finding that they must dictate their reports to assure increased reimbursement and for readability and completeness of the medical record. The Third edition of *Stedman's Dermatology & Immunology Words, Includes Rheumatology, Allergy, & Transplantation*, is just the right reference for medical transcriptionists who find themselves having to transcribe reports from specialties that are unfamiliar to them.

This book responds to the needs of these transcriptionists by covering terms from new and evolving areas in dermatology and immunology, including allergy and rheumatology, as well as organ transplantation. Additionally, the appendix sections have useful information to help the transcriptionist understand what is being dictated. There are illustrations, sample reports, lists of common terms by procedure, and a list of transplant organizations.

The explanatory notes in the front of the book show you how this book is designed and give you a good guideline on the different methods of finding the correct word.

Many thanks to Carrie Donathan, CMT, FAAMT, for assisting me as second editor. Her knowledge and experience add another layer of accuracy to this book. I appreciate the assistance of the editorial staff and the wordsearch abilities of the many medical language specialists who glean the most updated terms from medical journals and other publications.

Thanks to Steve Lichtenstein for his role as Associate Managing Editor and for coordinating the timeline and logistics.

It takes more than one or two people to create a useful and valuable reference book. Our team of professionals is dedicated to continue to publish the type of reference books that you will find useful for years

Sandy Kovacs, CMT, FAAMT

Publisher's Preface

Stedman's Dermatology & Immunology Words, Third Edition, offers an authoritative assurance of quality and exactness to the wordsmiths of the healthcare professions—medical transcriptionists, medical editors and copyeditors, health information management personnel, court reporters, and the many other users and producers of medical documentation.

We received many requests for updates to *Stedman's Dermatology & Immunology Words*. As the requests continued to accumulate, we realized that medical language professionals needed a current, comprehensive reference for these specialties.

In *Stedman's Dermatology & Immunology Words, Third Edition*, users will find thousands of terms related to dermatology, immunology, rheumatology, allergy, and transplantation. Included are terms for problems like acne, contact dermatitis, alopecia, eczematous dermatoses, autoimmune diseases, allergies, allergic asthma, rheumatologic disorders. Transplantation terms, including words for tissue engineering, HLA typing, and antirejection drug therapies, have been added for this edition. Included are terms for diagnostic and therapeutic procedures, new techniques, and lab tests, as well as equipment names and abbreviations with their expansions. The appendix sections provide anatomical illustrations with useful captions and labels; normal lab values; sample reports; common terms by procedure; and drugs listed by indication. For quick reference, we have also included lists of common allergens and transplant organizations.

This compilation of more than 80,000 entries, fully cross-indexed for quick access, was built from a base vocabulary of approximately 45,000 medical words, phrases, abbreviations, and acronyms. The extensive A-Z list was developed from the database of *Stedman's Medical Dictionary, 27th Edition*, and supplemented by terminology found in current medical literature (please see list of References on page xvii).

We at Lippincott Williams & Wilkins strive to provide you with the most up-to-date and accurate word references available. Your use of this Word Book will prompt new editions, which we will publish as often as updates and revisions justify. We welcome your suggestions for improvements, changes, corrections, and additions—whatever will make this Stedman's product more useful to you. Please complete the postpaid card at the back of this book or complete the Got a Good Word submission on www.stedmans.com.

Explanatory Notes

Medical transcription is an art as well as a science. Both approaches are needed to correctly interpret the dictation of a physician, whose language is a product of education, training, and experience. This variety in medical language means that there are several acceptable ways to express certain terms, including jargon. *Stedman's Dermatology & Immunology Words, Third Edition*, provides variant spellings and phrasings for many terms. These elements, in addition to complete cross-indexing, make *Stedman's Dermatology & Immunology Words, Third Edition*, a valuable resource for determining the validity of terms as they are encountered.

Alphabetical Organization

Alphabetization of main entries is letter by letter as spelled, ignoring punctuation, spaces, prefixed numbers, or other special characters. For example:

hydroxyproline
5-hydroxypropafenone
hydroxytoluene

Terms beginning with Greek letters show the Greek letter spelled out and listed alphabetically. For example:

alpha, α
    a. agonist
    a. blocking agent
    a. lipoprotein
    a. receptor

In subentry alphabetization, the abbreviated singular form or the spelled-out plural form of the noun main entry word is ignored.

Format and Style

All main entries are in **boldface** to expedite locating a sought-after term, to enhance distinction between main entries and subentries, and to relieve the textual density of the pages.

Irregular plurals and variant spellings are shown on the same line as the singular or preferred form of the word. For example:

scolex, pl. **scoleces**

curette, curet

Hyphenation

As a rule of style, multiple eponyms (e.g., Green-Kenyon corneal marker) are hyphenated. Also, hyphens have been added between a manufacturer and one or more eponyms (e.g., Vital-Metzenbaum dissecting scissors). Please note that in many cases, hyphenation is a question of style, not of accuracy, and thus is a matter of choice.

Possessives

Possessive forms have been dropped in this reference for the sake of consistency and conformance with the guidelines of the American Association for Medical Transcription (AAMT) and other groups. Please note, however, that in many cases, retaining the possessive, like hyphenating, is a question of style, not of accuracy, and thus is a matter of choice. To form the possessive of a word, simply add the apostrophe or apostrophe "s" to the end of the word.

Cross-indexing

The word list is in an index-like main entry-subentry format that contains two combined alphabetical listings:

(1) A *noun* main entry-subentry organization, which is typical of the A-Z section of medical dictionaries like *Stedman's*:

dermatosis
    acantholytic d.
    acquired d.
    ashy d.
    bullous d.

nail
    brittle n.
    convex n.
    parrot-beak n.
    reedy n.

(2) An *adjective* main entry-subentry organization, which lists words and phrases as you hear them. The main entries are the adjectives or modifiers in a multiword term. The subentries are the nouns around which the terms are constructed and to which the adjectives or modifiers pertain:

congenital
    c. ectodermal defects
    c. erythropoietic porphyrian.
    c. ichthyosiform erythoderma
    c. syphilis

nevus
    n. comedonicus
    n. fibrosus
    n. flammeus
    n. pigmentosus

This format provides the user with more than one way to locate and identify a multiword term. For example:

dissemination
    skin d.

skin
    s. dissemination

disease
    Quincke d.
    Raynaud d.

Quincke
    Q. disease
    Q. edema

It also allows the user to see together all terms that contain a particular descriptor, as well as all types, kinds, or variations of a noun entity. For example:

balloon
    b. laser angioplasty
    b. occlusion
    Blue Max b.
    Brandt cytology b.
    Express b.

angioplasty
    balloon laser a.
    complex a.
    a. guiding catheter
    high-risk a.
    transluminal coronary a.

Wherever possible, abbreviations are separately defined and cross-referenced. For example:

FUO
    fever of unknown origin

fever
    f. of unknown origin (FUO)

origin
    fever of unknown o. (FUO)

References

In addition to the manufacturers' literature we gather at various medical meetings, scientific reports from hospitals, and the lists created by our MT Editorial Advisory Board members from their daily transcription work, we used the following sources for new terms in *Stedman's Dermatology & Immunology Words, Third Edition*:

Books

Adelman DC, Casale TB, Corren J. Manual of Allergy and Immunology, 4th Edition. Philadelphia: Lippincott Williams & Wilkins, 2003.

Arndt KA, Bowers KE. Manual of Dermatologic Therapeutics, 6th Edition. Philadelphia: Lippincott Williams & Wilkins, 2002.

Austen KF, Frank MM, Atkinson JP, Cantor HI. Samter's Immunologic Diseases. Philadelphia: Lippincott Williams & Wilkins, 2001.

Bowden RA, Ljungman P, Paya C, eds. Transplant Infections. Philadelphia: Lippincott-Raven, 1998.

Cush JJ, Kavanaugh AF. Rheumatology: Diagnosis and Therapeutics. Baltimore: Lippincott Williams & Wilkins, 1999.

Drake E. Sloane's Medical Word Book, 4th Edition. Philadelphia: Saunders, 2002.

Emery RW, Miller LW, eds. Handbook of Cardiac Transplantation. Philadelphia: Hanley & Belfus, Inc., 1996.

Hall JC. Sauer's Manual of Skin Diseases, 8th Edition. Philadelphia: Lippincott Williams & Wilkins, 2000.

Handbook of Allergic Disorders. Philadelphia: Lippincott Williams & Wilkins, 2003.

Honsinger RW, Green GR, eds. Handbook of Drug Allergy. Philadelphia: Lippincott Williams & Wilkins, 2004.

Koopman WJ. Arthritis and Allied Conditions: A Textbook of Rheumatology, 14th Edition. Philadelphia: Lippincott Williams & Wilkins, 2000.

Koopman WJ, Boulware DW, Heudebert GR, eds. Clinical Primer of Rheumatology. Philadelphia: Lippincott Williams & Wilkins, 2003.

Lahita RG, ed. Textbook of the Autoimmune Diseases. Philadelphia: Lippincott Williams & Wilkins, 2000.

Lance LL. Quick Look Drug Book 2001. Baltimore: Lippincott Williams & Wilkins, 2001.

Maddrey WC, Schiff ER, Sorrell MF, eds. Transplantation of the Liver, 3rd Edition. Philadelphia: Lippincott Williams & Wilkins, 2001.

Odom RB, James WD, Berger TG. Andrews' Diseases of the Skin: Clinical Dermatology, 9th Edition. Philadelphia: Saunders, 2000.

Patterson R, ed. Allergic Diseases: Diagnosis and Management, 5th Edition. Philadelphia: Lippincott-Raven, 1997.

Paul WE. Fundamental Immunology, 5th Edition. Philadelphia: Lippincott Williams & Wilkins, 2003.

Ratz JL, ed. Textbook of Dermatologic Surgery. Philadelphia: Lippincott Williams & Wilkins, 1997.

Rietschel RL, Fowler JF, eds. Fisher's Contact Dermatitis, 5th Edition. Philadelphia: Lippincott Williams & Wilkins, 2001.

Scheman AL, Severson DL. Pocket Guide to Medications Used in Dermatology, 8th Edition. Philadelphia: Lippincott Williams & Wilkins, 2003.

Sheehan C. Clinical Immunology: Principles and Laboratory Diagnosis, 2nd Edition. Philadelphia: Lippincott-Raven, 1997.

Sontheimer RD, Provost TT, eds. Cutaneous Manifestations of Rheumatic Diseases. Philadelphia: Lippincott Williams & Wilkins, 2004.

Stedman's Medical Dictionary, 27th Edition. Baltimore: Lippincott Williams & Wilkins, 2000.

Vera Pyle's Current Medical Terminology, 8th Edition. Modesto, CA: Health Professions Institute, 2000.

Images

Barratt MA, Parkton, MD. From Stedman's Medical Dictionary, 27th Edition. Baltimore: Lippincott Williams & Wilkins, 2000.

Caldwell S, Pikesville, MD. From Stedman's Medical Dictionary, 27th Edition. Baltimore: Lippincott Williams & Wilkins, 2000.

Duckwall Productions, Baltimore, MD. From Stedman's Medical Dictionary, 27th Edition. Baltimore: Lippincott Williams & Wilkins, 2000.

Hardy NO, Westport, CT. From Chaffee EE, RN, MN & Greisheimer, MD, PhD. Basic Physiology and Anatomy, 3rd Edition. Philadelphia: JB Lippincott Company, 1974.

Hardy NO, Westport, CT. From Stedman's Medical Dictionary, 27th Edition. Baltimore: Lippincott Williams & Wilkins, 2000.

Idezuki H, Prinz. Surgical Diseases of the Pancreas, 3rd Edition. Baltimore, Lippincott Williams & Wilkins, 1997.

Kaplowitz N. Liver & Biliary Disease, 2nd Edition. Baltimore, Williams & Wilkins, 1996.

LifeART Emergency 4, CD-ROM. Baltimore, Lippincott Williams & Wilkins.

LifeART Nursing 1, CD-ROM. Baltimore, Lippincott Williams & Wilkins.

LifeART Pediatrics 1, CD-ROM. Baltimore, Lippincott Williams & Wilkins.

LifeART Super Anatomy Collection 3, CD-ROM. Baltimore, Lippincott Williams & Wilkins.

LifeART Super Anatomy Collection 7, CD-ROM. Baltimore, Lippincott Williams & Wilkins.

MediClip Clinical Cardiopulmonary, CD-ROM. Baltimore, Lippincott Williams & Wilkins.

Senkarik M, San Antonio, TX. Smeltzer SC & Bare BG. Brunner & Suddarth's Textbook of Medical Surgical-Nursing, 8th Edition. Philadelphia: JB Lippincott Company, 1996.

Ward L, Salt Lake City, UT. From Fuller J, RN, PhD & Schaller-Ayers J, RN, MNSc, PhD. A Nursing Approach, 2nd Edition. Philadelphia: J.B. Lippincott Company, 1994.

Willis, MC. Medical Terminology: The Language of Health Care. Baltimore: Williams & Wilkins, 1996.

Journals

The American Journal of Dermatopathology. Baltimore: Lippincott Williams & Wilkins, 1999-2000.

Archives of Dermatology. Chicago: American Medical Association, 1999-2004.

Arthritis & Rheumatism. New York: John Wiley & Sons, 1999-2000.

Current Opinions in Organ Transplantation. Philadelphia: Lippincott Williams & Wilkins, 1999-2000.

Immunology Today. London: Elsevier Science, 2000.

JCR: Journal of Clinical Rheumatology. Baltimore: Lippincott Williams & Wilkins, 2000-2004.

Journal of Allergy and Clinical Immunology. St. Louis, MO: Mosby, 1999-2000.

The Latest Word. Philadelphia: Saunders, 1999-2000.

Transplantation. Baltimore: Lippincott Williams & Wilkins, 1999-2004.

Websites

http://centerwatch.com/patient

http://edcenter.med.cornell.edu/CUMC_PathNotes/Dermpath/Dermpath_02.html

http://www.arthritis.org/answers/drugguide/default.asp

http://www.fda.gov/cder/rdmt/internetflap.htm

http://www.hpisum.com

http://www.kidney.org/recips/donor/

http://www.labspec.co.za/l_occu.htm

http://www.medicaledu.comp/absorptv.htm

http://www.mtdesk.com

http://www.mtmonthly.com

http://www.niaid.nih.gov/publications/transplant/glossary.htm

http://www.organdonor.gov/opo.htm

http://www.spwb.saunders.net

http://www.unicapinvitrosight.com/templates/Allergens.asp?id=2192

zhttp://www.virtualdrugstore.com

α
A
 anti-Sjögren syndrome A (anti-SSA)
 Aquasol A
 Aristocort A
 A and D Ointment
 hepatitis A (HA)
 A 2M
 protein kinase A (PKA)
 psoralen ultraviolet A (PUVA)
 secretory immunoglobulin A
 Sjögren syndrome A (SS-A)
2A
 cyclin-dependent kinase inhibitor
  2A (CDKN2A)
A5
 Peroxin A5
A10
 Peroxin A10
A-200
 A-200 Pyrinate
 A-200 Shampoo
Å
 angstrom
 Å unit
a
 a collarette of epidermis
 a disintegrin and matrilysin
  (ADAM)
5a8
 monoclonal antibody to CD4, 5a8
A1 test
AA, AL amyloidosis
AAD
 acroangiodermatitis
AADI
 anterior atlantodental interval
A-alpha nerve fiber
Aarskog-Scott syndrome
Aastrom Replicell System
AAV
 adeno-associated virus
 ANCA-associated vasculitis
Ab
 antibody
abacavir
abalone
Abbott HIVAG-1 monoclonal antigen
ABC
 ABC method
ABCD
 ABCD rule of dermatoscopy
 ABCD sign
Abelcet
Abelson murine leukemia virus

Abernethy sarcoma
aberrant
 a. glycosaminoglycan metabolism
 a. ribonucleic acid
abigne
AbioCor implantable replacement heart
abiotrophy
abirritant
ablastin
ablation
 transvenous endoluminal
  radiofrequency a.
ablative
abnormal
 a. DNA repair
 a. gut fermentation
 a. localization of immature
  precursors (ALIP)
 a. loricrin cross-linking
abnormality
 biochemical a.
 calcaneal a.
 calcinosis cutis, osteoma cutis,
  poikiloderma, and skeletal a.'s
  (COPS)
 a.'s of genitalia, retardation of
  growth, and deafness
 humoral a.
 immunochemical a.
 microvascular a.
 nail fold capillaroscopy a.
 nail fold capillary loop a.
 oral cavity a.
 pigmentary a.
 skeletal a.
abnutzung pigment
ABO
 ABO antigen
 ABO incompatibility
 ABO mismatch
ABO-incompatible kidney transplantation
abortive
 a. neurofibromatosis
 a. transduction
abortus
 Bacillus a.
ABPA
 ABPA panel
abradant
abrade
abraded wound
abrasion
 brush burn a.
 mechanical a.
 pleural a.

abrasive
Abreva
Abrikosov tumor
Abs
    CTLA-4-specific Abs
abscess
    brain a.
    Brodie a.
    cheesy a.
    cold a.
    conglobate a.
    crypt a.
    cutaneous a.
    Dubois a.
    eosinophilic a.
    filarial a.
    follicular a.
    gas a.
    intraepidermal a.
    metastatic tuberculous a.
    mixed aerobic/anaerobic a.
    Munro a.
    mycobacterial a.
    Paget a.
    pararenal a.
    paraspinal a.
    paraspinous a.
    Pautrier a.
    phlegmonous a.
    pneumococcic a.
    protozoal a.
    pulp a.
    pulpal a.
    pyemic a.
    pyogenic a.
    recurrent cutaneous a.
    spirillar a.
    staphylococcal a.
    stellate a.
    sterile a.
    strumous a.
    subepidermal a.
    subungual a.
    sudoriferous a.
    sudoriparous a.
    tuberculous a.
    verminous a.
abscessus
    Mycobacterium a.
absent
    a. dermal component
    a. reaction
    a. tonsil
Absidia
absolute
    a. blood eosinophil count (AEC)
    oak moss a.
absorbable mesh
absorbent ointment

Absorbine
    A. Antifungal Foot powder
    A. Jock Itch
    A. Jr. Antifungal
absorptiometry
    dual-beam photon a.
    photon a.
absorption
    cutaneous a.
    external a.
    nonspecific a.
    parenteral a.
    percutaneous a.
abtropfung
ABX-CBL monoclonal antibody
ACA
    anticardiolipin antibody
    ACA antibody
acacia
    a. tree
    a. tree pollen
Acaderm patch test
ACAID
    anterior chamber-associated immune
    deviation
acanthamebiasis
Acanthamoeba
    A. astronyxis
    A. castellani
    A. culbertsoni
    A. glebae
    A. hatchetti
    A. palestinensis
    A. polyphaga
    A. rhysodes
Acanthaster planci
Acanthocheilonema
    A. viteae
    A. viteae excretory-secretory antigen
acanthocyte
acanthoid
acantholysis
    pemphigus vulgaris a.
    suprabasilar a.
acantholytic
    a. dermatosis
    a. dyskeratoma
    a. dyskeratosis
    a. squamous cell carcinoma
acanthoma, pl. acanthomata, acanthomas
    a. adenoides cysticum
    basosquamous cell a.
    clear cell a.
    Degos a.
    epidermolytic a.
    a. fissuratum
    a. inguinale
    intraepidermal a.
    pale cell a.

pilar sheath a.
a. tropicum
a. verrucosa seborrheica
acanthorrhexis
acanthosis
a. palmaris
a. papulosa nigra
a. seborrheica
acanthotic epidermal proliferation
acarian
acariasis
demodectic a.
psoroptic a.
sarcoptic a.
acaricidal activity
acaricide
acarid
acaridiasis
Acarina
acarine dermatosis
acarinosis
A-Caro-25
acarodermatitis urticarioides
acaroid
acaroides
acarophobia
acarotoxic
Acarus
A. balatus
A. folliculorum
A. siro
acatalasemia
acatalasia
accelerated
a. phase (AP)
a. reaction
a. rejection
accelerator
Arthramel A.
A. cannula
Ac'cents permanent lash liner
Accents system
accentuation
acrosyringeal a.
follicular a.
perifollicular a.
accessory
a. auricle
a. molecule
a. muscle
a. tragus

accident
serum a.
accidental host
acclimatization
Accolate
accordion hand
Accuderm punch
Accuhair needle
AccuHist
A. PDX drops
A. PDX syrup
A. Pediatric drops
AccuProbe system
Accu-set System
AccuSite injectable gel
Accutane
AccuTrax peak flow meter
Accuzyme
A. enzymatic debrider
A. enzymatic debriding agent
ACD
ACD features of melanoma
ACE
angiotensin-converting enzyme
ACE IT
Ace bandage
Acedapsone
Acel-Imune
acellular pannus tissue
Acephen
acephylline
aceracear
acervuline
acetabular dysplasia
acetabuli
protrusio a.
acetabulum
acetamidine
acetaminophen
chlorpheniramine, phenylpropanolamine, and a.
a., chlorpheniramine, and pseudoephedrine
a. and diphenhydramine
a. and isometheptene mucate
a. and phenyltoloxamine
phenyltoloxamine, phenylpropanolamine, and a.
acetanilide
acetarsol
acetarsone
Acetasol HC Otic

NOTES

acetate
aluminum a.
betamethasone a. (BA)
cortisone a.
Cortone A.
cyproterone a. (CPA)
dexamethasone a.
Florinef A.
fludrocortisone a.
hydrocortisone a.
Hydrocortone A.
leuprolide a.
mafenide a.
m-cresyl a.
megestrol a.
methylprednisolone a. (MPA)
nafarelin a.
octreotide a.
paramethasone a.
pexiganan a.
phorbol myristate a. (PMA)
pirbuterol a.
pramoxine, camphor, zinc a.
sermorelin a.
acetazolamide
acetic
a. acid
a. acid, propanediol diacetate, and
hydrocortisone
acetin
acetone-insoluble antigen
acetonide
triamcinolone a. (TAA)
Acetoxyl
acetylation
a. of cellular protein
a. of serum protein
acetylcholine
a. depletion
a. receptor antibody (AChRAb)
acetylcholinesterase deficiency
acetylcysteine
acetyl ethyl tetramethyl tetralin (AETT)
acetylhydrolase
platelet-activating factor a. (PAF-
AH)
acetylsalicylic acid (ASA)
acetyltransferase
chloramphenicol a. (CAT)
Achard-Thiers syndrome
Achenbach syndrome
Aches-N-Pain
Achilles
A. bursitis
A. tendinitis
A. tendon
achlorhydria
Acholeplasma laidlawii
achondrogenesis type II

Achorion schoenleinii
AChRAb
acetylcholine receptor antibody
achromasia
achromatosis
achromia
consecutive a.
a. parasitica
a. unguium
achromians
incontinentia pigmenti a.
Achromobacter xylosoxidans
achromoderma
achromotrichia
Achromycin
A. Ophthalmic
A. topical
A. V
A. V Oral
acid
aberrant ribonucleic a.
acetic a.
acetylsalicylic a. (ASA)
adenylic a.
a. agglutination
all-trans-retinoic a. (ATRA)
aluminum acetate and acetic a.
amino a.
aminobenzoic a.
aminolevulinic a. (ALA)
5-aminolevulinic a.
aminosalicylic a.
amoxicillin and clavulanic a.
a. anhydride
anti-ribonucleic a. (anti-RNA)
arylalcoanoic a.
azelaic a.
battery a.
benzoic acid and salicylic a.
bichloracetic a.
boric a.
cantharic a.
chemiluminescent in situ
hybridization for detection of
cytomegalovirus
deoxyribonucleic a.
chenodeoxycholic a.
cholic a.
13-*cis*-retinoic a.
citric a.
clavulanic a.
coal tar and salicylic a.
delta-aminolevulinic a.
deoxyribonucleic a. (DNA)
dichloroacetic a.
docosahexaenoic a.
a. dye
eicosapentaenoic a.

enteric coated acetylsalicylic a.
  (ECASA)
essential fatty a. (EFA)
exogenous polyunsaturated fatty a.
fibric a.
flufenamic a.
folic a.
folinic a.
a. fuchsin
fusidic a.
gamma-linolenic a.
geniposidic a.
gluconic a.
glucuronic a.
glycolic a.
glycyl-transfer ribonucleic a.
gold 4-amino-2-mercaptobenzoic a.
guanylic a.
holmium ethylenediamine
  tetramethylene phosphonic a.
homogentisic a. (HGA)
hyaluronic a.
hydroperoxyeicosatetraenoic a.
hydrophobic ascorbic a.
hydroquinone USP and glycolic a.
hydroxyeicosatetraenoic a. (HETE)
5-hydroxyindoleacetic a.
iduronic a.
infectious nucleic a.
inosinic a.
kojic a.
lactic a.
L-ascorbic a.
linoleic a.
lipoteichoic a. (LTA)
malic a.
a. maltase
A. Mantle
A. Mantle creme
mefenamic a.
monochloroacetic a.
N-acetylneuraminic a.
nalidixic a.
octulosonic a.
oleic a.
omega-3, -6 fatty a.
paraaminobenzoic a. (PABA)
paraaminosalicylic a.
phytanic a.
plicatic a.
podophyllin and salicylic a.
pseudomonic a.

pyruvic a.
retinoic a.
ribonucleic a. (RNA)
salicylic acid and lactic a.
salicylic acid-lactic a. (SAL)
a. Schiff stain
serum uric a. (SUA)
a. skin
sodium citrate and citric a.
stearic a.
sulfuric a.
sulfur and salicylic a.
tartaric a.
Tc-dimercaptosuccinic a. (DMSA)
tenoxicam a.
tiaprofenic a.
ticarcillin and clavulanic a.
tranexamic a.
transfer ribonucleic a. (tRNA)
trichloroacetic a. (TCA)
tris-boric acid-
  ethylenediaminetetraacetic a. (TBE)
undecylenic a.
uric a.
zinc oxide, talc, carbolic acid,
  boric a.
Acidaminococcus fermentans
acidase
  antideoxyribonucleic a.
acidification
  endosomal a.
acidophilus
  Lactobacillus a.
  a. milk
acidosis
  lactic a.
  metabolic a.
  renal tubular a.
  respiratory a.
acid-Schiff
  periodic a.-S. (PAS)
  a.-S. test
acid-secreting gastric parietal cell
aciduria
  orotic a.
acinar cell
Acinetobacter
  A. anitratus
  A. calcoaceticus
  A. calcoaceticus-baumannii complex
  A. lwoffi
Acintomadura

NOTES

5

ACIP
    Advisory Committee on Immunization
      Practice
ACIS
    Automated Cellular Imaging System
      ACIS immunohistochemical stain
Acitin
acitretin
aCL
    anticardiolipin
      aCL antibody
ACLAb
    anticardiolipin antibody
Aclovate topical
acmes
    stadium a.
acne
    A. Aid cleansing bar
    a. albida
    apocrine a.
    a. arthritis
    a. artificialis
    a. atrophica
    a. bacillus
    bromide a.
    a. cachecticorum
    a. cheloidalis
    chlorine a.
    a. ciliaris
    ClearLight treatment for a.
    colloid a.
    comedo a.
    common a.
    a. conglobata
    conglobate a.
    a. cosmetica
    cystic a.
    a. cystica
    a. decalvans
    a. detergicans
    a. disseminata
    a. dorsalis
    epidemic a.
    a. erythematosa
    a. estivalis
    excoriated a.
    a. excoriée des jeunes filles
    a. frontalis
    a. fulminans
    a. generalis
    halogen a.
    a. hypertrophica
    a. indurata
    infantile a.
    a. inversa
    iodide a.
    keloid a.
    a. keloidalis (AK)
    a. keloidalis nuchae

    a. keratosa
    lupoid a.
    Mallorca miliary actinic a.
    a. mechanica
    mechanical a.
    a. medicamentosa
    menstrual a.
    a. mentagra
    miliary a.
    Mudd a.
    a. necrotica
    a. necrotica miliaris
    a. necroticans et exulcerans
     serpiginosa nasi
    neonatal a.
    a. neonatorum
    nodulocystic a.
    occupational a.
    oil a.
    papular a.
    a. papulosa
    petroleum a.
    picker's a.
    pomade a.
    premenstrual a.
    a. punctata
    pustular a.
    a. pustulosa
    pyogenic sterile arthritis, pyoderma
     gangrenosum and a. (PAPA)
    a. rosacea
    a. scrofulosorum
    a. seborrheica
    a. simplex
    steroid a.
    summer a.
    a. surgery
    a. syphilitica
    systemic a.
    tar a.
    a. tarsi
    a. telangiectodes
    a. tetrad
    trade a.
    tropical a.
    a. tropicalis
    a. urticata
    a. varioliformis
    a. venenata
    a. vulgaris
acneform, acneiform
    a. dermatitis
    a. eruption
    a. lesion
    a. syphilid
acneforme, acneiforme
acnegen
acnegenic
acneic

acneiform (*var. of* acneform)
acneiforma
    ulerythema a.
acneiforme (*var. of* acneforme)
acne-pustulosis-hyperostosis-osteitis
acnes
    Bacillus a.
    Corynebacterium a.
    Propionibacterium a.
acne-seborrhea complex
Acnex
acnitis
Acnomel
    A. Acne Mask
    A. BP 5
    A. cream
acomia
Acorn classification
acoustic reflex threshold
acquired
    a. biotin deficiency
    a. C1 inhibitor deficiency
    a. cornification disorder
    a. digital fibrokeratoma
    a. dyskeratotic leukoplakia
    a. generalized lipodystrophy
    a. hemolytic anemia
    a. hemolytic icterus
    a. hemophilia
    a. hypertrichosis lanuginosa
    a. hypogammaglobulinemia
    a. ichthyosis
    a. immunity
    a. immunodeficiency
    a. immunodeficiency syndrome-
        related virus (ARV)
    a. intrathymic tolerance
    a. leukoderma
    a. leukopathia
    a. melanocytic nevus
    a. partial face-sparing lipodystrophy
    a. pellicle
    a. perforating dermatosis
    a. progressive kinking of the hair
        (APKH)
    a. sensitivity
    a. trichoepithelioma
    a. vascular disorder
acquisita
    alopecia a.
    skin-dominated epidermolysis
        bullosa a.

acquisitum
ACR
    American College of Rheumatology
        ACR criteria
        ACR diagnostic criteria for SLE
        ACR diagnostic criteria for
            systemic lupus erythematosus
Acradinium-ester-labeled nucleic acid
    probe
acral
    a. arteriolar ectasia
    a. erythema
    a. fibrokeratoma
    a. persistent papular mucinosis
    a. vitiligo
Acremonium
acrex
acridine
acriflavine
acrisorcin
acritochromacy
acrivastine and pseudoephedrine
acroangiodermatitis (AAD)
acroasphyxia
acrocephalosyndactyly
acrochordon
acrochordonectomy
    Strother a.
acrocyanosis
    orthostatic a.
    remitting necrotizing a.
acrodermatitis
    a. chronica
    a. continua
    a. continua of Hallopeau
    a. enteropathica (AE)
    Hallopeau a.
    a. hiemalis
    papular a.
    a. papulosa infantum
    a. perstans
    pustular a.
    a. pustulosa
    a. vesiculosa tropica
acrodermatosis
acrodynia
acrodynic erythema
acrofacial vitiligo
acrogeria
acrohyperhidrosis
acrokeratoelastoidosis

NOTES

acrokeratosis
    a. neoplastica
    paraneoplastic a.
    a. paraneoplastica
    a. verruciformis
    a. verruciformis of Hopf
acrokeratotic poikiloderma
acrolein
acrolein-induced cystitis
acroleukopathy
acromegalic arthropathy
acromegaly
acromelalgia
acromelanosis progressiva
acromicria
acromioclavicular
    a. articulation
    a. degeneration
    a. joint
acromiodeltoideus
acroosteolysis
acropachy
    thyroid a.
acropachyderma
acroparesthesia
    Nothnagel-type a.
    Schultze a.
    Schultze-type a.
acropigmentatio
    a. reticularis
    a. reticular of Kitamura
acropigmentation
    a. of Dohi
    Kitamura reticulate a.
acropurpura
acropustulosis
    a. of infancy
    infantile a.
acroscleroderma
acrosclerosis
acrospiroma
    eccrine a.
    giant eccrine a.
    malignant clear cell a.
acrosyringeal accentuation
acrosyringium
acroterica
    morphea a.
acroteric morphea
Acrotheca aquaspera
acrotrophodynia
AcryDerm
    A. border island dressing
    A. hydrogel sheet
    A. Strands
    A. Strands filler
acrylate
acrylic acid allergy
acrylonitrile

Acsorex
act
    Bone Mass Measurement A.
    Coinage A.
    throwing a.
    Toxic Substance Control A.
Actagen
    A. Syrup
    A. Tablet
actamar
actarit
ACTH
    adrenocorticotropic hormone
    ACTH therapy
Acthar
ActHIB vaccine
Acticel wound dressing
Acticin Cream
Acticoat burn dressing
Acticort topical
Actiderm
actidione
Actifed
    A. Allergy Tablet
    A. 12 Hour
Actimmune
actin
    filamentous a.
    A. FSL
    A. monomer
actin-binding protein
Actinex topical
actinic
    a. burn
    a. cheilitis
    a. dermatitis
    a. elastosis
    a. granuloma
    a. keratosis
    a. lichen planus (ALP)
    a. light
    a. porokeratosis
    a. prurigo
    a. purpura
    a. reticuloid
    a. reticuloid syndrome
actinica
    cheilitis a.
    dermatitis a.
actinicity
actinicus
    lichen planus a.
actinism
actinobacillosis
Actinobacillus
    A. *actinomycetemcomitans*
    A. *equuli*
    A. *hominis*
    A. *lignieresii*

A. suis
A. ureae
actinodermatitis
actinodermatosis
actinoides
    Thysanosoma a.
actinolyte
Actinomadura
    A. madurae
    A. pelletieri
actinometer
actinometry
actinomycelial
Actinomyces
    A. bovis
    A. hominis
    A. israelii
    A. naeslundii
actinomycetemcomitans
    Actinobacillus a.
    a., Cardiobacterium hominis,
      Eikenella corrodens and Kingella
      kingae
actinomycetoma
actinomycin
actinomycoma
actinomycosis
    cervical a.
    cervicofacial a.
actinomycotic mycetoma
actinomycotin
actinoneuritis
actinophage
actinophytosis
actinoquinol sodium
actinotherapeutics
actinotherapy
    foil bath pulsed ultraviolet a.
    ultraviolet a.
action
    mechanism of a.
ActiPatch therapy
Actiprofen
**Actisorb Silver 220 antimicrobial
binding dressing**
activated
    a. charcoal
    a. macrophage
    a. partial thromboplastin time
      (APTT)
    a. vitamin K-dependent factor

activation
    complement a.
    immune a.
    lymphocyte a.
    melanocytic a.
    natural killer cell a.
    NK cell a.
activation-induced cell death (AICD)
activator
    plasminogen a.
    polyclonal a.
    a. protein 1 (AP1)
active
    a. anaphylaxis
    a. carrier
    A. Dry Lotion
    a. immunity
    a. immunization
    a. joint
    Labello A.
    a. nevus
    a. pinocytosis
    a. prophylaxis
    a. range of motion
    a. sensitization
    a. serum
    a. transport
Activella
activin
activity
    acaricidal a.
    adenosine triphosphatase a.
    amidolytic a.
    ATPase a.
    complement a.
    a.'s of daily living
    hyaluronidase a.
    IL-2 receptor-b and cytotoxic a.
    immunophilin isomerase a.
    increased sympathoadrenal a.
    kallikrein a.
    lymphocyte chemoattractant a.
    patient global assessment of
      disease a.
    physician global assessment of
      disease a.
    recombinational a.
    rheumatoid factor-like a. (RFLA)
    vitiligo disease a. (VIDA)
actomyosin
Actonel tablet
Actos

NOTES

Actron
Acu-Derm I.V./TPN dressing
Acu-Dyne
acuity
> LogMAR visual a.

Acular Ophthalmic
aculeatus
> *Ruscus a.*

acuminata
> verruca a.

acuminate
> a. papular syphilid
> a. wart

acuminatum, pl. **acuminata**
> papilloma a.
> verruca acuminata

acuminatus
> lichen ruber a.

acupuncture needle dermatitis
Acu-Razor blade
Acuson 128XT ultrasound
Acusyst-Xcell
> A.-X. monoclonal antibody
> A.-X. monoclonal antibody
>   culturing system

acuta
> parapsoriasis lichenoides et
>   varioliformis a.
> parapsoriasis varioliformis a.
> pityriasis lichenoides et
>   varioliformis a. (PLEVA)
> pustulosis vacciniformis a.
> urticaria a.

acute
> a. allergic urticaria
> a. anaphylactic reaction
> a. anterior poliomyelitis
> a. asthma attack
> a. atrophic oral candidiasis
> a. atrophic paralysis
> a. bronchopulmonary aspergillosis
>   panel
> a. bulbar poliomyelitis
> a. cellular xenograft rejection
> a. conjunctival chemosis
> a. contagious conjunctivitis
> a. crescentic glomerulonephritis
> a. cutaneous leishmaniasis
> a. decubitus ulcer
> a. disseminated histiocytosis
> a. disseminated myositis
> a. epidemic conjunctivitis
> a. epidemic leukoencephalitis
> a. epiglottitis
> a. febrile neutrophilic dermatosis
> a. follicular conjunctivitis
> a. generalized exanthematous
>   pustulosis (AGEP)
> a. hemorrhagic glomerulonephritis

> a. herpes zoster
> a. herpetic gingivostomatitis
> a. hypersensitivity pneumonitis
> a. idiopathic polyneuritis
> a. idiopathic thrombocytopenic
>   purpura
> a. infectious disease
> a. infectious nonbacterial
>   gastroenteritis
> a. interstitial nephritis
> a. intravascular hemolysis
> a. laryngotracheobronchitis
> a. lupus pneumonitis
> a. meningococcemia
> a. multifocal placoid pigment
>   epitheliopathy
> a. necrotizing encephalitis
> a. necrotizing ulcerative gingivitis
>   (ANUG)
> a. otitis media (AOM)
> a. paranasal sinusitis
> a. paronychia
> a. periorbital edema
> a. peritonitis
> a. phase protein
> a. phase reaction
> a. physiology and chronic health
>   evaluation
> a. primary hemorrhagic
>   meningoencephalitis
> a. pulmonary reaction
> a. radiation pneumonitis
> a. radiodermatitis
> a. rejection episode
> a. retroviral syndrome
> a. rheumatic arthritis
> a. rheumatoid arthritis
> a. rhinitis
> a. scalp cellulitis
> a. seroconversion syndrome
> a. transfusion reaction
> a. tubular necrosis
> a. vascular purpura

acutum
> ulcus vulvae a.

acutus
> pemphigus a.

acyclovir
acyl chain
ADA
> adenosine deaminase
> ADA deficiency

Adagen
adalimumab
ADAM
> a disintegrin and matrilysin

Adamantiades-Behçet syndrome
adamantinoma
Adams-Oliver syndrome

adapalene
    a. cream
    a. gel
Adapin
adaptor
    bi-luer lock a.
    ENTsol a.
ADASI
    Atopic Dermatitis Area and Severity
    Index
ADC
    apparent diffusion coefficient
ADCC
    antibody-dependent cellular cytotoxicity
addicted scrotum syndrome
Addison
    A. disease
    A. keloid
    A. morphea
    A. pigmentation
Addison-Gull disease
addisonian
    a. dermal pigmentation
    a. melanosis
addisonism
addition-deletion mutation
additive
    a. arthritis
    colloid a.
    food a.
    impermeant solution a.
    substrate solution a.
addressin
addressing ligand
adductor digiti quinti
adefovir
Aden
    A. fever
    A. ulcer
adenine arabinoside
adenitis
    Bartholin a.
    syphilitic inguinal a.
    vestibular a.
adeno-associated virus (AAV)
adenocarcinoma
    colonic a.
    eccrine a.
    Lucké a.
    sebaceous a.
adenoepithelioma

adenoidal facies
adenoidal-pharyngeal-conjunctival (A-P-C)
    a.-p.-c. virus
adenoid cystic carcinoma
adeno-like
    gallus a.-l. (GAL)
adenolipoma
adenolipomatosis
adenoma
    aggressive digital papillary a.
    (ADPA)
    apocrine a.
    papillary eccrine a.
    sebaceous a.
    a. sebaceum
adenomatoid
adenomatosis oris
adenopathy
    hilar a.
adenosatellite virus
adenosine
    a. deaminase (ADA)
    a. deaminase deficiency
    a. triphosphatase (ATPase)
    a. triphosphatase activity
adenosylcobalamin
adenoviral gene transfection
Adenoviridae
adenovirus (AdV)
    canine a. 1
    a. fiber knob
    gutless a.
    immunogenetic wild-type a.
adenovirus-induced steroid resistance
adenovirus-mediated gene transfer
adenovirus-reactive T cell
adenylate cyclase toxin
adenylic acid
adenylosuccinic acid synthetase
ADEPT
    antibody-directed enzyme prodrug
    therapy
adequate
    a. hydration
    a. urine output
adermal
adermia congenita
adermic
adermogenesis
Ad fiber-knob

NOTES

ADG
  adjustable-depth gauge
  ADG needle
adherence
  a. assay
  immune a.
  treatment a. (TA)
adherent mucus gel layer
adhesin
adhesin-receptor interaction
adhesion
  a. aid
  cell-cell a.
  corneocyte a.
  homophilic cell-cell a.
  integrin-mediated a.
  keratinocytic a.
  a. molecule
  a. molecule cascade
  a. phenomenon
  a. protein
  a. test
adhesional and glide friction
adhesive
  Biobrane a.
  a. capsulitis
  Dermabond topical skin a.
  Indermil tissue a.
  Indermil topical a.
  Scanpor acrylate a.
  a. serositis
adiaphoresis
adiaphoretic
adiaspiromycosis
Adie tonic pupil
adipectomy
adipofibroma
adipogenic
adipogenous
adipometer
adiponecrosis subcutanea neonatorum
adiposa
  blepharoptosis a.
  seborrhea a.
adiposalgia
adipose infiltration
adiposis dolorosa
adipositis
adiposity
  painful a.
adiposum
  sclerema a.
adjustable-depth
  a.-d. gauge (ADG)
  a.-d. gauge needle
adjuvant
  Freund incomplete a. (FIA)
  immunologic a.

  MPL vaccine a.
  a. vaccine
ADL 2-1294
Adlone Injection
ADM
  amyopathic dermatomyositis
administration
adnata
  alopecia a.
adnexal
  a. carcinoma
  a. tumor
adnexum, pl. **adnexa**
  ocular adnexa
adolescent eczema
adoptive
  a. immunity
  a. immunotherapy
Adoxa tablet
ADPA
  aggressive digital papillary adenoma
ADR
  adverse drug-induced reaction
adrenal
  a. cortex disorder
  hypothalamo-pituitary a.
  a. insufficiency
Adrenalin Chloride
adrenergic
  a. drug
  a. urticaria
adrenocortical
  a. failure
  a. insufficiency
adrenocorticosteroid therapy
adrenocorticotropic
  a. hormone (ACTH)
  a. hormone therapy
adrenoleukodystrophy
Adriamycin
Adrucil injection
ADS
  antibody-deficient syndrome
ADSI
  Atopic Dermatitis Severity Index
Adson
  A. test
  A. toothed forceps
adsorbed
  tetanus toxoid, a.
adsorbent
Adsorbotear Ophthalmic solution
adsorption
  immune a.
adsorptive voltametry
adult
  a. asthma
  a. bullous dermatosis
  a. eczema

latent autoimmune diabetes of a.'s (LADA)
a. T-cell leukemia/lymphoma (ATLL)
a. tuberculosis
adult/adolescent spectrum of HIV disease
adulterated rapeseed oil-associated toxic oil syndrome
adult-onset systemic Still disease
adultorum
scleredema a.
a. scleroderma
adult-type rheumatoid arthritis
AdV
adenovirus
Advair
Advanced Formula Oxy Sensitive Gel
advancement flap
adventitia
adventitial dermis
adventitious cyst
adverse
a. drug-induced reaction (ADR)
a. drug reaction
a. food reaction
Advia Centaur specific IgE assay
Advil
Children's A.
A. Cold & Sinus Caplets
Advisory Committee on Immunization Practice (ACIP)
advocate
patient a.
AE
acrodermatitis enteropathica
AEC
absolute blood eosinophil count
ankyloblepharon, ectodermal defect, and cleft lip and/or palate
AEC syndrome
Aedes albopictus
aegleria invadens
Aeroaid
aeroallergen
animal a.
mold a.
Aerobacter
aerobe
obligate a.
aerobic
AeroBid-M Oral Aerosol Inhaler

AeroBid Oral Aerosol Inhaler
aerobiology
Aerochamber nebulizer
aerodigestive
AeroEclipse Aerosol Delivery Device
aerofaciens
Eubacterium a.
aerogen
aerogenes
Pasteurella a.
aerogenesis
aerogenic tuberculosis
AeroHist Plus
aeroirritant
AeroKid syrup
Aerolate
A. III
A. Jr
A. SR
aerometric study
Aeromonas
A. caviae
A. hydrophila
A. septicemia
A. shigelloides
A. sobria
A. veronii
aerophil
aerophilic
aeroplankton
Aeroseb-Dex
Aeroseb-HC topical
aerosol
Brethaire Inhalation A.
DEY albuterol inhalation a.
Duo-Medihaler A.
Fluro-Ethyl A.
ipratropium bromide a.
monodisperse a.
Nasalide nasal A.
a. spray
Tilade Inhalation A.
Virazole A.
aerosolization
aerosolized pollutant exposure
AeroSonic personal ultrasonic nebulizer
AeroTech II nebulizer
AeroZoin
Aertemia Salinas sequence
aeruginosa
Pseudomonas a.
aestival (*var. of* estival)

NOTES

aestivale (*var. of* estivale)
aestivalis (*var. of* estivalis)
AETT
   acetyl ethyl tetramethyl tetralin
AEU
   allercoat enzyme allergosorbent unit
AF
   Diprolene AF
AF-1, -2 antigen
AFC
   antibody-forming cell
afferent
   a. arteriole
   a. nerve fiber
affinity
   a. antibody
   functional a.
   intrinsic a.
   a. labeling
   a. maturation
affinity-purified antiidiopeptide antibody
afibrinogenemia
A-Fil
Afipia felis
Aflexa
Africa
   Out of A.
African
   A. Burkitt lymphoma
   A. cutaneous Kaposi sarcoma
   A. endemic relapsing fever
   A. Gold
   A. hemorrhagic fever
   A. histoplasmosis
   A. honeybee
   A. horse sickness
   A. horse sickness virus
   A. lymphadenopathic Kaposi
     sarcoma
   A. meningitis
   A. swine fever
   A. swine fever virus (ASFV)
   A. tick typhus
   A. tick virus
   A. trypanosomiasis
Africanized honeybee sting
African-variety Kaposi sarcoma
Afrin
   A. Children's Nose drops
   A. Nasal Solution
   A. Tablet
Afrinol
AFS
   aldehyde-fuchsin stain
Aftate
aftosa
afzelii
   Borrelia a.

Ag
   antigen
   Aquacel Ag
AGA
   androgenetic alopecia
agalactiae
   Streptococcus a.
agammaglobulinemia
   Bruton a.
   secondary a.
   Swiss type a.
   transient a.
   X-linked a.
agar
   BCYE a.
   buffered charcoal yeast extract a.
   corn meal a.
   a. diffusion assay
   a. gel diffusion
   Kirby-Bauer a.
   Löwenstein-Jensen a.
   Mueller-Hinton a.
   Sabouraud a.
agarose gel
agency
   Regional Organ Procurement A.
     (ROPA)
Agenerase
agenesia
agenesis
   pilorum a.
   pulmonary a.
agent
   Accuzyme enzymatic debriding a.
   alkylating a.
   alpha-adrenergic blocking a.
   antibacterial a.
   antifibrinolytic a.
   antifoaming a.
   antihypertensive a.
   antihyperuricemic a.
   antiinfective a.
   antimalarial a.
   antipruritic a.
   antirheumatic a.
   antiviral a.
   azole antifungal a.
   Bittner a.
   chelating a.
   chemical a.
   chemotherapy a.
   cholinergic a.
   coloring a.
   comedolytic a.
   cooling a.
   covering a.
   cytoprotective a.
   cytotoxic a.
   delta a.

denaturing a.
depigmenting a.
dispersing a.
Eaton a.
emulsifying a.
entire body imaging a.
enzymatic debriding a.
epsilon-aminocaproic a.
F a.
fertility a.
foamy a.
gastroprotective a.
hemostatic a.
immunosuppressive a.
keratolytic a.
lactic dehydrogenase a.
LDH a.
LeukoScan diagnostic a.
macrolide antimicrobial a.
MS-1, -2 a.
nonantiinflammatory analgesic a.
noncorticosteroid antiinflammatory a.
Norwalk a.
Norwalk-like a.
Panafil enzymatic debriding a.
Panafil-White enzymatic
  debriding a.
pigmenting a.
prophylaxis a.
psychotropic a.
Reovirus-like a.
Santyl enzymatic debriding a.
sclerosing a.
topical hemostatic a.
transforming a.
virus-inactivating a.
Wor Ditchling a.
AGEP
  acute generalized exanthematous
    pustulosis
age pigment
age-related osteoporosis
agglutinate
agglutinating antibody
agglutination
  acid a.
  bacteriogenic a.
  cold a.
  cross a.
  false a.
  group a.
  immune a.

indirect a.
latex particle a.
mixed a.
nonimmune a.
passive a.
reversed passive latex a.
spontaneous a.
agglutinative
agglutinin
  blood group a.
  chief a.
  cold a.
  cross-reacting a.
  febrile a.
  flagellar a.
  group a.
  H a.
  immune a.
  incomplete a.
  major a.
  minor a.
  O a.
  partial a.
  plant a.
  saline a.
  serum a.
  somatic a.
  warm a.
  Yersinia pseudotuberculosis a.
agglutinogen
  blood group a.
  T a.
agglutinogenic
agglutinophilic
agglutinoscope
agglutogen
agglutogenic
aggrecanase-induced aggrecan neoepitope
aggrecan CS/KS
aggregate
  a. anaphylaxis
  IgG-RF complement a.
  immunoglobulin G rheumatoid
    factor complement a.
  link-protein-stabilized a.
  snowball a.
  snowbank a.
aggregated human IgG
aggregation
  familial a.
aggregometry
aggressin

NOTES

15

aggressive
> a. cell cluster
> a. digital papillary adenoma (ADPA)
> a. hepatitis
> a. infantile fibromatosis

aging
> photo a.
> premature a.

AgiSite alginate wound cover
agminata
agminated
> a. atypical nevus
> a. follicle
> a. lentiginosis

agminate folliculitis
agnails
agnogenic myeloid metaplasia (AMM)
agnus-castus
> *Vitex a.-c.*

agonist
> alpha-adrenergic a.
> beta-adrenergic a.
> bronchoactive a.
> histamine H$_1$ a.

agranulocytosis
> feline a.

agrarius
> *Apodemus a.*

agretope
agria
> protoporphyria prurigo a.
> prurigo a.

Agrimonia eupatoria
Agrimony
agrius
> lichen a.

Agrobacterium
> *A. radiobacter*
> *A. tumefaciens*

AH50 assay
AHR
> airway hyperresponsiveness

A-hydroCort
AI
> apo AI

AI-502
AIA
> aspirin-intolerant asthma

AICA-riboside
> aminoimidazole carboxamide-riboside

AICD
> activation-induced cell death

aid
> adhesion a.
> Compoz Nighttime Sleep A.
> Sleep A.
> Travel A.

AIDS
> lichenoid and granulomatous dermatitis of AIDS (LGDA)
> transfusion-associated AIDS (TA-AIDS)
> AIDS vaccine

Ailos nebulizer
ainhum
ainhumoides
> sclerodactylia annularis a.

AIR
> AIR max
> AIR min

air
> a. bronchogram
> a. cleaner
> a. coil
> cold dry a. (CDA)
> a. conditioning
> high-efficiency particulate a. (HEPA)
> liquid a.
> a. pollution
> a. pollution control
> a. spora
> a. trapping

airborne
> a. allergen
> a. contact dermatitis
> a. spore
> a. transmission

Airet
air-fluidized bed
airspace
> a. consolidation
> peripheral a.
> a. process

Airstrip composite dressing
AirWatch Asthma monitor
airway
> a. bacterial colonization
> cellular accumulation in the a.'s
> a.'s disease
> a. eosinophilia
> a. hyperresponsiveness (AHR)
> a. pressure release ventilation (APRV)
> a. reactivity
> a. resistance
> a. responsiveness
> a. smooth muscle (ASM)

Ajellomyces dermatitidis
AK
> acne keloidalis

Akabane virus
akamushi
> a. disease
> *Leptotrombidium a.*
> *Trombicula a.*

akari
    Rickettsia a.
AK-Chlor Ophthalmic
AK-Cide Ophthalmic
AKD
    atypical Kawasaki disease
AK-Dex Ophthalmic
AK-Dilate Ophthalmic solution
akeratosis
AK-Homatropine Ophthalmic
AK-Mycin
AK-Nefrin Ophthalmic solution
Akne-Mycin topical
AK-Neo-Dex Ophthalmic
AK-Poly-Bac Ophthalmic
AK-Pred Ophthalmic
Akrinol Cream
Akros extended care mattress
AkroTech mattress
AK-Spore
    AK-S. H.C. Ophthalmic Ointment
    AK-S. H.C. Ophthalmic suspension
    AK-S. H.C. Otic
AK-Sulf Ophthalmic
AK-Tate
AKTob Ophthalmic
AK-Tracin Ophthalmic
AK-Trol Ophthalmic
AKU
    alkaptonuria
Akwa Tears solution
ALA
    aminolevulinic acid
    ALA dehydratase deficiency
    porphyria
AlaBLOT kit
Ala-Cort topical
Aladdin infant flow system
alae nasi
alafacept
Alagille syndrome
Alamast
alanine aminotransferase
alanyl-transfer ribonucleic acid
  synthetase
alanyl-tRNA synthetase
Ala-Quin topical
alar ligament
Ala-Scalp topical
AlaSTAT
    A. allergy immunoassay system

    A. assay
    A. latex allergy test
alastrim
alastrimic
Alatest Latex-specific IgE allergen test
  kit
AlaTOP inhalant allergy screen
alba, pl. albae
    lepra a.
    linea a.
    miliaria a.
    morphea a.
    phlegmasia a.
    pityriasis a.
    stria a.
albedo unguium
albendazole sulfoxide
Albenza
albicans, pl. albicantes
    Candida a.
    linea a.
    Monilia a.
    stria a.
albida
    acne a.
albidum
    atrophoderma a.
albimanus
    Anopheles a.
albinism
    Amish a.
    autosomal dominant
     oculocutaneous a.
    brown oculocutaneous a.
    circumscribed a.
    complete imperfect a.
    complete perfect a.
    Cuna moon-child a.
    cutaneous a.
    Forsius-Eriksson-type ocular a.
    a. I, II
    localized a.
    minimal-pigment oculocutaneous a.
    Nettleship-Falls ocular a.
    Nettleship-Falls-type ocular a.
    ocular a. (OA)
    oculocutaneous a. (OCA)
    partial a.
    piebald a.
    red a.
    rufous oculocutaneous a.

NOTES

albinism *(continued)*
    temperature-sensitive
      oculocutaneous a.
    type (I, IA, IB, II)
      oculocutaneous a.
    type (I, II) ocular a.
    type (I-MP, I-TS)
      oculocutaneous a.
    tyrosinase-negative
      oculocutaneous a.
    tyrosinase-positive oculocutaneous a.
    tyrosinase-related oculocutaneous a.
    X-linked ocular a. (XOAN)
    yellow mutant a.
    yellow oculocutaneous a.
albinismus
    a. circumscriptus
    a. conscriptus
    a. universalis
albino
albinoidism
albinotic
alboatrum
    Verticillium a.
Albolene
albopictus
    Aedes a.
Albright
    A. dimpling sign
    A. disease
    A. hereditary osteodystrophy
    A. sign
    A. syndrome
albumin
    Bence Jones a.
    low plasma a.
    penicillin-penicilloyl human
      serum a. (PPO-HSA)
    Q a.
albumin-autoagglutinating factor
albus
    lichen a.
    Staphylococcus a.
albuterol
    a. sulfate
    a. sulfate syrup
Alcaligenes
    A. bookeri
    A. denitrificans
    A. faecalis
    A. odorans
    A. piechaudii
    A. xylosoxidans
ALCAT
    antigen leukocyte cellular antibody test
Alcian blue stain
alclometasone dipropionate
Alcock syndrome

alcohol
    benzyl a.
    camphor and a.
    cinnamic a.
    ethyl a.
    isopropyl a.
    a. pledget
    wool wax a.
alcoholic white shake lotion
alcohol-related liver disease (ALD)
Alcyonidrium
ALD
    alcohol-related liver disease
aldehyde
    cinnamic a.
aldehyde-fuchsin stain (AFS)
alder
    red a.
    a. tree
    a. tree pollen
aldesleukin
Aldrich syndrome
alefacept
alendronate sodium
Aleppo boil
aleukemic leukemia
Aleutian
    A. mink disease
    A. mink disease virus
Aleve
alexandrite laser
alexin unit
Alexion anticomplement C5a
ALEXlazr laser
Alezzandrini syndrome
alfa
    natural interferon a.
alfa-2a
    interferon a.-2a
alfa-2b
    interferon a.-2b
alfalfa
    a. grass
    a. weed pollen
alfa-n3
    interferon a.-n3
Alferon N
AlgiDerm
    A. alginate dressing
    A. alginate wound cover
    A. wound dressing
algid stage
alginate
    a. wound cover
    a. wound dressing
AlgiSite
    A. alginate dressing
    A. wound dressing
Algisorb wound dressing

alglucerase
algodystrophy
algofunctional Lequesne index
algorithm
    Dermatologic Diagnostic A.
    diagnostic a.
    Needleman-Wunsch a.
    problem-oriented a.
Algosteril
    A. alginate dressing
    A. alginate wound cover
Alibert
    A. disease
    A. keloid
    A. mentagra
Alibert-Bazin
    A.-B. syndrome
    A.-B. type mycosis fungoides
Alibour solution
alignment
    patellofemoral a.
Alimentum formula
ALIP
    abnormal localization of immature
    precursors
aliphatic
    a. hydrocarbon
    a. residue
aliquant
aliquot
alitretinoin
alizarin red S stain
Alkaban-AQ
alkaline phosphatase and pyrophosphate
alkalinization
alkalinizer
    urinary a.
alkali patch test
alkaloid
    Vinca a.
alkanolamineborate
alkaptonuria (AKU)
Alka-Seltzer Plus Cold Liqui-Gels
  Capsule
alkyl
    a. aryl ether
    a. phenoxyl polyethoxy ethanol
alkylamine
alkylating
    a. agent
    a. therapy
Alldress composite dressing

alleaceae
Allegra
Allegra-D
allele
    blank a.
    DR1 a.
    DR3 a.
    DR5 a.
    HLA a.
    a. HLA DQw7
    a. HLA-DR4
    a. HLA-DR7
    HLA-DRB1 a.
    a. HLA DRw53
    human leukocyte antigen a.
    a. human leukocyte antigen DQw7
    a. human leukocyte antigen DRw53
    null a.
    permissive MHC a.
    promotor a.
allelic
    a. exclusion
    a. polymorphism
Allelock
Aller-Aide
AllerCare allergy control product
Aller-Chlor Oral
allercoat enzyme allergosorbent unit
  (AEU)
Allercon Tablet
Allerderm Protective Glove System
Allerdryl
Allerest
    A. 12-Hour Nasal Solution
    A. Maximum Strength
Allerfrin
    A. Syrup
    A. Tablet
Allergan Ear drops
allergen
    airborne a.
    20-a. Hermal screening series
    avocational a.
    a. challenge
    a. contact
    environmental a.
    epidermal a.
    a. exposure
    flux a.
    a. immunotherapy
    inhalant a.
    a. inhalation challenge test

NOTES

allergen *(continued)*
    insect a.
    Lolium perenne a.
    Lol p a. (I-III)
    mammal a.
    occupational a.
    recombinant a.
Allergenco MK-3 spore trap
allergenic
    a. epitope
    a. extract
allergen-induced
    a.-i. asthma
    a.-i. mediator release
allergen-specific nasal challenge
allergic
    a. angiitis
    a. angioedema
    a. apostematous cheilitis
    a. asthma
    a. colitis
    a. conjunctivitis
    a. contact stomatitis
    a. coryza
    a. crease
    a. diathesis
    a. drug reaction
    a. eczema
    a. eczematous contact-type
      dermatitis
    a. encephalomyelitis
    a. eosinophilic gastroenteritis
    a. eosinophilic gastroenterocolitis
    a. extract
    a. eye disorder
    a. facies
    a. gap
    a. gold dermatitis
    a. granulomatosis
    a. granulomatous arteritis
    a. importance
    a. inflammation
    a. manifestation
    a. nonthrombocytopenic purpura
    a. orchitis
    a. phlyctenulosis
    a. rhinitis
    a. rhinobronchitis
    a. rhinoconjunctivitis
    a. salute
    a. sensitivity
    a. shiner
    a. urticaria
    a. vasculitis
allergin
allergist
allergization
allergize
allergized

allergoid
allergologic
allergologist
allergology
allergosis
allergy
    acrylic acid a.
    arthropod a.
    atopic a.
    bacterial a.
    Benylin for A.'s
    bitterwood a.
    car a.
    cat a.
    cerebral a.
    chironomid a.
    cold a.
    contact a.
    cow's milk a. (CMA)
    delayed a.
    dog a.
    drug a.
    durable-press a.
    dust a.
    A. Elixir
    food a.
    gelatin a.
    gold a.
    hereditary a.
    IgE-mediated food a.
    immediate a.
    immunoglobulin E-mediated food a.
    insect a.
    insulin a.
    intrinsic a.
    Japanese sargassum a.
    Küstner fish a.
    latent a.
    latex a.
    local anesthetic a.
    mice a.
    milk a.
    mite-snail combined a.
    nasal a.
    natural rubber latex a.
    nickel a.
    ocular a.
    peanut a. (PN)
    physical a.
    polyvalent a.
    propylene glycol a.
    A. Relief
    rodent a.
    Rowe elimination diet for
      food a.'s
    rubber a.
    seasonal a.
    a. skin test
    soy protein a.

spina bifida-associated latex a.
spontaneous a.
a. tablet
tree nut a. (TN)
universal a.
a. vaccine
Allergy/Sinus/Headache
Tavist A./S./H.
AllerMax Oral
Allernix
Allerphed Syrup
Allerprick needle
AllerSpray
Allescheria boydii
Allevyn
A. adhesive foam dressing
A. cavity foam dressing
A. island foam dressing
A. synthetic dressing
A. Thin dressing
A. tracheostomy foam dressing
Allfen-DM
all-fours maneuver
alligator skin
Allis forceps
Allium sativum
alloantibody
alloantigen
alloantigenicity
alloantigen-independent risk factor
alloatherogenesis
allochromasia
Allochrysine
AlloDerm
Cymetra micronized A.
A. processed tissue graft
A. universal dermal tissue graft
Allodermanyssus sanguineus
allogenic, allogeneic
a. antigen
a. bone marrow cell infusion
a. bone marrow transplantation
a. dendritic cell
a. effect
a. effect factor
a. graft
a. hematopoietic stem cell
transplantation (allo-HSCT)
a. inhibition
a. transplant
allograft
cardiac a.

double renal a.
heart a.
human small intestinal a.
a. irradiation
kidney a.
liver a.
lung a.
neonatal skin a.
a. pathology
a. rejection
allogroup
allo-HSCT
allogenic hematopoietic stem cell
transplantation
alloimmunization
AlloMune
allopeptide
donor a.
allophenic
alloplast
Alloprin
allopurinol
alloreactive cell
alloreactivity
cell a.
allosensitization
allotope
allotoxin
allotransplantation
cardiac a.
liver a.
allotrichia circumscripta
allotype
Am a.
Gm a.
InV a.
Km a.
latent a.
nominal a.
simple a.
a. suppression
allotypic
a. determinant
a. marker
Allovectin-7 DNA/lipid complex
Allpyral
allscale
all-trans-retinoic acid (ATRA)
allylamine
allyl isothiocyanate
Almeida disease
almond

NOTES

Alnus glutinosa
Alocort
aloe

Cortaid with A.
Dermtex HC with A.
Fruit of the Earth Moisturizing A.
A. Vesta antifungal ointment

aloetic
Alomide Ophthalmic
alone

pancreas transplant a. (PTA)

alopecia

a. acquisita
a. adnata
androgenetic a. (AGA)
a. androgenetica
a. capitis totalis
Celsus a.
cicatricial a.
a. cicatrisata
cicatrizing a.
a. circumscripta
congenital sutural a.
congenital triangular a.
a. disseminata
drug a.
drug-induced a.
favic a.
favid a.
female pattern a.
follicular a.
a. follicularis
a. furfuracea
a. generalisata
a. hereditaria
hot comb a.
Jonston a.
a. leprotica
a. liminaris
a. liminaris frontalis
lipedematous a.
lupus a.
male pattern a.
marginal a.
a. marginalis
a. marginata
mechanical a.
a. medicamentosa
moth-eaten a.
a. mucinosa
a., nail dystrophy, ophthalmic complication, thyroid dysfunction, hypohidrosis, ephelides and enteropathy, and respiratory tract infection (ANOTHER)
a. neoplastica
a. neurotica
noncicatrizing a.

nonscarring a.
a. orbicularis
patterned a.
physiologic a.
pityriasic a.
a. pityrodes
postmenopausal frontal fibrosing a.
postoperative pressure a.
postpartum a.
a. prematura
premature a.
a. presenilis
pressure a.
pseudopelade-type a.
roentgen a.
scarring vertex a.
a. seborrheica
senile a.
a. senilis
a. symptomatica
syphilitic a.
a. syphilitica
tick bite a.
toxic a.
a. toxica
traction a.
traumatic a.
a. traumatica
a. triangularis
a. triangularis congenitalis
a. universal areata
a. universalis
x-ray a.

alopecic
Aloprim Injection
Alora transdermal patch
ALP

actinic lichen planus
antileukoproteinase

alpha, α

a. adrenergic stimulation
a. cell
a. chain
a. chain disease
a., delta sleep anomaly
a. fetoprotein
a. Gal antibody
a. hemolysin
a. hydroxy acid lotion
interferon a. (IFN-alpha)
A. Keri lotion
a. lactalbumin
a. nerve fiber
PGF_2 a.
A. 1 pump
5 a. reductase
a. thalassemia
a. wave intrusion

alpha-adrenergic
    a.-a. agonist
    a.-a. blocking agent
alpha-amino-p-toluene sulfonamide
alpha$_2$-antiplasmin
alpha-antitrypsin
    serum a.-a.
alpha$_1$-antitrypsin (alpha$_1$-AT)
    a.$_1$-a. deficiency
    a.$_1$-a. deficiency panniculitis
alpha$_1$-AT
    alpha$_1$-antitrypsin
alpha-difluoromethylornithine
alpha-enolase
alpha-Gal epitope
alpha$_2$ globulin
alpha-glutathione S-transferase assay
alpha-heavy-chain disease
alpha-helix
alpha-interferon 3
Alpha-Keri
    A.-K. oil
    A.-K. soap
alpha-lactalbumin
alpha-latrotoxin
alpha-melanocyte-stimulating hormone (alpha-MSH)
alpha-methyldopa
alpha-MSH
    alpha-melanocyte-stimulating hormone
alpha$_2$-neuraminoglycoprotein
alpha-nonrapid eye movement sleep
alpha-NREM
    alpha-NREM sleep
alpha$_1$-proteinase deficiency
5-alpha-reductase inhibitor
alpha-1-thymosin
Alphatrex topical
alpha$_1$-trypsin inhibitor
Alphavirus
alphoides
    lepra a.
alphos
    lepra a.
alprazolam
AL protein
ALPS
    autoimmune lymphoproliferative syndrome
Alrex
AL-Rr Oral

ALS
    amyotrophic lateral sclerosis
    antilymphocyte serum
Alström syndrome
Alteon
alteration
    ecologic a.
    glucocorticoid-mediated stress-induced immune a.
    metabolic a.
    postinflammatory pigment a.
    red cell membrane a.
Alternaria
    A. alternata
    A. alternata fungus
    A. mold
    A. tenuis
alternariosis
alternata
    Alternaria a.
alternate-day therapy
alternative
    a. pathway of complement cascade
    a. polyadenylylation
alternifolia
    Melaleuca a.
Al-Test
Alti-Flunisoline
Altinac
aluminum
    a. acetate
    a. acetate and acetic acid
    a. chloride
    a. chloride hexahydrate
    a. chloride solution
    a. chlorohydrate
    a. density step scale
    a. Finn chamber
    a. lactate
    a. oxide
    a. salt
alum-precipitated
    a.-p. antigen
    a.-p. preparation
    a.-p. pyridine-extracted pollen extract
Alupent
Alustra
alvei
    Bacillus a.
    Hafnia a.

NOTES

23

alveolar
    a. capillary
    a. fluid clearance
    a. infiltration by histiocyte
    a. macrophage
    a. ventilation
    a. ventilation per minute
alveolar-arterial oxygen gradient
alveolar-lung parenchymal interface
alveolar-septal amyloidosis
alveoli (*pl. of* alveolus)
alveolitis
    diffuse fibrosing a.
    extrinsic allergic a.
    fibrosing a.
    occupational allergic a.
alveolointerstitial
alveolus, pl. **alveoli**
    ventilated a.
ALW
    arch-loop-whorl
alymphoplasia
    Nezelof type of thymic a.
    thymic a.
Alzet osmotic pump
Am
    Am allotype
    Am antigen
AMAD
    Assessment Measure for Atopic
    Dermatitis
amalgam
    dental a.
    a. tattoo
amalonaticus
    Citrobacter a.
amantadine hydrochloride
Amapari virus
amaranth
    green a.
Amaranthaceae
amaranth-chenopod
amastigotes
amatol
amber
    Baltic a.
Ambi
    A. 10
    A. Skin Tone
Ambi-100/55
Ambi-60/580
Ambi-60/580/30
AmBisome
Amblyomma
    A. americanum
    A. cajennense
    A. hebraeum
amboceptor unit
Amboyna button

ambrette
    musk a.
Ambrosia
    A. artemisiifolia
    A. psilostachya
    A. trifida
ambulans
    ulcus a.
ambulant erysipelas
Ambulator shoe
ambustiforme
    ulcus a.
ambustion
ambustionis
    dermatitis a.
amcinonide
Amcort Injection
amdinocillin
Ameba histolytica
amebiasis cutis
amebic
    a. granuloma
    a. ulcer
amebicide
ameboma
Amechol
amegakaryocytic thrombocytopenia (AT)
amelanosis
amelanotic
    a. melanoma
    a. nevus
amelioration
    leukapheresis-induced a.
ameloblastoma
    melanotic a.
    peripheral a.
    pigmented a.
America
    Dystrophic Epidermolysis Bullosa
    Research Association of A.
    (DEBRA)
    Infectious Disease Society of A.
    (IDSA)
    National Psoriasis Foundation/United
    States of A. (NPF/USA)
Americaine
American
    A. cockroach
    A. College of Rheumatology
    (ACR)
    A. College of Rheumatology
    criteria
    A. elm
    A. elm tree
    A. leishmaniasis
    A. mayapple
    A. Rheumatism Association (ARA)
    A. Rheumatism Association criteria

A. Society of Transplant Surgeons
A. trypanosomiasis
americana
    leishmaniasis a.
americanum
    Amblyomma a.
americanus
    Necator a.
Amerigel
    A. lotion
    A. topical ointment
    A. topical ointment hydrogel
      dressing
amerospore
Amersol
Amesec
A-methaPred injection
amethopterin
Amevive
amiantacea
    pityriasis a.
    tinea a.
amiantaceous crust
Amico
    A. extractor
    A. nail nipper
amicrobic
amide compound
amidolytic activity
amidophosphoribosyltransferase
amifloxacin
amikacin sulfate
Amikin injection
amine
    biogenic a.
amino
    a. acid
    a. acid-based low fat proprietary
      formula
    a. acid metabolism
    a. ethyl ethanolamine
aminoacetonitrile
aminoacyl-tRNA synthetase
aminobenzoate
    a. ester
    ethyl a.
aminobenzoic acid
aminoglutethimide
aminoglycoside
aminoimidazole
    a. carboxamide-riboside (AICA-
      riboside)

aminolevulinate
    topical methyl a.
aminolevulinic
    a. acid (ALA)
    a. acid HCl
    5-a. acid
Amino-Opti-E Oral
aminopenicillin
aminophylline, amobarbital, and
  ephedrine
aminopterin syndrome
Aminoquinoline
aminosalicylate sodium
aminosalicylic acid
aminosidine sulfate
aminosteroid
21-aminosteroid
aminotransferase
    alanine a.
amiodarone pigmentation
amiprilose
    a. HCl
    a. hydrochloride
Amish albinism
Ami-Tex LA
Amitril
amitriptyline hydrochloride
Amlexanox
AMM
    agnogenic myeloid metaplasia
ammonia
    a. dermatitis
    a. rash
ammoniated mercury
ammonium
    a. lactate
    quaternary a.
amnioma
A-mode ultrasound
amorolfine
amorphous
    a. parenchymal opacification
    a. substance
AMO Vitrax
amoxicillin/clavulanate (AMX/CL)
amoxicillin and clavulanic acid
Amoxil
Amp
    Jaa A.
amphimicrobe
amphiphysin
amphiregulin (AR)

NOTES

25

Amphocil
amphophilous
Amphotec
amphotericin
    a. B
    a. B cholesteryl sulfate complex
    a. B colloidal dispersion
    a. B lipid complex
    a. B lipid complex injection
    a. B liposomal formulation
amphotropic virus
ampicillin
    a. and probenecid
    a. and sulbactam
Ampicin Sodium
Ampilean
amplicon
    deoxyribonucleic acid a.
    DNA a.
Amplicor viral load test
amplification
    a. assay
    chirp-pulse a.
    HBV bDNA signal a.
    hepatitis B virus branched chain
      deoxyribonucleic acid signal a.
    human immunodeficiency virus
      DNA a.
    nucleic acid sequence based a.
      (NASBA)
Amplified Mycobacterium Tuberculosis
  Direct Test
amplifier host
Ampliwax PCR Gem
amprenavir
amprolium hydrochloride
amputating ulcer
amputation neuroma
amstelodamensis
    typhus degenerativus a.
amstelodami
    Aspergillus a.
Amvisc plus
AMX/CL
    amoxicillin/clavulanate
    AMX/CL suspension
Amycolatopsis orientalis
amyctic
amylin
    IAPP a.
amyloid
    a. A protein
    articular a.
    cutaneous a.
    a. degeneration
    a. disease
    a. fibril
    a. fibril protein
    a. P component

    primary a.
    a. Q
    secondary a.
    a. structure
    a. syndrome
    systemic a.
    a. tumor
amyloidogenic transthyretin (ATTR)
amyloidosis
    AA, AL a.
    alveolar-septal a.
    bullous a.
    cerebral a.
    a. cutis
    cystatin C a.
    dialysis-related a.
    endocrine a.
    familial a.
    fibrogen-associated a.
    focal a.
    gelsolin a.
    hemodialysis-associated a.
    hereditary cardiopathic a.
    heredofamilial a.
    immune-derived a.
    immunocyte-derived a.
    lichen a.
    lichenoid a.
    localized cutaneous a.
    lysozyme-associated a.
    macular a.
    mediastinal a.
    neuropathic a.
    nodular pulmonary a.
    nonneuropathic systemic a.
    oculoleptomeningeal a.
    parenchymal a.
    pleural a.
    polyneuropathic a.
    primary cutaneous a.
    primary localized a.
    primary systemic a.
    pseudotumoral mediastinal a.
    pulmonary a.
    secondary systemic a.
    secondary tumor-associated
      cutaneous a.
    systemic visceral a.
    tracheobronchial a.
    transthyretin a.
amyloidotic
    a. nephropathy
    a. polyneuropathy
amyopathic dermatomyositis (ADM)
amyotrophic
    a. lateral sclerosis (ALS)
    a. syphilitic myelitis
ANA
    speckled-pattern ANA

anabolic steroid
anabrosis
anabrotic
Anacardium
    A. melanorrhoea
    A. occidentale
Anacin
anaemicus (*var. of* anemicus)
anaerobe
    facultative a.
anaerobic
    a. bacterial arthritis
    a. *Bifidobacterium*
    a. cellulitis
Anaerobiospirillum
anaerobius
    Peptostreptococcus a.
anaesthetica
    lepra a.
Anaflex 750
Anafranil
anagen
    a. effluvium
    a. growth phase
anagrelide
Ana-Guard
Anahelp
anakinra
Ana-Kit
anal fissure
anallergic
analog, analogue
    purine a.
    semisynthetic a.
analogous
Analpram
analysis, pl. **analyses**
    antigenic a.
    displacement a.
    dual-fluorescence a.
    gait a.
    genome-side linkage a.
    genomic a.
    Griess a.
    heteroduplex a.
    immunofluorescence a.
    latent class a.
    Northern blot a.
    post hoc a.
    power spectral a.
    quantitative immunoglobulin a.
    saturation a.

    spectral a.
    ultrastructural a.
    univariate regression a.
    a. of variance (ANOVA)
    a. of variance test
    zymographic a.
analyte
analyzer
    digital dermoscopy a. (DDA)
    Electra 1000C coagulation a.
    Gemini automated centrifugal a.
    Malvern a.
    MiniOX 1A oxygen a.
    Opti 1 portable pH/blood gas a.
    SPART a.
    TDX a.
Anamine Syrup
anamnesis
anamnestic
    a. reaction
    a. response
ananaphylaxis
anaphylactic
    a. antibody
    a. crisis
    a. desensitization
    a. hypersensitivity reaction
    a. intoxication
    a. shock
    a. state
    a. syndrome
anaphylactica
    enteritis a.
anaphylactogen
anaphylactogenesis
anaphylactogenic
anaphylactoid
    a. crisis
    a. phenomenon
    a. purpura
    a. reaction
    a. shock
anaphylatoxin
    a. inactivator
    a. peptide
anaphylaxis
    active a.
    aggregate a.
    antiserum a.
    bird nest a.
    chronic a.
    complement-mediated a.

NOTES

anaphylaxis *(continued)*
    controlled a.
    drug a.
    eosinophil chemotactic factor of a.
      (ECF-A)
    fire ant a.
    food-associated exercise-induced a.
    generalized a.
    heterocytotropic a.
    homocytotropic a.
    Hymenoptera venom a.
    immediate active cutaneous a.
    inflammatory factor of a. (IF-A)
    inverse a.
    local a.
    passive cutaneous a. (PCA)
    penicillin-induced a.
    pharmacologic mediators of a.
    reversed passive a.
    slow-reacting factor of a. (SRF-A)
    slow-reacting substance of a. (SRS-A)
    systemic a.
    undifferentiated somatoform IA a.
    wheat-dependent, exercise-induced a.
      (WDEIA)
anaphylaxis-angioedema-frequent
    idiopathic a.-a.-f. (IA-A-F)
anaphylaxis-angioedema-infrequent
anaphylaxis-generalized-frequent
    idiopathic a.-g.-f. (IA-G-F)
anaphylaxis-generalized-infrequent
    idiopathic a.-g.-i. (IA-G-I)
anaphylaxis-questionable
    idiopathic a.-q. (IA-Q)
anaphylaxis-variant
    idiopathic a.-v. (IA-V)
anaphylotoxin
anaplasia
Anaplex Liquid
Anaprox
Ana-Sal HIV test
anatomical
    a. tubercle
    a. wart
anatoxic
anatoxin
anatripsis
anatriptic
Anatuss
Anavar
ANCA
    antineutrophil cytoplasmic antibody
    antineutrophil cytoplasmic autoantibody
ANCA-associated vasculitis (AAV)
ANCA-positive vasculitis (APV)
Ancef
anchor
    glycophosphatidylinositol a.

Ancobon
Ancotil
ancylostoma
    A. braziliense
    A. caninum
    a. dermatitis
    A. duodenale
ancylostomiasis
    cutaneous a.
    a. cutis
Anderson
    A. cascade impactor
    A. sampler
Anderson-Fabry disease
andersoni
    Dermacentor a.
Andersson lesion
Andes virus
Andrews disease
Androcur
androgen
androgen-dependent syndrome
androgenetica
    alopecia a.
androgenetic alopecia (AGA)
androstane
androstanediol
androstanedione
androstene
androstenedione
androsterone
anemia
    acquired hemolytic a.
    aregenerative a.
    Blackfan-Diamond a.
    chronic hemolytic a.
    congenital a.
    Cooley a.
    dermatopathic a.
    drug-related immunohemolytic a.
    equine infectious a.
    Fanconi a.
    fish tapeworm a.
    hapten mechanism of hemolytic a.
    hypochromic normocytic a.
    iron deficiency a.
    megaloblastic a.
    microangiopathic hemolytic a.
    neonatal a.
    a. neonatorum
    pernicious a.
    severe aplastic a. (SAA)
    sickle cell a.
anemic halo
anemicus, anaemicus
    nevus a.
anemone
    sea a.
anemophilous

anergic
    a. leishmaniasis
    a. T cell
AnergiX.RA
anergy
    cutaneous a.
    native a.
    natural a.
    negative a.
    nonspecific a.
    a. panel
    peripheral a.
    positive a.
    specific a.
    in vitro a.
Anestacon
anesthesia
    Madajet XL local a.
anesthetic
    eutectic mixture of local a.'s
      (EMLA)
    intradermal a.
    a. leprosy
    preoperative a.
    topical a.
anetoderma
    a. of Jadassohn
    Jadassohn a.
    Jadassohn-Pellizzari a.
    a. of prematurity
    Schweninger-Buzzi a.
    a. of Schweninger-Buzzi
    a. scleroatrophy
aneuploidy
    deoxyribonucleic acid a.
    DNA a.
aneurin hydrochloride
ANGEL
    angiolipoma, posttraumatic neuroma,
    glomus tumor, eccrine spiradenoma,
    and leiomyoma cutis
    ANGEL tumor
angel kisses lesion
Angelman syndrome
angel-wing deformity
angiectodes
    nevus a.
angiitis
    allergic a.
    choroidal a.
    Churg-Strauss a.
    granulomatous a.

    hypersensitivity a.
    leukocytoclastic a.
    a. livedo reticularis
    necrotizing a.
    nonnecrotizing a.
    systemic hypersensitivity a.
angina
    Bretonneau a.
    herpetic a.
    Ludwig a.
    Vincent a.
anginose scarlatina
angioblastic lymphadenopathy
angiocentric lymphoma
Angiocol
angiodermatitis
    disseminated pruriginous a.
angiodestructive lymphoma
angioedema
    allergic a.
    chronic a.
    episodic a.
    facial a.
    hereditary vibratory a.
    a. profile
    vibratory a.
angioedema-induced urticaria
angioedema-urticaria-eosinophilia
  syndrome
angioendothelioma
    endovascular papillary a.
angioendotheliomatosis
    malignant a.
    neoplastic a.
    a. proliferans
    proliferating systematized a.
    reactive cutaneous a. (RCA)
    systemic proliferating a.
angiofibroma contagiosum tropicum
angiogenesis
    a. factor
    a. inhibitor
angiogranuloma
angiography
angiohistiocytoma
    multinucleate cell a.
angioid streak
angioinvasive lesion
angiokeratoma
    circumscriptum a.
    a. corporis diffusum
    a. corporis diffusum universale

NOTES

angiokeratoma *(continued)*
    Fabry a.
    a. of Fordyce
    Fordyce a.
    localized a.
    a. of Mibelli
    Mibelli a.
    solitary a.
    verrucous a.
angiokeratosis, pl. **angiokeratoses**
angioleiomyoma
angiolipoma, posttraumatic neuroma, glomus tumor, eccrine spiradenoma, and leiomyoma cutis (ANGEL)
angiolupoid
angiolymphatic invasion
angiolymphoid hyperplasia
angioma
    capillary a.
    a. cavernosum
    cavernous a.
    cherry a.
    hereditary hemorrhagic a.
    infectious a.
    keratotic a.
    plane a.
    plexiform a.
    senile a.
    serpiginosum a.
    a. serpiginosum
    a. simplex
    spider a.
    stellate a.
    strawberry a.
    sudoriparous a.
    superficial a.
    tuberous a.
    tufted a.
angiomatodes
    nevus a.
angiomatoid Spitz nevus
angiomatosis
    bacillary a.
    cutaneomeningospinal a.
    diffuse dermal a.
    meningooculofacial a.
    Sturge-Weber encephalotrigeminal a.
    universal a.
angiomatous nevus
angiomyolipoma
angiomyoneuroma
angioneuromyoma
angioneurotic
    a. dermatosis
    a. edema
angioneurotica
    purpura a.

angioplasty
    percutaneous transfemoral renal a. (PTRA)
angioproliferative lesion
angiosarcoma (AS)
angiosperm
Angiostrongylus costaricensis
angiotensin-converting enzyme (ACE)
angle
    center-edge a.
    Laurin a.
    Lovibond a.
angry
    a. back phenomenon
    a. back reaction
    a. back syndrome
angstrom (A)
Angström unit (A unit)
angular
    a. cheilitis
    a. conjunctivitis
    a. stomatitis
anhidrosis
    thermal a.
    thermogenic a.
anhidrotic ectodermal dysplasia
anhydride
    acid a.
    phthalic a.
    terpine a.
    trimellitic a.
anhydrous
    a. facial foundation
    a. lanolin
    a. theophylline
ani
    pruritus a.
anicteric virus hepatitis
anidrosis
anidrotic
animal
    a. aeroallergen
    control a.
    conventional a.
    a. dander
    a. dander sensitivity
    a. hair
    Houssay a.
    normal a.
    a. scabies
    sentinel a.
    a. toxin
    a. virus
anion
    superoxide a.
anionic detergent
anisa
    Legionella a.
anisakiasis

Anisakis simplex
anise
anisum
    Pimpinella a.
anitratus
    Acinetobacter a.
Anitschkow myocyte
ankle
    anular atrophic connective tissue
      panniculitis of the a.
    retinaculum of a.
ankyloblepharon, ectodermal defect, and cleft lip and/or palate (AEC)
ankylosing
    a. enthesopathy
    a. hyperostosis
    a. spondylitis (AS)
ankylosis
    bony a.
    a. nonunions
anlage
Ann Arbor staging
annexin V
annual bluegrass
annular (*var. of* anular)
annulare
    erythema a.
    generalized granuloma a.
    localized granuloma a.
    perforating granuloma a.
    subcutaneous granuloma a.
annularis
    leukotrichia a.
    lichen planus a.
    lipoatrophia a.
    livedo a.
    psoriasis a.
annulata
    psoriasis a.
    thrix a.
annulatus, pl. **annulati**
    pilus a.
    pseudopilus a.
annulus (*var. of* anulus)
ano
    fistula in a.
anogenital
    a. disorder
    a. epidermal cyst
    a. pilar cyst
    a. sebaceous cyst
    a. squamous cell carcinoma

    a. vestibular cyst
    a. vestibular papilla
    a. wart
anomaly
    alpha, delta sleep a.
    DiGeorge a.
    Jordan a.
    morning glory a.
    nevoid a.
    reticulate pigmented a.
    Rieger a.
    sleep a.
anonychia
Anopheles
    A. albimanus
    A. freeborni
    A. funestus
    A. gambiae
anorectal herpes simplex virus infection
anorexia
anorexigenic
ANOTHER
    alopecia, nail dystrophy, ophthalmic complication, thyroid dysfunction, hypohidrosis, ephelides and enteropathy, and respiratory tract infection
    ANOTHER syndrome
ANOVA
    analysis of variance
    ANOVA test
anoxia
    focal a.
Ansaid Oral
anserina
    cutis a.
anserine bursitis
answer
    Herbal A.
ant
    a. bite
    black a.
    fire a.
    red imported fire a.
    a. sting
antagonism
    bacterial a.
antagonist
    calmodulin a.
    insulin a.
    interleukin-1 receptor a. (IL-1ra)
    leukotriene receptor a. (LTRA)

NOTES

antagonist *(continued)*
    nonselective adenosine receptor a.
    recombinant human interleukin-1
      receptor a.
antalgic gait
antazoline phosphate
Antazone
antecubital fossa
Antegren
antemortem
antenna, pl. **antennae**
Antense antitension device
anterior
    a. atlantodental interval (AADI)
    a. chamber-associated immune
      deviation (ACAID)
    a. interosseous nerve syndrome
    a. spinal artery syndrome
    a. synechia formation
    a. tarsal tunnel syndrome
    a. uveitis
anteriores
    limbi palpebrales a.
anteversion
    femoral a.
anthelix
    elastotic nodules of a.
anthelminthic
anthelmintic
anthelotic
anthema
anthesis
Anthopsis deltoidea
anthracic
anthracis
    Bacillus a.
anthracoid
anthraconecrosis
Anthra-Derm
Anthraforte
anthralin
anthramucin
anthranilate
Anthranol
anthrarobin
Anthrascalp
anthrax
    cutaneous a.
    a. toxin
anthropi
    Ochrobacterium a.
anthroponosis
anthroponotic cutaneous leishmaniasis
anthropophaga
    Cordylobia a.
anti-70K antibody
anti-A antibody
Anti-Acne
    A.-A. Control Formula

A.-A. Formula for Men
A.-A. Spot Treatment
antiadhesin antibody
anti-a-fodrin antibody
antiagglutinin
antialexin
antiallergic
anti-alpha-fodrin antibody
antianaphylaxis
antiandrogen
antianthrax serum
antiantibody
antiantitoxin
antiapoptotic
    a. effect
    a. molecule
antiarachnolysin
antiautolysin
anti-B4 blocked ricin
anti-B7-1 monoclonal antibody
antibacterial
    a. agent
    a. soap
    a. therapy
anti-B antibody
antibasement
    a. membrane antibody
    a. membrane nephritis
    a. membrane zone autoantibody
antibiogram
antibiont
antibiosis
antibiotic
    a. enterocolitis
    fluoroquinolone a.
    a. protein
    a. sensitivity
    a. sensitivity test
antibiotic-associated colitis
AntibiOtic Otic
antibiotic-resistant
anti-BMZ autoantibody
antibody (Ab)
    ABX-CBL monoclonal a.
    ACA a.
    acetylcholine receptor a. (AChRAb)
    aCL a.
    Acusyst-Xcell monoclonal a.
    affinity a.
    affinity-purified antiidiopeptide a.
    agglutinating a.
    alpha Gal a.
    anaphylactic a.
    anti-A a.
    antiadhesin a.
    anti-a-fodrin a.
    anti-alpha-fodrin a.
    anti-B a.
    antibasement membrane a.

anti-B7-1 monoclonal a.
antibody excess a.
anticardiolipin a. (ACA, ACLAb)
anti-CD3 a.
anti-CD4 a.
anti-CD18 humanized a.
anti-CD54 a.
anti-CD11a humanized
  monoclonal a.
antichemokine a.
antichromatin a.
anti-CMV a.
anticolon a.
anticyclic citrullinated peptide a.
anti-D anti-Rh a.
anti-DNA a.
anti-DNA-topoisomerase I a.
anti-dsDNA a.
anti-EA a.
anti-EBV a.
antiendomysial a.
anti-Epstein-Barr virus a.
anti-Fas a.
antifibrin a.
antifilaggrin a.
anti-GAD a.
anti-HA a.
anti-HAV a.
anti-HB$_e$ a.
anti-HB$_s$ a.
antihistone a.
antihistone-(H2A-
  H2B)/deoxyribonucleic acid
  complex a.
anti-HLA class I a.
antiidiotype a.
anti-IgA a. (IgE class)
anti-IgE humanized monoclonal a.
anti-Jo-1 a.
anti-Jp-1 a.
anti-70K a.
antikeratin a.
anti-Ku a.
anti-La a.
antilactoferrin a.
anti-La/SSB a.
antimelanocyte a.
anti-Mi-2 nuclear a.
antimitochondrial a.
anti-MPO a.
antimyosin a.
antineuronal a.

antineutrophil cytoplasmic a.
  (ANCA)
antinuclear matrix a.
antinucleosomal a.
antinucleosome a.
anti-P a.
antiparvovirus 19 a.
antipeptide a.
antiphospholipid a. (APA)
anti-PM-Scl a.
antipneumococcal a.
anti-Ri a.
antiribonucleoprotein a.
antiribosomal a.
antiribosomal-P a.
antiribosome a.
anti-RNA pol I a.
anti-RNP a.
anti-Ro a.
anti-Ro/SSA a.
antirubella a.
anti-S a.
anti-Scl-70 a.
antisignal recognition particle a.
anti-signal recognition particle a.
  (anti-SRP antibody)
anti-Sm a.
anti-Smith a.
antismooth muscle a.
antisperm a.
anti-SRP a.
anti-SSA a.
anti-SSB a.
antisynthetase a.
anti-Th a.
antithymocyte a.
antithyroid microsomal a.
antitopoisomerase I a.
anti-tTG a.
antityrosinase a.
anti-U1, -U3 RNP a.
anti-VEGF a.
anti-Yo a.
auto-antiidiotypic a.
autologous a.
avidity a.
basement membrane zone a.
Bexxar radiolabeled monoclonal a.
bispecific a.
bivalent a.
blocking a.
a. blocking assay

NOTES

antibody *(continued)*
  blood group a.
  BMZ a.
  BR96-doxorubicin monoclonal a.
  2C3 anti-VEGF a.
  CC49 monoclonal a.
  CD1a a.
  CD5 a.
  CD5+ a.
  CD10 a.
  CD18 a.
  CD19 a.
  CD20 a.
  CD21 a.
  CD22 a.
  CD24 a.
  CD28 a.
  CD29 a.
  CD38 a.
  CD43 a.
  CD44 a.
  CD49a a.
  CD49b a.
  CD49c a.
  CD49e a.
  CD49f a.
  CD54 a.
  CD106 a.
  CD3 monoclonal a.
  CD4 monoclonal a.
  CD8 monoclonal a.
  CD16 monoclonal a.
  CD25 monoclonal a.
  CD56 monoclonal a.
  CD69 monoclonal a.
  CD71 monoclonal a.
  cell-bound a.
  CF a.
  C100-3 hepatitis C virus a.
  chimeric a.
  chromatin a.
  cold a.
  cold-reactive a.
  a. combining site
  combining-site a.
  complement-fixing a.
  complete a.
  cross-reacting a.
  cryptosporidiosis a.
  cytophilic a.
  cytoplasmic antineutrophil
    cytoplasmic a. (C-ANCA)
  CytoTab polyclonal a.
  cytotropic a.
  daclizumab monoclonal a.
  a. deficiency
  a. deficiency disease
  Diffistat-G polyclonal a.
  direct fluorescent a. (DFA)

Donath-Landsteiner a.
a. dysfunction
E5 monoclonal a.
7E3 monoclonal antiplatelet a.
enhancing a.
Epstein-Barr virus-induced early a.
Escherichia coli polysaccharide a.
a. excess
Forssman a.
Gal a.
group A carbohydrate a.
Ha-1A monoclonal a.
hemagglutinating a.
a. to hepatitis B core antigen
  (HB$_c$Ab, HBcAb)
a. to hepatitis Be antigen (HB$_e$Ab,
  HBeAb)
a. to hepatitis B surface antigen
  (HB$_s$Ab, HBsAb)
heteroclitic a.
heterocytotropic a.
heterogenetic a.
heterophil a., heterophile a.
histone a.
histone-DNA a.
HIV neutralizing a.
homocytotropic a.
human anti-CMV a.
human anticytomegalovirus a.
humanized anti-CD3 monoclonal a.
human leukocyte a. (HLA)
humoral a.
hybrid a.
hybridoma a.
I-B1 radiolabeled a.
idiotype a.
IgA antiendomysial a.
IgA antigliadin a.
IgE a.
IgG a.
IgM anticardiolipin a.
immobilizing a.
ImmuRAIT-LL2 monoclonal a.
incomplete a.
indirect fluorescent a.
infliximab monoclonal a.
inhibiting a.
inhibition fluorescent a.
islet cell a. (ICA)
isophil a.
Jo-1 a.
LDP-02 humanized monoclonal a.
LeuTech radiolabeled a.
LymphoCide a.
lymphocytotoxic a.
MAb-170 monoclonal a.
MabThera monoclonal a.
Mi-2 a.
monoclonal a. (MoAb)

monoclonal antiendothelial cell a. (mAECA)
myositis-specific a.
native type anti-DNA a.
natural a.
neutralizing murine monoclonal antitumor necrosis factor a.
nonprecipitable a.
nonprecipitating a.
nonprecipitation a.
normal a.
nucleosome a.
OKT3 a.
Oncolym radiolabeled monoclonal a.
opsonizing a.
ornithine-ketoacid transaminase 3 a.
Orthoclone OKT3 anti-CD3 monoclonal a.
Orthomune monoclonal a.
Ovarex MAb monoclonal a.
palivizumab a.
panel-reactive a. (PRA)
panreactive monoclonal a.
percent reactive antibody/panel reactive a. (PRA)
perinuclear antineutrophil cytoplasmic a. (P-ANCA)
P-K a.
PM 81 monoclonal a.
polyclonal a.
polynucleotide a.
Prausnitz-Kustner a.
precipitating a.
preexisting a.
preformed a.
prophylactic a.
ProstaScint monoclonal a.
r24 a.
RATG polyclonal a.
reaginic a.
ReoPro monoclonal a.
Rituxan monoclonal a.
Scl-70 a.
serum antiglomerular-basement-membrane a.
single-stranded anti-DNA a.
SJ441 a.
skin-sensitizing a.
speckled-pattern antinuclear a.
Thomsen a.
thyroid-blocking a. (TBAB)

thyroid-stimulating a.
thyroid-stimulating hormone-displacing a.
thyroid-stimulating hormone receptor a.
thyroperoxidase a.
TI-23 cytomegalovirus monoclonal a.
treponema-immobilizing a.
treponemal a.
TSH-displacing a.
TSH receptor a. (TRAb)
type (I, IIb) antineuronal a.
univalent a.
U1 RNP a.
Vi a.
vitiligo a.
warm-reactive a.
Wassermann a.
WinRho SD a.
xenoreactive natural a. (XNA)
XMMEN-OE5 monoclonal a.
Y12 monoclonal a.
antibody-deficient syndrome (ADS)
antibody-dependent cellular cytotoxicity (ADCC)
antibody-directed enzyme prodrug therapy (ADEPT)
antibody-forming cell (AFC)
antibody-phage display
antibotulinus serum
antibromic
anti-C3 assay
anticalpastatin autoantibody
anticardiolipin (aCL)
  a. antibody (ACA, ACLAb)
  a. antibody syndrome
  a. autoantibody
anti-CD3
  a.-CD3 antibody
  SMART a.-CD3
anti-CD4 antibody
anti-CD11a
  a.-CD11a humanized monoclonal antibody
  a.-CD11a humanized monoclonal antibody for psoriasis
anti-CD18 humanized antibody
anti-CD54 antibody
anti-Centruroides antivenin
antichemokine antibody
anticholera serum

NOTES

anticholinergic drug
antichromatin antibody
alpha$_1$-antichymotrypsin
anti-CMV
    anticytomegalovirus
    anti-CMV antibody
anticoagulant
    circulating a.
anticolon antibody
anticomplement
anticomplementary
    a. factor
    a. serum
anticontagious
anticonvulsant
    hydantoin a.
anticrotalus serum
anticyclic citrullinated peptide antibody
anticytokine
anticytomegalovirus (anti-CMV)
anticytotoxin
anti-D
    a.-D anti-Rh antibody
    a.-D enzyme-linked immunosorbent
    assay
    a.-D immunoglobulin
Anti-Dandruff
    Neutrogena Healthy Scalp A.-D.
    Satinique A.-D.
    A.-D. Shampoo
antideoxyribonuclease B
antideoxyribonucleic acidase
antidepressant
    heterocyclic a.
    tricyclic a.
antidimer DNA
anti-DNA antibody
anti-DNase B
anti-DNA-topoisomerase I antibody
antidote
    H F a.
antidouble-stranded DNA
anti-dsDNA antibody
anti-Dsg1
anti-EA antibody
anti-EBV
    anti-Epstein-Barr virus
    anti-EBV antibody
anti-EGF receptor antibody for cancer
antielastase
antiendomysial antibody
antiendotoxin
    XXMEN-OE5 a.
antienzyme
antiepidermal growth factor receptor
  antibody for cancer
antiepithelial serum
anti-Epstein-Barr
    a.-E.-B. virus (anti-EBV)

    a.-E.-B. virus antibody
    a.-E.-B.-virus antibody
antiestrogenic
anti-Fas antibody
antifibrin antibody
antifibrinolytic agent
antifilaggrin antibody
antifoaming agent
antifungal
    Absorbine Jr. A.
    Breezee Mist A.
    EcoNail a.
    a. therapy
anti-GAD antibody
anti-GBM
    antiglomerular basement membrane
antigen (Ag)
    Abbott HIVAG-1 monoclonal a.
    ABO a.
    Acanthocheilonema viteae excretory-
      secretory a.
    acetone-insoluble a.
    AF-1, -2 a.
    allogenic a.
    alum-precipitated a.
    Am a.
    antibody to hepatitis B core a.
      (HB$_c$Ab, HBcAb)
    antibody to hepatitis Be a.
      (HB$_e$Ab, HBeAb)
    antibody to hepatitis B surface a.
      (HB$_s$Ab, HBsAb)
    Au a.
    Aus a.
    Australia a.
    autologous a.
    bacterial a.
    Be^a a.
    Becker a.
    Bi a.
    Bile a.
    bivalent a.
    blank a.
    blood group a.
    bullous pemphigoid a. (BPA)
    cancer-testis a.
    capsular a.
    carcinoembryonic a. (CEA)
    C carbohydrate a.
    CDE a.
    centromere a.
    Chido-Rodgers a.
    chlordiazepoxide a.
    cholesterinized a.
    Chr^a a.
    cicatricial pemphigoid a.
    class (I, II, III) a.
    cold-induced skin a.
    commercial a.

common acute lymphocytic leukemia a. (CALLA)
complete a.
conjugated a.
cytotoxic T lymphocyte a.-4 (CTLA-4)
D a.
delta a.
Dharmendra a.
Di a.
differentiation a.
Dsg3 a.
Duffy a.
ENA a.
endogenous a.
epidermolysis bullosa acquisita a.
Epstein-Barr nuclear a. (EBNA)
a. excess
exogenous a.
extractable nuclear a. (ENA)
Fas a.
Fer a.
flagellar a.
food a.
Forssman a.
Frei a.
Fy a.
G a.
Ge a.
glycophorin a.
Gm a.
Good a.
Gr a.
group a.'s
H a.
H-2 a.
He a.
heart a.
hepatitis A a. (HAA)
hepatitis-associated a. (HAA)
hepatitis B core a. (HB$_c$Ag, HBcAg)
hepatitis Be a.
hepatitis B surface a. (HB$_s$Ag, HBsAg)
heterogenetic a.
heterogenic enterobacterial a.
heterophil a.
heterophile a.
hexon a.
high molecular weight-melanoma-associated a. (HMW-MAA)

histocompatibility a.
HLA a.
Ho a.
homologous a.
Hu a.
human leukemia-associated a.
human leukocyte a. (HLA)
human leukocyte class II a. (HLA-DQ1)
human lymphocyte a.
human thymus lymphocyte a.
I a.
Ia a.
idiotypic a.
incomplete a.
a. interferon
InV group a.
isophile a.
Jk a.
Jo-1 a.
Jobbins a.
Js a.
K a.
KF-1 a.
KI a.
killer inhibitor receptor-human leukocyte a. (KIR-HLA)
Km a.
Kveim a.
Kveim-Stilzbach a.
La a.
Lan a.
LDA-1 a.
Le a.
a. leukocyte cellular antibody test (ALCAT)
leukocyte common a.
Levay a.
LH 7:2 a.
Lu a.
luminal a.
Ly a.
Lyb a.
lymphocyte function-associated a. (LFA)
lymphogranuloma venereum a.
Lyt a.
M a.
M$_1$ a.
Mas a.
melanoma-specific a.
microchimeric a.

NOTES

antigen *(continued)*
  Mitsuda a.
  mixed vespid a.
  MNS a.
  monoclonal antibody immobilization of neutrophil a.'s (MAINA)
  Mu a.
  multivalent a.
  mumps skin test a. (MSTA)
  noninherited maternal a. (NIMA)
  nonspecific cross-reacting a. (NCA)
  O a.
  oncofetal a.
  organ-specific a.
  Ot a.
  OVA a.
  ovalbumin a.
  OX-K proteus a.
  Oz a.
  P a.
  p24 a.
  pancreatic oncofetal a. (POA)
  partial a.
  P blood group a.
  penton a.
  peptide a.
  PM-Scl a.
  pollen a.
  polymerized a.
  polymyositis-scleroderma a.
  polysaccharide a.
  pp65(UL83) a.
  private a.
  proliferating cell nuclear a. (PCNA)
  proliferation-associated a.
  protein a.
  public a.
  QA a.
  R a.
  red cell a.
  Rh a.
  Rhus toxicodendron a.
  Rhus venenata a.
  ribonucleoprotein a.
  RNP a.
  Ro a.
  S a.
  sensitized a.
  shock a.
  sialoglycoprotein a.
  skin-specific histocompatibility a.
  Sm a.
  Smith a.
  soluble liver a. (SLA)
  somatic a.
  species-specific a.
  specific a.
  Stobo a.

  streptococcal M a.
  Streptococcus M a.
  Su a.
  surface a.
  Sw^a a.
  Swann a.
  synthetic a.
  T a.
  Tac a.
  T-dependent a.
  theta a.
  thymus-independent a.
  tissue-specific a.
  Tj a.
  Tr^a a.
  transplantation a.
  tumor a.
  tumor-associated transplantation a. (TATA)
  tumor-specific transplantation a. (TSTA)
  a. unit
  V a.
  Vel a.
  Ven a.
  very late activation a.
  vespid a.
  Vi a.
  viral capsid a.
  VLA-1 a.
  Vw a.
  Webb a.
  Wr^a a.
  Wright a. (Wr^a)
  Xg a.
  Yersinia a.
  YKL-40 a.
  Yt^a a.

antigen-1
  leukocyte factor a.-1 (LFA-1)
antigen-3
antigen-4
  very late a.-4 (VLA-4)
antigen-antibody
  complement-activating a.-a.
  a.-a. complex
  a.-a. reaction
antigen-binding
  a.-b. diversity
  single-chain a.-b. (SCA)
  a.-b. site
antigen-combining site
antigenemia
  cytomegalovirus a.
  a. test
antigenemically cross-reacting food
antigenic
  a. analysis
  a. antibody lattice formation

a. binding receptor
a. competition
a. complex
a. determinant
a. drift
a. modulation
a. shift
a. variation
antigenicity
antigen-nonspecific immune complex assay
antigen-presenting cell (APC)
antigen-recognition
antigen-sensitive cell
antigen-specific immune response
antigenuria
    pneumococcal a.
antiglobulin test
antiglomerular basement membrane (anti-GBM)
anti-HA antibody
anti-HAV antibody
anti-HB$_s$ antibody
anti-HB$_e$ antibody
anti-HCV seropositive
anti-*Helicobacter*
antihelminthic
antihemagglutinin
antihemolysin
antihemolytic
antihepatitis
    a. A virus
    a. C virus seropositive
antihidrotic
Antihist-1
antihistamine
    H$_1$, H$_2$ a.
    nonsedating a.
    oral a.
antihistaminic
Antihist-D
antihistone antibody
antihistone-(H2A-H2B)/deoxyribonucleic acid complex antibody
anti-HLA class I antibody
anti-hnRNP
antihormone
antihost reactivity
antihuman
    a. globulin
    a. globulin test
    a. parvovirus immunoglobulin G

antihyaluronidase
antihydriotic
antihypertensive agent
antihyperuricemic agent
antiidiotype
    a. antibody
    a. autoantibody
    a. vaccine
anti-IFN-gamma
    anti-interferon-gamma
    SMART a.-I.-g.
anti-IgA antibody
anti-IgE humanized monoclonal antibody
anti-IIb-IIIA mAB therapy
antiimmune body
antiimmunoglobulin E immunotherapy
antiinfective agent
antiinflammatory
    a. cytokine
    nonsteroidal a.
    a. therapy
anti-interferon-gamma (anti-IFN-gamma)
Anti-Itch gel
anti-Jo-1 antibody
anti-Jp-1 antibody
antikeratin antibody
antikidney serum nephritis
anti-Ku antibody
anti-La antibody
antilactoferrin antibody
anti-La/SSB antibody
antileukocidin
antileukoproteinase (ALP)
antileukotoxin
anti-Lewisite
Anti-LFA-1
antiluetic
antilymphocyte
    a. induction
    a. serum (ALS)
antilysin
antimalarial
    a. agent
    a. drug
antimelanocyte antibody
antimeningococcus serum
antimetabolite
anti-Mi-2 nuclear antibody
antimicrobial
    A. MPM wound cleanser
    a. spectrum

NOTES

antimicrobiology susceptibility testing
Antiminth
antimitochondrial antibody
antimonial drug therapy for
  leishmaniasis
antimony spot
anti-MPO
    antimyeloperoxidase
      anti-MPO antibody
antimuscarinic acetylcholine receptor
antimycobacterial
antimycotic
antimyeloperoxidase
antimyosin antibody
antinative DNA
antinauseant
antineoplastic
antineuronal antibody
antineurotoxin
antineutrophil
    a. cytoplasmic antibody (ANCA)
    a. cytoplasmic antibody-associated
      vasculitis (ANCA-associated
      vasculitis)
    a. cytoplasmic antibody-positive
      vasculitis (ANCA-positive
      vasculitis)
    a. cytoplasmic autoantibody
      (ANCA)
antinuclear
    a. antibody immunodiffusion
    a. antibody immunofluorescence
    a. antibody screening by enzyme
      immunoassay
    a. antibody screening test
    a. antibody titer
    a. autoantibody
    a. matrix antibody
antinucleosomal antibody
antinucleosome
    a. antibody
    a. autoantibody
antioxidant vitamin
anti-P antibody
antiparallel B-sheet conformation
antiparasitic
antiparvovirus 19 antibody
anti-PCAM
    antiplatelet endothelial cell adhesion
      molecule
Anti-Pelliculaire
    Shampooing A.-P.
antipeptide antibody
antiperinuclear
    a. autoantibody
    a. factor (APF)
antiperiodic
antiperspirant
antiphagocytic

antiphlogistic
antiphospholipid
    a. antibody (APA)
    a. antibody syndrome (APS)
antipill finish
antiplatelet endothelial cell adhesion
    molecule (anti-PCAM)
anti-PM-Scl antibody
antipneumococcal antibody
antipneumococcic
antipneumococcus serum
anti-Pr cold autoagglutinin
antiprecipitin
antiproliferative effect
antiproteasomal
antiprotein S
antipruritic
    a. agent
    a. therapy
    topical a.
antipsoriatic
antipsoric
antipyretic
antipyrine and benzocaine
antipyrotic
antirabies
    a. serum
    a. serum, equine origin
antiresorptive
antireticular cytotoxic serum
antiretroviral
antirheumatic
    a. agent
    a. drug
    a. therapy
anti-Ri antibody
antiribonucleoprotein (anti-RNP)
    a. antibody
antiribosomal antibody
antiribosomal-P antibody
antiribosome antibody
antiricin
anti-RNA
    anti-ribonucleic acid
      anti-RNA pol I antibody
anti-RNP
    antiribonucleoprotein
      a.-RNP antibody
anti-Ro antibody
anti-Ro/SSA antibody
antirotavirus IgA titer
antirubella antibody
anti-S antibody
antiscabetic
antiscabietic
anti-Scl-70 antibody
antiseborrheic
antisense
    a. compound

a. drug
a. nucleotide
a. oligodeoxynucleotide
a. phosphorothioate oligonucleotide
a. RNA
antisepsis
Anti-Sept bactericidal scrub solution
antiseptic
antiseptic-impregnated central venous catheter
antiserum, pl. **antisera**
a. anaphylaxis
blood group a.
heterologous a.
homologous a.
monospecific a.
monovalent a.
multivalent a.
nerve growth factor a.
NGF a.
polyvalent a.
Reenstierna a.
specific a.
anti-signal
a.-s. recognition particle (anti-SRP)
a.-s. recognition particle antibody (anti-SRP antibody)
antisignal recognition particle antibody
anti-Sjögren
a.-S. syndrome A (anti-SSA)
a.-S. syndrome B (anti-SSB)
anti-SM
anti-Smith
anti-Sm antibody
anti-Smith (anti-SM)
a.-S. antibody
antismooth muscle antibody
antisnakebite serum
antispasmodic
antisperm antibody
anti-SRP
anti-signal recognition particle
a.-SRP antibody
anti-signal recognition particle antibody
anti-SSA
anti-Sjögren syndrome A
a.-SSA antibody
anti-SSB
anti-Sjögren syndrome B
anti-SSB antibody
antistaphylococcic

antistaphylolysin
antisteapsin
antistreptococcic
antistreptokinase
antistreptolysin-O (ASLO, ASO)
antisubstance
antisudorific
antisynthetase
a. antibody
a. syndrome
antitac
antitetanus toxin
anti-Th antibody
antithrombin III
antithymocyte
a. antibody
a. globulin (ATG, ATGAM, Atgam)
antithyroid microsomal antibody
antitopoisomerase I antibody
antitoxic serum
antitoxigen
antitoxin
bivalent gas gangrene a.
bothropic a.
Bothrops a.
botulinum a.
botulism a.
bovine a.
Crotalus a.
despeciated a.
diphtheria a.
dysentery a.
gas gangrene a.
normal a.
pentavalent gas gangrene a.
plant a.
a. rash
scarlet fever a.
Staphylococcus a.
tetanus a.
tetanus-perfringens a.
a. unit
antitoxinogen
antitrypsin
anti-tTG antibody
antituberculosis
antituberculous therapy
antitumorigenesis
antitussive
antitype (II, IX) collagen autoantibody
antityphoid

NOTES

antityrosinase antibody
anti-U1, -U3 RNP antibody
anti-VEGF antibody
antivenene unit
antivenin
    anti-Centruroides a.
    black widow spider a.
    a. polyvalent
antivenom
    Latrodectus mactans a.
    tiger snake a.
Antivert
antiviral
    a. agent
    a. drug
    a. immunity
    a. therapy
anti-Yo antibody
Antrizine
antrostomy
Anturane
Anucort HC suppository
ANUG
    acute necrotizing ulcerative gingivitis
anular, annular
    a. atrophic connective tissue
      panniculitis of the ankle
    a. distribution of lesion
    a. elastolytic giant cell granuloma
    a. erythema
    a. erythematous plaque
    a. lichen planus
    a. lipoatrophy
    a. syphilid
anularity
anulus, annulus
    a. fibrosus
    a. migrans
Anuprep HC suppository
Anusol
    Anusol-HC1 topical
    A.-HC suppository
Anxanil Oral
AOM
    acute otitis media
aortic arch syndrome
aortitis
    idiopathic a.
AP
    accelerated phase
      CML AP
        chronic
          myelocytic/myelogenous/myeloid
          leukemia accelerated phase
AP1
    activator protein 1
APA
    antiphospholipid antibody

Apacet
APACHE
    A. II score
    A. II system
apatite
APC
    antigen-presenting cell
A-P-C
    adenoidal-pharyngeal-conjunctival
    A-P-C virus
APE
    aqueous pollen extract
APEC
    asymmetric periflexural exanthem of
    childhood
APECED
    autoimmune polyendocrinopathy-
    candidiasis-ectodermal dysplasia
    autoimmune polyendocrinopathy-
    candidiasis-ectodermal dystrophy
    APECED syndrome
Apert
    A. hirsutism
    A. syndrome
apertural pore rupture
ApexiCon
    A. E cream
    A. ointment
APF
    antiperinuclear factor
apheresis
APHLT
    auxiliary partial heterotopic liver
    transplantation
aphtha, pl. **aphthae**
    Bednar a.
    Behçet a.
    cachectic a.
    a. febriles
    herpetiform a.
    a. major
    Mikulicz a.
    a. minor
    a. tropicae
Aphthasol
aphthoid
aphthosis
    Touraine a.
aphthous
    a. genital ulcer
    a. oral ulcer
    a. stomatitis
Aphthovirus
aphylactic
aphylaxis
apical lobe fibrosis
apicoposterior segment
apiculus

apiospermum
   Monosporium a.
   Scedosporium a.
apis
   A. mellifera
   a. mellifera sting
   Spiroplasma a.
APKH
   acquired progressive kinking of the hair
aplasia
   a. cutis congenita
   gold-induced a.
   pure red cell a. (PRCA)
Apley
   A. grind test
   A. maneuver
Apligraf
   A. skin substitute
   A. tissue-engineered skin
Aplisol
apnea
   obstructive sleep a. (OSA)
   sleep a.
apneustic breathing
apo AI
Apo-Allopurinol
Apo-Amoxil
Apo-Ampi
Apo-ASA
ApoB
Apo-Beclomethasone
Apo-Cetirizine
Apo-Cimetidine
apocrine
   a. acne
   a. adenoma
   a. bromhidrosis
   a. carcinoma
   a. chromhidrosis
   a. cystadenoma
   a. differentiation
   a. epithelioma
   a. hidrocystoma
   a. malaria
   a. miliaria
   a. poroma
   a. retention cyst
   a. sweat gland
apocrinitis
Apodemus
   A. agrarius
   A. flavicollis

Apo-Diclo
Apo-Diflunisal
Apo-Doxy Tabs
Apo-Erythro E-C
Apo-Famotidine
Apo-Fluconazole
Apo-Flurbiprofen
Apo-Gain
Apo-Hydroxyzine
Apo-Ibuprofen
Apo-Indomethacin
Apo-Ipravent
Apo-Keto
Apo-Keto-E
apolipoprotein
APOLT
   auxiliary partial orthotopic liver transplant
   auxiliary partial orthotopic liver transplantation
Apo-Metronidazole
Apo-Minocycline
Apo-Nabumetone
Apo-Napro-Na
Apo-Naproxen
aponeurosis
   palmar a.
aponeurotic fibroma
Apo-Pen VK
apophylaxis
apophysial, apophyseal
   a. joint
Apo-Piroxicam
apoplexy
   cutaneous a.
Apo-Prednisone
apoptosis
   cellular inhibitor of a. (cIAP)
   crypt epithelial cell a.
   dysregulated lymphocytic a.
   lymphocytic a.
apoptosis-associated molecule
apoptotic
   a. bleb
   a. body
   a. cell
   a. index
   a. keratinocyte
Apo-Ranitidine
apostematosa
   cheilitis glandularis a.
Apo-Sulfinpyraz

NOTES

Apo-Sulin
Apo-Tetra
Apo-Zidovudine
apparatus
  Golgi a.
  internal hair a.
  Kidde a.
  LHE a.
  pilosebaceous a.
  spark-gap a.
  vacuum tube a.
apparent
  a. diffusion coefficient (ADC)
  a. leukonychia
appearance
  ball-in-claw a.
  cluster-of-grapes a.
  coral-head a.
  enamel paint spot a.
  finger-in-glove a.
  ground-glass a.
  hair-on-end a.
  hair-standing-on-end a.
  hidebound a.
  orange peel a.
  plucked chicken papules a.
  safety-pin a.
  slapped-cheek a.
  slapped-face a.
  stuck-on a.
  Swiss cheese a.
  tire-patch a.
  toxic a.
appendage
  epidermal a.
appendageal cord
appendicular
  a. disease
  a. tuberculosis
apple
  a. jelly nodule
  a. jelly papule of lupus vulgaris
appliance
  maxillary occlusal a.
  TheraSnore oral a.
applied kinesiology
approach
  CLIP replacement a.
appropriate culture
approximation
  zigzag a.
apraxia
  speech a.
Aprodine
  A. Syrup
  A. Tablet
apron pattern
aprotinin

APRV
  airway pressure release ventilation
APS
  antiphospholipid antibody syndrome
  autoimmune polyglandular syndrome
    APS type 1, 2
APTT
  activated partial thromboplastin time
apurpuric
APV
  ANCA-positive vasculitis
AQ
  Nasacort AQ
Aquacare
  A. moisturizer
  A. topical
Aquacel
  A. Ag
  A. AG wound dressing
  A. Hydrofiber dressing
  A. wound packing and dressing
Aquacort
aquagenic
  a. pruritus
  a. urticaria
Aqua Glycolic Lotion
AquaMEPHYTON injection
Aquanil lotion
Aquaphor
  A. Antibiotic topical
  A. gauze
aquaphorin 1, 2
Aquaphyllin
aquarium granuloma
AquaSite Ophthalmic solution
Aquasol
  A. A
  A. A & D
  A. E
  A. E Oral
Aquasorb
  A. hydrogel sheet
  A. transparent hydrogel dressing
aquaspera
  Acrotheca a.
  Rhinocladiella a.
AquaTar
aquatic exercises
aqueous
  a. epinephrine
  penicillin a.
  a. pollen extract (APE)
  a. solution
  a. vaccine
AR
  amphiregulin
ARA
  American Rheumatism Association
  ARA criteria

arabicum
elephantiasis a.
arabinoside
adenine a.
cytosine a.
arabum
elephantiasis a.
lepra a.
ara-C
arachidonic
a. acid cascade
a. acid metabolism
a. acid metabolite
a. acid pathway
arachnidism
necrotic a.
arachnodactylia
arachnodactyly
congenital contractural a.
contractural a.
arachnoideus
nevus a.
arachnophlebectomy
Miglin method for a.
a. needle
a. procedure
a. surgical device
Aralen phosphate with primaquine phosphate
Aramine
araneidism
araneosus
nevus a.
araneus
nevus a.
A-range
dihydroxyacetone-psoralen ultraviolet A-r. (DHA-PUVA)
psoralen ultraviolet A-r. (PUVA)
aranodactylia
Arava
arbor
a. vitae
a. vitae tree
arborescens
lipoma a.
arborize
arbovirus, arborvirus
arc
mercury a.

arcade
fibrous a.
vascular a.
arcanobacterial pharyngitis
Archeaopsylla erinacei
architecture
histologic a.
arch-loop-whorl (ALW)
arch-loop-whorl system
arciform distribution of lesion
Arcoxia
arcuate
arcuatus
Chortoglyphus a.
area
body surface a.
butterfly a.
Celsus a.
dermatomic a.
flexural a.
flush a.
Hof a.
intertriginous a.
Jonston a.
periocular a.
perioral a.
periorbital a.
total body surface a. (TBSA)
areata
alopecia universal a.
ophiasic alopecia a.
pseudoalopecia a.
areate
areatus
areflexic paraparesis
aregenerative anemia
arenaceous
Arenaviridae virus
Arenavirus
areola, pl. **areolae**
Chaussier a.
nevoid hyperkeratosis of nipple and a.
primary a.
vaccinal a.
areolar
areolate
Argasidae
Arg^{519}-Cys mutation in type II collagen
Argentine
A. hemorrhagic fever
A. hemorrhagic fever virus

NOTES

45

Argentinean hemorrhagic fever
Argentinian Study Group for
Prevention of Cardiac Insufficiency
(GESICA)
Argesic-SA
arginine codon
argininosuccinate synthetase deficiency
argininosuccinicaciduria
Arglaes
> A. antimicrobial barrier film
>   dressing
> A. powder

argon laser
argon-pumped tunable-dye laser
Argostideae
Argyll Robertson pupil
argyria
argyriasis
argyric
argyrism
Argyrol S.S.
argyrosis
Aria CPAP system
ARI Group I–IV filter
Aristocort
> A. A
> A. A topical
> A. Forte
> A. Forte injection
> A. Intralesional injection
> A. Intralesional suspension
> A. Oral
> Syrup of A.
> A. Tablet

Aristospan
> A. Intra-articular
> A. Intra-articular injection
> A. Intralesional
> A. Intralesional injection

Arizona
> A. ash
> A. ash tree
> A. coral snake
> A. cypress
> A. cypress tree

arizonae
> *Salmonella a.*

Arizona/Fremont
> A./F. cottonwood
> A./F. cottonwood tree

arm
> a. duration maneuver
> a. raises maneuver
> a. straighten maneuver

Arm-a-Med
> A.-a.-M. isoetharine
> A.-a.-M. Isoproterenol
> A.-a.-M. Metaproterenol

armamentarium
> cytotoxic a.

armandii
> *Clematis a.*

armed macrophage
Arndt-Gottron
> A.-G. disease
> A.-G. syndrome

arnica montana
Arning tincture
aromatic hydrocarbon
around-the-clock oral maintenance
bronchodilator therapy
arrangement
> chromosome a.
> corymbose a.
> lesion a.
> V-D-J gene a.

array
> reticulate a.

arrector, pl. arrectores
> a. pili muscle
> a. pilorum
> a. pilorum muscle
> a. pilus

arrest
> cardiorespiratory a.

arresting
> high-efficiency particulate a.
>   (HEPA)

Arrhenius-Madsen theory
arrhizus
> *Rhizopus a.*

arrhythmia
Arrow pneumothorax kit
arrowroot
Arroyo
> Whitewater A.

arsenic
> Mapharsen organic a.
> neoarsphenamine organic a.
> a. pigmentation
> a. trioxide
> tryparsamide organic a.

arsenical
> a. contact dermatitis
> a. keratosis

arsphenamine dermatitis
ArtAssist
> A. compression dressing/wrap
> A. leg compression dressing

Artecoll permanent wrinkle treatment
artefact (*var. of* artifact)
artefacta
> dermatitis a.

Artemisia
> *A. salina*
> *A. vulgaris*

artemisiifolia
> Ambrosia a.

Artemis vulgaris

Arteparon

arterial
> a. disorder
> a. hypoxemia
> a. spider
> a. ulcer

arterial-ecchymotic type Ehlers-Danlos syndrome

arteriole
> afferent a.

arteriopathy
> Takayasu a.

arteriosclerosis
> fibrotic a.
> a. obliterans

arteriosclerotic gangrene

arteriovenous
> a. block
> a. fistula
> a. shunt

arteritis
> allergic granulomatous a.
> cranial a.
> eosinophilic a.
> equine viral a.
> granulomatous a.
> intimal a.
> juvenile temporal a. (JTA)
> Takayasu a.
> temporal giant cell a.

Arterivirus

artery
> interlobular a.
> nutrient a.

Artha-G

arthralgia

Arthramel Accelerator

Arthraphate capsule

Arthrisin

arthrites pseudoseptiques et bacterides d'Andrews

arthritic tuberculosis

arthriticum
> erythema a.

arthritidis
> Mycoplasma a.

arthritis, pl. arthritides
> acne a.
> acute rheumatic a.

acute rheumatoid a.
additive a.
adult-type rheumatoid a.
anaerobic bacterial a.
atypical mycobacterial a.
axial psoriatic a.
bacterial a.
Borrelia-associated a.
brucella a.
burnt-out rheumatoid a.
Candida a.
candidal a.
carrageenan a.
chronic postrheumatic fever a.
crystal a.
crystal-induced a.
degenerative a.
dislocation a.
dysenteric a.
enterogenic reactive a.
enteropathic a.
enthesitis-related a.
erosive a.
familial granulomatous a.
familial recurrent a.
A. Foundation ibuprofen
A. Foundation Nighttime
A. Foundation Pain Reliever
fungal a.
glenohumeral a.
gonococcal a.
gouty a.
gram-negative bacilli a.
granulomatous idiopathic a.
hemochromatotic a.
hemorrhagic a.
herpes simplex virus a.
idiopathic destructive a. (IDA)
infectious a.
inflammatory a.
intestinal bypass a.
Jaccoud a.
juvenile chronic a.
juvenile idiopathic a. (JIA)
juvenile rheumatoid a. (JRA)
large-joint inflammatory a.
leukemic a.
lipopolysaccharide-induced a.
LPS-induced a.
lupus a.
Lyme a.
meningococcal a.

NOTES

arthritis *(continued)*
  monoarticular a.
  monoarticular antigen-induced a.
  mutilans a.
  a. mutilans
  neuropathic a.
  nongonococcal bacterial a.
  noninflammatory a.
  ochronotic a.
  oligoarticular seronegative
    rheumatoid a.
  ovalbumin-induced a.
  patellofemoral a.
  pauciarticular juvenile chronic a.
  pauciarticular juvenile rheumatoid a.
  peripheral a.
  phase (I, II) rheumatoid a.
  polyarticular gonococcal a.
  polyarticular juvenile rheumatoid a.
  polyarticular septic a.
  polymicrobial a.
  poststreptococcal reactive a. (PSRA)
  posttraumatic a.
  postvenereal reactive a.
  pseudocystic rheumatoid a.
  pseudoseptic a.
  psoriatic a.
  purulent a.
  pyogenic a.
  reactive a. (ReA)
  retinyl acetate-induced a.
  rheumatoid a. (RA)
  a. robustus
  rubella a.
  Salmonella a.
  sarcoid a.
  senescent a.
  septic a.
  seronegative a.
  seronegative rheumatoid a.
  seropositive rheumatoid a.
  sexually acquired reactive a.
    (SARA)
  Staphylococcus aureus a.
  suppurative a.
  systemic juvenile rheumatoid a.
  traumatic a.
  tuberculous a.
  unicondylar a.
  venereal-associated a.
  viral a.
  a. without deformity
  Yersinia a.
arthritis-pseudogout
  pyrophosphate a.-p. (Pap)
arthritogenic
  a. peptide
  a. protein
arthritogenicity

Arthro 7
Arthro-BST arthroscopic probe
arthrocentesis
arthrochalasia-type Ehlers-Danlos
  syndrome
arthrochalasis multiplex congenita
arthrodesis
arthrography
  double-contrast a.
arthrogryposis
  a. congenita, distal, type I, II
    syndrome
  distal a.
arthroophthalmopathy
  hereditary a.
Arthropan
arthropathia psoriatica
arthropathica
  psoriasis a.
arthropathy
  acromegalic a.
  cuff tear a.
  enteropathic a.
  facet joint a.
  gonococcal a.
  hemophilic a.
  Jaccoud a.
  myxedematous a.
  neuropathic a.
  ochronotic a.
  primary amyloidotic a.
  psoriatic a.
  pyrophosphate a.
  resorptive a.
  seronegativity, enthesopathy, a.
    (SEA)
arthropica
  psoriasis a.
arthropism
arthroplasty
  hybrid total a.
  Mayo modified total elbow a.
arthropod
  a. allergy
  a. bite
  a. dermatosis
  a. sting
arthropod-borne virus
arthroscope
  Citoscope-16 a.
  30-degree oblique a.
  Medical Dynamics 5990 needle a.
  Stryker a.
arthroscopic
  a. autologous chondrocyte
    transplantation
  a. débridement
arthroscopy
  needle a.

arthrosia
 exanthesis a.
arthrosis
 uncovertebral a.
arthrospore
arthrosteitis
 pustulotic a.
arthrotomy
Arthus
 A. phenomenon
 A. reaction
Arthus-type reaction
articular
 a. amyloid
 a. cartilage damage
 a. chondrocyte
 a. disease
 a. hyaline cartilage
 a. joint tissue catabolism
 a. leprosy
articulation
 acromioclavicular a.
 scapulothoracic a.
 sternoclavicular a.
articulorum
 eczema a.
Articulose-50 injection
artifact, artefact
 buffer a.
 crush a.
artificial
 a. active immunity
 a. nail
 a. passive immunity
 a. skin
 a. tears
artificialis
 acne a.
Artria
art/trs gene
arum plant
ARV
 acquired immunodeficiency syndrome-
  related virus
aryepiglottic fold
arylalcoanoic acid
AS
 angiosarcoma
 ankylosing spondylitis
A.S.
 Crysticillin A.S.

ASA
 acetylsalicylic acid
  MSD enteric-coated ASA
asaccharolyticus
 Peptostreptococcus a.
Asacol Oral
Asadrine
Asaphen
asbestos
 a. corn
 a. wart
Asboe-Hansen
 A.-II. disease
 A.-H. sign
ascariasis
ascaris
Ascaris lumbricoides
ascending lymphangitis
Ascher syndrome
asci (*pl. of* ascus)
ascites
 North American Study of treatment
  for Refractory A. (NASTRA)
Ascoli
 A. reaction
 A. test
 A. treatment
Ascomycetes
ascospore
Ascriptin
ascus, pl. **asci**
ASD
 adult/adolescent spectrum of HIV
  disease
asepsis
aseptic
 a. necrosis
 a. technique
Asepticator unit
ASFV
 African swine fever virus
ash
 Arizona a.
 green a.
 a. leaf spot
 Oregon a.
 a. tree
 a. tree pollen
 white a.
ashgray
 a. blister beetle
 a. blister beetle sting

NOTES

ash-leaf macule
ashsphere
ashy
    a. dermatitis
    a. dermatosis
    a. dermatosis of Ramirez
Asiatic
    A. cholera
    A. pill
asimadoline
Askin biopsy
Aslera
ASLO, ASO
    antistreptolysin-O
    ASLO test
    ASLO titer
ASM
    airway smooth muscle
    ASM 981 cream
Asmalix
ASO (*var. of* ASLO)
asparagine-linked oligosaccharide
asparagus
aspartic proteinase
aspen
    a. pollen
    a. tree
aspergilloma
aspergillosis
    disseminated a.
    invasive a.
    primary cutaneous a.
    pulmonary a.
    rhinocerebral a. (RA)
Aspergillus
    A. *amstelodami*
    A. *avenaceus*
    A. *caesiellus*
    A. *candidus*
    A. *carneus*
    A. *clavatus*
    A. *deltoidea*
    A. *flavus*
    A. *fumigatus*
    A. *nidulans*
    A. *niger*
    A. *oryzae*
    A. *osteomyelitis*
    A. *restrictus*
    A. *sydowi*
    A. *terreus*
    A. *ustus*
    A. *versicolor*
aspergillustoxicosis
aspirate
    nasopharyngeal a. (NPA)
aspiration
    a. biopsy

    myringotomy with a.
    recurrent a.
aspirator
aspirin
    Bayer Buffered A.
    enteric coated a.
    Extra Strength Bayer Enteric
      500 A.
    A. Free Anacin Maximum Strength
    musculoskeletal disorder enteric-
      coated a. (MSD enteric-coated
      ASA)
    A. Plus Stomach Guard
    Saint Joseph Adult Chewable A.
    a. sensitivity
    a. triad
Aspirin-Free Bayer Select Allergy Sinus Caplets
aspirin-induced papillary necrosis
aspirin-intolerant asthma (AIA)
aspirin-sensitive asthma
aspirin-tolerant asthma (ATA)
Asprimox
assassin
    a. bug
    a. bug bite
assay
    adherence a.
    Advia Centaur specific IgE a.
    agar diffusion a.
    AH50 a.
    AlaSTAT a.
    alpha-glutathione S-transferase a.
    amplification a.
    antibody blocking a.
    anti-C3 a.
    anti-D enzyme-linked
      immunosorbent a.
    antigen-nonspecific immune
      complex a.
    Borrelia burgdorferi DNA a.
    CH50 a.
    chemiluminescence a.
    chemokine a.
    Colorimeti A.
    competitive binding a.
    complement binding a.
    conglutinin a.
    Cotinine a.
    C1q a.
    Crithidia luciliae
      immunofluorescence a.
    cytotoxicity a.
    21-Day Cumulative Irritancy A.
    double antibody sandwich a.
    EAC rosette a.
    Ehrlich ascites carcinoma rosette a.
    electrophoretic mobility shift a.
      (EMSA)

enzyme-linked immunosorbent a.
(ELISA)
enzyme-linked immunospot a.
(ELISPOT)
Farr a.
FCXM a.
flow-cytometry cross match a.
FlowPRA beads a.
fluid-phase C1q-binding a.
hemolytic plaque a.
hepatitis B viral DNA a.
HIV DNA amplification a.
human androgen receptor a.
(HUMARA)
human immunodeficiency virus
deoxyribonucleic acid
amplification a.
hybrid capture a. (HCA)
immune adherence
immunosorbent a. (IAHIA)
immune complex a.
immunobead a.
immunochemical a.
immunodiffusion a.
immunofluorescence a.
immunoprecipitation a.
immunoradiometric a. (IRMA)
indirect a.
Jerne plaque a.
latex agglutination a.
leukocyte attachment a.
Limulus amebocyte lysate a.
lymphocyte function a.
murex hybrid capture a.
PCR a.
polyethylene glycol precipitation a.
polymerase chain reaction a.
precipitin a.
Premier H. pylori a.
proliferation a.
QPCR a.
quantitative complement a.
quantitative polymerase chain
reaction a.
Quickscreen a.
radioimmunoprecipitation a. (RIPA)
radioligand a.
radioreceptor a.
Raji cell radioimmune a.
RCR a.
recombinant immunoblot a. (RIBA)
replication-competent retrovirus a.

ribonuclease protection a. (RPA)
Roche Amplicor CMV DNA a.
sandwich a.
2-site immunoradiometric a.
skin-based a.
solid-phase C1q-binding a.
staphylococcal-binding a.
staphylococcal protein A binding a.
TaqMan a.
TIL cell a.
Treponema pallidum
hemagglutination a. (TPHA)
in vitro cytotoxic a.
assessment
gravimetric a.
A. Measure for Atopic Dermatitis
(AMAD)
Assess peak flow meter
Assmann tuberculous infiltrate
associate
microbial a.'s
associated macrophage
association
American Rheumatism A. (ARA)
a. constant
Cosmetic, Toiletries, and
Fragrance A.
associative reaction
astacoid rash
asteatode
asteatosis cutis
asteatotic
a. dermatitis
a. eczema
Astech peak flow meter
Astelin Nasal Spray
astemizole
Asteraceae
asteroid body
asteroides
Nocardia a.
asthenia
neurocirculatory a.
tropical anhidrotic a.
asthma
adult a.
allergen-induced a.
allergic a.
aspirin-intolerant a. (AIA)
aspirin-sensitive a.
aspirin-tolerant a. (ATA)
atopic a.

NOTES

asthma *(continued)*
    baker's a.
    brittle a.
    bronchial a.
    catechol-*O*-methyl transferase a.
    chronic a.
    COMT a.
    cough-variant a.
    Crocodile Bile Pill for A.
    drug-induced a.
    extrinsic a.
    fatal a.
    food a.
    frequent episodic a. (FA)
    functional abnormality in a.
    hay a.
    infrequent episodic a. (IA)
    intrinsic a.
    malignant potentially fatal a.
    Millar a.
    miller's a.
    mixed a.
    near-fatal a.
    nocturnal a.
    nonallergic a.
    occupationally induced a. (OA)
    occupational non-IgE-dependent a.
    persistent a. (PA)
    poorly reversible a.
    potentially fatal a.
    premenstrual exacerbation of a.
      (PMA)
    severe a. (SA)
    steroid-dependent a.
    subclinical a.
    summer a.
    A. Symptom Utility (ASU)
    A. Symptom Utility Index
    Trichophyton-induced a.
    variant a.
    virus-induced a.
    wine-induced a.
AsthmaCare Education: Intensive Training (ACE IT)
AsthmaHaler Mist
asthma-like symptom
AsthmaMentor peak flow meter
AsthmaNefrin
asthmatic
    a. bronchitis
    tight a.
asthmatica
    Tylophora a.
asthmaticus
    status a.
asthmogenic
AstraZeneca LP
astringent
    Clean & Clear Deep Cleaning a.

astrocyte
astrocytoma cell
astronyxis
    Acanthamoeba a.
Astroviridae virus
Asturian leprosy
asturiensis
    elephantiasis a.
ASU
    Asthma Symptom Utility
asymmetric
    a. distribution
    a. oligoarthritis
    a. oligoarthropathy
    a. periflexural exanthem of
      childhood (APEC)
    a. peripheral sensory neuropathy
    a. polyarthritis
asymptomatic
    a. cricoarytenoid synovitis
    a. pulmonary melanoma metastasis
asystolia
AT
    amegakaryocytic thrombocytopenia
ATA
    aspirin-tolerant asthma
Atabrine
Atarax Oral
atavism
    phylogenetic a.
ataxia
    cerebellar a.
    locomotor a.
    a. telangiectasia
    a. telangiectasia syndrome
ataxia-telangiectasia
A/Texas/36/91-like influenza
ATG
    antithymocyte globulin
    Enbrel plus ATG
ATGAM, Atgam
    antithymocyte globulin
    5 ATGAM antilymphocyte therapy
Athabascan, Athabaskan
    A. type of severe combined
      immunodeficiency disease
      (SCIDA)
atheroembolic disease
atheroembolus, pl. **atheroemboli**
atherogenicity
atheroma
atheromatosis cutis
atheromatous embolus
atherosclerosis
athlete's
    a. foot
    a. nodule
athletic nail
Athos laser

A

athrepsia
atlantoaxial
    a. joint
    a. subluxation
atlantodental dislocation
ATLL
    adult T-cell leukemia/lymphoma
atmoknesis
Atolone Oral
atonic ulcer
atopen
atopic
    a. allergy
    a. asthma
    A. Dermatitis Area and Severity Index (ADASI)
    a. dermatitis rash
    A. Dermatitis Severity Index (ADSI)
    a. eczema
    a. hand dermatitis
    a. hypersensitivity
    a. keratoconjunctivitis
    a. march
    a. reagin
    a. sensitivity
atovaquone
Atozine Oral
ATPase
    adenosine triphosphatase
    ATPase activity
ATRA
    all-trans-retinoic acid
Atra-Tain
atrepsy
atresia
    biliary a.
    junctional epidermolysis bullosa with pyloric a.
atretic meningocele
atria (*pl. of* atrium)
atrial conduction disturbance
atrichia
atrichosis
atrichous
atrioventricular (AV)
    a. block
Atrisone
atrium, pl. **atria**
    a. of infection
Atrohist
Atropair Ophthalmic

atrophedema
atrophia
    a. maculosa varioliformis cutis
    a. pilorum propria
atrophic
    a. candidiasis
    a. glossitis
    a. hyperkeratotic lesion
    a. lichen planus
    a. macule
    a. papulosis
    a. plaque
    a. rhinitis of swine
    a. stria
    a. white scar
atrophica
    acne a.
    hyperkeratosis figurata centrifuga a.
    macula a.
    morphea a.
    stria a.
atrophicae
    lineae striae a.
atrophicans
    dermatitis cruris pustulosa et a.
    epidermolysis bullosa a.
    folliculitis cruris a.
    keratosis pilaris a.
    lichen planus et acuminatus a.
    lichen sclerosus et a.
    pityriasis alba a.
atrophicus
atrophie
    a. blanche
    a. blanche lesion
    a. noire
atrophoderma
    a. albidum
    a. biotripticum
    a. diffusum
    follicular a.
    idiopathic a.
    neuritic a.
    a. neuriticum
    a. of Pasini and Pierini
    Pasini-Pierini idiopathic a.
    progressive idiopathic a.
    a. reticulatum
    a. reticulatum symmetricum faciei
    a. scleroatrophy
    senile a.
    a. striatum

NOTES

atrophoderma *(continued)*
    a. striatum et maculatum
    a. ulerythematosa
    a. vermicularis
    vermiculate a.
    a. vermiculatum
atrophodermatosis
atrophy
    blue a.
    Buchwald a.
    central papillary a.
    cigarette-paper a.
    diffuse a.
    a. of fat
    fat-replacement a.
    honeycomb a.
    intrinsic muscle a.
    linear a.
    macular a.
    optic a.
    papillary a.
    primary idiopathic macular a.
    skin a.
    syphilitic spinal muscular a.
    traction a.
    villous a.
    wucher a.
Atropine-Care Ophthalmic
atropine sulfate
Atropisol Ophthalmic
Atrovent
    A. Aerosol Inhalation
    A. Inhalation Solution
A/T/S
    A/T/S lotion
    A/T/S topical
attachment plaque
attack
    acute asthma a.
    drop a.
    syncopal a.
attenuant
attenuated
    a. live mumps virus vaccine
    a. poxvirus vector
    Rickettsia vaccine, a.
    a. tuberculosis
    a. virus
attenuate vaccinia virus
attenuation
attenuator
Attenuvax
ATTR
    amyloidogenic transthyretin
    ATTR Val30Met
Atuss-12DX extended release oral suspension
atypical
    a. erythema multiforme

    a. histiocytosis
    a. ichthyosiform erythroderma
    a. Kawasaki disease (AKD)
    a. lipoma
    a. measles
    a. mole
    a. mole syndrome
    a. mycobacterial arthritis
    a. mycobacterial colonization
    a. mycobacterial infection
    a. pityriasis rosea
    a. pneumonia
Au antigen
Auchmeromyia
audiometry
    screening a.
    threshold a.
audiovestibular dysfunction
audouinii
    Microsporum a.
Audouin microsporon
augmentation
    paraffin breast a.
    silicone breast a.
    a. therapy
augmented histamine test
augmenti
    stadium a.
Augmentin
Aujeszky
    A. disease
    A. disease virus
Aura
    A. Laser
    A. Laser system
aural
    a. fistula
    a. keratosis
Auralate
Auralgan
auranofin
aurantiasis cutis
Aureobasidium pullulans
aureotherapy
aureus
    methicillin-resistant
    Staphylococcus a. (MRSA)
    Staphylococcus a.
auriasis
auricle
    accessory a.
auricular
    a. chondritis
    chronic infantile neurological, cutaneous and a. (CINCA)
    a. perichondritis
auricular
auriculotemporal syndrome
aurid

aurochromoderma
Aurolate
aurothioglucose
    sodium a.
aurothiomalate
    sodium a.
Auroto
Aus antigen
Auspitz
    A. dermatosis
    A. sign
Australia antigen
Australian
    A. parrot droppings
    A. parrot feather
    A. parrot protein
    A. pine
    A. pine tree
    A. punch
    A. X disease
    A. X disease virus
    A. X encephalitis
australis
    Rickettsia a.
autacoid
autoagglutination
autoagglutinin
    anti-Pr cold a.
    cold a.
autoaggression
    systemic a.
autoallergen
autoallergic
autoallergization
autoallergy
autoamputate
autoanaphylaxis
autoantibody
    antibasement membrane zone a.
    anti-BMZ a.
    anticalpastatin a.
    anticardiolipin a.
    antiidiotype a.
    antineutrophil cytoplasmic a.
     (ANCA)
    antinuclear a.
    antinucleosome a.
    antiperinuclear a.
    antitype (II, IX) collagen a.
    brain-reactive a.
    cold a.
    Donath-Landsteiner cold a.

    hemagglutinating cold a.
    idiotype a.
    monoclonal a.
    muscarinic receptor a.
    myositis-associated a.
    myositis-specific a. (MSA)
    PARP a.
    plasma protein a.
    poly(ADP-ribose)polymerase a.
    warm a.
autoanticomplement
autoantigen
    a. collagen
    48-kd La a.
    52-kd Ro a.
    60-kd Ro a.
auto-antiidiotypic antibody
autochemotherapy
autoclasis
autocrine hormone
autocytolysin
autocytolysis
autocytotoxin
autodermic
autodigestion of connective tissue
autoeczematization
autoerythrocyte
    a. sensitivity
    a. sensitization
    a. sensitization syndrome
autogeneic graft
autogenous vaccine
autograft
autografting
    cultured epithelial a.
autogram
autographism
Autohaler
    Maxair A.
autohemagglutination
autohemolysin
autohemolysis
autoimmune
    a. atrophic gastritis
    a. blistering mucocutaneous disease
    a. chronic hepatitis
    a. disorder
    a. encephalomyelitis
    a. exocrinopathy
    a. hemolysis
    a. lymphoproliferative syndrome
    (ALPS)

NOTES

autoimmune *(continued)*
    a. neonatal thrombocytopenia
    a. neutropenia
    a. panhypopituitarism
    a. paraneoplastic syndrome
    a. phenomenon
    a. pituitary disease
    a. polyendocrinopathy-candidiasis-ectodermal dysplasia (APECED)
    a. polyendocrinopathy-canidiasis-ectodermal dystrophy
    a. polyglandular syndrome (APS)
    a. progenitor cell
    a. progesterone dermatitis
    a. response
    a. thrombocytopenic purpura
    a. type of reaction
autoimmunity
    cell-mediated a.
    kaleidoscope phenomenon of a.
autoimmunization
autoimmunocytopenia
autoinfection
autoinjector
autoinoculable
autoinoculation
autoisolysin
AuTolo
    A. Cure Process
    A. Cure Process wound treatment
autologous
    a. antibody
    a. antigen
    a. bone marrow transplant
    a. cultured epithelium
    a. graft
    a. mixed leukocyte reaction
    a. transplantation
autolyse
autolysin
autolysis
autolytic
autolyze
autoMACS
    automated magnetic cell sorting
automated
    A. Cellular Imaging System (ACIS)
    A. Cellular Imaging System immunohistochemical stain
    a. cytochemical system
    a. magnetic cell sorting (autoMACS)
Automeris
autonomic
    a. epilepsy flush
    a. imbalance syndrome
    a. nervous system
    a. urticaria

autonomous
autophagia
autophagic
autophagy
autophytica
    dermatitis a.
autoplast
autoplastic graft
autoplasty
autoradiography
autoreactive B cell
autoreinfection
autoreproduction
autosensitivity
    deoxyribonucleic acid a.
    DNA a.
autosensitization dermatitis
autosensitize
autosepticemia
autoserotherapy
autoserum therapy
autosomal
    a. codominant
    a. dominant
    a. dominant lamellar ichthyosis
    a. dominant oculocutaneous albinism
    a. dominant periodic fever syndrome
    a. recessive
    a. recessive ichthyosis
    a. recessive severe combined immunodeficiency disorder
    a. recessive trait
autosplenectomy
Auto Suture SFS stapler
autotherapy
autotoxicans
    horror a.
autotoxicus
    horror a.
autotransplant
autotransplantation
autovaccination
auxiliary
    a. partial heterotopic liver transplantation (APHLT)
    a. partial orthotopic liver transplant (APOLT)
    a. partial orthotopic liver transplantation (APOLT)
auxilytic
AV
    atrioventricular
    AV block
Avacor
Avanta implant
Avant Garde Shampoo
avascularity

avasculosus
　　nevus a.
AVC
　　AVC Cream
　　AVC suppository
Aveeno
　　A. Cleansing Bar
　　A. Moisture Cream
　　A. oatmeal bath
　　Oilated A.
　　regular A.
　　A. skin replenishing cleansing
　　　lotion
Aveeno/colloidal oatmeal bath
avellana
　　Corylus a.
Avelox
　　A. IV
　　A. tablet
avenaceus
　　Aspergillus a.
Aventyl
Aviadenovirus
avian
　　a. diphtheria
　　a. encephalomyelitis virus
　　a. erythroblastosis virus
　　a. infectious encephalomyelitis
　　a. infectious laryngotracheitis
　　a. infectious laryngotracheitis virus
　　a. influenza
　　a. influenza virus
　　a. leukosis
　　a. leukosis-sarcoma complex
　　a. leukosis-sarcoma virus
　　a. lymphomatosis
　　a. lymphomatosis virus
　　a. mite dermatitis
　　a. monocytosis
　　a. myeloblastosis
　　a. myeloblastosis virus
　　a. neurolymphomatosis virus
　　a. pneumoencephalitis virus
　　a. reticuloendotheliosis
　　a. sarcoma
　　a. sarcoma virus
　　a. viral arthritis virus
Avicine vaccine
avidin-biotin-peroxidase
　　a.-b.-p. complex method
　　a.-b.-p. staining

avidity
　　a. antibody
　　high a.
　　low a.
Avinza
Avipoxvirus
Avirax
avirulent
Avita acne cream
avitaminosis
avium
　　Mycobacterium a.
avium-intracellulare
　　Mycobacterium a.-i. (MAI)
Avlosulfon
avobenzone
avocado soybean unsaponifiable
avocational
　　a. allergen
　　a. intervention
Avogel hydrogel sheeting
avoidance
Avon Skin-So-Soft
Avosil scar gel
A-Wuhan/359/95-like influenza
axenic
axial
　　a. disease
　　a. involvement
　　a. psoriatic arthritis
　　a. type
axilla
　　ringworm of a.
axillaris
　　hidradenitis a.
　　tinea a.
　　trichomycosis a.
　　trichonocardiosis a.
axillary
　　a. Fox-Fordyce disease
　　a. freckling
　　a. hair
　　a. hyperhidrosis
　　a. nerve compression
　　a. nerve palsy
　　a. venom gland
axiltraction
axis
　　HPA a.
　　hypothalamic-pituitary adrenal a.
　　psycho-neuro-immuno-endocrine a.
　　a. of symmetry

NOTES

Axsain
Ayercillin
Ayndet moisturizing soap
AZA
    azathioprine
Azactam
Azadirachta indica
azalide
azapropazone
azar
    kala a.
azatadine maleate
azathioprine (AZA)
azathioprine-induced myelosuppression
azelaic
    a. acid
    a. acid cream
azelastine
    a. hydrochloride nasal spray
    a. hydrochloride ophthalmic solution
Azelex
azidothymidine (AZT)
azithromycin

Azlocillin
Azmacort
azobenzene dye
azodicarbonamide
azo dye
azole
    a. antifungal agent
    a. compound
azoospermia
azoprotein
azotemia
    progressive a.
AZT
    azidothymidine
aztreonam
azul
Azulfidine EN-tabs
azure lunula of nail
azurocidin
azurophil
    a. granule
    a. granule protein
Azzopardi phenomenon

B

amphotericin B
antideoxyribonuclease B
anti-DNase B
anti-Sjögren syndrome B (anti-SSB)
blood group-specific substances A and B
branched DNA signal amplication assay for hepatitis B
B cell
B cell fibroblast
chondroitin sulfate B
B fraction serum
granzyme B (GrB)
B lymphocyte
Nasahist B
Prevex B
Sjögren syndrome B (SS-B)
B virus

B1

B1 cell
nuclear lamin B1

B4

B4 blocked ricin
leukotriene B4 (LTB4)

B7

B7 costimulatory molecule
B7 protein

B19

human parvovirus B19
parvovirus B19
B19 virus

B60

HLA B60

B$_6$

vitamin B$_6$

b1

Hev b1
rubber elongation factor

b6

Hev b6
hevein

b$_{558}$

membrane-bound cytochrome b$_{558}$

B7:counterreceptor interaction

BA

betamethasone acetate

Babesia

B. bigemina
B. bovis
B. canis
B. divergens
B. equi
B. felis
B. major

B. microti
B. rodhaini

babesiosis

Babinski

B. sign
B. syndrome

Babinski-Vaquez syndrome

baboon syndrome

baby

blueberry muffin b.
carbon b.
collodion b.
B. Magic soap
Water B.'s

BABYbird respirator

Baby's Own Ointment

bacampicillin hydrochloride

Baccharus

Baciguent topical

bacillary angiomatosis

bacillary-barren tuberculids

Bacille Calmette-Guérin vaccine

bacilli (*pl. of* bacillus)

bacilliformis

Bartonella b.

bacillogenic sycosis

bacillosis

bacillus, pl. **bacilli**

b. abortus
acne b.
B. acnes
b. alvei
b. anthracis
b. anthracis toxin
Calmette-Guérin b.
B. Calmette-Guérin live
b. cereus
cholera b.
b. circulans
comma b.
Frish b.
fusiform b.
gram-negative b. (GNB)
gram-positive b. (GPB)
Hansen b.
Koch b.
b. laterosporus
lepra b.
b. licheniformis
b. megaterium
Park-Williams b.
b. polymyxa
b. pseudodiphtheriticum
b. pumilus
b. sphaericus

bacillus *(continued)*
  b. *stearothermophilus*
  b. *subtilis*
  vole b.
  Warthin-Starry-staining b.
  Whipple b.
bacitracin
  b., neomycin, and polymyxin b
  b., neomycin, polymyxin b, and
    hydrocortisone
  b., neomycin, polymyxin b, and
    lidocaine
  b. and polymyxin b
Bacit-Stat
Back-Ese M
Backhaus towel clip
back mice
backtitration
baclofen
bacoti
  Liponyssus b.
BacT/Alert Microbial Detection System
BACTEC
  BACTEC 550
  BACTEC 16B-17D
  BACTEC radiometry
  BACTEC system
bacteremia
  gram-negative b. (GNB)
  gram-positive b. (GPB)
  MAI b.
  Mycobacterium avium-
    intracellulare b.
  polymicrobial b.
  Pseudomonas aeruginosa b.
  puerperal b.
  vancomycin-resistant *Enterococcus*
    faecium b.
  VREF b.
bacteria (*pl. of* bacterium)
bacteria-free stage of bacterial
  endocarditis
bacterial
  b. allergy
  b. antagonism
  b. antigen
  b. arthritis
  b. conjunctivitis
  b. contamination
  b. disease
  b. endocarditis
  b. exotoxin
  b. hemolysin
  b. infection
  b. interference
  b. intertrigo
  b. macromolecule
  b. paronychia
  b. peptidoglycan

  b. phagocytosis test
  b. plaque
  b. pneumococcal pneumonia
  b. septicemia
  b. synergistic gangrene
  b. toxin
  b. translocation
  b. vaccine
  b. virus
bacterial-induced vascular damage
bacterially induced hemostatic disorder
bactericide
  specific b.
bacterid
  pustular b.
bacterioagglutinin
bacteriocide
bacteriocidin
bacteriocin factor
bacteriocinogen
bacteriocinogenic plasmid
bacteriogenic agglutination
bacteriolysin
bacteriolysis
  immune b.
bacteriolytic serum
bacteriolyze
bacteriopexy
bacteriophage
  defective b.
  filamentous b.
  b. immunity
  lambda b.
  mature b.
  b. phi-X174
  b. resistance
  temperate b.
  typhoid b.
  b. typing
  vegetative b.
  virulent b.
bacteriophagia
bacteriophagic
bacteriophagology
bacteriopsonin
bacteriosis
bacteriostasis
bacteriostat
bacteriostatic
bacteriotic
bacteriotoxic
bacteriotropic substance
bacteriotropin
bacterium, pl. **bacteria**
  Bordetella pertussis b.
  commensal bacteria
  coryneform b.
  facultative b.
  heterotopic plate count bacteria

HPC bacteria
lysogenic b.
pyogenic b.
resistant b.
bacteriuria
Bacteroides fragilis
Bacticort Otic
Bactigras
Bactine Hydrocortisone
Bactocill
    B. injection
    B. Oral
Bactolysins
BactoShield topical
Bactrim DS
Bactroban topical
Baculoviridae
baculovirus
Baelz disease
Baerensprung (*var. of* Barensprung)
Bäfverstedt syndrome
bag
    B. Balm lubricant/emollient
    2-L rubber b.
bagassosis
Baghdad
    B. boil
    bouton de B.
Bahia grass
Bairnsdale ulcer
baked tongue
Baker-Cummings punch
Baker cyst
baker's
    b. asthma
    b. dermatitis
    b. eczema
    b. itch
baking soda paste
BAL
    bioartificial liver
    bronchoalveolar lavage
    BAL therapy
Balamuthia mandrillaris
balanitis, pl. **balanitides**
    Candida b.
    b. circinata
    circinate b.
    b. circumscripta
    erosive *Candida* b.
    Follmann b.
    fusospirochetal b.

plasma cell b.
    b. plasmacellularis
    pseudoepitheliomatous keratotic and micaceous b.
    b. xerotica obliterans
    b. of Zoon
balanoposthitis
    streptococcal b.
balantidial
    b. colitis
    b. dysentery
Balantidium coli
balatus
    Acarus b.
bald
    b. cypress
    b. cypress tree
Baldex
baldness
    common b.
    congenital b.
    female pattern b.
    male pattern b.
    moth-eaten b.
    pubic b.
ball
    fungus b.
    b. of mucus
    red b.'s
ball-in-claw
    b.-i.-c. appearance
    b.-i.-c. pattern
Ballingall disease
ballistospore
balloon
    b. cell
    b. cell nevus
ballooning degeneration
balm
    Extra Strength B.
    b. of Gilead
Balminil Decongestant
balnea
    pruritus b.
balnei
    Mycobacterium b.
Balneol lotion
balneotherapy
Balnetar
Baló
    B. concentric encephalitis

NOTES

Baló *(continued)*
    B. concentric sclerosis
    B. concentric syndrome
Balpred
balsam
    Mecca b.
    b. of Peru
    b. of tolu
balsamic
Baltic amber
bamboo
    b. hair
    b. spine
banal-appearing nevomelanocyte
banal bacterial infection
banana roll
banana-shaped body
Bancroft filariasis
bancrofti
    Filaria b.
    Wuchereria b.
Bancroftian filariasis
band
    b. keratopathy
    longitudinal hyperpigmented b.
    marginal b.
    Muehrcke b.
bandage
    Ace b.
    Coban cohesive medium stretch b.
    Comperm tubular elastic b.
    Coplus cohesive medium stretch b.
    Crepe short stretch b.
    Elastomull elastic gauze b.
    Elset long stretch b.
    Gelocast b.
    Hamilton b.
    Hollister medial adhesive b.
    Hydron Burn B.
    Isoelast adhesive short stretch b.
    Isoplast adhesive short stretch b.
    4-layer b. (FLB)
    3M Clean Seals b.
    Nylexogrip cohesive long stretch b.
    2-octylcyanoacrylate topical b.
    Profore 4-layer b.
    b. sign
    Stegman-Tromovitch b.
    Tricoplast adhesive elastic b.
    TubiFast b.
    Ulcosan unna boot with inelastic
        zinc plaster b.
Band-Aid
    B.-A. composite dressing
    B.-A. Liquid
banding
Bandrowski base (BB)
Bang disease
banishing cream

bank
    gene b.
    New England Organ B. (NEOB)
Banker-type dermatomyositis
bankokerend
Bannayan-Riley-Ruvalcaba syndrome
Bannister disease
Bannwarth syndrome
Banophen
    B. Decongestant Capsule
    B. Oral
Banti syndrome
bar
    Acne Aid cleansing b.
    Aveeno Cleansing B.
    Fostex B.
    Olay Sensitive Skin b.
    PanOxyl B.
    Steel Bars high protein nutrition b.
    ZNP b.
Bara-Med
barba, pl. **barbae**
    folliculitis barbae
    pseudofolliculitis barbae (PFB)
    sycosis barbae
    tinea barbae
    trichophytosis barbae
Barbados leg
barbed
    b. hypostome
    b. stinger
barber
    b. pilonidal sinus
    B. psoriasis
    pustular psoriasis of the palms and
        soles of B.
barber's itch
Barbour-Stoenner-Kelly (BSK)
    B.-S.-K. broth
barbula hirci
Barc Liquid
Barcoo
    B. disease
    B. rot
Bard Absorption dressing
Bardet-Biedl
    B.-B. 1–5 syndrome
Bard-Parker blade
bare lymphocyte syndrome
Barensprung, Baerensprung
    B. erythrasma
barium sulfide
bark
    jambolan b.
    b. scorpion
    b. scorpion sting
barking cough
barley
Barmah Forest virus

barn
    b. dust
    b. itch
Barnett classification
Barraquer forceps
Barraquer-Simons syndrome
barrier
    blood-aqueous b.
    blood-ocular b.
    blood-retinal b.
    blood-urine b.
    b. cream
    b. function
    b. layer
    physical b.
    b. protective cream
    b. zone
Barriere-HC
Bart
    B. syndrome
    B. thalassemia
Bartholin adenitis
bartholinitis
Barth syndrome
Bartonella
    B. bacilliformis
    B. elizabethan
    B. henselae
    B. henselae detection
bartonellosis
Bart-Pumphrey syndrome
basal
    b. cell
    b. cell layer
    b. cell membrane
    b. cell nevus
    b. cell nevus syndrome
    b. cell papilloma
    b. lamina
    b. meningitis
    b. transalveolar fluid
basale
    stratum b.
basalis
    decidua b.
basaloid
    b. cell
    b. folliculolymphoid hyperplasia
Basan syndrome
base
    Bandrowski b. (BB)

    meningitis of the b.
    b. pair (bp)
basedoid
Basedow disease
basement
    b. membrane
    b. membrane zone (BMZ)
    b. membrane zone antibody
Basex syndrome
basic
    b. calcium phosphate crystal
    B. Clinical Scoring System
    b. fibroblast growth factor (bFGF)
    b. red 46
basic-region leucine-zipper (bZIP)
basidiobolae
    entomophthoramycosis b.
basidiobolomycosis
Basidiobolus ranarum
Basidiomycetes
basidiospore
basilar
    b. meningitis
    b. vasculopathy
basiliximab
basiloma terebrans
basis
    nonimmunologic b.
    B. soap
basket-weave vacuolization
basolateral transport
basophil
    b. degranulation test
    b. kallikrein
basophilic degeneration
basosquamous
    b. carcinoma
    b. cell acanthoma
BASOTEST
bastard measles
Bateman
    B. disease
    B. purpura
    B. syndrome
Bates-Jensen pressure ulcer status tool
bath
    B. AS Functional Index
    Aveeno/colloidal oatmeal b.
    Aveeno oatmeal b.
    coal tar b.
    colloidal oatmeal b.
    b. itch

NOTES

bath *(continued)*
>oil b.
>b. oil
>potassium permanganate b.
>b. pruritus
>starch b.
>stop b.
>tar b.

bathing-trunk nevus
bathtub refinisher's lung
battery
>b. acid
>b. patch testing

Baumgartner needle holder
bax gene
bayberry tree
Bayer
>B. Buffered Aspirin
>B. Low Adult Strength
>B. Select Pain Relief Formula

Bayle disease
bayonet hair
Bayou virus
bay sore
Bazex syndrome
Bazin
>B. disease
>B. ulcer

BB
>Bandrowski base

B1–B5
>Coxsackievirus B1–B5

Bb
>*Borrelia burgdorferi*

B/Beijing/184/93-like influenza
BC
>CML BC

B-Caro-T
B-cell
>B-c. antigen receptor
>B-c. chronic lymphocytic leukemia
>(B-CLL)
>B-c. differentiation/growth factor
>B-c. epitope
>B-c. growth factor-1
>B-c. growth factor-2
>B-c. lymphocytic leukemia
>B-c. lymphocytoma cutis
>B-c. lymphoma
>B-c. malignancy
>B-c. memory
>B-c. pseudolymphoma

BCG
>Pacis BCG
>TICE BCG
>BCG vaccine

bcl-2, -6 gene
BClear system

B-CLL
>B-cell chronic lymphocytic leukemia

BCNU
>bischloroethylnitrosourea
>topical BCNU

bcr-abl chimeric transcript
BCR/abl gene re-arrangement test
BCYE
>buffered charcoal yeast extract

BCYE agar
16B-17D
>BACTEC 16B-17D

Bdellovibrio
BDI
>burn depth indicator

bead
>Bio-Enza B.
>Sephadex B.

beaded hair
beading
beam
>electron b.
>Gaussian b.
>total skin electron b. (TSEB)

bean
>broad b.
>castor b.
>coffee b.
>green coffee b.
>kidney b.
>lava b.
>lima b.
>navy b.
>string b.

Be^a antigen
beard
>ringworm of b.

Bearn-Kunkel-Slater syndrome
Bearn-Kunkel syndrome
Beau line
beauty mark
Beaver
>B. blade
>B. ES miniblade

Beben
becaplermin
Bechterew syndrome
Becker
>B. antigen
>B. hairy hamartoma
>B. muscular dystrophy
>B. nevus

Beclodisk
Becloforte
beclomethasone dipropionate
Beclovent Oral Inhaler
Beconase AQ Nasal Inhaler
bed
>air-fluidized b.

Biologics Airlift b.
low air-loss b.
powder b.
b. rest
b. sore
tanning b.
bedbug
b. bite
b. disease transmission
Bednar
B. aphtha
B. tumor
bedsore
bee
b. glue
b. sting
sweat b.
b. venom
beech tree
beefsteak fungus
beefwood
Beepen-VK Oral
beet
sugar b.
beetle
ashgray blister b.
blister b.
piper b.
striped blister b.
Behçet
B. aphtha
B. disease
B. syndrome
Behring
B. law
B. serum
Beigel disease
beigelii
Trichosporon b.
bejel treponematosis
Bekhterev-Strümpell spondylitis
Belix Oral
bell
B. international unit
B. palsy
belladonna, phenobarbital, and ergotamine tartrate
Bellergal-S
belli
Isospora b.
bellows breathing

belly
crix b.
Bel-Phen-Ergot S
Belzer
B. solution
B. UW
Bena-D injection
Benadryl
B. Allergy/Cold Fastmelt
B. Children's Allergy Fastmelt
B. Decongestant Allergy Tablet
B. Injection
B. Oral
B. topical
Benahist injection
Ben-Allergin-50 Injection
Ben-Aqua
Bence
B. Jones albumin
B. Jones protein
Benefin
BeneJoint cream
Benemid
Ben-Gay patch
benign
b. dry pleurisy
b. dyskeratosis
b. familial chronic pemphigus
b. giant cell synovioma
b. hemangiopericytoma
b. hyperplasia
b. inoculation lymphoreticulosis
b. inoculation reticulosis
b. intracranial hypertension
b. junctional nevus
b. juvenile melanoma
b. lipoblastomatosis
b. lymphadenosis
b. lymphangioendothelioma
b. lymphocytic infiltrate of Jessner-Kanof
b. lymphocytoma cutis
b. migratory glossitis
b. monoclonal gammopathy
b. mucosal pemphigoid
b. papular acantholytic dermatosis
b. paroxysmal peritonitis
b. pemphigus vegetans
b. recurrent endothelioleukocytic meningitis
b. symmetric lipomatosis
b. systemic mastocytosis

NOTES

benign *(continued)*
   b. trichilemmoma
   b. tumor
benigna
   lymphadenosis cutis b.
   lymphogranulomatosis b.
   variola b.
benignum
   lymphogranuloma b.
Benisone
Benoject injection
Benoquin
benoxaprofen
Benoxyl
Bensal HP
benserazide
bent-fork deformity
bentonite
   b. flocculation test
   quaternium-18 b.
bentoquatam
Benuryl
Benylin
   B. for Allergies
   B. Cold
   B. Cough Syrup
   B. Decongestant
Benzac
   B. AC Gel
   B. AC Wash
   B. W
   B. W Gel
   B. W Wash
BenzaClin gel
Benzagel
5-Benzagel
10-Benzagel
benzalkonium chloride
Benzamycin Pak
Benzashave Cream
benzathine
   penicillin g b.
benzbromarone
benzene
benzethonium chloride
benzimidazole
benziodarone
benznidazole
benzoate
   benzyl b.
   betamethasone b.
   b. preservative
benzocaine
   antipyrine and b.
   b., butyl aminobenzoate, tetracaine,
      and benzalkonium chloride
   b., gelatin, pectin, and sodium
      carboxymethylcellulose
   Orabase with b.

Benzodent
benzodiazepine midazolam
benzoic acid and salicylic acid
benzoin
benzophenone
benzoyl
   b. peroxide
   b. peroxide and hydrocortisone
benzphetamine hydrochloride
benzyl
   b. alcohol
   b. benzoate
benzylamine
benzylpenicilloyl-polylysine
Beradinelli-Seip syndrome
bergamot
   oil of b.
Berger IgA nephropathy
Bergh forceps
beriberi
Berkeley scarifier
Berkow formula
berlock, berloque
   b. dermatitis
Bermuda
   B. grass
   B. grass pollen
   B. smut
Bernard-Soulier syndrome
Bernese periacetabular osteotomy
Berotec
berylliosis
beryllium
   b. dermatitis
   b. disease
   b. granuloma
Besnier
   B. disease
   B. lupus pernio
   B. protoporphyria
   B. prurigo
   prurigo gestationis of B.
Besnier-Boeck disease
Besnier-Boeck-Schaumann disease
Beta-2
beta, β
   b. carotene
   b. corynebacteriophage
   b. hemolysin
   b. hemolysis
   interferon b. (IFN-beta)
   b. lactoglobulin
   b. phage
   b. thalassemia trait
beta-adrenergic
   b.-a. agonist
   b.-a. stimulation
beta-carotene

beta-cell destruction
betacellulin (BTC)
beta-$_{1C}$ globulin
Betachron E-R
Betacort
Betaderm
Betadine First Aid Antibiotics +
   Moisturizer
betae
      Phoma b.
beta-$_{1E}$ globulin
beta-$_{1F}$ globulin
Betagel
betaglycan
beta-glycoprotein
   glycine-rich b.-g.
beta-glycoproteinase
   glycine-rich b.-g.
beta$_2$-glycoprotein I (beta$_2$-GPI)
beta$_2$-glycoprotein II
beta$_2$-GPI
   beta$_2$-glycoprotein I
beta-HCH
   beta-hexachlorocyclohexane
17-beta-hydroxysteroid dehydrogenase
   (17-beta-HSD)
beta-heavy-chain disease
beta-hemolytic
   b.-h. streptococcus
   b.-h. streptococcus infection
beta-hexachlorocyclohexane (beta-HCH)
3-beta-HSD
   3-beta-hydroxysteroid dehydrogenase
17-beta-HSD
   17-beta-hydroxysteroid dehydrogenase
3-beta-hydroxysteroid dehydrogenase (3-
   beta-HSD)
beta-interferon
beta-lactam
beta-lactamase
   CAZ b.-l.
   ceftizoxime b.-l.
beta-lactoglobulin
Betalene topical
beta-mannosidase deficiency
beta-melanocyte-stimulating hormone
betamethasone
   b. acetate (BA)
   b. benzoate
   b. and clotrimazole
   b. dipropionate
   b. mousse

   b. sodium phosphate and acetate
      suspension
   b. valerate
beta$_2$-microglobulin level
Betapen-VK Oral
beta-pleated sheet
Betaseron
beta-thalassemia intermedia
Betatrex topical
Beta-Val topical
betel pepper
Bethesda Conference on Cardiac
   Transplantation
Betimol Ophthalmic
Betnesol
Betnovate
Betulaceae
Betula verrucosa
betulus
      Carpinus b.
bexarotene gel
Bextra
Bexxar radiolabeled monoclonal
   antibody
bFGF
   basic fibroblast growth factor
BFL
   bird-fancier's lung
BFP
   biologic false positive
BGC
      BGC Matrix collagen
      BGC Matrix hydrocolloid
      BGC Matrix hydrocolloid dressing
BHAP
   bisheteroarylpiperazine
bhastrika breathing
bhiwanol dermatitis
Biafine
      B. RE
      B. WDE
biallelic polymorphism
Bi antigen
Biavax II
Biaxin
      B. Filmtab
      B. XL
bicarbonate (HCO$_3$)
   sodium b.
bichloracetic acid
bicho dos pes

NOTES

Bicillin
B. C-R
B. C-R 900/300 injection
B. L-A injection
bicipital
b. syndrome
b. tendinitis
Bicitra
biclonal
b. gammopathy
b. peak
BIDS
brittle hair, intellectual impairment,
decreased fertility, short stature
ichthyosis plus BIDS (IBIDS)
BIDS syndrome
Biederman sign
bieneusi
Enterocytozoon b.
Biernacki sign
Bier spot
Biett
collarette of B.
Biett collar
Bifidobacterium
anaerobic *B.*
Bi-Flex
Osteo B.-F.
biflora
Impatiens b.
bifonazole shampoo
bifurcati
pili b.
bifurcatus
pilus b.
bigemina
Babesia b.
biglycan
Big V
Biken-CAM vaccine
bilateral sensorineural deafness
bilayered skin substitute (BSS)
Bile antigen
bilevel positive airway pressure (BiPAP)
bilharzial granuloma
bilharziasis
bilharzioma
biliaire
masque b.
biliary
b. atresia
b. pruritus
biliostasis
bilious cholera
bilirubinemia
biloba
Ginkgo b.
Biltricide
bi-luer lock adaptor

bimodal immunofluorescent pattern
binary nomenclature
binding
b. constant
deoxyribonucleic acid b.
DNA b.
binomial theorem
bioactive lipid derivative
bioartificial liver (BAL)
bioassay
bioavailability
Biobrane
B. adhesive
B. glove
B. synthetic dressing
B. synthetic skin substitute
Biobrane/HF skin substitute
Biocef
biochemical
b. abnormality
b. biopsy
b. metastasis
biocidal
biocide
Bioclot test
Bioclusive
B. MVP transparent film
B. synthetic dressing
B. transparent dressing
biodermatology
Bio-Enza Bead
bioerodible mucoadhesive
biogenic amine
Biohist-LA
bioinformatics
Biolex
B. hydrogel dressing
B. impregnated gauze
B. wound cleanser
biologic
b. false positive (BFP)
b. hemolysis
b. therapy
biological
b. immunotherapy
b. standard unit
b. vector
Biologics Airlift bed
biomagnetic therapy
biometer
UV b.
Biomox
Bionaire Air Cleaner
Bionicare 1000 stimulator system
Bion Tears solution
Biopatch
B. antimicrobial dressing
B. foam dressing
biophylactic

B

biophylaxis
BioPress plate
biopsy
    Askin b.
    aspiration b.
    biochemical b.
    donor b.
    elliptical b.
    excisional b.
    fine-needle aspiration b. (FNAB)
    incisional b.
    International Society for Heart and
      Lung Transplant b.
    intestinal b.
    ISHLT b.
    lung b.
    lymph node b.
    muscle b.
    nasopharyngeal b.
    needle b.
    needle-core b. (NCB)
    open lung b.
    peroral intestinal b.
    punch b.
    renal b.
    scissors b.
    shave b.
    synovial b.
    tangential b.
    temporal artery b. (TAB)
    total b.
    transjugular hepatic b.
    wedge renal b.
bioreactor
    magnetic-resonance imaging-
      compatible hollow-fiber b.
    MRI-compatible hollow-fiber b.
BioSpan tissue expander
Bio-Tab Oral
Biotene
Biothrax
biotin deficiency
biotinidase
    b. deficiency
    b. enzyme
biotinylated antihuman IgG
biotoxin
biotripticum
    atrophoderma b.
Biotropine
biotropism
Biozyme-C

BiPAP
    bilevel positive airway pressure
biphasic response
biphosphonate
bipolar electrosurgery
bipolymer
Birbeck granule
birch
    red b.
    river b.
    b. tree
    b. tree pollen
bird
    b. egg syndrome
    b. nest anaphylaxis
bird-breeder's
    b.-b. disease
    b.-b. lung
bird-fancier's lung (BFL)
birdshot retinochoroidopathy
birefringent
    b. collagen bundle
    b. crystal
Birex
birminghamensis
    Legionella b.
Birnaviridae
Birnavirus
Birtcher hyfrecator
birthmark
    hemangioma b.
    strawberry b.
    vascular malformation b.
bischloroethylnitrosourea (BCNU)
bisheteroarylpiperazine (BHAP)
Bishop-Harmon ophthalmic forceps
Biskra
    bouton de B.
    B. button
Bismatrol
bismuth
    b. granule
    b. subgallate
    b. subsalicylate
Bisolvon
bispecific antibody
bisphosphonate
bitartrate
    hydrocodone b.
    levarterenol b.
    metaraminol b.
    norepinephrine b.

NOTES

bite

ant b.
arthropod b.
assassin bug b.
bedbug b.
black fly b.
black widow spider b.
brown recluse spider b.
cat flea b.
centipede b.
chigger b.
conenose bug b.
Congo floor maggot b.
copperhead snake b.
coral snake b.
cottonmouth snake b.
Ctenocephalides canis b.
Ctenocephalides felis b.
deer fly b.
dog flea b.
Eastern coral snake b.
fiddle-back spider b.
fly b.
giant desert centipede b.
Gila monster b.
Glossina b.
gnat b.
harvest mite b.
Heloderma suspectum b.
horsefly b.
human b.
insect b.
kissing bug b.
Latrodectus mactans b.
Loxosceles reclusa b.
midge b.
mite b.
moccasin snake b.
mosquito b.
northern rat flea b.
Nosopsyllus fasciatus b.
Oriental rat flea b.
b. pathology
Phlebotomus sandfly b.
pit viper b.
rat flea b.
rattlesnake b.
red bug b.
sand flea b.
sandfly b.
Scolopendra heres b.
sea snake b.
snake b.
spider b.
stable fly b.
Stomoxys b.
Texas coral snake b.
tick b.
Triatoma gerstaeckeri b.

Triatoma sanguisuga b.
tsetse fly b.
Tunga penetrans b.
violin-back spider b.
Xenopsylla cheopis b.
Yersinia pestis b.
biterminal coagulation
biting
b. insect
nail b.
b. reef worm
bitolterol mesylate
Bitot spot
bitter dock
bittersweet nightshade
bitterwood allergy
Bittner
B. agent
B. milk factor
B. virus
biundulant meningoencephalitis
bivalency
monogamous b.
bivalent
b. antibody
b. antigen
b. gas gangrene antitoxin
Bizzozero node
Björnstad syndrome
BK
BK viruria
BK virus
black
b. ant
B. Creek Canal virus
b. currant rash
b. dermatographia
b. dermogram
b. dot hair
b. dot tinea
b. dot tinea capitis
b. eschar
b. eye
b. fever
b. fly
b. fly bite
b. hairy tongue
b. heel
B. Lagoon virus
b. light fluorescent lamp
b. locust
b. locust tree
b. measles
b. mulberry
b. palm
b. pepper
b. piedra
b. ray lamp
b. rubber mix

b. seeds in wart
Sudan b.
b. sweat
b. toe
b. walnut
b. walnut tree pollen
b. widow spider
b. widow spider antivenin
b. widow spider bite
blackberry
black-dot ringworm
Blackfan-Diamond
B.-D. anemia
B.-D. Langerhans cell histiocytosis
blackhead
blackjack disease
black-legged tick
bladder toxicity
blade
Acu-Razor b.
Bard-Parker b.
Beaver b.
CLM articulating laryngoscope b.
Derma b.
Gillette Blue B.
blain
blanch
blanchable red lesion
blanche
atrophie b.
blanched cutaneous elevation
blanching
delayed b.
Blancophor, blankophore
bland
b. aerosolized liquid
b. occlusive disorder
blank
b. allele
b. antigen
blanket
cooling b.
blankophore (*var. of* Blancophor)
Blaschko
B. dermatitis
B. line
B. linear dermatosis
lines of B.
blast
b. cell

refractory anemia with excess b.'s
(RAEB)
b. transformation
blastema
blastic NK-cell lymphoma
blastoconidia
Candida b.
blastogenesis
blastogenetic
Blastomyces
B. brasiliensis
B. dermatitidis
blastomycetes
pathogenic b.
blastomycetica
erosio interdigitalis b.
blastomycetic dermatitis
blastomycosis
cutaneous b.
European b.
keloidal b.
North American b.
primary cutaneous b.
South American b.
blastomycosis-like pyoderma
blastomycotica
dermatitis b.
blastomycotic osteomyelitis
Blatin
B. sign
B. syndrome
Blau syndrome
bleached rubber syndrome
bleb
apoptotic b.
b. stapling
bleeding
punctate b.
BlemErase Lotion
Blemish Control
Blenderm patch technique
blennorrhagia
blennorrhagic
blennorrhagica
keratoderma b.
keratosis b.
blennorrhagicum
keratoderma b.
blennorrheal conjunctivitis
blennorrhea neonatorum
Blenoxane
bleomycin sulfate

NOTES

Bleph-10 Ophthalmic
Blephamide Ophthalmic
blepharitis
    mixed seborrheic-staphylococcal b.
    seborrheic b.
    staphylococcal b.
blepharochalasia
blepharochalasis
blepharochromidrosis
blepharoconjunctivitis
blepharoplasty scissors
blepharoptosis adiposa
bleuâtres
    tache b.
blind
    b. boil
    b. loop syndrome
    b. passage
blinding disease
blindness
    night b.
    river b.
blister
    b. beetle
    b. beetle dermatitis
    b. beetle sting
    blood b.
    central b.
    diabetic b.
    fever b.
    fly b.
    flying b.
    friction b.
    pressure b.
    b. serum
    subcorneal b.
    sucking b.
    water b.
BlisterFilm transparent film
blistering
    b. collodion
    b. dermatitis
    b. distal dactylitis
    b. lesion
    b. skin
Blis-To-Sol
Blizzard syndrome
Blocadren Oral
Bloch reaction
Bloch-Siemens-Sulzberger syndrome
Bloch-Sulzberger
    B.-S. disease
    B.-S. syndrome
block
    arteriovenous b.
    atrioventricular b.
    AV b.
    bundle branch b.

    stellate ganglion b.
    Sun Defense Lip B.
blockade
    costimulatory b.
    reticuloendothelial b.
    stellate ganglion b.
    virus b.
blockage
    mechanical vessel b.
    vessel b.
blocker
    H2 b.
blocking
    b. antibody
    b. vagal afferent fiber
    b. vagal efferent fiber
Blomia tropicalis
blood
    b. blister
    b. chemistry
    b. coagulation
    b. coagulation test
    b. eosinophilia
    b. fluke
    b. gas
    b. group
    b. group agglutinin
    b. group agglutinogen
    b. group antibody
    b. group antigen
    b. group antiserum
    b. grouping
    b. group-specific substances A and B
    b. group substance
    b. group system
    b. mononuclear cell (BMC)
    occult b.
    b. pH
    b. pressure
    b. progenitor cell
    b. serum
    b. transfusion
    b. transfusion therapy
    b. type
    umbilical cord b. (UCB)
    whole b.
    b. worm
blood-aqueous barrier
bloodborne
blood-filled slit-like space
blood-ocular barrier
blood-retinal barrier
bloodsucking
blood-urine barrier
Bloom syndrome
Bloom-Torre-Machacek syndrome
blossom
    orange b.

blot
- Southern b.
- Western b.

blotch
- palpebral b.

blousing garter dermatitis

blubber finger

blubbery lip

Bluboro
- B. powder
- B. solution

blue
- b. atrophy
- Bonney b.
- b. bottle sting
- b. grass
- b. grass pollen
- methylene b.
- b. mussel
- b. nail
- B. Peel skin health product
- b. rubber-bleb nevus
- b. rubber-bleb nevus syndrome
- Selsun B.
- B. + SpITZ nevus
- b. spot
- trypan b.

blueberry
- b. muffin baby
- b. muffin child
- b. muffin lesion

bluecomb
- b. disease of turkey
- b. virus

bluegrass
- annual b.
- Kentucky b.

blue-gray
- b.-g. lesion
- b.-g. pigmentation

blue-toe syndrome

bluetongue virus

Bluettes cotton knit-lined glove

blunt dissection

blunted villus

blush

blushing

BLU-U blue light photodynamic therapy illuminator

BMC
- blood mononuclear cell
- bone mineral content

BMCMC
- bone marrow-derived cultured mast cell

BMD
- bone mineral density

B-mode ultrasound

BMS
- bronchoscopic microsampling

BMT
- bone marrow transplant
- bone marrow transplantation

BMZ
- basement membrane zone
- BMZ antibody

BNLF-1 oncogene

board
- Data Safety Monitoring B. (DSMB)
- institutional review b. (IRB)

Bockenheimer syndrome

Bockhart
- B. folliculitis
- B. impetigo

Bodechtel-Guttmann disease

Bodian stain

body
- antiimmune b.
- apoptotic b.
- asteroid b.
- banana-shaped b.
- Bollinger b.
- Borrel b.
- caterpillar b.
- b. cavity-based B-cell lymphoma
- cigar b.
- ciliary b.
- Civatte b.
- colloid b.
- Cowdry intranuclear inclusion b. type A, B
- Cowdry type (A, B) inclusion b.
- Creola b.
- cytoid b.
- cytomegalic inclusion b.
- cytoplasmic inclusion b.
- Dohle inclusion b.
- Donovan b.
- b. dysmorphic disorder
- Farber b.
- fuchsin b.
- glass b.
- glomus b.
- Guarnieri b.

B

NOTES

body *(continued)*
    Halberstaedter-Prowazek b.
    Heinz b.
    Henderson-Paterson b.
    Howell-Jolly b.
    inclusion b.
    Joest b.
    lamellar b. (LB)
    Leishman-Donovan b.
    Lindner b.
    Lipschütz b.
    loose b.
    b. louse
    b. mass
    Medlar b.
    Miyagawa b.
    b. moisturizer
    molluscum b.
    Negri b.
    nuclear inclusion b.
    Odland b.
    Paschen b.
    polyhedral b.
    Prowazek b.
    Prowazek-Greeff b.
    psittacosis inclusion b.
    reticulate b.
    rice b.
    ringworm of b.
    round b.
    Russell b.
    Schaumann b.
    sclerotic b.
    b. somatotype
    b. surface area
    tingible b.
    trachoma b.
    vitreous b.
    b. wrap
    zebra b.
Boeck
    B. itch
    B. sarcoid
    B. sarcoidosis
    B. scabies
Boerhaave sweat gland
boggy swelling
Bohn nodule
boil
    Aleppo b.
    Baghdad b.
    blind b.
    botfly b.
    date b.
    Delhi b.
    Madura b.
    Oriental b.
    salt water b.

    sea water b.
    tropical b.
bois
    pian b.
Bolivian hemorrhagic fever
Bollinger
    B. body
    B. granule
bolster finger
Bombay phenotype
Bombus **sting**
bone
    b. culture
    b. death
    b. decay
    b. densitometry
    b. disease
    b. erosion
    b. felon
    b. formation marker
    b. fragility
    b. grafting
    b. loss prevention
    b. marrow-derived cultured mast cell (BMCMC)
    b. marrow edema syndrome
    b. marrow examination
    b. marrow reserve
    b. marrow transplant (BMT)
    b. marrow transplantation (BMT)
    B. Mass Measurement Act
    b. mineral content (BMC)
    b. mineral density (BMD)
    b. morphogenetic protein receptor
    b. resorption marker
    b. sialoprotein (BSP)
    b. turnover marker
bone-seeking substance
Bonferroni
    B. correction
    B. t test
Bonine
Boniva
Bonney blue
Bonviva
bony
    b. ankylosis
    b. erosion
    b. spur
bookeri
    Alcaligenes b.
Böök syndrome
Boolean operator
booster
    b. dose
    b. phenomenon
    b. response
boot
    Dome-Paste b.

gelatin compression b.
Unna b.
borax
Borda
melanotic prurigo of B.
border
coast of Maine b.
ill-defined b.
indurated b.
irregular b.
raised b.
vermilion b.
volcanic b.
borderline
b. lepromatous leprosy
b. malignant hemangiopericytoma
b. tuberculoid leprosy
Bordetella
B. parapertussis
B. pertussis
B. pertussis bacterium
Bordet-Gengou phenomenon
Borg
B. scale
B. score
boric acid
Borna
B. disease
B. disease virus
Bornholm
B. disease
B. disease virus
Borofax topical
Borrel body
Borrelia
B. afzelii
B. burgdorferi (Bb)
B. burgdorferi DNA assay
B. garinii
B. lonestari
B. lymphocytoma
B. recurrentis
Borrelia-associated arthritis
borreliacidal
borreliosis, pl. **borrelioses**
Lyme b.
Borrow
method of B.
BORSA strain
Borsieri
B. line
B. sign

Borst-Jadassohn type intraepidermal epithelioma
bortezomib
bosch yaw
bosentan
bossing
frontal b.
Bostock disease
Boston exanthema
botfly
b. boil
b. facultative myiasis
b. obligate myiasis
bothropic antitoxin
Bothrops antitoxin
Botox Cosmetic
Botryomyces caespitosus
botryomycosis
botryosum
Stemphylium b.
Botrytis cinerea
bottle
ENTsol Refillable B.
botulin
botulinum
b. A exotoxin
b. antitoxin
botulinus toxin
botulism
b. antitoxin
food-borne b.
wound b.
botulismotoxin
boubas
Bouchard node
Bouffardi
B. black mycetoma
B. white mycetoma
bougie
bougienage
Bouin solution
bound
total counts b. (TCB)
boundary
intron-exon b.
bouquet fever
Bourneville
B. disease
B. syndrome
Bourneville-Brissaud disease

NOTES

Bourneville-Pringle
    B.-P. disease
    B.-P. syndrome
bouton
    b. de Baghdad
    b. de Biskra
    b. d'Orient
boutonneuse fever
boutonnière deformity
bovine
    b. antitoxin
    b. collagen dermal implant
    b. colloid
    b. colostrum
    b. ephemeral fever
    b. herpes mammillitis
    b. leukosis virus
    b. mastitis
    b. papular stomatitis
    b. papular stomatitis virus
    pegademase b.
    b. rhinovirus
    b. rotavirus stain
    b. spongiform encephalopathy
    b. superoxide dismutase
    b. ulcerative mammillitis
    b. vaccinia mammillitis
    b. virus diarrhea
    b. virus diarrhea virus
    b. whey protein concentrate
bovis
    Actinomyces b.
    Babesia b.
    Mycobacterium b.
bowed finger
bowel bypass syndrome
Bowen
    B. disease
    B. disease of the glans penis
    B. precancerous dermatosis
bowenoid
    b. cell
    b. papulosis
Bowins suction
Bowman layer
box
    b. elder maple
    b. elder maple tree
    b. elder tree pollen
    b. jellyfish
    b. jellyfish sting
Box-Cox transformation
Boyden
    B. chamber
    B. chamber technique
boydii
    Allescheria b.
    Petriellidium b.
    Pseudallescheria b.

Boyd surgical light
bozemanii
    Legionella b.
BP
    bullous pemphigoid
    Acnomel BP 5
bp
    base pair
BPA
    bullous pemphigoid antigen
BPI protein
BQ Tablet
BR
    breathing reserve
BR96-doxorubicin monoclonal antibody
brace
    DonJoy b.
    Knight-Taylor b.
bracelet
    identification b.
brachial neuritis of Lyme disease
brachio-oto-renal syndrome
brachioplasty
brachioradial pruritus
brachydactyly
    b., mental retardation syndrome
    b., type B1, C, E syndrome
brachymetaphalangism
brachyonychia
brachytherapy
    endobronchial b.
bracket fungus
Braden score for skin integrity
bradykinin
braiding
    corn-row b.
brain
    b. abscess
    b. PGD$_2$ synthase
Brainerd diarrhea
brain-reactive autoantibody
branched DNA signal amplication assay for hepatitis B
branchial
    b. cleft
    b. cyst
    b. plexus
Brandy flap
B-range
    ultraviolet B.-r. (UVB)
Branhamella catarrhalis
branny
    b. desquamation
    b. scale
    b. tetter
Brasfield
    B. chest radiograph score
    B. scoring system

B

brasiliensis
  Blastomyces b.
  Hevea b.
  Nocardia b.
  Paracoccidioides b.
Brasivol
brawny
  b. edema
  b. induration
  b. tetter
Brazilian
  B. pemphigus
  B. rubber
  B. rubber tree
braziliense
  Ancylostoma b.
Brazil nut
breadloafing
BreakAway absorptive wound dressing
breakbone fever
breaker
  Castroviejo blade b.
breathe
  B. Right
  B. Right nasal strip
breathing
  apneustic b.
  bellows b.
  bhastrika b.
  intermittent positive pressure b.
    (IPPB)
  mouth b.
  Ondine curse, periodic b.
  pursed lips b.
  b. reserve (BR)
  sleep-disordered b.
breathlessness
Breda disease
bredeney
  Salmonella b.
breed
  short-haired b.
breeding
  random b.
Breezee Mist Antifungal
Brehmer
  B. method
  B. treatment
Brequinar sodium
Breslow
  B. thickness

  B. thickness in malignant
    melanoma
  B. thickness in melanoma staging
Brethaire Inhalation Aerosol
Brethine
  B. injection
  B. Oral
Bretonneau
  B. angina
  B. disease
Brett syndrome
Breuerton view of the hand
Brevibacterium
brevicaulis
  Scopulariopsis b.
Brevicon
brevis
  Demodex b.
Brevoxyl Gel
brewer's yeast
BRF
  Painaid BRF
Bricanyl
  B. injection
  B. Oral
bridge
  intercellular b.
  Wound-Span B. B.
bridou
brief metabolic remission
bright erythema
Brill disease
Brill-Zinsser disease
Brion-Kayser disease
bristle-worm dermatitis
brittle
  b. asthma
  b. hair, intellectual impairment,
    decreased fertility, short stature
    (BIDS)
  b. hair, intellectual impairment,
    decreased fertility, short stature
    syndrome
  b. nail
  b. nail syndrome
broad
  b. bean
  b. beta disease
  b. spectrum
broad-based rete ridge
broccoli

NOTES

Brocq
>B. disease
>B. erythrose peribuccale pigmentaire
>erythrose péribuccale pigmentaire
> of B.
>B. lupoid sycosis
>pseudopelade of B.
>B. pseudopelade

Brodie abscess
Brofed Elixir
Bromaline Elixir
Bromanate Elixir
Bromarest
Bromatapp
Bromavir
Brombay
brome
>b. grass
>b. grass pollen

bromelain
Bromfed
>B. Syrup
>B. Tablet

Bromfed-PD
Bromfenex PD
bromhexine
bromhidrosiphobia
bromhidrosis, bromidrosis
>apocrine b.
>eccrine b.

bromide
>b. acne
>ethidium b.
>b. intoxication
>ipratropium b.
>pancuronium b.

bromidism
>vegetating b.

bromidrosiphobia
bromidrosis (*var. of* bromhidrosis)
bromine
bromism
bromocriptine
bromoderma
bromohyperhidrosis
2-bromo-2-nitropropane-1,3-diol
bromovinyldeoxyuridine
Bromphen
>B. Elixir
>B. Tablet

brompheniramine
>b. maleate
>b. and phenylephrine
>b. and phenylpropanolamine
>b. and pseudoephedrine

bromsulfophthalein retention
Bronalide
bronchi (*pl. of* bronchus)

bronchial
>b. artery embolization
>b. asthma
>b. candidiasis
>b. chondritis
>b. epithelial cell
>b. epithelium
>b. hygiene
>b. hyperreactivity
>b. inhalation challenge test
>b. mucous membrane
>b. provocation
>b. provocation test
>b. smooth muscle
>b. smooth muscle tone
>b. stenosis
>b. toilet

bronchiectasis
>proximal b.

bronchiolitis obliterans
bronchitis
>asthmatic b.
>Castellani b.
>chronic b.
>infectious avian b.
>mild wheezy b. (MWB)
>wheezy b. (WB)

bronchoactive agonist
bronchoalveolar
>b. cell carcinoma
>b. lavage (BAL)

bronchoconstriction
bronchoconstrictor response
bronchodilatation
bronchodilation
>plateau b.

bronchodilator
>Inhal-Aid b.
>Maxi-Myst b.
>nebulized b.

bronchogenic
>b. carcinoma
>b. cyst

bronchogram
>air b.

bronchomoniliasis
bronchopleural fistula
bronchopneumonia
>eosinophilic b.

bronchoprotective subsensitivity
bronchorrhea
Broncho Saline
bronchoscope
>Dumon-Harrell b.
>fiberoptic b.

bronchoscopic microsampling (BMS)
bronchoscopy
>fiberoptic b.
>ultrasound-guided b.

B

bronchospasm
bronchovascular marking
bronchus, pl. bronchi
    lobar b.
    subsegmental b.
Bronitin Mist
Bronkaid Mist
Bronkephrine injection
Bronkodyl
Bronkometer
Bronkosol
bronopol
Brontex
Bronzage
    Huile Solaire B.
bronze
    b. diabetes
    b. hyperpigmentation
bronzed skin
bronzinum
    chloasma b.
Brooke
    B. disease
    B. tumor
Brooke-Spiegler syndrome
broom
    butcher's b.
bropirimine
Brotane
broth
    Barbour-Stoenner-Kelly b.
    BSK b.
    Quant b.
    b. test
    Todd-Hewitt b.
brown
    B. and Brenn stain
    b. moth larvae sting
    b. oculocutaneous albinism
    b. recluse spider
    b. recluse spider bite
    b. tumor
Brown-Adson forceps
brown-black lesion
Brown-Brenn stain
brown-spot syndrome
brown-tail
    b.-t. moth dermatitis
    b.-t. moth larva
    b.-t. moth sting
    b.-t. rash

brucei
    Trypanosoma b.
brucella
    b. arthritis
    B. canis
    B. card test
    b. dermatitis
    b. strain 19 vaccine
brucellar meningitis
brucellergin
brucellin
brucellosis
    chronic b.
brucellum
    erythema b.
Bruce septicemia
Bruch membrane
Bruck syndrome
Brugia
    B. malayi
    B. timori
brugian filariasis
Brugsch syndrome
brumptii
    Scopulariopsis b.
Brumpt white mycetoma
Brunati sign
Brunner gland
Bruns syndrome
Brunsting-Perry
    localized pemphigoid of B.-P.
    B.-P. pemphigoid
Brunsting-type dermatomyositis
brush
    b. border receptor
    b. burn
    b. burn abrasion
    rotating wire b.
Brussels sprout
Bruton
    B. agammaglobulinemia
    B. disease
    B. tyrosine kinase gene
bruxism
Brymill
    B. CryAc cryosurgical unit
    B. 30 cryosurgical unit
BSK
    Barbour-Stoenner-Kelly
    BSK broth
    BSK II medium

NOTES

BSLE
  bullous systemic lupus erythematosus
B5 solution
BSP
  bone sialoprotein
BSS
  bilayered skin substitute
BTC
  betacellulin
B-thalassemia syndrome
BTI-322
  humanized BTI-322
buaki
buba madre
bubas
bubble
  b. gum dermatitis
  b. hair
bubo, pl. **buboes**
  Frei b.
  gonorrheal b.
  indolent b.
  malignant b.
  nonvenereal b.
  pestilential b.
  primary b.
  satellite buboes
  strumous b.
  venereal b.
bubon d'emblée
bubonic plague
bubonulus
Bucast
buccalis
  psoriasis b.
buccarum
  morsicatio b.
Buchscher scleroderma
Buchwald atrophy
bucillamine
Buckley syndrome
buckwheat
Bucladin-S
buclizine
bud
  farcy b.
Budd-Chiari syndrome
Buehler method
Buerger disease
buffalo
  b. fly
  b. hump
buffer
  b. artifact
  HEPES b.
  hybridization b.
  Laemmli sample b.

buffered
  b. charcoal yeast extract (BCYE)
  b. charcoal yeast extract agar
Bufferin
buff puff
bug
  assassin b.
  conenose b.
  kissing b.
Buhler test
Buin
  Piz B.
bulb
  hair b.
bulbar
bulbosa
  myringitis b.
bulge-activation hypothesis of hair cycle
bulge sign
bulla, pl. **bullae**
  coma b.
  friction b.
  hemorrhagic b.
  intraepidermal b.
  pressure b.
  sausage-shaped b.
bullate
bullation
bullectomy
  transaxillary apical b.
bullosa
  cicatricial junctional
    epidermolysis b.
  Cockayne-Touraine epidermolysis b.
  dermatitis striata pratensis b.
  Dowling-Meara epidermolysis b.
  dystrophic epidermolysis b.
  Hallopeau-Siemens epidermolysis b.
  Herlitz epidermolysis b.
  impetigo contagiosa b.
  inherited epidermolysis b.
  junctional epidermolysis b. (JEB)
  Köbner epidermolysis b.
  Pasini epidermolysis b.
  purpura b.
  recessive dystrophic
    epidermolysis b. (RDEB)
  urticaria b.
bullosis diabeticorum
bullosum
  erythema multiforme b.
bullosus
  herpes circinatus b.
bullous
  b. amyloidosis
  b. congenital ichthyosiform
    erythroderma
  b. disease
  b. drug reaction

b. edema
b. erythema multiforme
b. fever
b. hemorrhagic pyoderma gangrenosum
b. hives
b. impetigo
b. impetigo of newborn
b. lichen planus
b. myringitis
b. pemphigoid (BP)
b. pemphigoid antigen (BPA)
b. pemphigoid-like eruption
b. skin lesion
b. staphylococcal impetigo
b. syphilid
b. systemic lupus erythematosus (BSLE)
bull's eye lesion
bumblebee sting
bump
    goose b.
    razor b.
bundle
    birefringent collagen b.
    b. branch block
bunion
    b. bursitis
    tailor b.
bunionette
Bunnell
    B. intrinsic tightness
    B. sign
bunny nose
Bunyamwera
    B. fever
    B. virus
Bunyaviridae
Bunyavirus
bunyavirus encephalitis
bupivacaine hydrochloride
Bupleurum
burgdorferi
    Borrelia b. (Bb)
buried subcutaneous stitch
Burkard
    B. sampling device
    B. spore trap
Burkholderia
    B. cepacia
    B. pseudomallei
Burkitt lymphoma

burn
    actinic b.
    brush b.
    chemical b.
    b. depth indicator (BDI)
    b. eschar
    first-degree b.
    full-thickness b.
    mask b.
    mat b.
    partial-thickness b.
    radiation b.
    road b.
    rope b.
    second-degree b.
    superficial b.
    thermal b.
    third-degree b.
burnetii
    Coxiella b.
burning
    b. mouth
    b. mouth syndrome
    b. tongue
    b. vulva syndrome
burnt-out rheumatoid arthritis
Burow
    B. solution
    B. triangle
burr
burrobrush
    white b.
burrow
burrowing hair
bursa, pl. **bursae**
    diarthrodial joint b.
    distended b.
    pes anserinus b.
bursectomy
bursitis
    Achilles b.
    anserine b.
    bunion b.
    fungal b.
    iliopectineal b.
    iliopsoas b.
    infrapatellar b.
    ischial b.
    ischiogluteal b.
    obturator internus b.
    olecranon b.
    prepatellar b.

NOTES

bursitis *(continued)*
    pump-bumps b.
    retrocalcaneal b.
    subacromial b.
    subdeltoid b.
    tendinitis b.
    traumatic b.
    trochanteric b.
bursography
burst
    oxidative b.
    phagocyte oxidative b.
    prednisone b.
    respiratory b.
    steroid b.
Buruli ulcer
burweed
Bury disease
Busacca nodule
Buschke
    B. disease
    B. scleredema
Buschke-Löwenstein
    B.-L. giant condyloma
    B.-L. tumor
    B.-L. variant of verrucous
      carcinoma
Buschke-Ollendorf
    B.-O. disease
    B.-O. sign
    B.-O. syndrome
buserelin
bush
    iodine b.
    rabbit b.
    b. yaw
bushy capillary
buski
    Fasciolopsis b.
buspirone
Busse-Buschke disease
Butacaine
butamben picrate
butanedione monoxime

butcher's
    b. broom
    b. tubercle
butenafine
    b. HCl
    b. HCl cream
    b. hydrochloride
Butesin
butoconazole
butorphanol
butoxide
    piperonyl b.
    pyrethrin and piperonyl b.
butterfly
    b. area
    b. eruption
    b. lung
    b. patch
    b. rash
    b. sign
buttocks
    perinatal gangrene of b.
button
    Amboyna b.
    Biskra b.
    Oriental b.
butyl methacrylate
butyrate
    hydrocortisone b.
butyrophilin
BV-ara-U
BvgAS regulon
BvgS protein
Bwamba
    B. fever
    B. virus
Bydramine Cough Syrup
bypass arthritis-dermatitis syndrome
byssinosis
bystander T cell
by-the-wind sailor dermatitis
Bywaters lesion
bZIP
    basic-region leucine-zipper

C

calphostin C
C carbohydrate antigen
Dalacin C
C fraction serum
C group virus
C protein
somatomedin C
C syndrome

C1

C1 esterase
C1 esterase inhibitor
C1 esterase inhibitor deficiency

C3

complement C3
C3 proactivator
C3 proactivator convertase
serum C3
C3 test

C4

complement C4
serum C4
C4 test

C100-3 hepatitis C virus antibody
C1qR radioassay
C3b receptor
C3/C4 receptor
C5b-C8 complex
C5b-C9 complex
CA

croup-associated
CA virus

C5a

Alexion anticomplement C5a

cabinet

Waldmann UV5000 c.

cable rash
cachectica

purpura c.

cachectic aphtha
cachecticorum

acne c.
melanoderma c.
melanosis c.

cachexia

rheumatoid c.
c. syndrome

Cachexon
cadaver donor transplantation
cadaverous
caddis fly
Cade oil
cadherin
CADR

Clean Air Delivery Rate

caecutiens

Onchocerca c.

Caenorhabditis
caerulea (*var. of* cerulea)
caesiellus

Aspergillus c.

caespitosus

Botryomyces c.

Cafatine
café-au-lait spot
café coronary syndrome
Cafergot
Cafetrate
caine mix
Cairns syndrome
cajennense

Amblyomma c.

Cajuput oil
Calabar swelling
Caladryl lotion
Calahist Clear
Calamatum
calamine lotion
calcaneal

c. abnormality
c. petechia
c. rudiment
c. spur

calcar
Calciferol

C. injection
C. Oral

calcific

c. periarthritis
c. tendinitis

calcification

metastatic c.
soft tissue c.
subcutaneous c.

calcifying

c. epithelioma
c. epithelioma of Malherbe

Calcijex
calcineurin inhibitor (CNI)
calcinosis

c. circumscripta
c. cutis
c. cutis, osteoma cutis,
poikiloderma, and skeletal
abnormalities (COPS)
c. cutis, Raynaud phenomenon,
esophageal motility disorder,
sclerodactyly, and telangiectasia
(CREST)

calcinosis *(continued)*
    c. cutis, Raynaud phenomenon, esophageal motility disorder, sclerodactyly, and telangiectasia syndrome
    dystrophic c.
    iatrogenic c.
    traumatic c.
    tumoral c.
    c. universalis
calciphylaxis
calcipotriene therapy
calcipotriol
calcitonin
    oral c.
    salmon c.
calcitonin-origin amyloid deposit
calcitriol
calcium
    c. carbonate crystal
    etidronate and c.
    fenoprofen c.
    c. gluconate
    c. hydroxyapatite crystal deposition disease
    leucovorin c.
    c. oxalate crystal
    c. pentosan polysulfate
    c. phosphate crystal deposition disease
    c. pyrophosphate crystal deposition disease
calcium-dependent transcription
calcoaceticus
    Acinetobacter c.
calcofluor stain
Calcort
CaldeCort
    C. Anti-Itch Topical Spray
    C. topical
Caldesene topical
Caldwell-Luc procedure
Caldwell syndrome
Calendula officinalis
Calgitrol calcium alginate wound dressing with maltodextrin
Caliciviridae virus
Calicivirus
California
    C. black-legged tick
    C. encephalitis (CE)
    C. peppertree tree
    C. virus
californica
    Torpedo c.
caliper
    dial c.
    Mitutoyo digital c.

CALLA
    common acute lymphocytic leukemia antigen
        CALLA positive
Calliphora
Calliphoridae
callositas
callosity
callous
Callus Salve
Calmette-Guérin
    C.-G. bacillus
    C.-G. vaccine
Calmette test
Calmex
calmodulin antagonist
Calmurid
Calm-X Oral
calor
    c. mordax
    c. mordicans
calorica
    dermatitis c.
caloric intake
caloricum
    erythema c.
caloris
    stadium c.
calotropis
Calotropis procera
Calpain
calphostin C
calreticulin
calvities
Calycophora dermatitis
Calymmatobacterium granulomatis
Camcreme ECG paste
Camellia sinensis
camera
    Starcam large field of view gamma c.
Campath 1H
Campbell-De Morgan spot
camp fever
Campho-Phenique
camphor
    c. and alcohol
    c., menthol and phenol
camphorated menthol
cAMP response element-binding (CREB)
camptodactyly
    congenital c.
Campylobacter
    C. fetus enteritis
    C. jejuni
    C. pylori
Canada blue grass
Canada-Cronkhite syndrome

canal
    external auditory c. (EAC)
    Sucquet-Hoyer c.
Canale-Smith syndrome
canaliculi
    pili triangulati et c.
    pili trianguli et c.
canaliculitis
canary
    c. feather
    c. grass
    c. grass pollen
    reed c.
canarypox virus
C-ANCA
  cytoplasmic antineutrophil cytoplasmic antibody
    C-ANCA titer
cancellous
cancer
    anti-EGF receptor antibody for c.
    antiepidermal growth factor receptor antibody for c.
    chimney sweep's c.
    Diagnostic and Neuronal Analysis of Skin C. (DANAOS)
    c. en cuirasse
    epidermoid c.
    European Organization for Research and Treatment of C. (EROTIC)
    c. immunology
    c. immunotherapy
    kangri c.
    nailbed c.
    nonmelanoma skin c. (NMSC)
    skin c.
    c. vaccination
cancericidal, cancerocidal
cancerophobia, cancerphobia
cancerous
cancer-testis antigen
cancrum oris
Candela laser
Candida
    C. *albicans*
    C. *albicans* IgG
    C. arthritis
    C. balanitis
    C. blastoconidia
    Candida infection
    C. folliculitis
    C. *glabrata*

    C. glossitis
    C. glossodynia
    C. granuloma
    C. *guillermondii*
    C. *inconspicua*
    C. infection
    C. intertrigo
    C. *kefyr*
    C. *krusei*
    C. leukoplakia
    C. *lipolytica*
    C. *lusitaniae*
    C. onychia
    C. osteomyelitis
    C. *parapsilosis*
    C. *parapsilosis* colonization
    C. paronychia
    C. *rugosa*
    C. septicemia
    C. skin test
    C. therapy
    C. *tropicalis*
candidal
    c. angular cheilitis
    c. arthritis
    c. infection
    c. leukoplakia
    c. osteomyelitis
    c. paronychia
candidemia
    nosocomial c.
candidiasis
    acute atrophic oral c.
    atrophic c.
    bronchial c.
    chronic atrophic c.
    chronic hyperplastic c.
    congenital c.
    cutaneous c.
    disseminated c.
    invasive c.
    localized mucocutaneous c.
    mucocutaneous c.
    neonatal systemic c.
    oral c.
    oropharyngeal c.
    osteoarticular c.
    systemic c.
    vulvovaginal c. (VVC)
candidid
candidosis
candiduria

C

NOTES

candidus
    Aspergillus c.
    strophulus c.
Candistatin
candle dripping
Caner-Decker syndrome
Canesten
canestick deformity
canimorsus
    Capnocytophaga c.
canine
    c. adenovirus 1
    c. distemper virus
    c. herpesvirus
    c. herpetovirus
    c. oral papilloma
caninum
    Ancylostoma c.
    Dipylidium c.
canis
    Babesia c.
    Brucella c.
    Ctenocephalides c.
    Demodex c.
    Ehrlichia c.
    hepatitis contagiosa c.
    Microsporum c.
    Toxocara c.
canities
    rapid c.
    c. segmentata sideropenica
    c. unguium
canium
    Neospora c.
canker
    c. sore
    water c.
Cann-Ease moisturizing nasal gel
cannonball pattern
Cannon curette
cannula
    Accelerator c.
    Cobra c.
    Cook c.
    Illouz c.
    Klein c.
    Lamprey c.
    Narins c.
    Pinto c.
canonical polyadenylylation
cantaloupe
cantharic acid
cantharidal collodion
cantharidin
cantharis, pl. **cantharides**
Cantharone
canthaxanthin

canthorum
    dystopia c.
    dystrophia c.
canthus, pl. **canthi**
    inner c.
    nasal c.
    outer c.
    temporal c.
2C3 anti-VEGF antibody
Cantle line
canyon ragweed
cao gio
cap
    cradle c.
capacity
    functional residual c. (FRC)
    inspiratory c. (IC)
    maximum breathing c. (MBC)
    nasal conditioning c. (NCC)
    slow vital c. (SVC)
    total lung c. (TLC)
    vital c. (VC)
Caparinia
Capastat sulfate
Capex Shampoo
capillariasis
capillaritis
capillaropathy
capillaroscopy
    nail fold c.
capillary
    alveolar c.
    c. angioma
    bushy c.
    c. fragility test
    c. hemangioma
    c. hemangioma of infancy
    c. malformation
    c. nevus
    c. resistance test
    synovial c.
capilli (*pl. of* capillus)
capillitii
    dermatitis papillaris c.
    pediculosis c.
capillorum
    defluvium c.
    defluxio c.
capillus, pl. **capilli**
Capim virus
capitate
capitatum-multangular-lunatum
capitis
    black dot tinea c.
    endothelioma c.
    epithelioma c.
    gray-patch tinea c.
    inflammatory tinea c.
    pediculosis c.

Pediculus humanus c.
pityriasis c.
pthiriasis c.
seborrhea c.
tinea c.
trichophytosis c.
vitiligo c.
Capitrol
Caplan
    C. nodule
    C. syndrome
caplet
    Advil Cold & Sinus C.
    Aspirin-Free Bayer Select Allergy
      Sinus C.
    Dimetapp Sinus C.
    Dristan Sinus C.
    Miles Nervine C.
    TripTone C.
Capnocytophaga canimorsus
capnometer
    Datex Normocap infrared c.
Capoten
capreomycin (CM)
    c. sulfate
caprin
caprine
    c. herpesvirus
    c. herpetovirus
Capripoxvirus
caproate
    hydroxyprogesterone c.
caps
    Drixoral Cough & Congestion
      Liquid C.
capsaicin oleoresin
capsicum
Capsicum frutescens
capsid
Capsin
capsomer
capsular
    c. antigen
    c. precipitation reaction
capsulatum
    Histoplasma c.
capsule
    Alka-Seltzer Plus Cold Liqui-
      Gels C.
    Arthraphate c.
    Banophen Decongestant C.
    Dapacin Cold C.

Dimetapp 4-Hour Liqui-Gel C.
Duadacin C.
Guaivent PD c.
Kaletra c.
lopinavir/ritonavir c.
Neoral soft gelatin c.
Poly-Histine-D C.
Prograf c.
Pseudovent PED c.
tacrolimus c.
Tenon c.
Ziprasidone c.
capsulitis
    adhesive c.
Captia
    C. test
    C. test for syphilis
captopril
Capzasin-P
Carac cream
car allergy
Caraparu virus
carate
carateum
    Treponema c.
carbacephem
carbamazepine
carbamide
Carba mix
carbapenem
Carbaryl
carbate
    dimethyl c.
carbenicillin
    Indanyl c.
carbide
    cobalt in tungsten c.
carbinoxamine and pseudoephedrine
Carbiset Tablet
Carbiset-TR Tablet
Carb-N-Sert needle holder
Carbocaine injection
Carbodec Syrup
Carbodex
    C. DM pediatric oral drops
    C. DM syrup
CarboFlex
carbohydrate intolerance
carbol-fuchsin solution
carbon
    c. arc lamp
    c. baby

C

NOTES

carbon *(continued)*
    c. dermatosis
    c. dioxide laser
    c. dioxide laser scanner system
    c. monoxide
carbovir
carboxamide
    imidazole c.
carboxamide-riboside
    aminoimidazole c.-r. (AICA-
      riboside)
carboxyhemoglobin (HbCO)
carboxymethylcellulose
    benzocaine, gelatin, pectin, and
      sodium c.
    c. sodium
carboxymethyllysine
carboxypeptidase
carbuncle
carbuncular
carbunculoid
carbunculosis
carcinoembryonic antigen (CEA)
carcinogen
carcinogenesis
carcinoid
    c. flush
    c. syndrome
    c. tumor
carcinoma, pl. **carcinomata**
    acantholytic squamous cell c.
    adenoid cystic c.
    adnexal c.
    anogenital squamous cell c.
    apocrine c.
    basosquamous c.
    bronchoalveolar cell c.
    bronchogenic c.
    Buschke-Löwenstein variant of
      verrucous c.
    cloacogenic c.
    c. cuniculatum
    cylindromatous c.
    de novo squamous cell c.
    eccrine c.
    Ehrlich ascites c. (EAC)
    c. en cuirasse
    epidermoid c.
    esophageal c.
    fibroepithelioma basal cell c.
    fibrosing basal cell c.
    genital squamous cell c.
    hair-matrix c.
    infiltrative basal cell c.
    infundibulocystic basal cell c.
    intermediate c.
    intraepidermal c.
    invasive squamous cell c.
    keloidal basal cell c.

    Lucké c.
    melanotic c.
    Merkel cell c.
    metatypical c.
    microcystic adnexal c. (MAC)
    morbilliform basal cell c.
    morpheaform basal cell c.
    mucinous eccrine c.
    nasopharyngeal c.
    nevoid basal cell c.
    nodular basal cell c.
    noduloulcerative basal cell c.
    ocular basal cell c.
    pigmented basal cell c.
    pilomatrix c. (PC)
    pilomatrixoma c.
    prickle-cell c.
    primary cutaneous adenoid cystic c.
    primary neuroendocrine c.
    pseudoglandular squamous cell c.
    reticulum cell c.
    sclerosing sweat duct c.
    sebaceous c.
    c. in situ
    in situ squamous cell c.
    spindle cell c. (SC)
    squamous cell c. (SCC)
    superficial basal cell c.
    sweat gland c.
    syringoid c.
    trabecular c.
    trichilemmal c.
    V-2 c.
    verrucous c.
carcinomatosa
    lymphangitis c.
    meningitis c.
carcinomatosis
carcinomatous dermatitis
Cardec-S Syrup
cardiac
    c. allograft
    c. allograft vascular disease
    c. allotransplantation
    c. complication
    c. glycoside
    c. pacemaker dermatitis
    c. rejection
    c. sarcoidosis
    C. Transplant Research Database
cardiocutaneous
    c. myxoma
    c. syndrome
cardio-facio-cutaneous syndrome
cardiolipin
cardiomyocyte transplantation
cardiomyopathy
    restrictive c.

cardiopulmonary
    c. lupus
    c. resuscitation
cardiorespiratory arrest
cardiotrophin 1
cardiovascular
    c. collapse
    c. involvement
Cardiovirus
Cardiovit AT-10 ECG/spirometry combination system
carditis
careless weed
Carey Coombs murmur
carindacillin
carinii
    Pneumocystis c.
Carlesta
Carmalt forceps
Carmol
    C. 10 body lotion
    C. 20 cream
    C. 40 gel
    C. HC cream
    C. Scalp Treatment
    C. scalp treatment kit
    C. scalp treatment lotion
    C. Shampoo
    C. topical
Carmol-HC topical
carmustine
carnauba-wax-like keratoderma
carneus
    Aspergillus c.
Carney
    C. complex
    C. syndrome
carnitine palmitoyltransferase deficiency
carob
Caroguard
Caroli disease
Carolina rinse solution
Carolon multi-layer stocking system
carotene
    beta c.
carotenemia
carotenoderma
carotenosis cutis
carotid intima-media wall thickness
carotinemia
carotinosis cutis
carpal to metacarpal ratio

carpet beetle dermatitis
carpet-tack scale
Carpinus betulus
carpometacarpal (CMC)
    c. joint
carprofen
CarraFilm
    C. transparent film
    C. wound dressing
CarraGauze impregnated gauze
carrageenan arthritis
carrageenin-induced footpad inflammation model
CarraSmart
    C. foam
    C. foam dressing
CarraSorb
    C. H
    C. H alginate wound cover
    C. H calcium alginate wound dressing
    C. hydrogel dressing
    C. M
Carrasyn
    C. hydrogel
    C. hydrogel wound dressing
Carrel patch
carrier
    active c.
    c. cell
    chronic c.
    contact c.
    convalescent c.
    healthy c.
    incubatory c.
    intermittent c.
    c. state
    c. strain
Carrión disease
carrionii
    Cladosporium c.
carrot
Carter black mycetoma
cartilage
    articular hyaline c.
    cricoid c.
    hyaline articular c.
    c. implant
    c. matrix protein
    c. oligomeric protein
    c. proteoglycan
    tensile strength of osteoarthritic c.

C

NOTES

cartilage-hair hypoplasia
cartilaginous collagen
Cartrofen
carumonam
caruncle, pl. carunculae
    trichosis carunculae
Casal
    C. collar
    C. necklace
cascade
    adhesion molecule c.
    alternative pathway of
      complement c.
    arachidonic acid c.
    caspase c.
    clotting c.
    complement activation c.
    complementary c.
    C. impactor
    inflammatory c.
    rejection c.
    terminal c.
caseating granuloma
caseation necrosis
case control study
casei
    Lactobacillus c.
casein
cashew
Casoni
    C. intradermal test
    C. reaction
    C. skin test
caspase
    c. 3, 8
    c. cascade
    c. inhibitor
casseii
    Penicillium c.
cassette
    susceptibility c.
CAST
    cellular antigen stimulation test
cast
    erythrocyte c.
    hair c.
    Minerva c.
    Night C. R
    spica c.
    total contact c.
Castaneda principle
Castellani
    C. bronchitis
    C. Natural Formula
    C. paint
    C. point
    C. treatment
castellani
    Acanthamoeba c.

Castle examination light
Castleman disease
castor bean
Castroviejo
    C. blade breaker
    C. blade holder
    C. forceps
    C. needle holder
CAT
    chloramphenicol acetyltransferase
    conventional asthma therapy
    CAT enzyme
cat
    c. allergy
    c. dander
    c. distemper virus
    c. epithelium
    c. flea
    c. flea bite
    c. hookworm
    panleukopenia virus of c.'s
catabolin isoform
catabolism
    articular joint tissue c.
Cataflam Oral
catalase-negative
catalysis
catalytic domain
catalyze
catamenial hemothorax
Catapres
cataract
    poikiloderma atrophicans and c.
    secondary c.
catarrhalis
    Branhamella c.
    herpes c.
    Moraxella c.
catarrhal jaundice
catatrichy
catcher's crouch
catecholamine
catechol-O-methyl
    c.-O-m. transferase (COMT)
    c.-O-m. transferase asthma
category
    TIM therapeutic c.
    topical immunomodulator
      therapeutic c.
caterpillar
    c. body
    c. dermatitis
    Io c.
    puss c.
    c. rash
    saddleback c.
    c. sting
    stinging c.

catfish
>   saltwater c.
>   c. sting

cathepsin
>   c. D, G, L
>   c. K mRNA

catheter
>   antiseptic-impregnated central
>   venous c.
>   double-balloon triple lumen c.
>   P.A.S. Port c.
>   pheresis c.

catholysis

Cath-Secure tape

cati
>   *Toxocara c.*

cationic compound

catkin

Catrix wound dressing

cat-scratch disease (CSD)

cattail pollen

cattle
>   ephemeral fever of c.
>   infectious papilloma of c.
>   malignant catarrh of c.
>   papular stomatitis virus of c.
>   c. plague
>   c. plague virus
>   c. wart
>   winter dysentery of c.

Catu virus

cauda equina syndrome

cauliflower

causalgia

causative

caustic

cauterant

cauterization

cauterize

cautery
>   chemical c.
>   gas c.

cavernosum
>   angioma c.
>   lymphangioma c.

cavernosus
>   nevus c.

cavernous
>   c. angioma
>   c. hemangioma
>   c. lymphangioma

>   c. sinus
>   c. sinusoid

caviae
>   *Aeromonas c.*
>   *Nocardia c.*

caviar tongue

Cavilon barrier ointment

cavitary

cavitation

cavity
>   Cutinova c

cayenne
>   mal de C.
>   c. pepper-like macule
>   c. pepper spot

CAZ beta-lactamase

Cazenave
>   C. disease
>   C. lupus
>   C. vitiligo

C3bBb receptor

C4b receptor

CBT
>   cognitive-behavior therapy

CC49 monoclonal antibody

CCD
>   charged-couple device

CCE
>   chronic cutaneous erythematosus

CCHF
>   Congo-Crimean hemorrhagic fever

C3-coated
>   C.-c. cell
>   C.-c. erythrocyte

CCR2
>   chemokine receptor C.

CCR5
>   chemokine receptor C.

CCS
>   Composite cultured skin

C&D
>   curettage and desiccation
>   cystoscopy and dilation

CD3 monoclonal antibody

CD4+
>   CD4+ helper/inducer cell
>   CD4+ Measure
>   CD4+ T cell subset

CD4
>   CD4 cell
>   CD4 count

C

NOTES

CD4 (*continued*)
    CD4 human recombinant soluble rCD4
    CD4 human truncated-365 AA polypeptide
    CD4 immunoglobulin G, recombinant human
    CD4 monoclonal antibody
    CD4 T cell subset
    CD4 T-lymphocyte count

CD5
    CD5 antibody
    CD5 cell

CD5+ antibody

CD8
    CD38 on CD8
    CD8 cell
    CD8 monoclonal antibody
    CD8 T cell subset

CD8+ T cell
CD11a
CD11b
CD11c
CD14
CD15
CD30+ cutaneous lymphoma
CD38
    CD38 antibody
    CD38 on CD8

CD40
    CD40 ligand gene
    CD40 soluble protein

CD43 antibody
CD44
    CD44 antibody
    CD44 Hyaluronic acid receptor

CD49a antibody
CD49b antibody
CD49c antibody
CD49e antibody
CD49f antibody
CD54 antibody
CD56+ lymphoma
CD56 monoclonal antibody
CD57
    DAKO CD57

CD69 monoclonal antibody
CD71 monoclonal antibody
CD106 antibody
CD10 antibody
CD16 monoclonal antibody
CD18 antibody
CD19 antibody
CD1a antibody
CD20 antibody
CD21 antibody
CD22 antibody
CD24 antibody
CD25 monoclonal antibody

CD26/vitronectin receptor
CD28
    CD28 antibody
    CD28 protein

CD29 antibody
CD4/CD8 ratio
CDA
    cold dry air

CDC
    complement-dependent-cytotoxic
    complement-dependent cytotoxicity

C7D deficiency
CDE
    chlordiazepoxide
    CDE antigen

CDKN2A
    cyclin-dependent kinase inhibitor 2A
    CDKN2A mutation

cDNA
    PGHS-1, -2 cDNA
    cDNA probe

CDP 870
CDR
    CDR grafting

CE
    California encephalitis
    coefficient of error

CEA
    carcinoembryonic antigen

CeaVac
Ceclor
cedar
    Japanese c.
    mountain c.
    red c.
    salt c.
    Western red c.

CeeNU Oral
cefaclor
cefadroxil monohydrate
Cefadyl
cefamandole nafate
Cefanex
cefazolin sodium
cefditoren pivoxil
cefepime
cefixime
Cefizox
cefmenoxime
cefmetazole sodium
Cefobid
cefodizime
cefonicid sodium
cefoperazone sodium
ceforanide
cefotaxime sodium
cefotetan
cefoxitin sodium
cefpiramide

cefpodoxime proxetil
cefprozil
ceftazidime
ceftibuten
Ceftin Oral
ceftizoxime
    c. beta-lactamase
    c. sodium
ceftriaxone sodium
Cefzil
CEL
   Celsior
celandine
Celebrex
celecoxib cell
celery
Celestoderm
Celestone
    C. Oral
    C. Phosphate Injection
    C. Soluspan
celiac
    c. disease
    c. sprue
cell
    acid-secreting gastric parietal c.
    acinar c.
    adenovirus-reactive T c.
    c. adhesion protein
    allogenic dendritic c.
    alloreactive c.
    c. alloreactivity
    alpha c.
    anergic T c.
    antibody-forming c. (AFC)
    antigen-presenting c. (APC)
    antigen-sensitive c.
    apoptotic c.
    astrocytoma c.
    autoimmune progenitor c.
    autoreactive B c.
    B c.
    B1 c.
    balloon c.
    basal c.
    basaloid c.
    blast c.
    blood mononuclear c. (BMC)
    blood progenitor c.
    bone marrow-derived cultured
      mast c. (BMCMC)
    bowenoid c.

bronchial epithelial c.
bystander T c.
carrier c.
C3-coated c.
CD4 c.
CD5 c.
CD8 c.
CD4+ helper/inducer c.
CD8+ T c.
celecoxib c.
chronic inflammatory c.
ciliated epithelial c.
circulating B c.
Clara c.
clear c.
cleaved giant c.
common lymphoid progenitor c.
conjunctival goblet c.
contrasuppressor c.
corneal epithelial c.
cuboidal c.
cytolytic effector c.
cytomegalic c.
cytoplasmic islet c.
cytotoxic T c.
Daudi lymphoma c.
daughter c.
dendritic epidermal c.
c. deposition
disorder of phagocytic c.
Dorothy Reed-Sternberg c.
c. dose
double negative c.
Downey c.
effector c.
end c.
endomysial mononuclear c.
endothelial c.
enterochromaffin c.
Epicel autologous skin c.
epidermal Langerhans c.
epithelioid c.
extravillous cytotrophoblast c.
fibroblast-like spindle c.
foam c.
foreign body giant c.
Friend erythroleukemia c.
frozen-thawed red c.
germinative c.
giant c.
goblet c.
granular c.

C

NOTES

cell *(continued)*
  grape c.
  hairy c. (HC)
  HeLa c.
  helper T c.
  hematopoietic progenitor c. (HPC)
  hematopoietic stem c.
  high endothelial venule c.
  homozygous typing c.
  horny c.
  HPC c.
  human skin nurse c. (HSNC)
  human umbilical vein endothelial c.
    (HUVEC)
  hybrid c.
  hyperplastic mucus-secreting
    goblet c.
  I c.
  IgE-sensitized c.
  IgM-coated c.
  immunoblastic sarcoma of B, T c.
  immunocompetent c.
  immunoglobulin E-sensitized c.
  immunoglobulin M-coated c.
  immunoglobulin-secreting c.
  immunologically activated c.
  immunologically competent c.
  inclusion c.
  inducer c.
  inflammatory c.
  innocent bystander c.
  c. interaction gene
  intestinal epithelial c. (IEC)
  intracytoplasmic inclusion c.
  intraepithelial mast c.
  islet alpha c.
  JKA c.
  Jurkat c.
  K c.
  keratinized c.
  killer c.
  Kulchitsky c.
  Kupffer c.
  LAK c.
  c. lamina
  lamina propria immune c.
  Langerhans c.
  Langhans c.
  lazy NK c.
  LE c.
  lepra c.
  Leroy I c.
  Leu-3+ helper T c.
  leuko-poor red blood c.
  c. line
  Lipschütz c.
  lupus erythematosus c.
  lymph c.
  lymphoid c.
  lymphokine-activated c. (LAK)
  lymphoplasmacytoid lymphoma c.
  lymphoreticular c.
  M c.
  Madin-Darby bovine kidney c.
  mast c.
  maturation B c.
  MDBK c.
  mediator c.
  Merkel c.
  mesenchymal progenitor c.
  mesothelial c.
  metaplastic mucus-secreting c.
  microchimeric c.
  mononuclear c.
  monotonous c.
  monster c.
  morula c.
  Mott c.
  mucosal mast c.
  multifocal Langerhans c.
  multinucleated giant c. (MGC)
  multipotent hematopoietic c.
  myeloid stem c.
  naive B c.
  natural killer c.
  neoplastic c.
  nests of nevus c.'s
  nevus c.
  nevus c., A-, B-, C-type
  NK c.
  nonadherent c.
  non-B c.
  nonlymphocytic c.
  nuclear factor of activated T c.
    (NFAT)
  nucleated endothelial c.
  null c.
  nurse c.
  OKT c.
  Ortho-Kung T c.
  osteoblast-lineage c.
  Paget c.
  pagetoid c.
  palisade c.
  pannus c.
  pepsinogen-secreting zymogenic c.
  peripheral blood mononuclear c.
    (PBMC)
  peripheral blood progenitor c.
    (PBPC)
  peripheral blood stem c. (PBSC)
  pig aortic endothelial c. (PAEC)
  pigmented spindle c. (PSC)
  plasma c.
  pluripotential c.
  polyclonal B c.
  polymorphonuclear c.

porcine fetal lateral ganglionic
  eminence c.
pre-B c.
preformed granule-associated
  mast c.
prickle c.
Primed c.
progenitor lymphoid c.
C. Proliferation kit
proliferative c.
proximal tubular epithelial c.'s
  (PTEC)
pull c.
pyknotic c.
quantitation of B c.
Raji c.
red blood c.
Reed-Sternberg c.
regulatory CD4+ T c.
responder T c.
reticuloendothelial c.
retinal pigment epithelial c. (RPE)
rheumatoid synovial macrophage-
  like/dendritic c.
rosette-forming c.
rosettes of c.
satellite c.
scavenger c.
Schwann c.
sensitized c.
Sézary c.
sheath c.
sheets of nevus c.'s
sinusoidal c.
small noncleaved c. (SNC)
spindle c.
spindle-shaped c.
squamous c.
stem c.
c. strain
stromal c.
suicide c.
suppressor c.
c. surface expression
surface Ig-expressing B c.
c. surface marker
syngeneic c.
synovial lining c. (SLC)
synovia T c.
T c.
tanned red c.
target c.

Tart c.
tartrate-resistant acid phosphatase
  positive c.
Tc1, Tc2 c.
T cytotoxic c. (Tc)
TDTH c.
Tg c.
Th1 c.
Th2 c.
T-helper c. (Th)
T-helper type 2 c. (Th2)
T-helper type 3 c. (Th3)
thymic epithelial c.
thymus nurse c.
TIL c.
Tm c.
Touton giant c.
c. transformation
transiently amplifying c. (TAC)
TRAP-positive c.
T-suppressor c.
tumor-infiltrating lymphocyte c.
type II alveolar c.
unifocal Langerhans c.
Unna c.
veiled c.
Vero c.
virus-infected c.
virus-transformed c.
Warthin-Finkeldey c.
white blood c. (WBC)
cell-bound antibody
cell-cell
  c.-c. adhesion
  c.-c. interaction
CellCept
Cellex-C
cell-mediated
  c.-m. autoimmunity
  c.-m. hypersensitivity
  c.-m. immunity (CMI)
  c.-m. immunologic drug reaction
Cellufresh
cellular
  c. accumulation in the airways
  c. adoptive immunotherapy
  c. antigen stimulation test (CAST)
  c. blue nevus
  c. casts in urine
  c. diapedesis
  c. immune deficiency syndrome
    (CIDS)

NOTES

cellular *(continued)*
    c. immune panel
    c. immune theory
    c. immunity deficiency syndrome
    c. immunodeficiency with abnormal
      immunoglobulin synthesis
    c. inhibitor of apoptosis (cIAP)
    c. pannus
    c. xenograft rejection
    c. xenotransplantation
cellularis
    plasma c.
cellulite
cellulitis
    acute scalp c.
    anaerobic c.
    demarcated c.
    dissecting c.
    eosinophilic c.
    epizootic c.
    gaseous c.
    perianal streptococcal c.
    phlegmonous c.
    streptococcal c.
cellulose
    hydroxypropyl c.
    oxidized c.
cellulosic/cuprophan
Celluvisc
CELO
    chicken embryo lethal orphan
    CELO virus
celonychia
Celovirus
celsi
    kerion c.
Celsior (CEL)
Celsus
    C. alopecia
    C. area
    C. kerion
    C. papule
    C. vitiligo
Cel-U-Jec Injection
cement
    c. dermatitis
    c. line
cemented
    finger-packing doughy c.
cementoma
Cenafed Plus Tablet
CENP-B
    scleroderma autoantigen CENP-B
Centany
center
    C.'s for Disease Control and
      Prevention
    microtubule organizing c.
    necrotic c.

center-edge angle
centimorgan (cM)
centipede
    c. bite
    giant desert c.
central
    c. blister
    c. clearing
    C. European tick-borne encephalitis
      virus
    c. fibrinoid necrosis
    c. papillary atrophy
    c. polypurine tract (cPPT)
    c. pruritus
    c. Recklinghausen disease type II
    c. stratum
    c. type neurofibromatosis
centrifugal lipoatrophy
centrifugation
    density gradient c.
    discontinuous plasma-Percoll
      gradient c.
centrifugum
    leukoderma acquisitum c.
    ulerythema c.
centroblast
centrofacial
    c. lentiginosis
    c. plaque
centromere antigen
Centruroides
    C. exilicauda
    C. exilicauda sting
    C. sculpturatus
    C. sculpturatus sting
    C. vittatus
    C. vittatus sting
Centurion
    C. SiteGuard
    C. SiteGuard MVP
    C. SiteGuard MVP transparent film
    C. SorbaView
    C. SorbaView composite dressing
cepacia
    Burkholderia c.
cephalexin monohydrate
cephalhematoma
cephalic
    c. brainlike heterotopia
    c. histiocytosis
    c. pustulosis
cephalocele
    rudimentary c.
cephalooculocutaneous telangiectasia
cephalosporin
    third-generation c.
Cephalosporium
cephalothin sodium
cephamycin

cephapirin sodium
cephradine
Ceplene
Ceptaz
ceramidase deficiency
ceramide-S1P rheostat
Ceratopogonidae
cercaria, pl. cercariae
cercarial dermatitis
cerea
    seborrhea c.
cerebellar ataxia
cerebelliformis
    nevus c.
cerebral
    c. allergy
    c. amyloidosis
    c. macula
    c. malaria
cérébrale
    tache c.
cerebri
    pseudotumor c.
cerebritis
    lupus c.
cerebrospinal
    c. fever
    c. meningitis
    c. rhinorrhea
cerebrotendinous xanthomatosis
Ceredase injection
cereolysin
cereus
    Bacillus c.
cerevisiae
    Saccharomyces c.
Cerezyme
Cerose-DM
Certican
Certified Decongestant
Cerubidine
cerulea, caerulea, pl. ceruleae
    macula c.
ceruloplasmin
cerumen
Cerumenex ear drops
ceruminal
ceruminoma
ceruminous gland
cervical
    c. acceleration-deceleration
      syndrome

    c. actinomycosis
    c. lymph node swelling
    c. patagium
    c. vertebra
cervicitis
cervicofacial
    c. actinomycosis
    c. rhytidectomy
cervicothoracic kyphosis
cestodic tuberculosis
Cetacaine
Cetacort topical
Cetamide Ophthalmic
Cetaphil soap
Cetapred Ophthalmic
cetirizine
cetyl
    c. alcohol-coal tar distillate
    c. palmitate
cevimeline HCl
CF
    complement-fixing
    CF antibody
    CF test
c-fos protein
CH50 assay
Chaetomium globosum
chafe
chaffeensis
    Ehrlichia c.
Chagas disease
chagasic
chagoma
Chagres virus
chagrin
    peau de c.
chain
    acyl c.
    alpha c.
    glycosaminoglycan c.
    heavy c.
    hemolytic c.
    homology of c.
    IgG heavy c.
    immunoglobulin delta c.
    immunoglobulin epsilon c.
    immunoglobulin G heavy c.
    immunoglobulin heavy c.
    immunoglobulin mu c.
    invariant c.
    J c.
    kappa light c.

C

NOTES

chain *(continued)*
    lambda light c.
    light c.
    myosin light c.
    polypeptide c.
chair-rise maneuver
chalazion, pl. **chalazia**
    c. clamp
    c. knife
chalazodermia
chalk
    steroid c.
challenge
    allergen c.
    allergen-specific nasal c.
    c. diet
    dinitrochlorobenzene c.
    direct c.
    food ingestion c. (FICH)
    histamine c.
    methacholine bronchoprovocation c.
    nasal allergen c. (NAC)
    open food c. (OFC)
    oral c.
    oral food c. (OFC)
    c. test
chalone
chamber
    aluminum Finn c.
    Boyden c.
    Finn c.
    Van der Bend c.
chamber-scarification test
chamomile
    German c.
Chanarin-Dorfman syndrome
chancre
    erosive c.
    fungating c.
    hard c.
    hunterian c.
    indurated c.
    mixed c.
    monorecidive c.
    c. recidive
    c. redux
    Ricord c.
    Rollet c.
    soft c.
    sporotrichositic c.
    sporotrichotic c.
    sulcus c.
    syphilis c.
    tuberculous c.
    tularemic c.
chancriform
    c. pyoderma
    c. syndrome
chancroid

chancroidal
chancrous
change
    clinical c.
    eczematous c.
    environmental c.
    fibrinoid c.
    formula c.
    histologic c.
    hormonal c.
    mitral valve prolapse, aortic
      anomalies, skeletal changes, and
      skin c.'s (MASS)
    nail c.
    nonspecific climatic c.
    oil drop c.
    perigranulomatous fibrotic c.
    pigment c.
    polyneuropathy, organomegaly,
      endocrinopathy, monoclonal
      gammopathy, and skin c.'s
      (POEMS)
    psoriatic nail c.
    respiratory c.
    symmetric reticulonodular x-ray c.
    synovial fluid c.
    tinctorial c.
    vacuolar c.
channel
    voltage-gated potassium c.
Chantemesse reaction
Chaoul tube
chaparral
chappa
chapped
chapping
CHAQ
    Childhood Health Assessment
      Questionnaire
characteristic
    lesion surface c.
charcoal
    activated c.
Charcot joint
Charcot-Leyden crystal
chard
    Swiss c.
charged-couple device (CCD)
Charlin syndrome
Charlouis disease
Chase-Sulzberger phenomenon
chat
    langue au c.
Chauffard-Still syndrome
Chauffard syndrome
Chaussier areola
cheat grass pollen
cheek
    c. chewing

c. cosmetic
c. phenomenon
cheek-based 2-stage flap
cheese washer's lung
cheesy abscess
cheilectomy procedure
cheilitis, chilitis
  actinic c.
  c. actinica
  allergic apostematous c.
  angular c.
  candidal angular c.
  commissural c.
  contact c.
  c. exfoliativa
  c. glandularis
  c. glandularis apostematosa
  c. granulomatosa
  c. granulomatosa impetiginous
  granulomatous c.
  impetiginous c.
  Miescher granulomatous c.
  migrating c.
  c. mycotic venenata
  solar c.
  Volkmann c.
cheilosis
cheiroarthropathy
  diabetic c.
cheiropompholyx (*var. of*
  chiropompholyx)
chelating agent
chelator
  intracellular calcium c.
chelerythrine chloride
Chelex resin
chelicera, pl. **chelicerae**
Chelidonium majus
cheloid
cheloidalis
  acne c.
  folliculitis c.
chelonae
  Mycobacterium c.
chemabrasion
cheme
chemexfoliation
chemical
  c. agent
  c. burn
  c. cautery
  c. depilatory

c. dermatitis
c. grouping
c. hemostasis
c. hypersensitivity syndrome
c. leukoderma
c. meningitis
c. panniculitis
c. peel
c. peeling
c. prophylaxis
c. stimulus
c. sunscreen
chemicocautery
chemiluminescence assay
chemiluminescent
  c. DNA
  c. in situ hybridization for
    detection of CMV DNA
  c. in situ hybridization for
    detection of cytomegalovirus
    deoxyribonucleic acid
chemistry
  blood c.
chemoattract
chemoattractant
chemocautery
chemoembolization
  transarterial c. (TACE)
chemoimmunology
chemokine
  c. assay
  macrophage-derived c. (MDC)
  c. receptor CCR2
  c. receptor CCR5
  secondary lymphoid tissue c. (SLC)
  thymus and activation-regulated c.
    (TARC)
chemokinetic factor
chemonucleolysis
chemonucleosis
  chymopapain c.
chemoprophylaxis
chemoresistance
chemorrhexis
chemosis
  acute conjunctival c.
chemosurgery
  Mohs c.
chemotactic
  c. factor
  c. peptide

C

NOTES

chemotaxis
    eosinophilic c.
    impaired neutrophil c.
    leukocyte c.
    neutrophil c.
chemotechnique
chemotherapeutic index
chemotherapy
    c. agent
    combination c.
    interleukin-2 adjunctive c.
    Mohs fresh-tissue c.
chenodeoxycholic acid
Chenopodiaceae
Chenopodium
cheopis
    Xenopsylla c.
cherry
    c. angioma
    c. hemangioma
    c. spot
chest
    c. cold
    c. percussion and vibration
    "silent" c.
Chevron nail
Chewables
    Dimetapp C.
chewing
    cheek c.
Cheyletiella **infestation**
Cheyne-Stokes respiration
chicken
    c. embryo lethal orphan (CELO)
    c. embryo lethal orphan virus
    c. feather
    c. pox
chickenpox
    c. immune globulin (human)
    c. immunoglobulin
    c. vaccine
    c. virus
chiclero ulcer
Chido-Rodgers antigen
chief agglutinin
Chiesi powder inhaler
chigga
chigger
    c. bite
    c. dermatitis
    c. flea
chigoe
chikungunya virus
chilblain
    c. lupus
    c. lupus erythematosus
    c. lupus erythematosus of
      Hutchinson
    necrotized c.

chilblain-like erythema
CHILD
    congenital hemidysplasia with
      ichthyosiform erythroderma and limb
      defects
    CHILD syndrome
child, pl. **children**
    blueberry muffin c.
    chronic granulomatous disease of
      children
    Cuna moon c.
    linear IgA bullous disease in
      children
    Self-Perception Profile for children
childbed fever
childhood
    asymmetric periflexural exanthem
      of c. (APEC)
    c. bullous dermatosis
    chronic bullous dermatosis of c.
    c. eczema
    C. Health Assessment Questionnaire
      (CHAQ)
    linear IgA bullous dermatosis of c.
    c. myositis
    papular acrodermatitis of c. (PAC)
    polyarteritis in c.
childhood-type tuberculosis
Child-Pugh score
children (*pl. of* child)
Children's
    C. Advil
    C. Advil Suspension
    C. Depression Inventory
    C. Motion Sickness liquid
    C. Motrin Suspension
    C. Silfedrine
Child-Turcotte-Pugh
    C.-T.-P. classification
    C.-T.-P. score
chilitis (*var. of* cheilitis)
CHIME
    coloboma of the eye, heart defect,
      ichthyosiform dermatosis, mental
      ratardation and ear defect
    CHIME syndrome
chimera
chimeric antibody
chimerism
    hematopoietic c.
    hepatocellular c.
    leukocyte c.
    mixed hematopoietic c.
chimney sweep's cancer
chinensis
    Potentilla c.
Chinese
    C. elm

C. elm tree
C. restaurant syndrome
Chiou equation
ChIP
    chromatin immunoprecipitation
chip
    DNA microarray c.
    protein c.
Chiron bDNA viral load test
Chironex
    C. fleckeri
    C. fleckeri sting
chironomid allergy
chiropompholyx, cheiropompholyx
chirp-pulse amplification
chi sequence
Chisholm scale
Chisolm scale
chi-square test
chitin
chitinases
chive
Chlamydia
    C. disease
    C. pneumoniae
    C. psittaci
    C. trachomatis
chlamydial
    c. inclusion conjunctivitis
    c. infection
    c. urethritis
Chlamydiazyme II
chlamydospore
chlamydosporum
    Fusarium c.
Chlo-Amine Oral
chloasma
    c. bronzinum
    c. faciei
    c. gravidarum
    c. hepaticum
    melanoderma c.
    c. periorale virginium
    c. phthisicorum
    c. traumaticum
chloracne
chloracnegens
Chlorafed Liquid
chloral hydrate
chlorambucil

chloramine
    c. T
    taurine c.
chloramphenicol
    c. acetyltransferase (CAT)
    c. acetyltransferase enzyme
    c., polymyxin b, and
        hydrocortisone
    c. and prednisolone
ChloraPrep
Chloraseptic
Chlorate Oral
chlorcyclizine
chlordiazepoxide (CDE)
    c. antigen
Chloresium
    C. Soln wound cleanser
    C. solution
chlorhexidine gluconate
chloride
    Adrenalin C.
    aluminum c.
    benzalkonium c.
    benzethonium c.
    benzocaine, butyl aminobenzoate,
        tetracaine, and benzalkonium c.
    chelerythrine c.
    ethyl c.
    ferric c.
    Gebauer ethyl c.
    liquid ethyl c.
    methacholine c.
    methylbenzethonium c.
    methylrosaniline c.
    polyvinyl c. (PVC)
    stearalkonium ammonium c.
    sweat c.
    c. sweat test
    vinyl c.
chlorine acne
chlorocarbon
2-chlorodeoxyadenosine
chlorofluorocarbon
chloroform
chloroguanide hydrochloride
chlorohydrate
    aluminum c.
chloroma
Chloromycetin
chloroprocaine hydrochloride
Chloroptic Ophthalmic
Chloroptic-P Ophthalmic

C

NOTES

6-chloropurine
chloroquine
    c. phosphate
    c. and primaquine
    c. therapy
chloroquine-mepacrine (CM)
chloroquine-quinine (CQ)
chlorosis
chlorothiazide diuretic
chloroxine
Chlorphed
Chlorphed-LA Nasal Solution
chlorpheniramine
    Efidac/24 c.
    c. maleate
    c., phenylephrine, and codeine
    c., phenylephrine, and
      dextromethorphan
    c., phenylephrine, and
      phenylpropanolamine
    c., phenylephrine, and
      phenyltoloxamine
    c., phenylpropanolamine, and
      acetaminophen
    c., phenyltoloxamine,
      phenylpropanolamine, and
      phenylephrine
    c. and pseudoephedrine
    c., pyrilamine, phenylephrine, and
      phenylpropanolamine
chlorpromazine hydrochloride
chlorpropamide flush
chlorprothixene
chlortetracycline hydrochloride
Chlor-Trimeton
    C.-T. 4 Hour Relief Tablet
    C.-T. Injection
Chlor-Tripolon
    C.-T. Decongestant
    C.-T. N.D.
chocolate
cholangiocarcinoma
cholangiohepatoma
cholangiolitic hepatitis
cholangitis
    primary sclerosing c. (PSC)
    sclerosing c.
Choledyl
cholera
    Asiatic c.
    c. bacillus
    bilious c.
    European c.
    hog c.
    c. infantum
    c. morbus
    c. nostras
    c. sicca
    c. toxin

    typhoid c.
    c. vaccine
cholerae
    Vibrio c.
choleraesuis
    Salmonella c.
choleragen
choleraic
cholera-red reaction
cholerica
    vox c.
Cholesky model
cholestasis
    sickle ell intrahepatic c.
cholestatic hepatitis
cholesteatoma
cholesterinic molluscum
cholesterinized antigen
cholesteroderma
cholesterol
    c. crystal
    c. embolus
    low-density lipoprotein c. (LDL-C)
    very-low-density lipoprotein c.
cholesterolosis
    c. cutis
    extracellular c.
cholestyramine
cholic acid
choline
    c. magnesium trisalicylate
    c. salicylate
cholinergic
    c. agent
    c. response
    c. urticaria
cholinogenic dermatosis
chondrification
chondrin pellet
chondritis
    auricular c.
    bronchial c.
chondroadherin
chondrocalcinosis
    hydroxyapatite c.
chondrocyte
    articular c.
    c. cytoskeletal actin polymerization
    c. mitochondrial oxidative
      phosphorylation
    c. proteoglycan synthesis
    c. sponge
chondrocytic chondrolysis
chondrodermatitis
    c. helicis nodularis
    nodular c.
    c. nodularis chronica helicis
chondrodysplasia
    lethal c.

c. punctata
c. punctata dysplasia
c. punctata syndrome
thanatophoric diastrophic c.
twisted c.
chondrogenesis
chondroid syringoma
chondroitin
c. sulfate
c. sulfate B
c. sulfate/dermatan sulfate (CS/DS)
chondrolysis
chondrocytic c.
chondroma
chondromalacia patellae
chondromatosis
chondroprogenitor
chondroprotective drug
chondrosarcoma
chorda tympani syndrome
chorea
Sydenham c.
choreal
choriomeningitis
lymphocytic c. (LCM)
chorionic human recombinant gonadotropin
Chorioptes
chorioretinitis
choristoma
phakomatous c.
choroidal angiitis
choroiditis
Chortoglyphus arcuatus
Chr^a antigen
Christmas
C. tree pattern
C. tree test
Christopher spot
Christ-Siemens-Touraine syndrome
ChromaMeter CR-200 handheld colorimeter
chromate dermatitis
chromatica
trichomycosis c.
chromatin
c. antibody
c. immunoprecipitation (ChIP)
chromatism
chromatogenous

chromatography
gas c.
high-performance liquid c. (HPLC)
chromatophore nevus of Naegeli
chromatophorotropic
chromatosis
chrome
c. holes on the hand
c. patch test
c. sore
c. ulcer
chromhidrosis, chromidrosis
apocrine c.
eccrine c.
chromic gut suture
chromidrose plantaire
chromidrosis (*var. of* chromhidrosis)
chromobacteriosis
chromoblastomycosis
chromogenic
chromomycosis
chromonychia
chromophage
chromophore
chromophototherapy
chromosomal translocation
chromosome
c. arrangement
c. 6, class III MHC
c. number
Philadelphia c. (Ph)
c. 6q
c. walking
X c.
yeast artificial c. (YAC)
chromotherapy
chromotrichia
chromotrichial
chronic
c. acral dermatitis
c. allograft rejection
c. anaphylaxis
c. angioedema
c. anterior poliomyelitis
c. asthma
c. atrophic candidiasis
c. atrophic vulvitis
c. autoimmune thyroiditis
c. blood loss
c. bronchitis
c. brucellosis
c. bullous dermatosis of childhood

C

NOTES

chronic *(continued)*
c. carrier
c. cold agglutinin disease
c. conjunctivitis
c. cutaneous erythematosus (CCE)
c. cutaneous leishmaniasis
c. cyclosporine nephropathy
c. diarrhea
c. discoid lupus erythematosus
c. eczema
c. Epstein-Barr virus infection
c. erythema multiforme
c. familial giant urticaria
c. fatigue syndrome
c. fibroid tuberculosis
c. graft dysfunction
c. graft-versus-host disease
c. granulomatous disease of children
c. hemolytic anemia
c. hemosideric dermatosis
c. hereditary lymphedema
c. histiocytosis
c. hyperplastic candidiasis
c. hypersensitivity pneumonitis
c. idiopathic thrombocytopenic purpura
c. infantile neurological, cutaneous and auricular (CINCA)
c. infantile neurological, cutaneous and auricular syndrome
c. inflammatory cell
c. inflammatory disease
c. interstitial lung disease
c. ITP
c. jejunal inflammation
c. monoarthritis
c. mucocutaneous candidiasis syndrome
c. multifocal osteomyelitis
c. myelocytic/myelogenous/myeloid leukemia accelerated phase (CML AP)
c. myeloid leukemia (CML)
c. nephrotoxicity
c. otitis media
c. pain syndrome
c. papular dermatitis
c. paranasal sinusitis
c. paronychia
c. parvovirus B19 infection
c. phase shoulder impairment
c. posterior basic meningitis
c. postrheumatic fever arthritis
c. radiodermatitis
c. T-cell leukemia
c. tophaceous gout
c. undermining burrowing ulcer
c. undermining ulcer of Meleney

c. urticaria
c. widespread pain
chronica
acrodermatitis c.
keratosis lichenoides c.
mycosis cutis c.
c. parapsoriasis lichenoid
pityriasis lichenoides c. (PLC)
purpura pigmentosa c.
urticaria c.
chronicum
erythema c.
chronicus
genital lichen simplex c.
Chrysalin
chrysanthemum
chrysarobin
chrysiasis
chrysoderma
Chrysomyia
chrysorrhoea
Euproctis c.
Chrysosporium pruinosum
chrysotherapy
church spire pattern
Churg-Strauss
C.-S. angiitis
C.-S. granulomatosis
C.-S. syndrome (CSS)
C.-S. vasculitis
C.-S. vasculopathy
chylidrosis
chyloderma
chylomicronemia
chylomicron metabolism
chylous
chyluria
chymase
chymopapain chemonucleosis
chytide
CI
confidence interval
CI gene
CI-1004
cIAP
cellular inhibitor of apoptosis
Ciarrocchi disease
CIC
circulating immune complex
Cica-Care topical gel sheeting
cicatrices *(pl. of* cicatrix)
cicatricial
c. alopecia
c. horn
c. junctional epidermolysis bullosa
c. pemphigoid (CP)
c. pemphigoid antigen
c. pemphigoid disease
c. stenosis

cicatrisata
   alopecia c.
cicatrix, pl. **cicatrices**
   hypertrophic c.
   vicious c.
cicatrization
   exuberant c.
cicatrizing alopecia
ciclopirox
   c. olamine
   c. topical solution
CID
   combined immunodeficiency disease
cidal effect
Cidecin
cidofovir
CIDS
   cellular immune deficiency syndrome
CIE
   counterimmunoelectrophoresis
cigar body
cigarette-paper
   c.-p. atrophy
   c.-p. scar
   c.-p. scarring
   c.-p. wrinkling
cigarette smoke
ciguatera poisoning
cilastatin
   imipenem and c.
ciliaris
   acne c.
   tylosis c.
ciliary
   c. beat frequency
   c. body
   c. disorder
   c. neurotrophic factor
ciliated epithelial cell
ciliate dysentery
ciliorum
   defluxio c.
   tinea c.
Ciloxan Ophthalmic
CIM
   cutaneous intolerance to mechlorethamine
cimetidine
Cimex
   C. hemipterus
   C. lectularius
Cimicidae
cimicosis

CINCA
   chronic infantile neurological, cutaneous
   and auricular
   CINCA syndrome
cincinnatiensis
   Legionella c.
cinecienta
   dermatosis c.
cine computed tomography
cinerea
   Botrytis c.
cinnabar red spot
cinnamate
cinnamic
   c. alcohol
   c. aldehyde
cinnamon
Cinobac Pulvules
cinoxacin
cinoxate
Cipro
   C. injection
   C. Oral
ciprofloxacin hydrochloride
circadian
   c. cortisol
   c. function
circinata
   balanitis c.
   impetigo c.
   pityriasis c.
   psoriasis c.
   tinea c.
circinate
   c. balanitis
   c. psoriasis
   c. syphilitic erythema
circinatum
   erythema c.
circinatus
   favus c.
CircPlus leg compression dressing
circuit
   heart-lung c.
   immunoregulatory c.
Circulaire aerosol drug delivery system
circulans
   Bacillus c.
circular plasmid DNA
circulating
   c. anticoagulant
   c. antiepidermal BMZ IgG

NOTES

circulating *(continued)*
    c. B cell
    c. immune complex (CIC)
Circulon
    C. leg compression dressing
    C. System Step 1, 2 venous ulcer
      kit
circumflexa
    ichthyosis linearis c. (ILC)
circumscribed
    c. albinism
    c. myxedema
    c. neurodermatitis
    c. precancerous melanosis of
      Dubreuilh
circumscripta
    allotrichia c.
    alopecia c.
    balanitis c.
    calcinosis c.
    osteoporosis c.
    poliosis c.
circumscriptum
    c. angiokeratoma
    lymphangioma c.
circumscriptus
    albinismus c.
cirrhosis
    HCV-related c.
    hepatitis C virus-related c.
    primary biliary c. (PBC)
    xanthomatous biliary c.
cirrhotic lacrimal gland
cisplatin
13-*cis*-retinoic acid
cistern
    Pecquet c.
cisternae
    lymphatic c.
Citanest
    C. Forte
    C. Plain
Citoscope-16 arthroscope
Citracal
citrate
    daunorubicin c.
    piperazine c.
    saline sodium c. (SSC)
    c. synthase (CS)
    c. synthesis (CS)
citric acid
citrine skin
Citrobacter
    C. amalonaticus
    C. diversus
    C. freundii
citronellal
citronella oil
citrullination

citrullinemia
    neonatal c.
Citrus Red dermatitis
Civatte
    C. body
    C. disease
    poikiloderma of C.
    C. poikiloderma
CJD
    Creutzfeldt-Jakob disease
c-jun
    c-j. N-terminal kinase
    c-j. protein
c-kit
    soluble c-k. (sc-kit)
CKR5 mutation
cladiosis
cladosporioides
    Cladosporium c.
cladosporiosis
Cladosporium
    C. carrionii
    C. cladosporioides
    C. herbarum fungus
    C. mansoni
    C. werneckii
Claforan
clamdigger's itch
clamp
    chalazion c.
    Crile c.
    Dardik c.
    Desmarres c.
    Hirsch mucosal c.
    Providence c.
    Serrefine c.
Clara cell
Claravis
clarifier
clarithromycin
Claritin
    C. Extra
    C. Hives Relief
    C. RediTab
Claritin-D 24-Hour
Clark
    C. level (I–V)
    C. malignant melanoma
      classification
Clark-Elder malignant melanoma
  classification
Clarke-type electrode
clasmatocyte
class
    functional c. II–IV
    HLA c. 1
    Ig c.
    c. (I, II, III) antigen

c. II invariant chain-derived peptide (CLIP)
immunoglobulin c.
MHC c. I, II
c. switch

classic
c. allergy symptom
c. neurofibromatosis
c. pathway
c. type Ehlers-Danlos syndrome

classical pathway (CP)
classification
Acorn c.
Barnett c.
Child-Turcotte-Pugh c.
Clark-Elder malignant melanoma c.
Clark malignant melanoma c.
Durie and Salmon multiple myeloma c.
Eichenholtz c.
Elder c.
European-American Lymphoma c.
FAB c.
French-American-British c.
Gell and Coombs c.
ILO pneumoconiosis c.
Jopling c.
Lancefield c.
Lever and Schamberg-Lever c.
Loesche c.
Lukes-Collins non-Hodgkin lymphoma c.
Lund-Browder c.
morphologic c.
Nalebuff c.
Rappaport c.
REAL c.
Revised European-American Lymphoma c.
Ridley c.
Runyon c.
Rye c.
Shimada histopathologic c.
Steinbrocker c.
TIM drug c.
topical immunomodulator drug c.
transplant rejection c.
Walter Reed c.

clastothrix
claudication
jaw c.
neurogenic c.

c. of tongue
vascular c.

clavatus
Aspergillus c.

clavi (*pl. of* clavus)
clavicular sign
clavulanate
clavulanic acid
clavus, pl. **clavi**
interdigital c.
c. syphiliticus

claw
c. foot
c. nail

clawing
c. deformity
rheumatoid c.

Clay-Adams stain
clean
C. Air Delivery Rate (CADR)
C. & Clear Deep Cleaning astringent
C. & Clear Invisible Clearasil Clearstick
Dey-Wash skin wound c.

cleaner
air c.
Bionaire Air C.
unclassified air c.

Cleanmix DNA purification kit
cleanser
Antimicrobial MPM wound c.
Biolex wound c.
Chloresium Soln wound c.
Clinical Care wound c.
ClinsWound wound c.
Constant-Clens wound c.
Curaklense wound c.
Curasol wound c.
Debrisan wound c.
Dermagran wound c.
DermaMend wound c.
Dey-Wash skin wound c.
DiaB Klenz wound c.
Elta Dermal wound c.
Gentell wound c.
Hyperion wound c.
Iamin wound c.
lipid-free c.
Lobana wound c.
MicroKlenz wound c.
MPM antimicrobial wound c.

NOTES

cleanser *(continued)*
  Neutrogena fresh foaming c.
  Optipore Sponge wound c.
  Perineal Skin C.
  Plexion c.
  Puri-Clens wound c.
  Purpose c.
  Restore wound c.
  Rosula aqueous c.
  SAF-Clens wound c.
  Sea-Clens wound c.
  SeptiCare wound c.
  Shur-Clens wound c.
  SkinTegrity wound c.
  soap-free c.
  Techni-Care wound c.
  UltraKlenz wound c.
  Zoderm c.
cleansing
  c. cream
  Fostex Medicated C.
clear
  c. acanthoma
  C. Away Disc
  C. By Design
  C. By Design Gel
  C. Caladryl Spray
  Calahist C.
  c. cell
  c. cell papulosis
  c. cells scattered in a buckshot
    fashion
  C. Confident antifungal topical
    lotion
  Dimetapp C.
  c. hidradenoma
  C. Pore Treatment
  c. syringoma
clearance
  alveolar fluid c.
  creatinine c.
  immune complex c.
  measure mucociliary c. (MMC)
  mucociliary c.
Clearasil
  C. B.P. plus
  C. Maximum Strength
  C. Pads
clear-cut granuloma
clearing
  central c.
ClearLight treatment for acne
ClearSite
  C. hydrogel sheet
  C. impregnated gauze
Clearstick
  Clean & Clear Invisible
    Clearasil C.

cleavage
  collagenase-mediated c.
  granzyme B-mediated c.
  lines of c.
  metal-catalyzed oxidative c.
cleaved giant cell
cleft
  branchial c.
  lucent c.
clefting
  ectrodactyly, ectodermal, c. (EEC)
  suprabasal c.
cleidocranial dysplasia
clemastine
  c. fumarate
  c. and phenylpropanolamine
Clematis armandii
Cleocin
  C. HCl Oral
  C. hydrochloride
  C. Pediatric
  C. Pediatric Oral
  C. Phosphate Injection
  C. T
  C. T topical
  C. Vaginal
Clickhaler
clicking
  palatal c.
climacterica
  keratoderma c.
climactericum
  keratoderma c.
  keratosis c.
climatotherapy
Clinac BPO gel
Clinda-Derm topical
Clindagel topical gel
clindamycin/benzoyl
  c. peroxide
  c. peroxide gel
clindamycin phosphate topical gel
Clindoxyl
clinic
clinical
  C. Care wound cleanser
  c. change
  c. gout
  c. hyperthyroidism
  c. judgment
  c. manifestation
  c. myocarditis
  c. transplant coordinator (CTC)
Clinicel silicon gel-filled cushion
Clinique
  C. Antiacne Soap
  C. antibacterial soap
  C. Continuous Coverage
Clinoril

ClinsWound wound cleanser
clioquinol and hydrocortisone
CLIP
    class II invariant chain-derived peptide
        CLIP replacement approach
clip
    Backhaus towel c.
ClipTip reusable sensor
CLKTx
    combined liver and kidney
        transplantation
CLM articulating laryngoscope blade
cloacae
    Enterobacter c.
cloacogenic carcinoma
clobetasol
    c. dipropionate
    C. E Cream
    c. propionate
    c. propionate foam
    c. propionate lotion
Clobex lotion
clock-face pattern
Clocort Maximum Strength
Cloderm topical
clodronate-containing liposome
clofazimine palmitate
clofibrate
clomipramine
Clomycin
clonal
    c. deletion theory
    c. expansion
    c. ignorance
    c. selection theory
clonality
    T-cell c.
clonazepam
Cloncorchis sinensis
clone
    vector-transfected cell c.
clonidine hydrochloride
clonorchiasis
clonospecific oligoprobe hybridization
clonotype
clopidogrel
clorazepate
Clorpactin WCS-90
closed
    c. accordion sign
    c. comedo

    c. patch test
    c. wet dressing
closed-space infection
clostridia
clostridial myonecrosis
Clostridium difficile test (CLOtest)
closure
    lazy-S c.
    S-shaped c.
    The VAC Vacuum Assisted C.
    Velcro c.
CLOtest
    Clostridium difficile test
clothes louse
clothing
    c. dermatitis
    FrogWear sunscreen c.
    Solumbra sunscreen c.
    sunscreen c.
Clotrimaderm
clotrimazole
    betamethasone and c.
clotrimazole/betamethasone dipropionate
  lotion
Clot Stop drain
clotting cascade
Cloudman melanoma
Clouston syndrome
clove oil
clover
    sweet c.
cloxacillin sodium
Cloxapen
Clr deficiency
clubbed finger
clubbing
    idiopathic c.
    nail c.
    c. of nail
club hair
cluster
    aggressive cell c.
    seborrheic keratosis c.
cluster-of-grapes appearance
Clutton joint
CM
    capreomycin
    chloroquine-mepacrine
cM
    centimorgan
CMA
    cow's milk allergy

NOTES

CMC
  carpometacarpal
    CMC syndrome
CMED
  Cytoxan, methotrexate, etoposide,
    dexamethasone
CMI
  cell-mediated immunity
    Multitest CMI
CMIS
  common mucosal immune system
CML
  chronic myeloid leukemia
    CML AP
    CML BC
    CML CP
CMS AccuProbe 450 system
CMV
  cytomegalovirus
    Copalis ToRC automated antibody
      assay for CMV
c-myc
    c-m. gene
    c-m. protooncogene
CNI
  calcineurin inhibitor
cnidoblast
cnidosis
coadministration
coagglutinin
coagulase-positive micrococcus
coagulation
    biterminal c.
    blood c.
    disseminated intravascular c. (DIC)
    c. factor Va
    c. meshwork
    sepsis-induced disseminated
      intravascular c.
coagulopathy
    consumption c.
coal
    c. tar
    c. tar bath
    c. tar, lanolin, and mineral oil
    c. tar and salicylic acid
coalescence
coalescing
Coamatic protein C test
co-amoxiclav
coarse
    c. breath sounds
    c. facies
    c. rale
    c. surface
    c. texture
coast
    Ebola Ivory C.
    c. erysipelas

    c. of Maine border
    c. sage
coated tongue
cobalamin deficiency
cobalt
    c. dermatitis
    c. dichloride
    c. in tungsten carbide
cobalt-chrome head
Coban
    C. cohesive medium stretch
      bandage
    C. dressing
    C. wrap
Cobas Amplicor CMV Monitor test
cobblestoning
Cobb syndrome
cobra
    C. auto-gamma counter
    C. cannula
    c. hemotoxin
    c. venom cofactor
cocarde reaction
cocardiform
cocci (*pl. of* coccus)
coccidioidal
    c. granuloma
    c. osteomyelitis
Coccidioides immitis
coccidioidin skin test
coccidioidomycosis
    cutaneous c.
    disseminated c.
coccidiosis
coccogenic sycosis
coccus, pl. **cocci**
    gram-negative cocci
    gram-positive cocci
Cochin sore
Cochran-Mantel-Haenszel test
cockatiel feather
Cockayne syndrome
Cockayne-Touraine epidermolysis bullosa
cocklebur weed pollen
cockroach
    American c.
    German c.
cockscomb ulcer
cocktail
    immunosuppressant c.
cock-up deformity
cocoa
coconut
codeine
    chlorpheniramine, phenylephrine,
      and c.
codfish vertebra
Codiclear
coding joint

codominant
    autosomal c.
codon
    arginine c.
coefficient
    apparent diffusion c. (ADC)
    diffusion c.
    c. of error (CE)
    intraclass correlation c. (ICC)
    Kendall correlation c.
    c. of variation (CV)
coelenterate sting
coenzyme
    3-hydroxy-3-methylglutaryl c. A
    (HMG-CoA)
Coe virus
cofactor
    cobra venom c.
coffee bean
Coffin-Lowry syndrome
Coffin-Siris syndrome
Coflex flexible wrap
Cogan syndrome
Cogentin
cognate
    c. interaction
    c. recognition
cognitive-behavioral technique
cognitive-behavior therapy (CBT)
coherence therapy
Coherent UltraPulse CO$_2$ laser
Co-Hist
cohort
    Hopkins lupus c.
    c. study
coil
    air c.
    c. gland
    secretory c.
coimmunoprecipitate
Coinage Act
coincidental symptom
coin-rubbing dermatitis
coin-sized lesion
COL1A1 gene
COLAP
    colonoscopic allergen provocation
    COLAP test
CO$_2$ laser
COL2A1 type II procollagen gene
ColBenemid
colchicine and probenecid

cold
    c. abscess
    c. agglutination
    c. agglutinin
    c. air testing
    c. allergy
    C. & Allergy Elixir
    c. antibody
    c. autoagglutinin
    c. autoantibody
    Benylin C.
    chest c.
    c. cream
    c. dry air (CDA)
    c. exposure
    c. gangrene
    c. hemagglutinin disease
    c. hemolysin
    c. ischemia
    c. ischemia time
    c. laser treatment
    Ornex C.
    c. panniculitis
    c. quartz lamp
    c. quartz radiation
    c. reflex urticaria
    rose c.
    c. sore
    c. stage
    c. steel debulking
    c. storage (CS)
    c. ulcer
    c. virus
cold-dependent
    c.-d. dermographism
    c.-d. disorder
Coldec D extended release tablet
Cold-Eezer Plus
cold-induced
    c.-i. cell injury
    c.-i. necrosis
    c.-i. skin antigen
    c.-i. urticaria
    c.-i. vasospasm
Coldloc-LA
cold-reactive antibody
Coleman microinfiltration system
Coleoptera
Coley toxin
coli
    Balantidium c.

NOTES

coli *(continued)*
  Escherichia c.
  c. granuloma
colic
  infantile c.
colicin
colicinogeny
coliphage
colistimethate sodium
colistin
  c., neomycin, and hydrocortisone
  c. sulfate
colitis
  allergic c.
  antibiotic-associated c.
  balantidial c.
  collagenous c.
  dietary protein-induced c.
  milk-induced c.
  pseudomembranous c.
  ulcerative c.
colitose
collaboration
  Multicenter Airway Research C.
    (MARC)
  T cell-B cell c.
  C. Transplant Study
collacin
collagen
  Arg^{519}-Cys mutation in type II c.
  autoantigen c.
  BGC Matrix c.
  cartilaginous c.
  conformational kinks in c.
  c. CS
  Cys-containing type II c.
  c. denaturation
  Fibracol c.
  c. fibril
  fibrillar c.
  hyCure c.
  hydroxylysine content of c.
  c. implant
  c. implantation
  injectable c.
  c. injection
  intimal c.
  Matrix c.
  Medifil c.
  c. polymer
  short-chain type X c.
  Skin Temp c.
  type (I–XI, XIV) c.
  c. vascular disease
  c. vascular serologic test
  Woun'Dres c.
  Zyderm II c.
  Zyplast c.

collagenase
  c. inhibitor
  polymorphonuclear leukocyte c.
  type IV c.
  type V c.
collagenase-mediated cleavage
collagenization
collagenolysis
collagenolytic enzyme
collagenoma
collagenosis
  reactive perforating c. (RPC)
collagenous
  c. colitis
  c. fibroma
collapse
  cardiovascular c.
collar
  Biett c.
  Casal c.
  c. of pearls
  c. of Venus
collarette of Biett
collastin
CollaTape
collateral damage
collectin
collection
  gravitational particle c.
  isokinetic c.
Colles fracture
colli
  erythromelanosis follicularis faciei
    et c.
  fibromatosis c.
  leukoderma c.
  melanoleukoderma c.
  pterygium c.
Collier needle holder
collimated bema handpiece (CBH-1) for
  laser surgery
collimator
  fan-beam c.
Collins
  C. dynamometer
  C. solution
colliquativa
  tuberculosis cutis c.
colliquative
  c. degeneration
  c. sweat
collodion
  c. baby
  blistering c.
  cantharidal c.
  flexible c.
  hemostatic c.
  iodized c.
  c. membrane

salicylic acid c.
styptic c.
colloid
  c. acne
  c. additive
  c. body
  bovine c.
  c. cyst
  c. degeneration
  c. milium
  c. pseudomilium
colloidal
  c. oatmeal
  c. oatmeal bath
colloidalis conglomerata
Collyrium Fresh Ophthalmic
coloboma, heart anomaly, ichthyosis, mental retardation, and ear abnormality syndrome
colocalization
cologne
colonic adenocarcinoma
colonization
  airway bacterial c.
  atypical mycobacterial c.
  Candida parapsilosis c.
colonoscopic
  c. allergen provocation (COLAP)
  c. allergen provocation test
colony
  myeloid c.
colophony
color
  constitutive skin c.
  facultative skin c.
  inducible skin c.
  lesion c.
  pale c.
  variegated c.
Colorado
  C. microdissection needle
  C. tick fever (CTF)
coloration
colored alcoholic shake lotion
colorimeter
  ChromaMeter CR-200 handheld c.
Colorimeti Assay
coloring agent
Colorists
ColorZone tape
colostrum
  bovine c.

colpate
colporate
Columbia
  C. Antiseptic powder
  C. S. K. virus
column
  RNeasy spin c.
columnar
  c. epithelium
Coly-Mycin
  C.-M. M Parenteral
  C.-M. S Oral
  C.-M. S Otic drops
coma bulla
Combantrin
CombiDERM
  C. ACD hydrocolloid
  C. ACD hydrocolloid dressing
combi-effect
combination
  c. chemotherapy
  c. skin
combined
  c. antibody and cellular deficiency
  c. immunodeficiency disease (CID)
  c. immunodeficiency syndrome
  c. liver and kidney transplantation (CLKTx)
  measles, mumps and rubella vaccines, c.
  c. nevi
  penicillin g, benzathine and procaine, c.
  rubella and mumps vaccines, c.
combining site
combining-site antibody
combion test
Combi test
Combivir
Combo
  FP/Salm C.
    flucatisone propionate/salmeterol
combustionis
  dermatitis c.
Comby sign
comedo, pl. **comedones, comedos**
  c. acne
  closed c.
  comedones epidermal nevus
  c. extraction
  comedones extractor
  c. nevus

NOTES

comedo *(continued)*
    open c.
    solar c.
comedocarcinoma
comedogenic
comedolytic agent
comedones *(pl. of* comedo)
comedonicus
    c. nevus
    nevus unilateralis c.
comedos *(pl. of* comedo)
Comfeel
    C. hydrocolloid
    C. hydrocolloid dressing
    C. synthetic dressing
    C. Ulcus dressing
Comfort Tears solution
comma bacillus
commensal bacteria
commercial antigen
commissural cheilitis
committee
    International Knee
      Documentation C. (IKDC)
    National Vaccine Advisory C.
      (NVAC)
common
    c. acne
    c. acute lymphocytic leukemia
      antigen (CALLA)
    c. acute lymphocytic leukemia
      antigen positive
    c. baldness
    c. blue nevus
    c. cold virus
    c. lymphoid progenitor cell
    c. mucosal immune system (CMIS)
    c. opsonin
    c. peroneal nerve
    c. reed
    c. reed grass
    c. striped scorpion
    c. striped scorpion sting
    c. variable unclassifiable
      immunodeficiency
    c. wart
commune
    integumentum c.
communicable disease
compacta Jeanselmei pedrosoi
compactum
    Fonsecaea c.
    Hormodendron c.
    stratum c.
Companion 314 nasal CPAP system
comparative genomic hybridization
compartment load distribution
compatibility
compatible

Compeed Skin protector dressing
Comperm tubular elastic bandage
competence
    immunological c.
competition
    antigenic c.
competitive binding assay
competitor DNA
complement
    c. activation
    c. activation cascade
    c. activity
    c. binding assay
    c. C3
    c. C4
    c. chemotactic factor
    component of c.
    c. deficiency
    c. deviation
    c. sequence
    serum c. C1–C9
    c. system
    c. test
    total hemolytic c.
    c. unit
complement-activating antigen-antibody
complementarity
complementary
    c. and alternative medicine
      treatment
    c. cascade
    c. strand
complementation
complement-dependent-cytotoxic (CDC)
complement-dependent cytotoxicity
    (CDC)
complement-fixation
    c.-f. reaction
    c.-f. test
complement-fixing (CF)
    c.-f. antibody
complement-mediated
    c.-m. anaphylaxis
    c.-m. host defense process
    c.-m. tumor cell immunopurging
complete
    c. antibody
    c. antigen
    c. blood count
    c. imperfect albinism
    c. perfect albinism
    c. transduction
complex
    Acinetobacter calcoaceticus-
      baumannii c.
    acne-seborrhea c.
    Allovectin-7 DNA/lipid c.
    amphotericin B cholesteryl
      sulfate c.

amphotericin B lipid c.
antigen-antibody c.
antigenic c.
avian leukosis-sarcoma c.
Carney c.
C5b-C8 c.
C5b-C9 c.
circulating immune c. (CIC)
cytolytic macromolecular c.
desmosome-tonofilament c.
DNA-carrier c.
EAHF c.
elastomeric c.
epithelioid combined nevi
  Carney c. (ECN-CC)
feline leukemia-sarcoma virus c.
gene c.
Ghon c.
Golgi c.
GP ib-IX c.
H-2 c.
heterodimeric c.
heterooligomeric c.
HLA c.
hyaluronate-polylysine c.
IgG c.
immune c. (IC)
insulin-like growth factor BP3 c.
killer inhibitor receptor-human
  leukocyte antigen c.
KIR-HLA c.
C. 15 lotion
major histocompatibility c. class I,
  II
membrane attack c. (MAC)
membranolytic attack c. (MAC)
Merkel-cell-neurite c.
Mycobacterium avium c. (MAC)
peptidoglycan-polysaccharide c.
phosphatidylserine-prothrombin c.
popliteal-arcuate c.
primary c.
c. regional pain syndrome (CRPS)
semimembranosus c.
triangular fibrocartilage c. (TFCC)
tuberous sclerosis c. (TSC)

complexion
T zone c.

complication
cardiac c.
delayed c.

immunologic c.
nonimmunologic c.

component
absent dermal c.
amyloid P c.
c. of complement
glenoid c.
leuko-poor blood c.
matrix c.
secretory c.
serum amyloid A, P c.
spliceosomal c.
ultrastructural c.

composite
C. cultured skin (CCS)
c. graft

compound
amide c.
antisense c.
azole c.
cationic c.
c. cyst
mercurial c.
c. nevus
ornithine carbamyl transferase c.
psoralen c.
saligenin c.
sulfhydryl c.
C. W
C. W plus

Compoz
C. gelcap
C. Nighttime Sleep Aid

compress
cool c.
ice c.

compression
axillary nerve c.
suprascapular nerve c. (SSC)
vertebral artery c.
in vitro mechanical c.

Comprilan wrap
computed tomography (CT)
computer-assisted arthritis detection
computerized tomodensitometry
COMT
catechol-O-methyl transferase
COMT asthma

Comtrex
concanamycin A
concanavalin A-stimulated T^H cell line
  supernatant

C

NOTES

concentrate
 bovine whey protein c.
 E-Toxa-Clean C.
 hyperimmune bovine colostrum
  IgC c.
 leukocyte c.
 parvum bovine Ig c.
 platelet c.
concentration
 femtomolar c.
 grass pollen c.
 intradermal test c.
 median effective c. (EC50)
 minimal bactericidal c. (MBC)
 minimal inhibitory c. (MIC)
 minimum inhibitory c. (MIC)
 prick test c.
concentricum
 Trichophyton c.
concomitant
 c. condition
 c. immunity
concrete seborrhea
condition
 concomitant c.
 Fordyce c.
 isocapnic c.
 nondenaturing c.
 seborrheic dermatitis-like c.
 severe chronic allergic c.
conditional-lethal mutant
conditionally lethal mutant
conditioned hemolysis
conditioner
conditioning
 air c.
 myeloablative c.
condom dermatitis
condyloma, pl. **condylomata**
 Buschke-Löwenstein giant c.
 flat c.
 giant c.
 c. lata
 condylomata lata
 c. latum
 c. planus
 pointed c.
condylomatosis
condylomatous
Condylox
cone
 keratosic c.
conenose, cone-nose
 c. bug
 c. bug bite
Conex
conferta
 urticaria c.

confetti macule
Confide HIV test
confidence interval (CI)
configuration
 lesion c.
 string of pearls c.
confirmation
 tissue c.
confluent
 c. measles
 c. and reticulate papillomatosis
confocal laser scanning microscopy
Conformant
 C. contact layer sheet
 C. wound dressing
conformation
 antiparallel B-sheet c.
conformational
 c. determinant
 c. kinks in collagen
congelationis
 dermatitis c.
congelation urticaria
congeneric
congenita
 adermia c.
 aplasia cutis c.
 arthrochalasis multiplex c.
 cutis marmorata telangiectatica c.
 dyskeratosis c.
 hyperkeratosis universalis c.
 keratosis universalis c.
 melanosis diffusa c.
 pachyonychia c.
 type II pachyonychia c.
congenital
 c. anemia
 c. aplasia of thymus
 c. baldness
 c. camptodactyly
 c. candidiasis
 c. circumscribed hypomelanosis
 c. contractural arachnodactyly
 c. cytomegalovirus
 c. depigmentation
 c. disorder
 c. dysphagocytosis
 c. ectodermal defect
 c. ectodermal dysplasia
 c. elephantiasis
 c. fascial dystrophy
 c. generalized fibromatosis
 c. generalized phlebectasia
 c. giant pigmented nevus
 c. hemidysplasia
 c. hemidysplasia with ichthyosiform
  erythroderma and limb defects
  (CHILD)

c. hemidysplasia with ichthyosiform erythroderma and limb defects syndrome
c. HIV infection
c. human immunodeficiency virus infection
c. hypomelanotic macule
c. Lyme disease
c. rubella
c. rubella syndrome
c. sebaceous gland hyperplasia
c. self-healing reticulohistiocytosis
c. sutural alopecia
c. syphilis
c. telangiectatic erythema
c. total lipodystrophy
c. toxoplasmosis
c. triangular alopecia
c. varicella
congenitale
hemangioma c.
keratoma malignum c.
poikiloderma c.
Thomson poikiloderma c.
congenitalis
alopecia triangularis c.
erythroderma ichthyosiformis c.
Congess
C. Jr
C. Sr
Congestac ND
Congestaid
Congestant D
Congest-Eze
congestion
nasal c.
Tylenol Sinus Severe C.
Vicks 44D Cough & Head C.
congestivum
erythema c.
conglobata
acne c.
conglobate
c. abscess
c. acne
conglomerata
colloidalis c.
elastosis colloidalis c.
conglutination
conglutinin assay
Congo
C. floor maggot

C. floor maggot bite
C. red stain
Congo-Crimean hemorrhagic fever (CCHF)
congolensis
Dermatophilus c.
congruence
joint c.
conidium, pl. **conidia**
conjugated
c. antigen
c. estrogen
c. hapten
conjugation
conjugative plasmid
conjunctiva, pl. **conjunctivae**
lepra conjunctivae
limbi c.
conjunctival
c. goblet cell
c. injection
c. testing
conjunctivitis
acute contagious c.
acute epidemic c.
acute follicular c.
allergic c.
angular c.
bacterial c.
blennorrheal c.
chlamydial inclusion c.
chronic c.
gonococcal c.
herpes simplex c.
infantile purulent c.
limbal vernal c.
lymphogranuloma venereum c.
Moraxella c.
seasonal allergic c. (SAC)
toxicogenic c.
vernal c.
viral c.
Connaught flu
connective
c. tissue
c. tissue nevus
c. tissue panniculitis
c. tissue proteinase
connector
transmembrane c.
connexin hemichannel

C

NOTES

conniventes
valvulae c.
connori
Nosema c.
conorii
Rickettsia c.
Conradi disease
Conradi-Hünermann syndrome
consciousness
disturbance of c.
conscriptus
albinismus c.
consecutive achromia
consensus sequence
consistency
lesion c.
consolidation
airspace c.
patchy airspace c.
progressive acinar c.
constant
association c.
binding c.
diffusion c.
dissociation c.
intrinsic association c.
c. region
Constant-Clens wound cleanser
constitutional
c. hirsutism
c. reaction
c. ulcer
constitutive skin color
consumption
c. coagulopathy
maximal oxygen c.
Contac
C. Allergy Formula
C. Cold Non-Drowsy
contact
allergen c.
c. allergy
c. carrier
c. cheilitis
c. dermatitis
C. Dermatitis Research Group
c. dermatoconjunctivitis
c. eczema
c. hypersensitivity
c. leukoderma
c. metastasis
c. photodermatitis
c. photosensitization
c. poison
c. urticaria
contactant
irritant c.
occupational allergic c.
contact-layer wound dressing

contact-type dermatitis
contagion
immediate c.
mediate c.
contagiosa
impetigo c.
keratosis follicularis c.
sycosis c.
contagiosum
ecthyma c.
epithelioma c.
erythema c.
contagiosus
pemphigus c.
contagious
c. disease
c. ecthyma
c. ecthyma (pustular dermatitis)
virus of sheep
c. pustular dermatitis
c. pustular stomatitis virus
contagiousness
contagium
contaminant
contaminate
contamination
bacterial c.
content
bone mineral c. (BMC)
high liquid c.
moisture c.
total body bone mineral c.
Contergan
contig
continua
acrodermatitis c.
continued fever
continuous
c. low-flow oxygen
c. passive motion
c. positive airway pressure (CPAP)
continuous-wave
c.-w. dye laser surgery
c.-w. laser
contortus
Haemonchus c.
contraceptive dermatitis
contraction
epitope c.
MHC c.
myosin heavy chain c.
wound c.
contractural arachnodactyly
contracture
Dupuytren c.
flexion c.
waxy c.
contralateral sign
contransfection

contrast effect
contrasuppression
contrasuppressor cell
Contreet
 C. Antimicrobial Barrier Dressing
 C. hydrocolloid nonadhesive foam
  dressing
contributory irritant
control
 air pollution c.
 c. animal
 Blemish C.
 c. of emotional factor
 Lamis PressureFuse automatic
  pressure c.
 Lander Dandruff C.
 mite c.
 mold c.
 odor c.
 Oxy C.
 c. protein
 Shaklee Dandruff C.
controlled
 c. anaphylaxis
 c. cough
controller
 Maalox H2 Acid C.
 Pepcid AC Acid C.
contusiforme
 erythema c.
contusiformis
 dermatitis c.
 erythema c.
contusion
Contuss XT
conus
 tinea c.
convalescence serum
convalescent
 c. carrier
 c. serum
 c. stage
conventional
 c. animal
 c. asthma therapy (CAT)
conversion
 index of marrow c. (IMC)
convertase
 C3 proactivator c.
 furin c.
convex nail
convoluted foam mattress

convulsion
 theophylline-induced c.
ConXn
COOH-terminal peptide
Cook cannula
cookei
 Ixodes c.
cool compress
Cooley anemia
CoolGlide aesthetic laser system
coolie itch
cooling
 c. agent
 c. blanket
 rapid c.
CoolSpot skin-cooling device
CoolTouch 1320nm laser system
Coombs
 C. serum
 C. test
coordinator
 clinical transplant c. (CTC)
CO-Oximeter module
Copalis ToRC automated antibody
 assay for CMV
Copaxone
Cophene-B injection
copious sputum
Coplus cohesive medium stretch
 bandage
copper
 c. bromide laser
 c. deficiency
 c. deposition
 c. dermatitis
 c. itch
 c. metabolism
 c. vapor laser
copperhead
 c. snake
 c. snake bite
Coppertone
 C. Lipkote
 C. Oil-Free
 C. Skin Selects
 C. Sport
 C. Sunscreen
 C. Waterproof Sunblock
copra
 c. itch
 c. mite dermatitis
coprecipitation

NOTES

coproantibodies
coproporphyria
    erythropoietic c. (ECP)
    hereditary c. (HCP)
coproporphyrin
coproporphyrinogen
COPS
    calcinosis cutis, osteoma cutis,
      poikiloderma, and skeletal
      abnormalities
    COPS syndrome
Co-Pyronil 2 Pulvules
coral
    c. cut
    c. dermatitis
    fire c.
    c. snake
    c. snake bite
coral-head appearance
Corbus disease
cord
    appendageal c.
    C. Blood Registry
    umbilical c.
Cordran
    C. SP
    C. SP topical
    C. tape
Cordyceps
Cordylobia anthropophaga
core
    c. decompression
    c. window
Corgard
Coricidin D
corii
    sclerosis c.
corium
    superficial c.
corkscrew
    c. hair
    c. spirochete
Corlett pyosis
Cormax Ointment
corn
    asbestos c.
    hard c.
    c. meal agar
    seed c.
    c. smut
    soft c.
cornea, pl. corneae
    herpes c.
    ichthyosis sebacea corneae
corneal
    c. epithelial cell
    c. opacification
    c. transplantation
    c. ulcer

corneocyte
    c. adhesion
    c. desquamation
Corneometer
corneous
corner stitch
corneum
    Nosema c.
    stratum c. (SC)
corneus
    c. hypertrophicus
    lichen obtusus c.
cornification
    c. disorder
    normal c.
    type 1-24 c.
cornified
    c. cell envelope
    c. layer
cornmeal
cornoid lamella
corn-row braiding
cornual
cornuate
cornu cutaneum
corona
    c. phlebectasia
    c. seborrheica
    c. veneris
    zona c.
coronal view
coronary
    c. fistula
    c. vasculitis
Coronaviridae virus
coronavirus
coronoid fossa
corporis
    pediculosis c.
    Pediculus c.
    pthiriasis c.
    seborrhea c.
    tinea c.
    trichophytosis c.
corps ronds
cor pulmonale
corpuscle
    Hassall c.
    Hayem c.
    Meissner c.
    molluscum c.
    Negri c.
    Vater-Pacini c.
    Wagner-Meissner tactile c.
Corque topical
correction
    Bonferroni c.
    Frechet 3-flap slot c.
    Tukey post-hoc c.

corrosive
　c. poison
　c. ulcer
corset
　lumbar c.
Cort
　S-T C.
Cortacet
CortaGel topical
Cortaid
　C. Maximum Strength
　C. Maximum Strength topical
　C. with Aloe
　C. with Aloe topical
Cortate
Cortatrigen Otic
Cort-Dome topical
Cortef
　C. Feminine Itch
　C. Feminine Itch topical
Cortenema
cortex of hair
Corticaine cream
corticale
　Cryptostroma c.
cortical fusi
corticosteroid
　fluorinated c.
　inhaled c. (ICS)
　parenteral c.
　c. rosacea
　synthetic depot c.
　systemic c.
　topical c.
corticotrope
corticotropin
Corticoviridae
Cortifoam
Cortin topical
cortisol
　circadian c.
　urinary free c. (UFC)
cortisone acetate
Cortisporin
　C. Ophthalmic Ointment
　C. Ophthalmic Suspension
　C. Otic
　C. Topical Cream
　C. Topical Ointment
cortivazol
Cortizone-10 topical
Cortoderm

Cortone
　C. Acetate
　C. Acetate injection
　C. Acetate Oral
Corylus avellana
corymbiform
corymbose
　c. arrangement
　c. syphilid
corynebacteria
corynebacteriophage
　beta c.
Corynebacterium
　C. *acnes*
　C. diphtheriae
　C. minutissimum
coryneform bacterium
Coryphen
coryza
　allergic c.
Coryzavirus
CO Sleuth
Cosmederm-7
Cosmegen
cosmesis
cosmetic
　c. allergy test
　Botox C.
　cheek c.
　c. dermatitis
　eyelash c.
　eyelid c.
　c. intolerance syndrome
　lip c.
　C., Toiletries, and Fragrance
　　Association
　undercover c.
cosmetica
　acne c.
cosmetician
cosmeticus
　status c.
cosmetologist
cosmetology
cosmid
costa
　erisipela de la c.
　erysipelas de la c.
　C. Simple Scoring System
costal fringe
costaricensis
　Angiostrongylus c.

NOTES

C

Costello syndrome
costimulation
costimulatory
    c. blockade
    inducible c. (ICOS)
    c. molecule
    c. receptor
costovertebral-girdle joint
Cotinine assay
cotriggering hypothesis
Cotrim DS
cotrimoxazole
cotton
    defoliating c.
    defoliation of c.
    c. glove
    c. linter
    c. roll stomatitis
cottonmouth
    c. snake
    c. snake bite
cottonseed
cottonwood
    Arizona/Fremont c.
    c. tree
    c. tree pollen
cotton-wool
    c.-w. patch
    c.-w. spot
cough
    barking c.
    controlled c.
    Diphen C.
    dry c.
    huff c.
    nonproductive c.
    reflex c.
    Silphen C.
    whooping c.
coughing
    paroxysm of c.
cough-variant asthma
Coulter
    C. counter
    C. ICD-Prep test
coumarin necrosis
council
    Medical Research C. (MRC)
count
    absolute blood eosinophil c. (AEC)
    CD4 c.
    CD4 T-lymphocyte c.
    complete blood c.
    hemolysis, elevated liver enzymes,
     low platelet c.
    high mole c.
    lymphocyte subset c.
    peripheral blood c.
    reticulocyte c.

    WBC c.
    white blood c. (WBC)
countenance
    Hippocratic c.
counter
    Cobra auto-gamma c.
    Coulter c.
    scintillation c.
    Top-Count microplate
     scintillation c.
counterimmunoelectrophoresis (CIE)
counterirritant
counterirritation
counterregulatory effect
countervailing
coup
    c. de sabre
    c. d'ongle
coupling
    rhodopsin-type c.
Covaderm composite wound dressing
covariate
cover
    AgiSite alginate wound c.
    AlgiDerm alginate wound c.
    alginate wound c.
    Algosteril alginate wound c.
    CarraSorb H alginate wound c.
    Curasorb Zinc alginate wound c.
    Dermacea alginate wound c.
    FyBron alginate wound c.
    Gentell alginate wound c.
    Kalginate alginate wound c.
    Maxorb alginate wound c.
    PolyMem alginate wound c.
    Restore alginate wound c.
    SeaSorb alginate wound c.
    Sorbsan alginate wound c.
    Tegagen HG, HI alginate
     wound c.
coverage
    Clinique Continuous C.
covering agent
Coverlet composite dressing
Covermark corrective makeup
Cover-Roll gauze
coverslip
Cover-Strip wound closure strip
Covertell composite dressing
cow
    c. dander
    c. milk allergy (CMA)
Cowden disease
Cowdria ruminantium
Cowdry
    C. intranuclear inclusion body type
    A, B
    C. type (A, B) inclusion body

cowl
  monk's c.
cow-milk protein intolerance
cowpox virus
cow's
  c. mild-sensitive enteropathy
  c. milk
  c. milk allergy (CMA)
COX
  cyclooxygenase
  COX enzyme
COX-1
  cyclooxygenase-1
  COX-1 enzyme
  COX-1 inhibitor
COX-2
  cyclooxygenase-2
  COX-2 inhibitor
Cox
  C. organism
  C. regression
coxarthrosis
Coxiella burnetii
COX/LO inhibitor
Cox-Mantel test
Coxsackie
  C. B virus
  C. encephalitis
Coxsackievirus B1–B5
Cox-Spjotvoll method
CP
  cicatricial pemphigoid
  classical pathway
  CML CP
  CP disease
CPA
  cyproterone acetate
CPAP
  continuous positive airway pressure
  NightBird nasal CPAP
C-peptide secretion
CPM
  continuous passive motion
  CPM machine
C-polysaccharide
  pneumococcal C.-p. (CPS)
cPPT
  central polypurine tract
CPS
  pneumococcal C-polysaccharide
CQ
  chloroquine-quinine

C1q
  C1q assay
  C1q deficiency
  C1q immune complex detection
  C1q receptor
C-R
  Bicillin C-R
crab
  c. grass
  c. hand
  c. larvae irritation
  c. louse
  c. yaw
crabro
  Vespula c.
cracked
  c. heel
  c. lip
crackle
  end-inspiratory c.
  inspiratory "Velcro" c.
  Velcro c.
crackled hair
cradle cap
Crandall syndrome
cranial
  c. arteritis
  c. neuropathy
cranialis
  hyperostosis c.
craniocarpotarsal syndrome
cranio-carpo-tarsal syndrome
craniocervical junction
craniosynostosis
  c. Adelaide type syndrome
  c. type (1, 2) syndrome
craquelé
  eczema c.
  erythema c.
  onychia c.
crateriform ulcer
craw-craw, kra-kra
crazy paving dermatosis
C-reactive
cream
  Acnomel c.
  Acticin C.
  adapalene c.
  Akrinol C.
  ApexiCon E c.
  ASM 981 c.
  AVC C.

NOTES

C

123

cream *(continued)*
 Aveeno Moisture C.
 Avita acne c.
 azelaic acid c.
 banishing c.
 barrier c.
 barrier protective c.
 BeneJoint c.
 Benzashave C.
 butenafine HCl c.
 Carac c.
 Carmol 20 c.
 Carmol HC c.
 cleansing c.
 Clobetasol E C.
 cold c.
 Corticaine c.
 Cortisporin Topical C.
 Cutivate c.
 Cytolex c.
 DiabetiDerm Deep Moisturizing c.
 Differin c.
 diflorasone diacetate c.
 docosanol c.
 doxepin hydrochloride c.
 ELA-Max c.
 Eldopaque Forte c.
 Elidel c.
 Elimite C.
 EMLA c.
 Eucerin c.
 Exact C.
 facial undercover c.
 Finevin c.
 Flex-Power Performance Sports c.
 Florone c.
 fluorouracil c.
 Glyquin c.
 hydrocortisone acetate c.
 hydroquinone c.
 hydroquinone c.
 HydroSkin c.
 Ivarest c.
 Ivy Soothe c.
 Kinerase c.
 Kinerase N6-furfuryladenine skin c.
 Kwell C.
 Lamisil topical c.
 Lasan c.
 Lidakol c.
 LipoTECA c.
 Locilex pexiganan acetate c.
 Locilex topical c.
 Lotrimin AF C.
 Lustra c.
 masoprocol c.
 Maximum Strength Desenex
  Antifungal C.
 Mentax c.

 MetroCream topical c.
 Micanol c.
 Naftin c.
 Neosporin C.
 Neutrogena hand c.
 Neutrogena Healthy Skin anti-
  wrinkle c.
 nonoxynol-9 c.
 Noritate c.
 oil-in-water c.
 pimecrolimus c.
 podophyllotoxin c.
 Pramosone c.
 Prevex Diaper Rash c.
 Prudoxin c.
 Psorion C.
 Renova c.
 Rosac c.
 Solaquin Forte c.
 SSD C.
 Stokoguard outdoor c.
 Sween C.
 tazarotene c.
 Tazorac c.
 terbinafine hydrochloride c.
 tretinoin c.
 triamcinolone c. (TAC)
 Tri-Luma c.
 Unibase c.
 Vaniqa c.
 water-washable c.
 Zanfel c.
 Zetone c.
 Zoderm c.
 Zonalon Topical c.

crease
 allergic c.
 earlobe c.
 palmar c.

creatinine
 c. clearance
 c. kinase

creatininemia

CREB
 cAMP response element-binding
  CREB protein

creeping
 c. eruption
 c. myiasis
 c. ulcer
 c. vesiculation

CREG
 cross-reactive antigen group
  CREG mismatch

creme
 Acid Mantle c.
 Fungoid HC c.
 Gormel c.

Novasome c.
Vite E c.
Creola body
creosote
Crepe short stretch bandage
crepey poikiloderma
crepitans
    peritendinitis c.
crepitant
crepitation
crepitus
crescentic glomerulonephritis
CREST
    calcinosis cutis, Raynaud phenomenon,
     esophageal motility disorder,
     sclerodactyly, and telangiectasia
     CREST syndrome
Cresylate
Creutzfeldt-Jakob disease (CJD)
Cricket recording pulse oximeter
cricoarytenoid joint
cricoid cartilage
Crigler-Najjar
    C.-N. syndrome
    C.-N. syndrome type 1
Crile clamp
Crile-Wood needle holder
Crimean-Congo
    C.-C. hemorrhagic fever
    C.-C. hemorrhagic fever virus
crinis, pl. **crines**
crinium
    fragilitas c.
    nodositas c.
crisis, pl. **crises**
    anaphylactic c.
    anaphylactoid c.
    scleroderma renal c. (SRC)
criteria
    ACR c.
    American College of
     Rheumatology c.
    American Rheumatism
     Association c.
    ARA c.
    Hardonk c.
    Jones c.
    O'Duffy c.
    Paulus c.
    Paulus composite score c.
    Resnick c.
    Sackett c.

Sapporo c.
Steinbrocker c.
WHO c.
World Health Organization c.
Crithidia
    C. luciliae
    C. luciliae immunofluorescence
     assay
criticus
    status c.
crix belly
Crixivan
crocodile
    C. Bile Pill for Asthma
    c. skin
Crohn disease
Crolom Ophthalmic solution
cromoglycate
    PMS-Sodium C.
    sodium c.
cromolyn sodium
Cronkhite-Canada syndrome
crop
    seborrheic keratosis c.
cross
    c. agglutination
    c. infection
    Maltese c.
    c. reaction
    c. sensitization
    C. Top replacement oxygen sensor
cross-antigenicity
cross-desensitization
crossectomy
cross-link
    c.-l. hydroxylysylpyridinoline
    pyridinoline c.-l.
    urine pyridinoline collagen c.-l.
cross-linked N-telopeptide
cross-linking
    abnormal loricrin c.-l.
cross-match
    flow cytometry c.-m. (FCXM)
    negative c.-m.
cross-matching
cross-match-positive recipient
Cross-McKusick-Breen syndrome
cross-presentation
cross-priming pathway
cross-reacting
    c.-r. agglutinin

NOTES

cross-reacting *(continued)*
    c.-r. antibody
    c.-r. material
cross-reaction
cross-reactive
    c.-r. antigen group (CREG)
    c.-r. antigen group mismatch
    c.-r. idiotype
cross-reactivity
cross-sensitivity
cross-sensitization
cross-tachyphylaxis
cross-talk
Crotalidae
Crotalus antitoxin
Crotamiton
crouch
    catcher's c.
croup
croup-associated (CA)
    c.-a. virus
croupous membrane
Crouzon
    C. disease
    C. syndrome
Crowe-Dickermann syndrome
Crowe sign
Crow-Fukase syndrome
crowned dens syndrome
crown of Venus
CRPS
    complex regional pain syndrome
cruenta
    ephidrosis c.
Cruex topical
crural fold
cruris
    epidermophytosis c.
    tinea c.
    trichophytosis c.
crurum
    erythrocyanosis c.
crush artifact
crust
    amiantaceous c.
    milk c.
    oyster-shell c.
crustacean
crustaceous eruption
crusta lactea
crusted
    c. excoriation
    c. ringworm
    c. scabies
    c. tetter
crustosum
    eczema c.
cruzi
    Trypanosoma c.

Cryac
crymophilic
crymophylactic
cryoanesthesia
cryobiology
Cryocrit
Cryo/Cuff
cryofibrinogenemia
cryogen
cryoglobulin
cryoglobulinemia
    essential mixed c.
    familial c.
    mixed c.
    purpura c.
cryolysis
cryopathy
cryophilic
cryophylactic
cryoprecipitable
cryoprecipitagogue
cryoprecipitate
cryoprecipitation
cryoprotein
cryospray
Cryostat
cryosurgery
Cryo-Surg liquid nitrogen spray unit
cryotherapy
cryotolerant
crypt
    c. abscess
    c. epithelial cell apoptosis
    c. epithelial cell dropout
    c. hyperplasia
cryptic epitope
cryptococcal meningoencephalitis
cryptococcica
    folliculitis decalvans c.
cryptococcosis
Cryptococcus neoformans
cryptogenic infection
Cryptomeria japonica
cryptoplasmic
cryptopyic
cryptosporidiosis antibody
***Cryptosporidium* oocyst**
Cryptostroma corticale
cryptostromosis
cryptotoxic
cryptotrichotillomania
crystal
    c. arthritis
    basic calcium phosphate c.
    birefringent c.
    calcium carbonate c.
    calcium oxalate c.
    Charcot-Leyden c.
    cholesterol c.

dehydrate c.
c. deposition disease
hematoidin c.
hemoglobin c.
lipid liquid c.
monosodium urate monohydrate c.
oxalate c.
plate-like c.
potassium permanganate c.
c. rash
c. violet
c. violet vaccine
xanthine c.
crystal-induced arthritis
crystallina
miliaria c.
uridrosis c.
variola c.
crystallopathy
Crysticillin
C. A.S.
C. A.S. injection
CS
citrate synthase
citrate synthesis
cold storage
collagen CS
invariant chain CS
CSD
cat-scratch disease
CSD skin test
CS/DS
chondroitin sulfate/dermatan sulfate
decorin CS/DS
fibromodulin CS/DS
seglycin CS/DS
versican CS/DS
Csillag disease
CS/KS
aggrecan CS/KS
CSS
Churg-Strauss syndrome
CT
computed tomography
thin-section CT
C-Tanna-12D
CTC
clinical transplant coordinator
Ctenocephalides
C. canis
C. canis bite

C. felis
C. felis bite
C-terminal homolog
C-terminus
CTF
Colorado tick fever
CTF virus
CTI
cutaneous tolerance index
CTLA-4
cytotoxic T lymphocyte antigen-4
CTLA-4 soluble protein
CTLA-4-specific Abs
CTNS gene
CTX
cyclophosphamide
ctx
Cytoxan
Cuban itch
Cubicin powder for IV
cubital tunnel syndrome
cuboidal cell
cucumber
sea c.
cuff
rotator c.
c. tear arthropathy
cuff-tear arthropathy shoulder
cuirasse
cancer en c.
carcinoma en c.
culbertsoni
Acanthamoeba c.
Culex
Culicidae
culicosis
Cullen sign
culprit organism
cultivated
c. barley grass
c. barley smut
c. corn grass
c. corn smut
c. oat grass
c. oat smut
c. rye grass
c. rye smut
c. wheat grass
c. wheat smut
cultivation
culture
appropriate c.

NOTES

culture *(continued)*
>bone c.
>elective c.
>enrichment c.
>fungal c.
>mixed lymphocyte c. (MLC)
>Nicolle-Novy-MacNeal c.
>organ c.
>stool c.

cultured
>c. autologous melanocyte
>c. epithelial autografting
>c. thymic epithelium

cumini
>*Syzygium c.*

cumulative
>c. insult dermatitis
>c. toxicity

Cuna
>C. moon child
>C. moon-child albinism

cunicular
cuniculatum
>carcinoma c.
>epithelioma c.

cuniculi
>*Encephalitozoon c.*

cuniculus
Cunninghamella **pathogen**
Cupressaceae pollinosis
Cuprimine
curable serous meningitis
Curaderm
>C. hydrocolloid
>C. hydrocolloid dressing

Curafil
>C. hydrogel dressing
>C. impregnated gauze

Curafoam
>C. foam dressing
>C. wound dressing

Curagel
>C. Hydrogel dressing
>C. Hydrogel sheet

Curaklense wound cleanser
Curasol
>C. hydrogel dressing
>C. impregnated gauze
>C. wound cleanser

Curasorb
>C. calcium alginate dressing
>C. Zinc alginate dressing
>C. Zinc alginate wound cover

curate
CureLight
>C. Broadband red light
>C. lamp

curettage
>c. and desiccation (C&D)
>liposuction-assisted c.

curette, curet
>Cannon c.
>Fox c.
>Heath c.
>Meyhoeffer c.
>Piffard c.
>Reu c.
>Skeele c.

curettement
Curious Experiences Survey
Curity ABD absorptive dressing
Curling ulcer
curly dock weed pollen
currant
currens
>larva c.

current
>d'Arsonval c.
>direct galvanic c.
>Oudin c.
>vacuum tube cutting c.

Curschmann spiral
Curth-Maklin cornification disorder
Curtinova hydrocolloid dressing
curve
>dose-response c.
>epidemic c.

Curvularia lunata
Cushing
>C. disease
>C. syndrome

cushingoid facies
cushion
>Clinicel silicon gel-filled c.
>Ficoll c.
>SkareKare silicon gel-filled c.

Custodiol HTK solution
cut
>coral c.

cutanea
>sclerosis c.

cutaneomeningospinal angiomatosis
cutaneous
>c. abscess
>c. absorption
>c. albinism
>c. amyloid
>c. ancylostomiasis
>c. anergy
>c. anthrax
>c. apoplexy
>c. B-cell lymphocytic leukemia
>c. B-cell lymphoma
>c. blastomycosis
>c. candidiasis
>c. ciliated cyst

c. coccidioidomycosis
c. diphtheria
c. drug eruption
c. dyschromia
c. ectasia
c. elastosis
c. focal mucinosis
c. gangrene
c. graft-versus-host reaction
c. histoplasmosis
c. horn
c. hyperpigmentation
c. intolerance to mechlorethamine
(CIM)
c. larva migrans
c. leukocytoclastic vasculitis
c. lupus
c. lupus erythematosus
c. manifestation
c. mastocytosis
c. melanoma
c. meningioma
c. muscle
c. myelofibrosis
c. necrotizing vasculitis
c. necrotizing venulitis
c. neoplasia
c. neurogenic inflammation
c. nodule
c. polyarteritis nodosa
c. polyarthritis
c. pseudolymphoma
c. purpura
c. pustular lesion
c. sarcoidosis
c. sign
c. sinus
c. sporotrichosis
c. surgeon
c. tag
c. tolerance index (CTI)
c. toxoplasmosis
c. tuberculin test
c. tuberculosis
c. tumor
c. ulcer
cutaneous-subcutaneous nodule
cutaneum
cornu c.
sebum c.
cutaneus
nodulus c.

cutem
cuticle
c. of hair
c. of inner root sheath
cuticularization
Cutifilm
C. Plus
C. Plus composite dressing
Cutinova
C. Cavity
C. Cavity filler
C. Cavity wound filling material
C. foam dressing
C. Hydro
C. Hydro dressing
C. Thin hydrocolloid
C. Thin hydrocolloid dressing
cutireaction test
cutis
amebiasis c.
amyloidosis c.
ancylostomiasis c.
angiolipoma, posttraumatic neuroma,
glomus tumor, eccrine
spiradenoma, and leiomyoma c.
(ANGEL)
c. anserina
asteatosis c.
atheromatosis c.
atrophia maculosa varioliformis c.
aurantiasis c.
B-cell lymphocytoma c.
benign lymphocytoma c.
calcinosis c.
carotenosis c.
carotinosis c.
cholesterolosis c.
cysticercosis c.
diphtheria c.
dystrophic calcinosis c.
endothelioma c.
hemangioma hypertrophicum c.
histiocytoma c.
c. hyperelastica
hypertrophicum c.
idiopathic calcinosis c.
c. laxa
leiomyoma c.
leukemia c.
lymphadenosis benigna c.
lymphocytoma c.
c. marmorata

C

NOTES

cutis *(continued)*
    c. marmorata telangiectatica congenita
    membranous aplasia c.
    metastatic calcinosis c.
    neuroma c.
    osteoma c.
    osteosis c.
    c. pendula
    c. pensilis
    c. rhomboidalis nuchae
    sarcomatosis c.
    sulci c.
    T-cell lymphocytoma c.
    c. testacea
    tuberculosis fungosa c.
    tuberculosis verrucosa c.
    c. unctuosa
    c. vera
    verrucosa c.
    c. verticis gyrata
cutisector
Cutivate
    C. cream
    C. topical
cutter
    C. insect repellent
    motorized c.
cutting
    c. fluid
    c. oil dermatitis
CV
    coefficient of variation
Cw6
    HLA Cw6
CW dye laser
CyA
    cyclosporine
cyanhidrosis
cyaniventris
    Dermatobia c.
cyanoacrylate
cyanocobalamin deficiency
cyanohidrosis
cyanosis
    pernio c.
cyanotic
cycle
    bulge-activation hypothesis of hair c.
    gait c.
    itch-scratch-lichenification c.
    leukapheresis c.
    purine nucleotide c.
cycler
    thermal c.
cyclic
    c. citrullinated peptide
    c. guanosine monophosphate

    c. neutropenia
    c. nucleotide adenosine monophosphate
    c. polypeptide
    c. urticaria
cyclin-dependent
    c.-d. kinase inhibitor 2A (CDKN2A)
    c.-d. kinase inhibitor 2A mutation
cyclizine hydrochloride
Cyclocort topical
cycloheximide
Cyclomen
cyclomethicone
cyclooxygenase (COX)
    c. enzyme
    c. pathway
    c. product
cyclooxygenase-1 (COX-1)
cyclooxygenase-2 (COX-2)
cyclophilin A
cyclophosphamide (CTX)
cyclophosphamide-prednisone
cycloplegic
Cycloprox
cycloserine
cyclosporine (CyA)
    c. A
    c. capsules modified
    high c.
    intermediate c.
    low c.
    c. maintenance therapy
    c. microemulsion
cyclosporine-induced neurotoxicity
Cyclotech dosing device
cylindroma
cylindromatous carcinoma
Cymetra micronized AlloDerm
Cynodon dactylon
cynomolgus macaque tissue
cypress
    Arizona c.
    bald c.
    Italian c.
    Monterey c.
cyproheptadine hydrochloride
cyproterone acetate (CPA)
Cyrano defect
Cys-containing type II collagen
CysLT1
CysLT2
cyst
    adventitious c.
    anogenital epidermal c.
    anogenital pilar c.
    anogenital sebaceous c.
    anogenital vestibular c.
    apocrine retention c.

Baker c.
branchial c.
bronchogenic c.
colloid c.
compound c.
cutaneous ciliated c.
dermoid c.
desmoid c.
epidermal c.
epidermoid cyst
epithelial c.
eruptive vellus hair c.
false c.
Favre-Racouchot c.
follicular infundibular c.
follicular isthmus c.
hair c.
implantation c.
inclusion c.
jaw c.
keratinous c.
milia c.
mucinous c.
mucous c.
multilocular thymic c. (MTC)
myxoid c.
parasitic c.
parvilocular c.
pheomycotic c.
pilar c.
piliferous c.
pilonidal c.
popliteal c.
preauricular c.
proliferating pilar c.
proliferating trichilemmal c.
pseudohorned c.
renal c.
retention c.
sebaceous c.
sequestration c.
subchondral c.
synovial c.
thyroglossal c.
trichilemmal c.
unicameral c.
unilocular c.
vanilla-fudge c.
vestibular c.
cystadenoma
apocrine c.

cystatin
c. C
c. C amyloidosis
c. C-origin amyloid deposit
cysteamine
cysteine
c. proteinase
c. proteinase inhibitor
cysteinyl leukotriene, LTC$_4$
cystic
c. acne
c. deformation
c. fibrosis test
c. hidradenoma
c. hygroma
c. lymphatic malformation
cystica
acne c.
cysticercosis cutis
cysticidal
cysticum
acanthoma adenoides c.
epithelioma adenoides c.
lymphangioma c.
cystide
cystis
cystitis
acrolein-induced c.
hemorrhagic c.
cystoscopy and dilation (C&D)
cystous
Cystoviridae
cytapheresis
cytarabine hydrochloride
cytase
cytoadhesion
cytochalasin B, D
cytochrome
c. C
c. deficiency
c. P450
c. P-450-3A4
cytocidal
cytodiagnosis
CytoGam
cytogenic technique
cytogram
cytoid body
cytoimmunologic monitoring
cytokine
antiinflammatory c.
IL-1, -2, -3, -4, -10, -13 c.

C

NOTES

cytokine *(continued)*
    IL-1-beta c.
    monocyte-derived c.
    motif-bearing c.
    pleiotropic c.
    c. production
    proinflammatory c.
    c. synthesis inhibitory factor
    TH1 c.
    TNF mRNA c.
Cytolex cream
cytology
cytolysin
cytolysis
cytolytic
    c. effector cell
    c. macromolecular complex
cytomegalic
    c. cell
    c. inclusion body
cytomegalovirus (CMV)
    c. antigenemia
    congenital c.
    c. disease
    c. immune globulin intravenous,
      human
    c. retinitis
    tissue-invasive c. (TI-CMV)
cytometer
    Epics Elite flow c.
    FACSCalibur flow c.
    FACScan flow c.
cytometric indirect immunofluorescence
cytometry
    flow c.
cytopathogenic virus
cytophagic
    c. histiocytic panniculitis
    c. lobular panniculitis
cytophagous
cytophagy
cytophil group
cytophilic antibody
cytophylactic
cytophylaxis
cytoplasm
cytoplasmic
    c. antineutrophil cytoplasmic
      antibody (C-ANCA)

    c. granule
    c. inclusion
    c. inclusion body
    c. islet cell
    c. plaque
cytoprotective agent
cytoryctes
Cytosar-U
cytosine arabinoside
cytoskeletal
    c. protein
    c. scaffold
cytoskeleton
cytosolic
CytoTab polyclonal antibody
cytotoxic
    c. agent
    c. armamentarium
    c. drug
    c. immunologic drug reaction
    c. immunosuppressive therapy
    c. T cell
    c. test
    c. T lymphocyte antigen-4 (CTLA-
      4)
cytotoxicity
    antibody-dependent cellular c.
      (ADCC)
    c. assay
    complement-dependent c. (CDC)
    natural killer-mediated c.
    NK cell-mediated c.
cytotoxin
cytotoxin-positive stain
cytotropic
    c. antibody
    c. antibody test
cytotropism
Cytovene
Cytovene-IV
Cytoxan (ctx)
    C. injection
    C., methotrexate, etoposide,
      dexamethasone (CMED)
    C. Oral

D

D antigen
Aquasol A & D
Congestant D
Coricidin D
D deficiency factor
Sleep-Eze D

D₂

prostaglandin D_2 (PGD2)
d4T, didehydrothymidine
DA

DA pregnancy test
Daae disease
Dab-o-Matic
Dabska tumor
dacarbazine (DTIC)
daclizumab monoclonal antibody
DaCosta syndrome
dacryoadenitis
dacryocystitis
dacryocystorhinostomy
dactinomycin
dactyledema
Dactylis glomerata
dactylitis

blistering distal d.
distal d.
multidigit d.
septic d.
d. strumosa
syphilitic d.
d. tuberculosa
tuberculous d.
dactylolysis spontanea
dactylon

Cynodon d.
dactyloscopy
daisy

oxeye d.
Dakar bat virus
DAKO CD57
Dakrina Ophthalmic solution
Dalacin

D. C
D. T
D. Vaginal
Dalalone

D. D.P.
D. L.A.
Dale reaction
dalfopristin
Dalmane
damage

articular cartilage d.
bacterial-induced vascular d.

collateral d.
extravillous trophoblastic d.
immunologic organ d.
d. index score
musculotendinous d.
residual thermal d. (RTD)
sun and chemical combination d.
toxic organ d.
damaged joint progression
dammini

Ixodes d.
DANAOS

Diagnostic and Neuronal Analysis of
Skin Cancer
danazol
Danbolt-Closs syndrome
dandelion
dander

animal d.
cat d.
cow d.
dog d.
inhaled d.
d'Andrews

arthrites pseudoseptiques et
bacterides d'A.
Dandruff Treatment Shampoo
dandy fever
Dane particle
Danex
Dan-Gard
Danielssen-Boeck

D.-B. disease
D.-B. sarcoidosis
Danielssen disease
Danocrine
Danysz

D. effect
D. phenomenon
Dapa
Dapacin Cold Capsule
dapsone (DDS)

d. topical gel
Dapsone Pharmacokinetics
dapsone/pyrimethamine
daptomycin
Daraprim
DAR breathing system
Dardik clamp
Darier

morbus D.
D. sign
Darier-Roussy sarcoid
Darier-White disease
dark dot disease

darkfield
> d. examination of tissue smear
> d. microscopy

darkly pigmented macule
dark-staining nodule
Darrach procedure
d'Arsonval current
dartos
> tunica d.

D'Assumpeau rhytidoplasty marker
dasycarpus
> *Dictamnus d.*

data
> D. Safety Monitoring Board
>   (DSMB)
> x-ray crystallographic d.

database
> Cardiac Transplant Research d.

date
> d. boil
> d. fever

Datex Normocap infrared capnometer
datura plant
Daudi lymphoma cell
daughter cell
daunorubicin
> d. citrate
> d. hydrochloride

DaunoXome
Davidsohn differential test
da Vinci Surgical system
Davis
> D. and Geck systemic plastic
>   reconstruction P3 or PS3 needle
> D. and Geck systemic PR and
>   PRE P3 or PS3 needle

Dawbarn sign
Dawson encephalitis
3-day
> 3-d. fever
> 3-d. measles

21-Day Cumulative Irritancy Assay
daylight sign
Daypro
DayQuil Sinus with Pain Relief
2-day ultrarush protocol
DBI
> documented bacterial infection

D&C dye
DCL
> disseminated cutaneous leishmaniasis

DCTD
> diffuse connective tissue disease

DDA
> digital dermoscopy analyzer

ddC
> zalcitabine

ddc
> dideoxycytidine

D-Di
> D-dimer

ddI
> didanosine

D-dimer (D-Di)
DDS
> dapsone

DE
> Ru-Tuss DE

de
> d. facto
> D. Morgan spot
> d. novo
> d. novo pyrimidine synthesis
> d. novo squamous cell carcinoma
> d. Quervain disease
> d. Quervain stenosing tenosynovitis
> d. Quervain syndrome
> D. Sanctis-Cacchione syndrome

deacylation
dead
> d. finger
> d. space:tidal volume ratio

dead-end host
deafness
> abnormalities of genitalia,
>   retardation of growth, and d.
> bilateral sensorineural d.
> keratitis d.
> lentigines, electrocardiographic
>   defects, ocular hypertelorism,
>   pulmonary stenosis, abnormalities
>   of genitalia, retardation of
>   growth, d. (LEOPARD)
> nerve d.

deallergize
deamidated
> d. gliadin
> d. gliadin peptide

deaminase
> adenosine d. (ADA)
> myoadenylate d.

death
> activation-induced cell d. (AICD)
> bone d.
> d. domain
> donor brain d.
> fetal d.

Debacterol
DEBRA
> Dystrophic Epidermolysis Bullosa
>   Research Association of America

Debré phenomenon
débridement
> arthroscopic d.
> Papain enzymatic d.

debrider
> Accuzyme enzymatic d.
> Panafil enzymatic d.

Panafil-White enzymatic d.
Santyl enzymatic d.
debris
phagocytosable d.
subungual d.
Debrisan
D. topical
D. wound cleanser
Debrox drops
debulking
cold steel d.
DEC
diethylcarbamazine
Decadron
D. and Hexadrol
D. Injection
D. Oral
D. Phosphate
D. Phosphate Respihaler
D. Phosphate Turbinaire
Decadron-LA
Decaject-LA
decalvans
acne d.
folliculitis d.
keratosis follicularis spinulosa d.
porrigo d.
tinea d.
decalvant
decamer
decamethonium
decarboxylase
glutamic acid d. (GAD)
d. inhibitor
decarboxylation
Decaspray
decay
bone d.
decidua
d. basalis
d. parietalis
decidual tissue
deciduous skin
Declomycin
Decofed Syrup
decompensation
decompression
core d.
Decon
Par D.
Deconamine
D. SR

D. Syrup
D. Tablet
deconditioning
motor d.
physical d.
decongestant
Balminil D.
Benylin D.
Certified D.
Chlor-Tripolon D.
d. nasal spray
New D.
d. nose drops
d. tablet
topical d.
Deconsal II
Decontabs
decorin CS/DS
decoy DNA
decreased
d. fertility, short stature
d. renal function
decrementi
stadium d.
decubation
decubital gangrene
decubitus ulcer
dedifferentiated
Deelman effect
deep
d. felon
d. hemangioma
d. mycosis
d. penetrating nevus
deep-seated
d.-s. pustule
d.-s. vesicle
deer
d. fly
d. fly bite
d. fly disease
d. fly fever
d. hair
d. tick
DEET
diethyltoluamide
Deet
defect
congenital ectodermal d.
congenital hemidysplasia with ichthyosiform erythroderma and limb d.'s (CHILD)

D

NOTES

135

defect *(continued)*
Cyrano d.
gene d.
host d.
human host defense d.
human nude d.
humoral d.
immunoregulatory d.
limb d.
neuroectodermal d.
opsonophagocytic d.
retardation and ear d.
scleral d.
standing cutaneous cone d.
T-cell d.
tricone d.
defective
d. bacteriophage
d. interfering (DI)
d. interfering particle
d. phage
d. probacteriophage
d. prophage
d. virus
Defen-LA
defense
immunological d.
d. mechanism
defensin
defervesce
defervescence
defervescentiae
stadium d.
defervescent stage
defibrination syndrome
deficiency
acetylcholinesterase d.
acquired biotin d.
acquired C1 inhibitor d.
ADA d.
adenosine deaminase d.
alpha$_1$-antitrypsin d.
alpha$_1$-proteinase d.
antibody d.
argininosuccinate synthetase d.
beta-mannosidase d.
biotin d.
biotinidase d.
carnitine palmitoyltransferase d.
C7D d.
ceramidase d.
C1 esterase inhibitor d.
C1r d.
cobalamin d.
combined antibody and cellular d.
complement d.
copper d.
C1q d.
cyanocobalamin d.

cytochrome d.
essential fatty acid d.
factor (D, H, I) d.
familial alpha-lipoprotein d.
familial apoprotein CII d.
folic acid d.
genetic C2 d.
glucose-6-phosphatase d.
growth hormone d.
HGPRT d.
histamine-releasing factor d.
HRF d.
hyaluronidase d.
hypoxanthine-guanine
  phosphoribosyltransferase d.
IgA d.
IL-12p40 d.
IL-2 receptor alpha chain
  (CD25) d.
immune d. (ID)
immunity d.
immunological d.
interferon gamma receptor d.
iron d.
Jak3 d.
juvenile biotin d.
leukocyte adhesion d. (LAD)
leukocyte adhesion d. type 1
  (LAD1)
leukocyte adhesion d. type 2
  (LAD2)
leukocyte adhesion d. type 3
  (LAD3)
leukocyte adhesion d. type 4
  (LAD4)
lipoprotein lipase d.
mannan-binding lectin d.
MHC antigen d.
MHC class (I, II) d.
MPO d.
multiple sulfatase d.
myeloperoxidase d.
myoadenylate deaminase d.
myophosphorylase d.
neonatal biotin d.
neutrophil-specific (secondary)
  granule d.
niacin d.
opsonic d.
ornithine transcarbamylase d.
pantothenic acid d.
phagocytic d.
phosphotransferase d.
placental sulfatase d.
p56 Lck d.
primary cell-mediated d.
primary immune d. (PID)
prolidase d.
properdin d.

protein C d.
purine nucleoside phosphorylase d.
pyridoxine d.
pyridoxol d.
pyruvate kinase d.
riboflavin d.
secondary antibody d.
secretory component d.
selective antipolysaccharide
  antibody d. (SPAD)
selenium d.
severe combined immune d.
  (SCID)
specific antibody d. (SAD)
steroid sulfatase d.
thiamine d.
tocopherol d.
tyrosine aminotransferase d.
vitamin A d.
vitamin B d.
vitamin B_1 d.
vitamin B_5 d.
vitamin B_6 d.
vitamin B_{12} d.
vitamin C d.
vitamin D d.
vitamin E d.
vitamin K d.
ZAP-70 d.
zinc d.
deflazacort
deflexion
  hip d.
deflorescence
defluvium
  d. capillorum
  d. unguium
defluxio
  d. capillorum
  d. ciliorum
defluxion
defoliating cotton
defoliation of cotton
deformans
  spondylosis d.
deformation
  cystic d.
deformity
  angel-wing d.
  arthritis without d.
  bent-fork d.
  boutonnière d.

canestick d.
clawing d.
cock-up d.
flexion d.
habit tic d.
opera-glass d.
pencil and cup d.
piano-key d.
postosteotomy d.
saddle nose d.
swan-neck d.
trap-door d.
violin d.
zigzag d.
defurfuration
degenerated microfilaria
degeneration
  acromioclavicular d.
  amyloid d.
  ballooning d.
  basophilic d.
  colliquative d.
  colloid d.
  elastoid d.
  elastotic d.
  epithelial d.
  fatty d.
  fibrinous d.
  glenohumeral d.
  granular d.
  hepatolenticular d.
  hyaline d.
  liquefaction d.
  malignant d.
  mucinous d.
  mucoid d.
  myxomatous d.
  paraneoplastic subacute cerebellar d.
  reticular d.
  sternoclavicular joint d.
  unilateral macular d.
degenerativa
  melanosis corii d.
degenerative
  d. arthritis
  d. collagenous plaque
  d. tendinopathy
Degos
  D. acanthoma
  D. disease
  malignant papillomatosis of D.
  D. syndrome

D

NOTES

Degos-Delort-Tricot syndrome
degradation
    postmortem core protein d.
degradomics
degranulation
    goblet cell d.
    piecemeal d. (PMD)
degreasing properties
30-degree oblique arthroscope
dehaptenation
dehiscence
Dehist injection
dehumidification
dehumidifier
dehydrate crystal
dehydration
dehydroemetine
dehydroepiandrosterone sulfate (DHEAS)
dehydrogenase
    3-beta-hydroxysteroid d. (3-beta-HSD)
    17-beta-hydroxysteroid d. (17-beta-HSD)
    inosinic acid d.
    lactate d.
    lactic d. (LDH)
    uridine diphosphoglucose d.
Deinococcus radiodurans
DEJ
    dermal-epidermal junction
Dejerine-Sottas disease
Deknatel wound tape
Del
    D. Aqua-5 Gel
    D. Aqua-10 Gel
delavirdine
Delaxin
delayed
    d. allergy
    d. anagen release
    d. blanching
    d. complication
    d. graft function (DGF)
    d. hypersensitivity (DH)
    d. hypersensitivity immunologic drug reaction
    d. hypersensitivity skin testing
    d. nasal response (DYNR)
    d. patch test reading
    d. pressure urticaria
    d. systemic reaction
    d. tanning
    d. telogen release
    d. transfusion reaction
    d. xenograft rejection (DXR)
delayed-type
    d.-t. hypersensitivity (DTH)
    d.-t. hypersensitivity response
Delcort topical

deletion
    homozygous autosomal recessive d.
    tolerance through d.
Delhi
    D. boil
    D. sore
deliensis
    Trombicula d.
delitescence
delivery
    drug d.
delling
DELM imaging system
Del-Mycin topical
delta, δ
    d. agent
    d. antigen
    d. antigen hepatitis
    Galton d.
    d. sleep
    d. virus
delta-aminolevulinic acid
Delta-Cortef Oral
Deltasone
    D. Dosepak
    D. Oral
Delta-Tritex topical
deltoidea
    Anthopsis d.
    Aspergillus d.
delusion of parasitosis
demarcated
    d. cellulitis
    d. reaction
demarcation
Demarquay sign
Dematiaceae
dematiaceous fungus
Demazin
d'emblée
    bubon d.
    mycosis fungoides d.
    syphilis d.
demeclocycline hydrochloride
dementia
    transmissible d.
Demerol
demodectic
    d. acariasis
    d. mange
Demodex
    D. brevis
    D. canis
    D. equi
    D. folliculorum
demodice
demodicidosis
demodicosis
DeMorgan hemangioma

Demulen
demyelinating
denaturation
    collagen d.
denaturing agent
Denavir ointment
dendritic
    d. epidermal cell
    d. macrophage
    d. morphology
dendriticum
    Dicrocoelium d.
dendritiform
dendrocyte
dendrocytoma
    myxoid dermal d.
dengue
    d. facies
    hemorrhagic d.
    d. hemorrhagic fever
    d. shock syndrome
    d. virus
denileukin diftitox
denitrificans
    Alcaligenes d.
Dennie
    D. infraorbital fold
    D. line
    D. sign
Dennie-Marfan syndrome
Dennie-Morgan
    D.-M. infraorbital fold
    D.-M. line
    D.-M. sign
Denorex
densa
    lamina d.
    sublamina d.
dense-deposit disease
densitometry
    bone d.
density
    bone mineral d. (BMD)
    fixed charge d.
    d. gradient bone marrow progenitor enrichment
    d. gradient centrifugation
dental
    d. amalgam
    d. fistula
    d. plaque

    d. sinus
    d. sinus tract
dentatus
    Stephanurus d.
denticola
    Treponema d.
dentifrice
dentinogenesis imperfecta
dentocariosa
    Rothia d.
denture
    d. epulis
    d. stomatitis
denture-sore-mouth syndrome
denudation of pustule
denude
denuded
Denys-Leclef phenomenon
deodorant dermatitis
deodorized mineral spirits, propylene glycol, fatty acid soap
2′-deoxyadenosine
deoxycholate
2-deoxy-D-glucose
deoxynucleoside
deoxypyridinoline
deoxyribonuclease (DNase)
    fibrinolysin and d.
    human recombinant d.
deoxyribonucleic
    d. acid (DNA)
    d. acid amplicon
    d. acid aneuploidy
    d. acid autosensitivity
    d. acid binding
    d. acid hybridization
deoxyribose
deoxyspergualin (DSG)
deoxyvirus
Depakene
Depakote
Depen
dependent edema
Dependovirus
DEPex
dephosphorylation
depigmentation
    congenital d.
    d. therapy
depigmenting agent
depigmentosus
    nevus d.

D

NOTES

depilate
depilation
depilatory
    chemical d.
depletion
    acetylcholine d.
depMedalone Injection
depocorticosteroid
    intraarticular d.
Depoject Injection
depolymerize
Depo-Medrol Injection
Depopred Injection
deposit
    calcitonin-origin amyloid d.
    cystatin C-origin amyloid d.
    glycosphingolipid d.
    immune d.
    immunoglobulin light chain-origin
      amyloid d.
    2-microglobulin-origin amyloid d.
    prion protein-origin amyloid d.
    protein origin amyloid d.
    transthyretin-origin amyloid d.
deposition
    cell d.
    copper d.
    fibrin d.
    hemosiderin d.
    hydroxyapatite crystal d.
    nonlinear IgA d.
    silicone d.
    urate d.
depot reaction
depth
    optical penetration d. (OPD)
depulization
Dercum disease
derivative
    bioactive lipid d.
    ergotamine d.
    piperidine d.
    purified protein d. (PPD)
    undecylenic acid and d.'s
    valproic acid and d.'s
derivative-standard
    purified protein d.-s. (PPD-S)
DERM
    Dermatology Education by Recall of
    Mnemonics
Derma
    D. blade
    FotoFinder D.
    D. Instruments
    D. K laser
    D. 20 laser system
    D. Soap
Dermablend makeup
Dermabond topical skin adhesive

dermabrader
    HydroBrader irrigating/aspirating d.
    Iverson d.
    sandpaper d.
dermabrasion
    diamond fraise d.
Dermacea
    D. alginate dressing
    D. alginate wound cover
Dermacentor
    D. andersoni
    D. occidentalis
    D. variabilis
Dermacne
Dermacomb topical
Dermacort topical
Dermaflex
    D. Gel
    D. HC
Derma-Gel hydrogel sheet
Dermagraft
    D. dermal substitute
    D. skin device
    D. skin substitute
    D. wound healing device
Dermagraft-TC skin substitute
Dermagran
    D. hydrogel dressing
    D. impregnated gauze
    D. ointment
    D. ointment/dressing
    D. wound cleanser
dermagraphy
dermahemia
Dermaide
dermal
    d. duct tumor
    Elta D.
    d. hypoplasia
    d. leishmanoid
    d. lesion
    d. lymphatic
    d. melanocytosis
    d. microvascular unit
    d. muscle
    d. papilla
    D. Regeneration Template
    d. system
    d. tuberculosis
    d. venular hyperpermeability
dermalaxia
dermal-epidermal junction (DEJ)
DermaMend
    D. cavity foam dressing
    D. foam wound dressing
    D. hydrogel dressing
    D. island foam dressing
    D. wound cleanser
dermametropathism

dermamyiasis linearis migrans oestrosa
Dermanail
DermaNet
    D. contact layer sheet
    D. contact layer wound dressing
Dermanyssus gallinae
Dermaphot system
Dermapor glove
DermaPulse
Dermarest
    D. Dricort
    D. Dricort topical
DermaScan
DermaSeptic device
Derma-Smoothe/FS topical
Derma-Smoothe Oil
DermaSof gel sheeting
Dermasone
DermAssist
    D. filler
    D. Glycerin
    D. Glycerin hydrogel dressing
    D. hydrocolloid
    D. hydrocolloid dressing
    D. hydrocolloid dressing material
    D. impregnated gauze
    D. transparent film
    D. wound filling material
dermatalgia
Dermatell
    D. hydrocolloid
    D. hydrocolloid dressing
    D. hydrocolloid dressing material
DermaTemp DT-1000 infrared
  temperature scanner
dermatic
dermatica
    zona d.
dermatitic
dermatitidis
    Ajellomyces d.
    Blastomyces d.
dermatitis, pl. **dermatitides**
    acneform d.
    actinic d.
    d. actinica
    acupuncture needle d.
    airborne contact d.
    allergic eczematous contact-type d.
    allergic gold d.
    d. ambustionis
    ammonia d.

ancylostoma d.
arsenical contact d.
arsphenamine d.
d. artefacta
ashy d.
Assessment Measure for Atopic D.
  (AMAD)
asteatotic d.
atopic hand d.
autoimmune progesterone d.
d. autophytica
autosensitization d.
avian mite d.
baker's d.
berlock d.
beryllium d.
bhiwanol d.
Blaschko d.
blastomycetic d.
d. blastomycotica
blister beetle d.
blistering d.
blousing garter d.
bristle-worm d.
brown-tail moth d.
brucella d.
bubble gum d.
d. bullosa striata pratensis
by-the-wind sailor d.
d. calorica
Calycophora d.
carcinomatous d.
cardiac pacemaker d.
carpet beetle d.
caterpillar d.
cement d.
cercarial d.
chemical d.
chigger d.
chromate d.
chronic acral d.
chronic papular d.
Citrus Red d.
clothing d.
cobalt d.
coin-rubbing d.
d. combustionis
condom d.
d. congelationis
contact d.
contact-type d.
contagious pustular d.

D

NOTES

dermatitis *(continued)*

    contraceptive d.
    d. contusiformis
    copper d.
    copra mite d.
    coral d.
    cosmetic d.
    d. cruris pustulosa et atrophicans
    cumulative insult d.
    cutting oil d.
    deodorant d.
    Dermo-Jet nickel d.
    desquamative d.
    detergent d.
    dhobie mark d.
    dialysis d.
    diaper d.
    diving suit d.
    dried fruit d.
    durable-press allergic contact d.
    dyshidrotic d.
    d. dysmenorrhoeica
    earlobe allergic d.
    eczematoid d.
    endogenous d.
    Engman d.
    eosinophilic d.
    epoxy resin d.
    Erysipelothrix d.
    d. erythematosa
    erythematous macular d.
    d. escharotica
    d. estivalis
    ethylenediamine d.
    d. excoriativa infantum
    d. exfoliativa
    d. exfoliativa epidemica
    d. exfoliativa infantum
    d. exfoliativa neonatorum
    exfoliative d.
    exudative discoid and lichenoid d.
    eyeglass frame d.
    eyelid d.
    d. factitia
    factitial d.
    factitious d.
    familial rosacea-like d.
    feather hydroid d.
    fiberglass d.
    fire coral d.
    fire sponge d.
    flea-collar d.
    florid d.
    Florida seaweed d.
    follicular nummular d.
    d. gangrenosa
    d. gangrenosa infantum
    genital atopic d.
    glove d.

    gold d.
    hearing aid d.
    d. hemostatica
    d. hiemalis
    housewives' d.
    d. hypostatica
    indirect coelenterate d.
    industrial d.
    d. infectiosa eczematoides
    infectious eczematoid d.
    infectious eczematous d.
    infectious labial d.
    insect d.
    interdigital d.
    irritant contact d. (ICD)
    irritant hand d.
    Jacquet erosive diaper d.
    Japanese hot foot d.
    juvenile plantar d. (JPD)
    karaya gum d.
    Korean yellow moth d.
    Leiner d.
    lichenified d.
    lichenoid contact d.
    livedoid d.
    Lynghya d.
    machine-worker d.
    mango d.
    marine d.
    meadow d.
    meadow-grass d.
    d. medicamentosa
    metal d.
    moth d.
    mother d.
    d. multiformis
    mycotic d.
    napkin d.
    nasal cannula d.
    nasal solar d.
    neck d.
    nematode d.
    neomycin d.
    nickel hand d.
    d. nodosa
    d. nodularis necrotica
    nonspecific d.
    nose-pad d.
    nummular eczematous d.
    nutritional deficiency d.
    nylon stocking d.
    Objective Severity Assessment of
      Atopic d. (OSAAD)
    occupational contact d.
    occupational rubber d.
    ocular atopic d.
    onion mite d.
    oozing d.
    Paederus d.

paper d.
d. papillaris capillitii
papular d.
papulosquamous d.
paraphenylenediamine d.
parthenium d.
d. pediculoides ventricosus
pellagra-associated d.
pellagroid d.
Pelodera d.
perfume d.
periocular d.
perioral d.
periorbital d.
periorificial d.
permanent-press finish clothing d.
photoallergic contact d. (PACD)
photocontact d.
photoingestant d.
photoirritant contact d. (PICD)
photosensitive nonscarring d.
photosensitivity d.
phototoxic contact d.
phototoxic textile d.
phytophototoxic d.
pigmentary atopic d.
pigmented purpuric lichenoid d.
plant d.
plantar d.
poison bun sponge d.
poison ivy d.
poison oak d.
poison sumac d.
poppers' d.
popsicle d.
d. pratensis striata
precancerous d.
primary irritant d.
proliferative d.
propylene glycol d.
protein contact d.
Pseudomonas cepacia d.
psoriasiform d.
d. psoriasiformis nodularis
purple sail d.
purpuric pigmented lichenoid d.
radiation d.
ragweed oil d.
rat mite d.
rebound d.
red feed d.
red moss d.

red sponge d.
red tide d.
d. repens
rhabditic d.
rhus d.
Rockwool d.
roentgen-ray d.
rosaceaform d.
rubber additive d.
sandal strap d.
Schamberg d.
schistosomal d.
schistosome cercarial d.
scombroid d.
sea anemone d.
sea cucumber d.
sea louse d.
sea nettle d.
sea urchin d.
seaweed d.
seborrheic d.
d. seborrheica
Severity Scoring of Atopic D. (SCORAD)
shoe dye d.
shoe-leather d.
d. simplex
Six-Area, Six-Sign Atopic D. (SASSAD)
d. skiagraphica
skin bends d.
soap d.
soapfish d.
solar d.
d. solaris
sponge spicule d.
starfish d.
d. stasis
stasis d.
stethoscope d.
stinging coral d.
stinging water d.
stomal d.
d. striata pratensis bullosa
subcorneal pustular d.
suction-socket prosthetic d.
sweaty sock d.
swimmer's d.
systemic contact d.
T-cell-mediated delayed type hypersensitivity d.
tetramethylthiuram d.

D

NOTES

dermatitis *(continued)*
  textile d.
  tinea d.
  Toxicodendron d.
  traumatic d.
  traumatica d.
  trefoil d.
  trunk d.
  tulip bulb d.
  uncinarial d.
  urostomy d.
  d. vegetans
  Velella velella d.
  d. venenata
  d. verrucosa
  verrucose d.
  vesicular d.
  weeping d.
  x-ray d.
dermatitis-arthritis-tenosynovitis syndrome
dermatoalloplasty
dermatoarthritis
  lipoid d.
dermatoautoplasty
Dermatobia
  D. cyaniventris
  D. hominis
dermatobiasis
dermatoblepharitis
dermatocele
dermatocellulitis
dermatochalasia
dermatochalasis
dermatoconiosis
dermatoconjunctivitis
  contact d.
dermatocyst
dermatodynia
dermatodysplasia verruciformis
dermatofibroma protuberans
dermatofibrosarcoma protuberans (DFSP)
dermatofibrosis
  d. lenticularis
  d. lenticularis disseminata
dermatogenic torticollis
dermatoglyph
dermatoglyphic
dermatoglyphics
dermatograph
dermatographia
  black d.
  urticarial d.
  white d.
dermatographic
dermatographism
dermatography
dermatoheliosis

dermatoheteroplasty
dermatohistopathology
dermatohomoplasty
dermatoid
Dermatologic Diagnostic Algorithm
dermatologist
dermatology
  D. Education by Recall of Mnemonics (DERM)
  D. Teachers Exchange Group (DTEG)
Dermatology-Specific Quality of Life (DSQL)
dermatolysis palpebrarum
dermatoma
dermatomal
  d. distribution
  d. superficial telangiectasia
  d. zoster
dermatome
  Duval disposable d.
  Reese d.
  Tanner-Vandeput mesh d.
dermatomegaly
dermatomic area
dermatomycosis
  d. furfuracea
  d. microsporina
  d. pedis
  d. trichophytina
dermatomyoma
dermatomyositis (DM)
  amyopathic d. (ADM)
  Banker-type d.
  Brunsting-type d.
  juvenile d. (JDMS)
  d. sine myositis
dermatoneurosis
dermatonosology
Dermatop
dermatopathia pigmentosa reticularis
dermatopathic
  d. anemia
  d. lymphadenitis
  d. lymphadenopathy
dermatopathology
dermatopathy
dermatophagia
Dermatophagoides
  D. farinae
  D. microceras
  D. pteronyssinus
dermatophilosis
Dermatophilus congolensis
dermatophone
dermatophylaxis
dermatophyte
  d. fungal infection
  d. infection

dermatophytid
  erysipelas-like d.
  d. reaction
Dermatophytin
Dermatophytin-O
dermatophytosis furfuracea
dermatoplastic
dermatoplasty
  Thompson d.
dermatopolymyositis
dermatopolyneuritis
dermatorrhagia
dermatorrhea
dermatorrhexis
dermatosclerosis
dermatoscope
  handheld d.
dermatoscopy
  ABCD rule of d.
  d. using epiluminescent microscopy
dermatosis, pl. **dermatoses**
  acantholytic d.
  acarine d.
  acquired perforating d.
  acute febrile neutrophilic d.
  adult bullous d.
  angioneurotic d.
  arthropod d.
  ashy d.
  Auspitz d.
  benign papular acantholytic d.
  Blaschko linear d.
  Bowen precancerous d.
  carbon d.
  childhood bullous d.
  cholinogenic d.
  chronic hemosideric d.
  d. cinecienta
  crazy paving d.
  dermolytic bullous d.
  digitate d.
  fall d.
  flaky paint d.
  gonorrheal d.
  Gougerot-Blum d.
  hand d.
  ichthyosiform d.
  IgA d.
  industrial d.
  inflammatory d.
  intraepidermal neutrophilic IgA d.
  juvenile plantar d.

  lichenoid chronic d.
  linear IgA bullous d. (LABD)
  meadow-grass d.
  d. medicamentosa
  menstrual d.
  neutrophilic intraepidermal IgA d.
  occupational d.
  papulosa nigra d.
  d. papulosa nigra
  persistent acantholytic d.
  pigmented purpuric lichenoid d.
  progressive pigmentary d.
  pruritic d.
  pustular d.
  radiation d.
  rhythmical d.
  Schamberg progressive pigmented
    purpuric d.
  seborrheic d.
  skin-dominated linear IgA
    bullous d.
  spring d.
  subcorneal pustular d.
  summer d.
  temperature-dependent d.
  transient acantholytic d. (TAD)
  ulcerative d.
  Unna d.
  vascular d.
  vulvar d.
dermatosparaxis type
dermatotherapy
dermatothlasia
dermatothlasis
dermatotropic
dermatoxenoplasty
dermatozoiasis
dermatozoon, pl. **dermatozoa**
dermatozoonosis
dermatrophia
Dermazine shampoo
dermic
Dermicel tape
DermiCort
dermis
  adventitial d.
  papillary d.
  periadnexal d.
  reticular d.
  upper d.
dermite
dermitis

D

NOTES

DermMaster system
dermoepidermal
    d. interface
    d. junction
    d. nevus
dermogram
    black d.
    geriatric d.
    pediatric d.
dermographia
dermographism
    cold-dependent d.
    white d.
dermohypodermal
dermoid
    d. cyst
    inclusion d.
    sequestration d.
Dermo-Jet nickel dermatitis
Dermolate topical
dermolysis
dermolytic bullous dermatosis
dermonecrotic
dermoneurosis
dermonosology
dermopanniculosis formans
dermopathy
    diabetic d.
    nephrogenic fibrosing d.
    restrictive d.
dermophlebitis
dermoplasty
dermoscopy using epiluminescent microscopy
dermostenosis
dermostosis
dermosyphilopathy
dermotoxin
dermotropic
dermotuberculin reaction
Dermovan
Dermovate
Dermoxyl
Dermtex
    D. HC with Aloe
    D. HC with Aloe topical
Derm-Vi Soap
DES
    diethylstilbestrol
desaturation
Desbuquois syndrome
descarboethoxyloratadine
Desenex
    Prescription Strength D.
desensitization
    anaphylactic d.
    epithelial lining fluid d. (ELFD)
    heterologous d.
    homologous d.

    massive-dose d.
    penicillin d.
desensitize
desert
    d. ragweed
    d. sore
desetope
desiccant
desiccation
    curettage and d. (C&D)
    mucous d.
desiccative
Desiclovir
design
    Clear By D.
    Morrey-Coonrad d.
desipramine
Desitin topical
Desjardins forceps
desloratadine tablet
Desmarres
    D. clamp
    D. retractor
desmin
desmoglein (Dsg)
    recombinant d. (rDsg)
desmoglein-1 (Dsg1)
desmoglein-3 (Dsg3)
desmoid
    d. cyst
    d. tumor
desmolysis
desmon
desmoplastic
    d. malignant melanoma
    d. Spitz nevus
    d. trichilemmoma
    d. trichoepithelioma
desmorrhexis
desmosome
desmosome-tonofilament complex
Desocort
Desogen
DesOwen topical
desoximetasone
despeciated
    d. antitoxin
    d. serum
despeciation
desquamans
    herpes d.
desquamate
desquamating
desquamation
    branny d.
    corneocyte d.
    furfuraceous d.
    generalized d.
    lamellar d.

membranous d.
peribronchial d.
plantar d.
d. of pustule
siliquose d.
desquamative
d. dermatitis
d. gingivitis
d. interstitial pneumonitis
desquamativum, pl. desquamativa
erythema d.
erythroderma d.
Desquam-E gel
Desquam-X
D.-X gel
D.-X Wash
destruction
beta-cell d.
oligodendrocyte d.
polymorphonuclear leukocyte-
dependent tissue d.
destructor
Lepidoglyphus d.
desynchronized sleep
detection
Bartonella henselae d.
computer-assisted arthritis d.
C1q immune complex d.
hepatitis B DNA d.
hepatitis C RNA d.
hepatitis C virus antibody d.
Ki-67 marker d.
Lyme disease DNA d.
Mycobacterium tuberculosis d.
myelin-associated glycoprotein
antibody d.
detergens
detergent
anionic d.
d. dermatitis
superfatted synthetic d.
synthetic d. (syndet)
detergicans
acne d.
determinant
allotypic d.
antigenic d.
conformational d.
genetic d.
d. group
idiotypic antigenic d.
isoallotypic d.

Kern d.
Km allotypic d.
Oz isotypic d.
sequential d.
determination
fecal fat d.
IgG subclass d.
detersive
detoxicate
detoxication
detoxification
detoxified toxin
detoxify
detritus
tissue d.
Deuteromycetes
DEV
duck embryo origin vaccine
development
Treg d.
Devergie disease
deviation
anterior chamber-associated
immune d. (ACAID)
complement d.
immune d.
standard d. (SD)
ulnar d.
device
AeroEclipse Aerosol Delivery D.
Antense antitension d.
arachnophlebectomy surgical d.
Burkard sampling d.
charged-couple d. (CCD)
CoolSpot skin-cooling d.
Cyclotech dosing d.
Dermagraft skin d.
Dermagraft wound healing d.
DermaSeptic d.
electrocoagulation biterminal d.
Endopearl bioabsorbable d.
extracorporeal assist d.
extracorporeal liver assist d.
(ELAD)
Flexi-Trak skin anchoring d.
flutter d.
gravimetric d.
Handisol phototherapy d.
Hexascan Mark (I, II) model
robotic scanning d.
Jacobson resonator d.
Orion d.

D

NOTES

device *(continued)*
    Osteomark NTx point-of-care d.
    over-the-door d.
    Panosol II home phototherapy d.
    Prosorba column d.
    pulse oximetry d.
    Skinscan d.
    SkinTech medical tattooing d.
    SomnoStar apnea testing d.
    stratum corneum hydration d.
    supportive d.
    Tanner mesher d.
    Telangitron d.
    ThermaCool TC radiofrequency d.
    Thoratec ventricular assist d.
    tissue-engineered polymer d.
    Tru-Area Determination
      measuring d.
    Vacu-Aide portable suction d.
    Venture demand oxygen delivery d.
    Vitrasert intraocular d.
Devic syndrome
DeVilbiss Pulmon-Aid nebulizer
devil grip
devil's
    d. bite lesion
    d. pinch
Devrom
dew
    d. itch
    D. sign
Dewar flask
Dexacidin Ophthalmic
Dexacort Phosphate Turbinaire
dexamethasone (DXM)
    d. acetate
    Cytoxan, methotrexate, etoposide, d.
      (CMED)
    neomycin, polymyxin b, and d.
    d. sodium phosphate
    d. suppression test (DST)
    tobramycin and d.
Dexasone L.A.
Dexasporin Ophthalmic
Dexchlor
dexchlorpheniramine maleate
Dexone LA
Dexon suture
Dexotic
dextran 1
dextranomer granule
dextromethorphan
    chlorpheniramine, phenylephrine,
      and d.
    pseudoephedrine and d.
    d. tannate, phenylephrine tannate,
      pyrilamine tannate
dextrose
    tetracaine with d.

DEY albuterol inhalation aerosol
Dey-Dose
    D.-D. Isoproterenol
    D.-D. Metaproterenol
Dey-Drop Ophthalmic solution
Dey-Lute isoetharine
Dey-Wash
    D.-W. skin wound clean
    D.-W. skin wound cleanser
DF2 septicemia
DFA
    direct fluorescent antibody
    DFA test
DFA-TP
    direct fluorescent antibody test for
      Treponema pallidum
    direct fluorescent antibody for
      Treponema phagedenis
D/Flex
DFSP
    dermatofibrosarcoma protuberans
DFU
    dideoxyfluorouridine
DGF
    delayed graft function
DH
    delayed hypersensitivity
DHA
    dihydroacetone
    dihydroxyacetone
DHA-paclitaxel
    Taxoprexin D.-p.
DHA-PUVA
    dihydroxyacetone-psoralen ultraviolet A-
    range
Dharmendra antigen
DHEAS
    dehydroepiandrosterone sulfate
D.H.E. 45 injection
d'Herelle phenomenon
dhobie
    d. itch
    d. mark
    d. mark dermatitis
DHS
    DHS Tar
    DHS zinc
DHT
    dihydrotestosterone
    domino heart transplantation
DI
    defective interfering
    HAQ DI
    DI particle
DiaB
    D. Gel
    D. Klenz wound cleanser
diabetes
    bronze d.

lipoatrophic d.
d. mellitus
posttransplant d.
tacrolimus-associated d.
type (1, 1A, 1B, 2) d.

diabetic
d. blister
d. cheiroarthropathy
d. dermopathy
d. foot ulcer
d. gangrene
d. hand syndrome
d. muscle infarction (DMI)
nonobese d. (NOD)
D. Skin Therapy
d. stiff-hand syndrome

diabetica
neurotabes d.

diabeticorum
bullosis d.
eczema d.
necrobiosis lipoidica d.
xanthoma d.
xanthosis d.

DiabetiDerm Deep Moisturizing cream
diabetogenic
DiabGel hydrogel dressing
diacerein
diacetate
diflorasone d.

diacylglycerol
diadermic
diagnosis
differential d.
EIA d.
electrodermal d.
problem-oriented d.

diagnostic
d. algorithm
d. diphtheria toxin
d. Interview Schedule
D. and Neuronal Analysis of Skin
Cancer (DANAOS)
d. principle
d. surgical therapy
d. test

dial
d. caliper
D. soap

dialkylthioreas
dialysate

dialysis
d. dermatitis
equilibrium d.

dialysis-related amyloidosis
diameter
mass median aerodynamic d.
(MMD)

Diamine
D. T.D.
D. T.D. Oral

diamond
d. fraise
d. fraise dermabrasion
d. fraise dermabrasion instrument
D. Jaw needle holder
d. skin

Diamox
Di antigen
Diaparene
diapedesis
cellular d.

diaper
d. dermatitis
d. granuloma
d. rash
d. rash intertrigo

diaphoresis
diaphoretic
diaphragmatic
d. hernia
d. pleurisy

diaphysis
diapnoic
diarrhea
bovine virus d.
Brainerd d.
chronic d.
prolonged d.
weanling d.

diarthrodial joint bursa
diary
diet d.

diascope
diascopy
Diasonic ultrasound
diastase-resistant
diastrophic dysplasia
diathesis, pl. **diatheses**
allergic d.
hemorrhagic d.

diathsique
prurigo d.

D

NOTES

diazepam
Diazo paper
Dibenzyline
Dibucaine
dibutylester
    squaric acid d. (SADBE)
DIC
    disseminated intravascular coagulation
    sepsis-induced DIC
dichloride
    cobalt d.
dichloroacetic acid
dichlorodifluoromethane and
   trichloromonofluoromethane
dichlorofluoromethane
dichlorotetrafluoroethane
    ethyl chloride and d.
Dick
    D. method
    D. reaction
    D. test
    D. test toxin
diclazuril
diclofenac
    d. sodium
    d. sodium gel
dicloxacillin sodium
Dicrocoelium dendriticum
Dictamnus dasycarpus
Dictyocaulus viviparus
dictyospore
didanosine (ddI)
didehydrothymidine
    d4T, d.
2'-3'-dideoxyadenosine
dideoxycytidine (ddc)
dideoxyfluorouridine (DFU)
dideoxynucleoside
DIDMOS
    drug-induced delayed multiorgan
    hypersensitivity syndrome
        DIDMOS syndrome of Sontheimer
        and Houpt
Didrex
Didrocal
Didronel
DIDS
    Dermatology Index of Disease Severity
didymospore
diet
    challenge d.
    d. diary
    elemental d.
    elimination d.
    Feingold d.
    few-foods d.
    gluten-free d. (GFD)
    hypoallergenic d.
    lactovegetarian d.

    low-fiber, fat-limited exclusion d.
     (LOFFLEX)
    low-phenylalanine d.
    low-tyrosine d.
    Sippy d.
    Zen macrobiotic d.
dietary
    d. protein enterocolitis
    d. protein-induced colitis
    d. protein-induced enterocolitis
    d. protein proctitis
Dieterle stain
diethylcarbamazine (DEC)
diethyldithiocarbamate
diethylstilbestrol (DES)
diethyltoluamide (DEET)
difference
    geographic d.
differential
    d. diagnosis
    d. expression pattern
    d. gene expression
    d. gene subtraction
differentiation
    d. antigen
    apocrine d.
    sebaceous d.
    trichilemmal d.
    tricholemmal d.
Differin
    D. cream
    D. gel
DiffGAM bovine anti-*Clostridium*
  difficile* immunoglobulin
difficile
Diffistat-G polyclonal antibody
Diff-Quik stain
diffusa
    leishmaniasis tegumentaria d.
    psoriasis d.
diffuse
    d. atrophy
    d. connective tissue disease
    (DCTD)
    d. cutaneous leishmaniasis
    d. cutaneous mastocytosis
    d. dermal angiomatosis
    d. erythema
    d. fibrosing alveolitis
    d. histiocytic reaction
    d. hyperkeratosis of palms and
    soles
    d. idiopathic skeletal hyperostosis
    (DISH)
    d. infantile fibromatosis
    d. infiltrative lymphocytosis
    d. infiltrative lymphocytosis
    syndrome
    d. inflammation

d. interstitial fibrosis of the lung
d. interstitial lung disease (DILD)
d. lepromatous leprosy
d. leprosy of Lucio
d. phlegmon
d. plane
d. plane xanthoma
d. progressive systemic sclerosis
d. proliferative glomerulonephritis
d. pulmonary infiltrate
d. reflectance spectroscopy (DRS)
d. scleritis
d. scleroderma
d. staining
diffusion
agar gel d.
d. coefficient
d. constant
gel d.
d. of the lunula
diffusum
angiokeratoma corporis d.
atrophoderma d.
keratoma d.
papilloma d.
diflorasone
d. diacetate
d. diacetate cream
Diflucan
D. injection
D. Oral
diflunisal
diftitox
denileukin d.
DiGeorge
D. anomaly
D. syndrome
digestion
intracellular d.
digit
drummer d.
rudimentary supernumerary d.
sausage d.
supernumerary d.
digital
d. dermoscopy analyzer (DDA)
d. fibrokeratoma
d. fibromatosis
d. ischemia
D. Medical Systems
d. mucinous pseudocyst

d. nerve
d. sympathectomy
d. whorl
digitalis
herpes d.
digitata
verruca d.
digitate
d. dermatosis
d. wart
Digitrapper MkIII sleep monitor
dihomogamm
dihydrate
dihydroacetone (DHA)
dihydrochloride
histamine d.
dihydrocodeine
dihydroergotamine mesylate
dihydrostreptomycin
dihydrotestosterone (DHT)
dihydroxyacetone (DHA)
d. self-tanning lotion
dihydroxyacetone-psoralen ultraviolet A-range (DHA-PUVA)
dihydroxy leukotriene, LTB4
3,4-dihydroxyphenylalanine (DOPA)
dihydroxypropyl theophylline
Dihyrex Injection
Dilantin
dilated
d. pore
d. pore of Winer
d. venule
dilation
cystoscopy and d. (C&D)
DILD
diffuse interstitial lung disease
Dilocaine
Dilor
diloxanide furoate
diluent
dilute
d. lyophilized allergen extract
d. Russell viper venom time
dilution
Dimaphen
D. Elixir
D. Tablet
Dimedrine
dimeglumine
dimenhydrinate

D

NOTES

151

dimension
>double gel diffusion precipitin test in one d.
>gel diffusion precipitin test in one d.
>single gel diffusion precipitin test in one d.

2-dimensional immunoelectrophoresis
dimer
dimeric
Dimericine
Dimetabs Oral
Dimetane
>D. Decongestant Elixir
>D. Extentabs
>D. Oral

Dimetapp
>D. Chewables
>D. Clear
>D. Extentabs
>D. 4-Hour Liqui-Gel Capsule
>D. Sinus Caplets
>D. Tablet

dimethicone
dimethyl
>d. carbate
>d. carbate butopyropoxyl insect repellent
>d. phthalate insect repellent

dimethylgloxime nickel spot test
dimidiatum
>*Scytalidium d.*

diminished breath sounds
dimorphic fungi
dimorphous leprosy
dimple sign
dimpling
Dinate Injection
dinitrochlorobenzene (DNCB)
>d. challenge

dinoflagellate toxin
dinucleotide
diode
>d. laser
>light-emitting d. (LED)

dioecious
Diomycin
Diopred
dioxide
>partial pressure of carbon d. (PCO$_2$)
>solid carbon d.
>sulfur d. (SO$_2$)
>titanium d.

dioxybenzone
DIP
>distal interphalangeal

Dipentum

Dipetalonema
>*D. perstans*
>*D. streptocerca*

diphasic milk fever
Diphenacen-50 Injection
Diphen Cough
diphencyprone (DPCP)
Diphenhist
diphenhydramine
>acetaminophen and d.
>d. hydrochloride
>parenteral d.
>d. and pseudoephedrine

diphenidol hydrochloride
Diphenylan Sodium
diphenylcyclopropenone
diphenylhydantoin
diphosphate
diphosphonate
>technetium d.

diphtheria
>d. antitoxin
>d. antitoxin unit
>avian d.
>cutaneous d.
>d. cutis
>false d.
>fowl d.
>d. and tetanus toxoid
>d., tetanus toxoid, and whole-cell pertussis vaccine and *Haemophilus* b conjugate vaccine
>d. toxin
>d. toxoid, tetanus toxoid, and pertussis vaccine (DTP)

diphtheriae
>*Corynebacterium d.*

diphtheria-pertussis-tetanus (DPT)
diphtheric desert sore
diphtheritic
>d. membrane
>d. ulcer

diphtheroid
diphtherotoxin
Diphyllobothrium latum
diplococcin
diplopia
Diprolene
>D. AF
>D. AF topical
>D. Glycol

dipropionate
>alclometasone d.
>beclomethasone d.
>betamethasone d.
>clobetasol d.

Diprosone topical

dipstick
    d. method
    d. technique
Dipylidium caninum
dipyridamole
direct
    d. agglutination test
    d. amplification test
    d. challenge
    d. Coombs test
    d. fluorescent antibody (DFA)
    d. fluorescent antibody test
    d. fluorescent antibody test for
       Treponema pallidum (DFA-TP)
    d. fluorescent antibody for
       Treponema phagedenis (DFA-TP)
    d. galvanic current
    d. histamine releaser
    d. immunofluorescence
    Mycobacterium tuberculosis D. (MTD)
    d. sequencing
directory
    Haines d.
dirithromycin
Dirofilaria immitis
dirofilariasis
    subcutaneous d.
disability
    hemarthritic d.
    hemarthrotic d.
    work d.
disaccharide intolerance
Disalcid
disc, disk
    Clear Away D.
    Durapore membrane d.
    EMLA anesthetic d.
    hair d.
    d. herniation
    d. rupture
    d. sensitivity method
    d. space infection
disciform thickening
discoid
    distinctive exudative d.
    exudative d.
    d. LE
    d. lesion
    d. lupus
    d. rash

discoidea
    psoriasis d.
discoides
    lupus erythematosus d.
    psoriasis d.
discoloration
    oil-spot d.
discontinuous
    d. plasma-Percoll gradient centrifugation
    d. sterilization
discordant
    d. cellular xenograft
    d. organ xenograft
discreta
    porokeratosis plantaris d.
discrete
    d. edge
    d. pit
    d. synovitis
    d. umbilicated papule
discrimination
    self-nonself d.
disease
    acute infectious d.
    Addison d.
    Addison-Gull d.
    adult-onset systemic Still d.
    airways d.
    akamushi d.
    Albright d.
    alcohol-related liver d. (ALD)
    Aleutian mink d.
    Alibert d.
    Almeida d.
    alpha chain d.
    alpha-heavy-chain d.
    amyloid d.
    Anderson-Fabry d.
    Andrews d.
    antibody deficiency d.
    appendicular d.
    Arndt-Gottron d.
    articular d.
    Asboe-Hansen d.
    Athabascan type of severe combined immunodeficiency d. (SCIDA)
    atheroembolic d.
    atypical Kawasaki d. (AKD)
    Aujeszky d.
    Australian X d.

D

NOTES

disease *(continued)*
autoimmune blistering
  mucocutaneous d.
autoimmune pituitary d.
axial d.
axillary Fox-Fordyce d.
bacterial d.
Baelz d.
Ballingall d.
Bang d.
Bannister d.
Barcoo d.
Basedow d.
Bateman d.
Bayle d.
Bazin d.
Behçet d.
Beigel d.
beryllium d.
Besnier d.
Besnier-Boeck d.
Besnier-Boeck-Schaumann d.
beta-heavy-chain d.
bird-breeder's d.
blackjack d.
blinding d.
Bloch-Sulzberger d.
Bodechtel-Guttmann d.
bone d.
Borna d.
Bornholm d.
Bostock d.
Bourneville d.
Bourneville-Brissaud d.
Bourneville-Pringle d.
Bowen d.
brachial neuritis of Lyme d.
Breda d.
Bretonneau d.
Brill d.
Brill-Zinsser d.
Brion-Kayser d.
broad beta d.
Brocq d.
Brooke d.
Bruton d.
Buerger d.
bullous d.
Bury d.
Buschke d.
Buschke-Ollendorf d.
Busse-Buschke d.
calcium hydroxyapatite crystal
  deposition d.
calcium phosphate crystal
  deposition d.
calcium pyrophosphate crystal
  deposition d.
cardiac allograft vascular d.

Caroli d.
Carrión d.
Castleman d.
cat-scratch d. (CSD)
Cazenave d.
celiac d.
central Recklinghausen d. type II
Chagas d.
Charlouis d.
Chlamydia d.
chronic cold agglutinin d.
chronic graft-versus-host d.
chronic inflammatory d.
chronic interstitial lung d.
Ciarrocchi d.
cicatricial pemphigoid d.
Civatte d.
cold hemagglutinin d.
collagen vascular d.
combined immunodeficiency d.
  (CID)
communicable d.
congenital Lyme d.
Conradi d.
contagious d.
Corbus d.
Cowden d.
CP d.
Creutzfeldt-Jakob d. (CJD)
Crohn d.
Crouzon d.
crystal deposition d.
Csillag d.
Cushing d.
cytomegalovirus d.
Daae d.
Danielssen d.
Danielssen-Boeck d.
Darier-White d.
dark dot d.
deer fly d.
Degos d.
Dejerine-Sottas d.
dense-deposit d.
de Quervain d.
Dercum d.
Devergie d.
diffuse connective tissue d.
  (DCTD)
diffuse interstitial lung d. (DILD)
DNA probe test for Lyme d.
dog d.
Dohle d.
Dowling-Degos d.
Dubois d.
Duhring d.
Dukes d.
Duncan d.
Dupuytren d.

Durand-Nicholas-Favre d.
Dutton d.
endocrine d.
end-stage organ d.
end-tidal cardiac d. (ETCO$_2$)
Engman d.
Epstein d.
exanthematous d.
exudative papulosquamous d.
Fabry d.
Fabry-Anderson d.
Farber d.
Favre-Racouchot d.
fibrosing d.
fifth d.
Filatov-Dukes d.
Finkelstein d.
first d.
Flegel d.
fly-borne d.
food-borne d.
food-induced respiratory d.
foot-and-mouth d. (FMD)
forced air system d.
Fordyce d.
Forestier d.
Fothergill d.
Fournier d.
fourth d.
Fox d.
Fox-Fordyce d.
Francis d.
Freiberg d.
Friend d.
fungal d.
furuncular d.
fusospirochetal d.
gamma-heavy-chain d.
gasping d.
Gaucher d.
genetic d.
Gerhardt d.
Gerhardt-Mitchell d.
Gianotti-Crosti d.
Gibert d.
Gilchrist d.
glycogen storage d.
Gorham d.
Gougerot and Blum d.
Gougerot-Blum d.
Gougerot-Sjögren d.
graft vessel d. (GVD)

granulomatous d.
Graves d.
Greenhow d.
Griesinger d.
Grover d.
Gumboro d.
Günther d.
gut-associated lymphoid d.
GVH d.
Habermann d.
Hailey-Hailey d. (HHD)
Hallopeau d.
hand-foot-and-mouth d.
Hand-Schüller-Christian d.
Hansen d.
hard pad d.
Hartnup d.
Hashimoto d.
Hashimoto-Pritzker d.
heavy-chain d. (HCD)
Hebra d.
helminthic parasitic d.
hemoglobin C, S d.
hemolytic sickle cell d.
hepatobiliary d.
hereditary d.
heritable connective tissue d.
Herlitz d.
hidebound d.
Hirschsprung d.
His-Werner d.
HLA class 1 associated d.
Hodgkin d.
hoof-and-mouth d.
Horton d.
Hunermann d.
Hurler d.
Hurst d.
Hyde d.
idiopathic cold agglutinin d.
idiopathic eczematous d.
immune complex d.
immune-mediated d.
immunobullous d.
immunodeficiency d.
immunologic inflammatory d.
immunoproliferative small
  intestinal d. (IPSID)
inclusion body d.
infarctive inflammatory d.
infectious d. (ID)
inflammatory bowel d. (IBD)

NOTES

155

disease *(continued)*
    inflammatory lung d.
    interstitial lung d. (ILD)
    intraepidermal blistering d.
    iron storage d.
    Isambert d.
    island d.
    isocyanate d.
    itchy red bump d.
    Jadassohn d.
    Jakob-Creutzfeldt d.
    Jessner-Kanof d.
    jodbasedow d.
    Jüngling d.
    Kalischer d.
    Kanzaki d.
    Kaposi d.
    Kashin-Beck d.
    Kawasaki d. (KD)
    Kellgren d.
    Ketron-Goodman d.
    kidney d.
    Kienböck d.
    Kikuchi d.
    Kimura d.
    kinky-hair d.
    Kobberling-Duncan d.
    Köbner d.
    Köhler d.
    Krabbe d.
    Kyasanur Forest d.
    Kyrle d.
    Lafora d.
    Lancereaux-Mathieu d.
    Landouzy d.
    Lane d.
    large artery d.
    Larrey-Weil d.
    Legg-Calvé-Perthes d.
    Legionnaires d.
    Leicester d.
    Leiner d.
    Leloir d.
    Lemierre d.
    Letterer-Siwe d.
    Lewandowski-Lutz d.
    Leyden d.
    Lhermitte-Duclos d.
    linear IgA d. (LAD)
    lipid storage d.
    lipochrome histiocytosis d.
    livedo-patterned d.
    liver d.
    Lobo d.
    Lortat-Jacobs d.
    Lou Gehrig d.
    lumpy skin d.
    lung d.
    Lutz-Miescher d.

Lutz-Splendore-Almeida d.
Lyell d.
Lyme d. (stage 1–3)
lymphocytic d.
lymphoproliferative d.
MacIsaac d.
Madelung d.
Majocchi d.
malignant neoplastic d.
mammary Paget d.
maple bark d.
maple-bark stripper's d.
Marburg virus d.
Marek d.
margarine d.
Marie-Strümpell d.
market men d.
McArdle d.
mechanobullous d.
Meleda d.
metabolic bone d.
Mibelli d.
Mikulicz d.
Milian d.
Milroy d.
Milton d.
Mitchell d.
mixed connective tissue d. (MCTD)
Mkar d.
Mondor d.
Morvan d.
Moschcowitz d.
mosquito-borne d.
Mseleni d.
Mucha d.
Mucha-Habermann d.
mucocutaneous d.
mucosal d.
mu-heavy chain d.
multicentric d.
mycoplasma d.
myeloproliferative d.
Nasu-Hakola d.
National Institute of Arthritis and Metabolic D.'s (NIAMD)
neonatal-onset multisystem inflammatory d. (NOMID)
neoplastic d.
Nettleship d.
Neumann d.
neurodegenerative d.
neuroectodermal melanolysomonal d.
neuropathic joint d.
neuropsychiatric d.
neutral lipid storage d.
Newcastle d. (ND)
Niemann-Pick d.

nodular sclerosing Hodgkin d.
  (NSHD)
nonneoplastic d.
obliterative airway d.
obstructive liver d.
occupational immunologic lung d.
  (OLD)
Ockelbo d.
ocular immune d.
ocular inflammatory d.
Ofuji d.
Ohara d.
"oid-oid" d.
orbital inflammatory d.
orphan d.
Osler d.
Osler-Weber-Rendu d.
overlap d.
Paget d.
parasitic d.
Parkinson d.
patellofemoral d.
Paxton d.
pelvic inflammatory d. (PID)
perforating d.
perna d.
Pette-Döring d.
Peyronie d.
phytanic acid storage d.
pigeon breeder's d.
pink d.
Plaut-Vincent d.
polycystic ovary d.
polyglandular autoimmune
  endocrine d.
Pompe d.
Poncet d.
porcupine d.
Posada-Wernicke d.
postthrombotic d.
posttransplantation
  lymphoproliferative d. (PTLD)
posttransplant lymphoproliferative d.
  (PTLD)
poultry handler's d.
Preiser d.
primary pulmonary parenchymal d.
Pringle d.
proliferative inflammatory d.
protozoal parasitic d.
psychocutaneous d.
Puente d.

pulmonary venoocclusive d.
  (PVOD)
pulseless d.
Quincke d.
Quinquaud d.
Ranikhet d.
Rayer d.
Raynaud d.
reactive airways d.
Recklinghausen d. type I
Reclus d.
Refsum d.
Reiter d.
Rendu-Osler-Weber d.
restrictive lung d.
reticulohistiocytosis d.
rheumatic heart d.
rheumatoid d.
Ribas-Torres d.
rippling muscle d.
Ritter d.
Robinson d.
Robles d.
Roitter d.
Rosai-Dorfman d.
Rosenbach d.
Roth-Bernhardt d.
Rubarth d.
runt d.
Rust d.
salivary gland virus d.
sandworm d.
saprophytic d.
Schamberg d.
Schenck d.
Scheuermann d.
Schilder d.
Schönlein d.
Scraple d.
secondary d.
Senear-Usher d.
seropositive d.
serum d.
Sever d.
severe combined
  immunodeficiency d. (SCID)
sexually transmitted d. (STD)
shimamushi d.
sickle cell d. (SCD)
silicone particle d.
sinopulmonary d.
sixth venereal d.

D

NOTES

disease *(continued)*
Sjögren d.
skinbound d.
slow virus d.
Sneddon-Wilkinson d.
specific d.
spirochetal d.
sponge diver d.
sponge fisherman d.
SS hemoglobin d.
staging classification for
  Hodgkin d.
Stanton d.
startle d.
stellate patterned d.
sternoclavicular d.
Sticker d.
Still d.
Strümpell d.
Sulzberger-Garbe d.
Sutton d.
Sweet d.
Swift d.
swine vesicular d.
Sylvest d.
d. syndrome
systemic autoimmune d.
systemic febrile d.
Takahara d.
Takayasu d.
Tangier d.
Tarui d.
Taylor d.
Tay-Sachs d.
T-cell and B-cell severe combined
  immunodeficiency d.
T-cell-mediated autoimmune d.
Teschen d.
Theiler d.
Thiemann d.
third d.
TI-CMV d.
traumatically induced
  inflammatory d.
tropical d.
tsutsugamushi d.
twentieth century d.
type I glycogen storage d.
Underwood d.
undifferentiated connective tissue d.
  (UCTD)
Unna d.
Unna-Thost d.
Urbach-Oppenheim d.
Urbach-Wiethe d.
vagabond's d.
vagrant's d.
valvular d.
van Buchem d.

varicella d.
vasoocclusive d.
vector-borne d.
venereal d.
venoocclusive d.
vesiculobullous d.
Vidal d.
Vincent d.
vinyl chloride d.
viral d.
virus X d.
VOD d.
Voerner d.
von Economo d.
von Gierke glycogen storage d.
von Recklinghausen d.
von Willebrand d. (vWD)
von Zumbusch d.
Wardrop d.
Wassilieff d.
wasting d.
Weber-Christian d. (WCD)
Weber-Cockayne d.
Weil d.
Well d.
Werlhof d.
Werther d.
Wesselsbron d.
Whipple d.
white spot d.
Whitmore d.
Whytt d.
Willan d.
Wilson d.
Winkler d.
winter vomiting d.
Witkop-Von Sallman d.
wood-pulp worker's d.
Woringer-Kolopp d.
X-linked lymphoproliferative d.
  (XLP)
yellow d.
Zahorsky d.
Zoon d.
Zumbusch d.
disease-syphilis
venereal d.-s. (VDS)
disequilibrium
linkage d.
DISH
diffuse idiopathic skeletal hyperostosis
disinfectant
phenolated d.
Sactimed-I-Sinald d.
disinfection
disintegrin proteinase
disjunctum
stratum d.
disk *(var. of* disc)

Diskhaler
  Flutide D.
  D. inhaler
Diskus inhaler
dislocation
  d. arthritis
  atlantodental d.
  peroneal tendon d.
dismutase
  bovine superoxide d.
disodium
  lobenzarit d.
  ticarcillin d.
disorder
  acquired cornification d.
  acquired vascular d.
  adrenal cortex d.
  allergic eye d.
  anogenital d.
  arterial d.
  autoimmune d.
  autosomal recessive severe
    combined immunodeficiency d.
  bacterially induced hemostatic d.
  bland occlusive d.
  body dysmorphic d.
  ciliary d.
  cold-dependent d.
  congenital d.
  cornification d.
  Curth-Maklin cornification d.
  dysesthesia d.
  elemental d.
  genetic d.
  hematologic d.
  hemostatic d.
  hereditary vascular d.
  heritable d.
  ICE d.
  immune complex d.
  immune-mediated coagulation d.
  immunodeficiency d.
  immunoglobulin-complexed
    enzyme d.
  immunologic d.
  immunoproliferative d.
  keratitis-deafness cornification d.
  ligamentous d.
  lymphoreticular d.
  median nerve d.
  meniscal d.
  metabolic d.

  mineral-related nutritional d.
  mitochondrial respiratory chain d.
    (MRCD)
  National Institute of Arthritis,
    Musculoskeletal and Skin D.'s
    (NIAMS)
  neurologic d.
  neuromuscular junction d.
  nevi with architectural d. (NAD)
  nutritional d.
  ocular inflammatory d.
  pancreatic d.
  papulosquamous d.
  partial combined
    immunodeficiency d.
  periarticular d.
  peripheral nerve entrapment d.
  d. of phagocytic cell
  pituitary d.
  posttransplantation
    lymphoproliferative d. (PTLD, PT-
    LPD)
  posttransplant lymphoproliferative d.
    (PTLD)
  primary immunodeficiency d.
  proliferation d.
  psychophysiologic d.
  rheumatic d.
  secondary psychiatric d.
  severe combined
    immunodeficiency d. (SCID)
  thyroid d.
  unilateral hemidysplasia
    cornification d.
  upper airway d. (UAD)
  vascular d.
dispar
  Lymantria d.
disperse dye
dispersing agent
dispersion
  amphotericin B colloidal d.
displacement
  d. analysis
  odontoid process d.
display
  antibody-phage d.
Dispos-a-Med Isoproterenol
disruption
  gene d.
  LTA$_4$ hydrolase gene d.

D

NOTES

dissecans
glossitis d.
osteochondritis d.
dissecting
d. cellulitis
d. cellulitis of scalp
d. perifolliculitis
d. scissors
dissection
blunt d.
d. cellulitis of scalp
selective sentinel lymph node d.
(SSLND)
sharp d.
d. tubercle
dissector
Luikart d.
disseminata
acne d.
alopecia d.
dermatofibrosis lenticularis d.
neurodermatitis d.
osteitis fibrosa cystica d.
porokeratosis palmaris plantaris
et d.
tuberculosis cutis follicularis d.
tuberculosis cutis miliaris d.
disseminated
d. aspergillosis
d. candidiasis
d. coccidioidomycosis
d. cutaneous gangrene
d. cutaneous leishmaniasis (DCL)
d. encephalomyelitis
d. gonococcal infection
d. herpes simplex
d. herpes zoster
d. intravascular coagulation (DIC)
d. Kaposi sarcoma
d. lupus erythematosus
d. neurodermatitis
d. pagetoid reticulosis
d. pruriginous angiodermatitis
d. recurrent infundibulofolliculitis
d. sporotrichosis
d. strongyloidiasis
d. superficial actinic porokeratosis
(DSAP)
d. tuberculosis
d. vaccinia
dissemination
skin d.
xanthoma d.
disseminatum
keratoma d.
xanthoma d. (XD)
disseminatus
lupus erythematosus d. (LED)

dissemine
neurodermite d.
disseminées parapsoriasis en plaques
dissociation constant
distal
d. arthrogryposis
d. dactylitis
d. dystrophy
d. interphalangeal (DIP)
d. intestinal obstruction syndrome
d. nail matrix
d. onycholysis
d. radicular joint (DRUJ)
d. splenorenal shunt (DSRS)
Distaval
distemper virus
distended bursa
distensae
striae cutis d.
distention
striaelike epidermal d.
distichia
distichiasis
distillate
cetyl alcohol-coal tar d.
Tar D.
distinctive exudative discoid
distortum
Microsporum canis, var d.
distress
respiratory d.
distribution
asymmetric d.
compartment load d.
dermatomal d.
lesion d.
linear d.
pattern of d.
shawl d.
Sips d.
districhiasis
distrix
disturbance
atrial conduction d.
d. of consciousness
microcirculatory d.
sleep d.
dithiothreitol (DTT)
Dithranol
ditiocarb
**Ditropan XL oxybutynin chloride
extended-release tablet**
diubiquitin
diuretic
chlorothiazide d.
loop d.
diutinum
scleredema d.

divergens
    Babesia d.
diversiloba
    Rhus d.
diversilobum
    Toxicodendron d.
diversity
    antigen-binding d.
diversus
    Citrobacter d.
diving suit dermatitis
division (I–IV) lesion
Dizac injection
Dizmiss
dizygotic
DLI
    donor lymphocyte infusion
DM
    dermatomyositis
    Guaifenex DM
    Iobid DM
    Iohist DM
    Maxiphen DM
DMax
    DMax Pediatric oral drops
    DMax syrup
DMDM hydantoin
D-Med Injection
DMI
    diabetic muscle infarction
DMSA
    Tc-dimercaptosuccinic acid
DNA
    deoxyribonucleic acid
    DNA amplicon
    DNA aneuploidy
    antidimer DNA
    antidouble-stranded DNA
    antinative DNA
    DNA autosensitivity
    DNA binding
    chemiluminescent DNA
    chemiluminescent in situ
      hybridization for detection of
      CMV DNA
    circular plasmid DNA
    competitor DNA
    decoy DNA
    episomal DNA
    DNA gyrase
    HBV DNA
    HLA-G DNA

    DNA homology
    human cloned DNA
    DNA hybridization
    DNA hybridization test
    improper repair of DNA
    DNA microarray chip
    naked plasmid DNA
    PCR for HIV DNA
    DNA polymerase
    DNA probe test
    DNA probe test for Lyme disease
    DNA repair
    single-stranded DNA
    DNA topoisomerase I
    DNA vaccination
    DNA vaccine
    DNA virus
DNA-anti-DNA system
DNA-binding test
DNA-carrier complex
DNA-chain terminator
DNase
    deoxyribonuclease
DNCB
    dinitrochlorobenzene
Doak
    D. Oil
    Tar D.
Doan's
    D. Backache Pill
    Extra Strength D.
    D., Original
dock
    bitter d.
    tall d.
    yellow d.
docosahexaenoic acid
docosanol cream
documented
    d. bacterial infection (DBI)
    d. viral infection (DVI)
dodecamer
dog
    d. allergy
    d. dander
    d. disease
    d. distemper virus
    d. epithelium
    d. fennel
    d. flea
    d. flea bite

D

NOTES

dog (*continued*)
    nonshedding d.
    d. tapeworm
Dogger Bank itch
Dohi
    acropigmentation of D.
Dohle
    D. disease
    D. inclusion body
dolastatin
dolens
    phlegmasia alba d.
***Dolichorespula* sting**
Dolobid
dolor
Dolorac
dolorimeter scoliosis
dolorosa
    adiposis d.
    neurolipomatosis d.
    tubercula d.
domain
    catalytic d.
    death d.
    Fas-associating protein with
      death d. (FADD)
    immunoglobulin d.
    pleckstrin homology d.
    silencer of death d. (SODD)
Domeboro
    Otic D.
Dome-Paste boot
domesticus
    Glycyphagus d.
dominant
    autosomal d.
    lamellar d.
    d. phenotype
domino
    d. heart transplantation (DHT)
    d. procedure
Domiphen
Donath-Landsteiner
    D.-L. antibody
    D.-L. cold autoantibody
    D.-L. syndrome
d'ongle
    coup d.
Donizetti potion
DonJoy brace
donor
    d. allopeptide
    d. biopsy
    d. brain death
    extended criteria d. (ECD)
    heart-beating d. (HBD)
    identical twin d.
    living d. (LD)
    d. lymphocyte infusion (DLI)

    marginal d.
    matched related d. (MRD)
    matched unrelated d. (MURD)
    nonheart-beating d. (NHBD)
    d. sclera
    universal d.
donor-recipient plug exchange
donor-related warm ischemia
donor-specific
    d.-s. tolerance
    d.-s. transfusion (DST)
donor-transmitted lymphoma
Donovan body
donovani
    Leishmania d.
Donovania granulomatis
donovanosis
DOPA
    3,4-dihydroxyphenylalanine
dopa
    d. radiation
    d. reaction
    d. stain
dopamine
dopa-oxidase
Doppler
    Laserflo laser D.
    D. ultrasound
d'orange
    peau d.
Dorcol
Dorfman-Chanarin syndrome
d'Orient
    bouton d.
Dormarex 2 Oral
Dormex
Dormin Oral
Dorothy Reed-Sternberg cell
dorsal
    d. scapular nerve entrapment
    d. surface
    d. wrist tenosynovitis
dorsalis
    acne d.
    tabes d.
dorsi
    elastofibroma d.
dorsoradial subluxation
Dortu phlebectomy hook
dory flop
Doryx Oral
dose
    booster d.
    cell d.
    erythema d.
    infecting d. (ID)
    L d.
    L+ d.
    lethal d. (LD)

Lf d.
Lr d.
maintenance d.
minimal erythema d. (MED)
minimal infecting d. (MID)
minimal lethal d. (MLD)
minimal phototoxic d. (MPD)
minimal reacting d. (MRD)
minimum effective naproxen d. (MEND)
sensitizing d.
shocking d.

Dosepak
Deltasone D.
Medrol D.

dose-related effect
dose-response curve
dosimeter
Rosenthal-French d.

dosing
once daily d. (ODD)
pulse d.

dot
Trantas d.'s

double
d. antibody immunoassay
d. antibody method
d. antibody precipitation
d. antibody sandwich assay
d. drug treatment
d. gel diffusion precipitin test in one dimension
d. immunodiffusion
d. immunodiffusion in agarose gels test
d. negative cell
d. renal allograft

double-balloon triple lumen catheter
double-contrast arthrography
double-crush syndrome
double-edge nail
double-hook Tyrell skin hook
double-sandwich IgM ELISA
doublestaining
fluorescent treponemal antibody absorption d. (FTA-ABS)

Douche
Yeast-Gard Medicated D.

doughnut wart
Douglas
D. fir
D. fir tree

douloureux
tic d.

Dove soap
Dovonex
dowager hump
dowicide
Dowicil 200
Dowling-Degos disease
Dowling-Meara epidermolysis bullosa
down
malignant d.
D. syndrome

Downey cell
down-regulation
downstream mediator
doxepin
d. HCl
d. hydrochloride cream

Doxil
doxofylline
doxorubicin
liposomal d.

Doxy-200
Doxy-Caps
Doxychel
D. injection
D. Oral

Doxycin
doxycycline
d. hyclate tablet
d. pleurodesis

Doxy-Tabs
Doxytec
D.P.
Dalalone D.P.

DPAP interactive airway management system
DPCP
diphencyprone

d-penicillamine
DPI
dry power inhaler

DPOC
placebo-controlled oral challenge testing

DPT
diphtheria-pertussis-tetanus

DQB1
major histocompatibility complex class II allele DRB1, DRB3, DRB4, DRB5, and DQB1

DQw1

D

NOTES

163

DQw7
    allele HLA DQw7
    allele human leukocyte antigen
      DQw7
Dr.
    D. Scholl's Athlete's Foot
    D. Scholl's Maximum Strength
      Tritin
DR1 allele
DR3 allele
DR5 allele
dracontiasis
dracunculiasis, dracunculosis
Dracunculus medinensis
dragon
    Minor Blue D.
drain
    Clot Stop d.
drainage
    enteric pancreatic d.
    paranasal sinus d.
    percussion and postural d.
    percutaneous abscess and fluid d.
      (PAFD)
    postural d.
    thoracic duct d. (TDD)
Draize Repeat Insult patch test
Dramamine
    D. II
    D. Oral
Dramilin Injection
drawer sign
Drechslera
Dreiser functional index score
Drenison
DRESS
    drug rash with eosinophil and systemic
      symptom
    DRESS syndrome of Bocquet and
      Roujeau
dressing
    AcryDerm border island d.
    Acticel wound d.
    Acticoat burn d.
    Actisorb Silver 220 antimicrobial
      binding d.
    Acu-Derm I.V./TPN d.
    Airstrip composite d.
    AlgiDerm alginate d.
    AlgiDerm wound d.
    alginate wound d.
    AlgiSite alginate d.
    AlgiSite wound d.
    Algisorb wound d.
    Algosteril alginate d.
    Alldress composite d.
    Allevyn adhesive foam d.
    Allevyn cavity foam d.
    Allevyn island foam d.

    Allevyn synthetic d.
    Allevyn Thin d.
    Allevyn tracheostomy foam d.
    Amerigel topical ointment
      hydrogel d.
    Aquacel AG wound d.
    Aquacel Hydrofiber d.
    Aquacel wound packing and d.
    Aquasorb transparent hydrogel d.
    Arglaes antimicrobial barrier
      film d.
    ArtAssist leg compression d.
    Band-Aid composite d.
    Bard Absorption d.
    BGC Matrix hydrocolloid d.
    Biobrane synthetic d.
    Bioclusive synthetic d.
    Bioclusive transparent d.
    Biolex hydrogel d.
    Biopatch antimicrobial d.
    Biopatch foam d.
    BreakAway absorptive wound d.
    CarraFilm wound d.
    CarraSmart foam d.
    CarraSorb H calcium alginate
      wound d.
    CarraSorb hydrogel d.
    Carrasyn hydrogel wound d.
    Catrix wound d.
    Centurion SorbaView composite d.
    CircPlus leg compression d.
    Circulon leg compression d.
    closed wet d.
    Coban d.
    CombiDERM ACD hydrocolloid d.
    Comfeel hydrocolloid d.
    Comfeel synthetic d.
    Comfeel Ulcus d.
    Compeed Skin protector d.
    Conformant wound d.
    contact-layer wound d.
    Contreet Antimicrobial Barrier D.
    Contreet hydrocolloid nonadhesive
      foam d.
    Covaderm composite wound d.
    Coverlet composite d.
    Covertell composite d.
    Curaderm hydrocolloid d.
    Curafil hydrogel d.
    Curafoam foam d.
    Curafoam wound d.
    Curagel Hydrogel d.
    Curasol hydrogel d.
    Curasorb calcium alginate d.
    CURASORB Zinc alginate d.
    Curity ABD absorptive d.
    Curtinova hydrocolloid d.
    Cutifilm Plus composite d.
    Cutinova foam d.

Cutinova Hydro d.
Cutinova Thin hydrocolloid d.
Dermacea alginate d.
Dermagran hydrogel d.
DermaMend cavity foam d.
DermaMend foam wound d.
DermaMend hydrogel d.
DermaMend island foam d.
DermaNet contact layer wound d.
DermAssist Glycerin hydrogel d.
DermAssist hydrocolloid d.
Dermatell hydrocolloid d.
DiabGel hydrogel d.
DuoDerm CGF hydrocolloid d.
DuoDerm SCB leg compression d.
DuoDerm synthetic d.
Dyna-Flex leg compression d.
Elastoplast elastic d.
Elta Dermal hydrogel d.
Epi-lock wound d.
ExuDerm hydrocolloid d.
Exu-Dry absorptive d.
Fibracol collagen-alginate d.
Flexzan foam wound d.
foam d.
FortaDerm wound d.
FyBron alginate wound d.
Gelocast Unna boot leg
  compression d.
gel wound d.
Gentell alginate wound d.
Gentell foam wound d.
Gentell hydrogel d.
GraftCyte gauze wound d.
Handages d.
hyCure collagen hemostatic
  wound d.
Hydrasorb foam wound d.
Hydrocol hydrocolloid d.
hydrocolloid d.
hydrofiber d.
hydrogel d.
HydroMed wound d.
hydrophilic polymer d.
HyFil hydrogel d.
Hypergel hydrogel d.
Hyperion Advanced alginate d.
Hyperion bordered hydrocolloid d.
Hyperion hydrophilic wound gel
  hydrogel d.
Hyperion thin hydrocolloid d.
Iamin Gel wound d.

Iamin hydrogel d.
Inerpan d.
Intelligent d.
IntraSite hydrogel d.
Iodoflex absorptive d.
Iodosorb absorptive d.
island wound d.
Kalginate alginate d.
Kaltostat alginate d.
Lyofoam A, C, T foam d.
Lyofoam Extra foam d.
Maxorb alginate wound d.
Medipore Dress-it d.
Mepiform self-adherent silicone d.
Mepilex Transfer d.
Mepitel contact-layer wound d.
Mepore absorptive d.
Mesalt debridement d.
Mitraflex Plus foam d.
Mitraflex SC foam d.
Mitraflex wound d.
MPM composite d.
MPM hydrogel d.
MultiPad absorptive d.
nonocclusive d.
Normlgel hydrogel d.
N-Terface contact layer wound d.
Nu-Derm hydrocolloid d.
Nu Gauze d.
Nu-Gel hydrogel wound d.
Nu-Gel synthetic d.
Oasis wound d.
occlusive d.
Omniderm synthetic d.
open wet d.
OpSite Flexigrid adhesive d.
OpSite Plus composite d.
OpSite postop composite d.
OpSite semipermeable d.
OsmoCyte pillow wound d.
Owens Surgical d.
Panoplex hydrogel d.
plastic adhesive d.
Polyderm foam d.
PolyMem alginate d.
PolyMem foam d.
polymer film d.
polymer foam d.
Polyskin II d.
Primaderm d.
Primapore absorptive wound d.
Primer leg compression d.

D

NOTES

dressing *(continued)*
  Pro-Clude transparent film
    wound d.
  ProCyte transparent adhesive
    film d.
  Profore leg compression d.
  Promogran matrix wound d.
  PuraPly wound d.
  RepliCare hydrocolloid d.
  Reston foam wound d.
  Reston hydrocolloid d.
  Restore alginate d.
  Restore hydrocolloid d.
  Restore hydrogel d.
  Royl-Derm wound hydrogel d.
  Saf-Gel hydrogel d.
  SeaSorb alginate wound d.
  semipermeable d.
  SignaDress sterile hydrocolloid d.
  Silon wound d.
  Siloskin d.
  silver and cadexomer iodine-based
    wound d.
  SiteGuard MVP transparent
    adhesive film d.
  SkinTegrity hydrogel d.
  SofSorb absorptive d.
  SoftCloth absorptive d.
  Sof-Wick d.
  SoloSite hydrogel d.
  SorbaView wound d.
  Sorbsan alginate d.
  Sorbsan wound d.
  StrataSorb composite wound d.
  SurePress leg compression d.
  Synthaderm wound d.
  Tegaderm semipermeable d.
  Tegaderm transparent d.
  Tegagel hydrogel d.
  Tegagen HG alginate wound d.
  Tegagen HI alginate d.
  Tegapore contact-layer wound d.
  Tegasorb synthetic d.
  Tegasorb Thin hydrocolloid d.
  Telfa composite d.
  Telfamax absorptive d.
  Tendersorb ABD absorptive d.
  Tenderwrap leg compression d.
  Thera-Boot leg compression d.
  d. therapy
  THINSite with BioFilm hydrogel
    topical wound d.
  Tielle absorptive d.
  tie-over bolster d.
  Triad hydrocolloid d.
  Ultec hydrocolloid d.
  Uniflex polyurethane adhesive
    surgical d.
  Unna-Flex leg compression d.

  Unna-Pak leg compression d.
  Vari/Moist wound d.
  Veingard d.
  Ventex composite d.
  Viasorb composite d.
  Viasorb wound d.
  Vigilon d.
  water-impermeable, nonsilicone-based
    occlusive d.
  wet d.
  Woun'Dres hydrogel d.
  Wound Span Bridge II d.
  Zipzoc Stocking leg compression d.
dressing/sheet
  Tegagel d.
dressing/wrap
  ArtAssist compression d.
Dricort
  Demarest D.
Dri-Ear Otic
dried
  d. fruit dermatitis
  d. human serum
drift
  antigenic d.
drip
  postnasal d. (PND)
dripping
  candle d.
Drisdol Oral
Dristan
  D. Long Lasting Nasal solution
  D. Sinus Caplets
Drithocreme HP
Dritho-Scalp
drive
  hypoxic ventilatory d. (HVD)
Drixomed
Drixoral
  D. Cough & Congestion Liquid
    Caps
  D. Non-Drowsy
  D. Syrup
DR/MLC cell marker
dronabinol
drop
  AccuHist PDX d.'s
  AccuHist Pediatric d.'s
  Afrin Children's Nose d.'s
  Allergan Ear d.'s
  Carbodex DM pediatric oral d.'s
  Cerumenex ear d.'s
  Coly-Mycin S Otic d.'s
  Debrox d.'s
  Decongestant nose d.'s
  DMax Pediatric oral d.'s
  Mallazine Eye d.'s
  Moisture Ophthalmic d.'s
  Myapap d.'s

Patanol eye d.'s
RO-Eye d.'s
Rondec d.'s
Triaminic Oral Infant d.'s
Tri-P Oral Infant d.'s
drop attack
droplet
 d. infection
 d. nucleus
drop-like psoriasis
dropout
 crypt epithelial cell d.
dropping
 Australian parrot d.'s
 pigeon d.'s
dropsy
 epidemic d.
Drotic Otic
drowsiness
Droxia
DRS
 diffuse reflectance spectroscopy
drug
 adrenergic d.
 d. allergy
 d. alopecia
 d. anaphylaxis
 anticholinergic d.
 antimalarial d.
 antirheumatic d.
 antisense d.
 antiviral d.
 d. challenge testing
 chondroprotective d.
 cytotoxic d.
 d. delivery
 d. eruption
 d. hypersensitivity
 immunophilin-binding d.
 immunosuppressive d.
 d. interaction
 d. intolerance
 ISAtx247 immunosuppressive d.
 large-molecular-weight d.
 lysosomotropic antimalarial d.
 MR d.
 muscle-relaxant d.
 myorelaxant d.
 noncross-reactive d.
 nonsteroidal antiinflammatory d.
  (NSAID)
 orphan d.

 d. overdose
 d. rash
 d. rash with eosinophil and
  systemic symptom (DRESS)
 rauwolfia d.
 d. reaction
 second-line d. (SLD)
 simple d.
 slow-acting antirheumatic d.
  (SAARD)
 sulfa d.
 uricosuric d.
drug-associated erythema multiforme
drug-fast
drug-induced
 d.-i. acanthosis nigricans
 d.-i. alopecia
 d.-i. asthma
 d.-i. bullous photosensitivity
 d.-i. delayed multiorgan
  hypersensitivity syndrome
  (DIDMOS)
 d.-i. delayed multiorgan
  hypersensitivity syndrome of
  Sontheimer and Houpt
 d.-i. depression of immune system
 d.-i. erythema
 d.-i. lupus
 d.-i. lymphadenopathy
 d.-i. photodermatitis
 d.-i. pneumonia
 d.-i. progressive symptom sclerosis
 d.-i. purpura
 d.-i. SLE syndrome
 d.-i. systemic lupus erythematosus
 d.-i. thrombocytopenia
drug-related
 d.-r. immunohemolytic anemia
 d.-r. myopathy
DRUJ
 distal radicular joint
drummer digit
DRw53
 allele HLA DRw53
 allele human leukocyte antigen
  DRw53
dry
 d. cough
 d. cutaneous leishmaniasis
 D. Eye Therapy solution
 d. flush
 d. gangrene

NOTES

D

167

dry *(continued)*
    d. ice
    d. leprosy
    d. lip
    d. mouth
    Peri-Strips D.
    d. power inhaler (DPI)
    d. skin
    d. surface
    d. tetter
dry-ice slush
dryness
    excessive d.
Dryox
    D. Gel
    D. Wash
Drysol
drywall sanding screen
DS
    Bactrim DS
    Cotrim DS
    Septra DS
    Sulfatrim DS
    Tolectin DS
    Uroplus DS
DSAP
    disseminated superficial actinic
      porokeratosis
DSG
    deoxyspergualin
Dsg
    desmoglein
Dsg1
    desmoglein-1
Dsg3
    desmoglein-3
    Dsg3 antigen
Dsg1/3 ELISA kit
DSMB
    Data Safety Monitoring Board
DSQL
    Dermatology-Specific Quality of Life
DSRS
    distal splenorenal shunt
DST
    dexamethasone suppression test
    donor-specific transfusion
d4T
    Zerit
DTEG
    Dermatology Teachers Exchange Group
DTH
    delayed-type hypersensitivity
DTIC
    dacarbazine
DTIC-Dome
DTP
    diphtheria toxoid, tetanus toxoid, and
      pertussis vaccine

DTT
    dithiothreitol
Duac topical gel
Duadacin Capsule
dual-beam photon absorptiometry
dual-fluorescence analysis
dual-function enzyme
dual kidney transplant
Dual-Luciferase assay method
duazomycin
Dubois
    D. abscess
    D. disease
    D. sign
duboisii
    Histoplasma d.
Dubreuilh
    circumscribed precancerous
      melanosis of D.
    D. elastoma
    D. precancerous melanosis
    precancerous melanosis of D.
Ducas and Kapetanakis pigmented
purpura
Duchenne muscular dystrophy
duck
    d. embryo origin vaccine (DEV)
    d. feather
    d. hepatitis virus
    d. influenza virus
    d. plague
    d. plague virus
ducreyi
    Haemophilus d.
Ducrey test
duct
    eccrine d.
    Pecquet d.
ductopenia
ductopenic rejection
Duffy
    D. antigen
    D. blood antibody type
    D. blood group
Duhring
    D. disease
    D. pruritus
Dukes disease
Dulbecco modified eagle's medium
dulcamara
dumas
dumdum fever
dumoffii
    Legionella d.
Dumon-Harrell bronchoscope
Duncan
    D. disease
    D. syndrome

d'Unna
  Pate d.
Dunnett multiple comparison test
Dunnigan syndrome
DUO
  TheraPress D.
duodenale
  Ancylostoma d.
DuoDerm
  D. CGF hydrocolloid dressing
  D. hydroactive gel for wound
    hydration
  D. SCB
  D. SCB leg compression dressing
  D. synthetic dressing
DuoFilm Solution
Duoforte
Duo-Medihaler Aerosol
DuoNeb
DuoPlant
Duotip-Test
Duo-Trach
duovirus
Duplex T
duplication
  1q d.
Dupuytren
  D. contracture
  D. disease
durable-press
  d.-p. allergic contact dermatitis
  d.-p. allergy
Durafedrin
Dura-Gest
Duralone Injection
dural sinus thrombosis
Duralutin injection
Duramist plus
Durand-Nicholas-Favre disease
Duranest injection
Durapore membrane disc
DuraScreen sunscreen
duration
  D. Nasal solution
  d. of treatment
Duratuss
dura twist skin hook
Dura-Vent/DA
Duricef
**Durie and Salmon multiple myeloma
  classification**
Durrax

durum
  fibroma d.
  heloma d.
  papilloma d.
  ulcus d.
dust
  d. allergy
  barn d.
  grain d.
  house d.
  d. mite
  mushroom d.
dustborne
Dutton
  D. disease
  D. relapsing fever
Duval disposable dermatome
Duvenhaga virus
DVI
  documented viral infection
Dwelle Ophthalmic solution
DXM
  dexamethasone
DXR
  delayed xenograft rejection
Dycill
Dyclone
dyclonine hydrochloride
dye
  acid d.
  azo d.
  azobenzene d.
  D&C d.
  disperse d.
  food d.
  injectable d.
  d. laser
Dymenate Injection
dymple
Dynabac
Dyna-Care pressure pad system
Dynacin
  D. Oral
  D. tablet
Dyna-Flex leg compression dressing
Dyna-Hex topical
dynamometer
  Collins d.
Dynapen
DYNR
  delayed nasal response
Dy-o-Derm

NOTES

D

Dyonics
>D. basket forceps
>D. Dyosite office arthroscopy system
>D. InteliJet fluid management system
>D. suction punch

dyphylline
dysarthria
dysautonomia
>familial d.

dysbaric
dysbetalipoproteinemia
>familial d.

dyschondroplasia with hemangioma
dyschroia
dyschromatosis symmetrica
dyschromia
>cutaneous d.

dyschromicum
dyscornification
>hypergranulotic d.

dyscrasia
dysenteriae
>*Shigella flexneri* d.
>viral d.

dysenteric arthritis
dysentery
>d. antitoxin
>balantidial d.
>ciliate d.
>scorbutic d.
>Sonne d.
>spirillar d.
>sporadic d.

dysesthesia disorder
dysfunction
>antibody d.
>audiovestibular d.
>chronic graft d.
>emotional d.
>erectile d.
>esophageal d.
>immunologic d.
>intestinal mucosal d.
>meibomian gland d.
>multiple organ system d. (MOSD)
>myocardial d.
>neuroimmune d.
>phagocyte d.
>sensorineural d.
>small airways d.
>Study of Left Ventricular D.
>temporomandibular d. (TMD)
>vascular d.

dysfunctional gut syndrome
dysgammaglobulinemia

dysgenesis
>gonadal d.
>reticular d.

dyshidria
dyshidrosis, dyshydrosis, dysidrosis
>lamellar d.
>sole d.
>trichophytic d.

dyshidrotic
>d. dermatitis
>d. eczema

dysidria
dysidrosis (*var. of* dyshidrosis)
dyskeratinization
dyskeratoma
>acantholytic d.
>focal acantholytic d.
>warty d.

dyskeratosis
>acantholytic d.
>benign d.
>d. congenita
>focal acantholytic d.
>malignant d.
>transient acantholytic d.

dyskeratotic keratinocyte
dyskinetic cilia syndrome
dyslipoidosis
dysmenorrhoeica
>dermatitis d.

dysmetabolism
>tryptophan d.

dysmorphobia
dysmorphogenesis
dysmucopolysaccharidosis
>fibrocytic d.

Dysne-Inhal
dysostosis, pl. **dysostoses**
>mandibulofacial d.

dyspareunia
dyspeptic
dysphagia
dysphagocytosis
>congenital d.

dyspigmentation
dysplasia
>acetabular d.
>anhidrotic ectodermal d.
>autoimmune polyendocrinopathy-candidiasis-ectodermal d. (APECED)
>chondrodysplasia punctata d.
>cleidocranial d.
>congenital ectodermal d.
>diastrophic d.
>ectodermal d.
>familial white folded mucosal d.
>fibrous d.
>hidrotic ectodermal d.

hypohidrotic ectodermal d. (HED)
Kniest d.
late-onset spondyloepiphyseal d.
lymphopenic thymic d.
mandibuloacral d.
mesodermal d.
metaphysial d.
multiple epiphyseal d.
neutrophil d.
otospondylometaphyseal d.
  (OSMED)
polyostotic fibrous d.
Rapp-Hodgkin ectodermal d.
sphenoid d.
spondyloepiphysial d. (SED)
thymic d.

dysplastic
d. nevus
d. nevus syndrome

dyspnea
dyspneic
dysprosium ferric hydroxide
dysproteinemia
dysproteinemic purpura
dysraphism
spinal d.

dysregulated lymphocytic apoptosis
dysregulation
immune d.

dyssebacia
dyssynchrony
thoracoabdominal d.

dysthymia
dystopia canthorum
dystrophia
d. canthorum
d. unguium

dystrophic
d. calcinosis
d. calcinosis cutis
d. epidermolysis bullosa
d. epidermolysis bullosa,
  albopapuloid variant
D. Epidermolysis Bullosa Research
  Association of America (DEBRA)
d. palmoplantar hyperkeratosis

dystrophica
elastosis d.
epidermolysis bullosa d.

dystrophin
dystrophy
autoimmune polyendocrinopathy-
  candidiasis-ectodermal d.
  (APECED)
Becker muscular d.
congenital fascial d.
distal d.
Duchenne muscular d.
Emery-Dreifuss d.
epidermolysis bullosa with
  muscular d.
fascioscapulohumeral d.
intermittent hair-follicle d.
lamellar d.
limb-girdle d.
medial canaliform d.
median canaliform d.
median nail d.
merosin deficiency d.
muscular d.
10-nail d.
20-nail d.
oculopharyngeal d.
reflex sympathetic d. (RSD)

D

NOTES

E

> Aquasol E
> Florone E
> E rosette

E₁

> prostaglandin E$_1$ (PGE$_1$)

E₂

> prostaglandin E$_2$ (PGE$_2$)
> purine-stimulated prostaglandin E$_2$ (PGE$_2$)

E5 monoclonal antibody

EAC

> Ehrlich ascites carcinoma
> external auditory canal
> EAC rosette
> EAC rosette assay

EAHF

> EAHF complex

EAR

> early allergic response
> early asthmatic response

ear

> middle e.
> Otocalm E.
> e. pit
> sugarcane e.

Earle L fibrosarcoma

earlobe

> e. allergic dermatitis
> e. crease
> e. sign of nickel sensitivity

early

> e. allergic response (EAR)
> e. asthmatic response (EAR)
> e. congenital syphilis
> e. latent syphilis
> e. reaction
> e. yaw

early-phase

> e.-p. reaction (EPR)
> e.-p. response

EARTS

> European Anti-ICAM Renal Transplant Study

EASI

> Eczema Area and Severity Index

Easprin

eastern

> E. coral snake
> E. coral snake bite
> e. equine encephalitis (EEE)
> E. tick-borne rickettsiosis

easy bruising syndrome

Eaton

> E. agent
> E. agent pneumonia

Eaton-Lambert syndrome

EB

> Epstein-Barr
> EB nuclear antigen test
> EB simplex
> EB viral capsid antigen test
> EB virus

ebastine

EBMT

> European Group for Bone Marrow Transplantation

EBNA

> Epstein-Barr nuclear antigen
> EBNA IgG ELISA test

Ebola

> E. hemorrhagic fever
> E. Ivory Coast
> E. virus

EB-specific IgM test

EBV

> Epstein-Barr virus
> EBV glycoprotein gp110
> EBV infection

EC

> Euro-Collins
> EC solution

E-C

> Apo-Erythro E-C

EC50

> median effective concentration

ECASA

> enteric coated acetylsalicylic acid
> entericcoated acetylsalicylic acid

ECAT 951/33 PET scanner

ECBO

> enteric cytopathogenic bovine orphan
> ECBO virus

eccentrica

> hyperkeratosis e.
> keratoderma e.
> poliosis e.

ecchymoma

ecchymosed

ecchymosis

> old e.
> Roederer e.

ecchymotic

> e. mark
> e. rash

ECCL

> encephalocraniocutaneous lipomatosis

eccrine
    e. acrospiroma
    e. adenocarcinoma
    e. angiomatous hamartoma
    e. bromhidrosis
    e. carcinoma
    e. chromhidrosis
    e. duct
    e. epithelioma
    e. hidradenitis
    e. hidrocystoma
    e. metaplasia
    e. poroma
    e. spiradenoma
    e. squamous syringometaplasia
    e. sweat gland
    e. syringofibroadenoma
    e. tumor
ECD
    extended criteria donor
ECF-A
    eosinophil chemotactic factor of
    anaphylaxis
echidninus
    Laelaps e.
echinococcosis
Echinococcus
    E. granulosus
    E. multilocularis
echinoderm
ECHO
    enteric cytopathogenic human orphan
    ECHO virus
echocardiography
echo sign
echoviral exanthema
echovirus
eclabium
ECLAM
    European Consensus Lupus Activity
    Measure
eclipse
    e. period
    e. phase
ECLM
    European Confederation for Laboratory
    Medicine
ECM
    erythema chronicum migrans
ECM-degrading proteinase
ECMO
    enteric cytopathogenic monkey orphan
    ECMO virus
ECN-CC
    epithelioid combined nevi Carney
    complex
EcoCheck oxygen monitor
ecologic alteration
E-Complex-600

EcoNail antifungal
econazole nitrate
Econopred Plus Ophthalmic
Ecostatin
ecotaxis
Ecotrin
ecotropic virus
ECP
    erythropoietic coproporphyria
    extracorporeal photophoresis
ecphyma
ECSO
    enteric cytopathogenic swine orphan
    ECSO virus
ectasia
    acral arteriolar e.
    cutaneous e.
    papillary e.
    sacral root sheath e.
    senile e.
    spider e.
Ectasule
ecthyma
    e. contagiosum
    contagious e.
    e. gangrenosum
    e. infectiosum
ecthymatiform
ecthymatous syphilid
ectoantigen
ectoderm
ectodermal
    e. dysplasia
    e. groove
ectodermatosis
ectodermogenic neurosyphilis
ectodermosis erosiva pluriorificialis
ectogenous
ectoparasite
ectopic
    e. cutaneous schistosomiasis
    e. keratinization
    e. sebaceous gland
Ectosone
ectothrix infection
ectotoxin
ectozoon
ectrodactyly, ectodermal, clefting (EEC)
ectromelia virus
eculizumab
eczema
    adolescent e.
    adult e.
    allergic e.
    E. Area and Severity Index
     (EASI)
    e. articulorum
    asteatotic e.
    atopic e.

baker's e.
childhood e.
chronic e.
contact e.
e. craquelé
e. crustosum
e. diabeticorum
dyshidrotic e.
e. epilans
e. epizootica
e. erythematosum
flexural e.
follicular nummular e.
hand e.
e. herpeticum
housewives' e.
e. hypertrophicum
idiopathic late-onset e.
infantile e.
e. intertrigo
intertrigo e.
lichenoid e.
e. madidans
e. marginatum
e. neuriticum
nummular e.
e. nummulare
nutritional deficiency e.
orbicular e.
e. papulosum
e. parasiticum
e. pustulosum
e. rubrum
e. scrofuloderma
seborrheic e.
e. seborrhoeicum
e. siccum
e. solare
e. squamosum
e. stasis
stasis e.
topical e.
tropical e.
e. tyloticum
e. vaccinatum
varicose e.
e. verrucosum
e. vesiculosum
weeping e.
winter e.
xerotic e.

eczematid
exsiccation e.
eczematization
eczematize
eczematodes
impetigo e.
eczematogenic
eczematogenous
eczematoid
e. dermatitis
e. pruritic plaque
e. seborrhea
eczematoides
dermatitis infectiosa e.
eczematous
e. change
e. lesion
e. patch
e. PMLE
e. polymorphous light eruption
e. reaction
edema
acute periorbital e.
angioneurotic e.
brawny e.
bullous e.
dependent e.
e. of feet
e. of hand
hemorrhagic e.
hereditary angioneurotic e. (HAE, HANE)
hysterical e.
indolent nonpitting e.
inflammatory e.
intercellular e.
intracellular e.
laryngeal e.
massive cerebral e.
Milton e.
e. neonatorum
noninflammatory e.
palpebral e.
periodic e.
persistent e.
pitting e.
Quincke e.
remitting seronegative symmetrical synovitis with pitting e. (RS3PE)
e. toxin (ET)
Yangtze e.
edematous

E

NOTES

edge
>discrete e.
>e. effect

Edmonston-Zagreb vaccine
edobacomab
EDSS
>expanded disability status scale

education
>patient e.

Edwardsiella
EEC
>ectrodactyly, ectodermal, clefting
>ectodermal dysplasia, ectrodactyly and
>>cleft lip and/or palate
>EEC syndrome

EEE
>eastern equine encephalitis
>EEE virus

E.E.S. Oral
EEU
>environmental exposure unit

EF
>eosinophilic fasciitis

EFA
>essential fatty acid

Efalith ointment
efalizumab
efavirenz
Efedron
effect
>allogenic e.
>antiapoptotic e.
>antiproliferative e.
>cidal e.
>contrast e.
>counterregulatory e.
>Danysz e.
>Deelman e.
>dose-related e.
>edge e.
>first-pass drug e.
>graft-versus-leukemia e.
>isomorphic e.
>Köbner e.
>Koebner effect
>light-sparing e.
>Lyon e.
>nongenomic glucocorticoid e.
>Overhauser e.
>postanesthetic e.
>postpartum e.
>prepriming e.
>proinflammatory e.
>secondary e.
>side e.
>squeeze e.
>steal e.
>tattooing e.
>tendonesis e.

>Tindall e.
>veto e.
>virostatic e.

effector
>e. cell
>e. molecule
>nephritogenic e.
>e. pathway

Effersyl
efficacy
efficiency
>hair removal e. (HRE)
>sleep e.

effluvium
>anagen e.
>short anagen telogen e.
>telogen e.

effort syndrome
effusion
>joint e.
>parapneumonic e.

Efidac/24 chlorpheniramine
eflornithine hydrochloride
Efodine
Efudex topical
EGF
>epidermal growth factor

egg-passage
>rabies vaccine, Flury strain e.-p.

eggplant
egg shell nail
Ehlers-Danlos
>E.-D. syndrome
>E.-D. syndrome, arterial-ecchymotic
>>type
>E.-D. syndrome, arthrochalasia type
>E.-D. syndrome, classic type
>E.-D. syndrome, fibronectin-deficient
>>type
>E.-D. syndrome, Gravis type
>E.-D. syndrome, human
>>dermatosparaxis type
>E.-D. syndrome, hypermobile type
>E.-D. syndrome, kyphoscoliosis type
>E.-D. syndrome, Mitis type
>E.-D. syndrome, ocular-scoliotic
>>type
>E.-D. syndrome, periodontitis type
>E.-D. syndrome, vascular type

Ehrlich
>E. ascites carcinoma (EAC)
>E. ascites carcinoma rosette assay
>E. phenomenon
>E. postulate
>E. side-chain theory

Ehrlichia
>*E. canis*
>*E. chaffeensis*

E. ewengii
E. sennetsu
ehrlichiosis
human granulocytic e.
EIA
enzyme-linked immunoassay
EIA diagnosis
Eichenholtz classification
eicosanoid inhibition
eicosapentaenoic acid
Eikenella
EI.U
ELISA unit
ekiri
EKV
erythrokeratoderma variabilis
elacin
ELAD
extracorporeal liver assist device
ELAD artificial liver
ELAM-1
endothelial leukocyte adhesion molecule-1
ELA-Max cream
elapid
Elapidae
Elase-Chloromycetin topical
Elase topical
elastase
neutrophil e.
polymorphonuclear leukocyte e.
Pseudomonas e.
elastic
e. fiber
e. fiber stain
e. recoil
e. skin
e. tissue
e. wrap
elastica
helminthiasis e.
elastic-fiber fragmentation
elasticity
sputum viscosity and e.
elasticum
localized acquired cutaneous pseudoxanthoma e.
periumbilical perforating pseudoxanthoma e.
pseudoxanthoma e. (PXE)
elasticus
Lewandowsky nevus e.

Elastikon elastic tape
elastin
elastofibroma dorsi
Elasto-Gel hydrogel sheet
elastohydrodynamic lubrication
elastoid degeneration
elastolysis
generalized e.
middermal e.
elastolytic giant cell granuloma
elastoma
Dubreuilh e.
juvenile e.
Miescher e.
elastomer
thermoplastic e. (TPE)
elastomeric
e. complex
e. pump
Elastomull elastic gauze bandage
Elastoplast elastic dressing
elastorrhexis
elastosis
actinic e.
e. colloidalis conglomerata
cutaneous e.
e. dystrophica
linear focal e.
nodular e.
perforating calcific e.
senile e.
solar e.
thermal e.
elastotic
e. degeneration
e. nodules of anthelix
e. stria
elastoviscosity
elastoviscous solution
Elavil
elbow
golfer's e.
Little League e.
Mayo classification of rheumatoid e.
tennis e.
transplant e.
Elbowlift suspension pad
Eldecort topical
elder
marsh e.

E

NOTES

elder *(continued)*
　　rough marsh e.
　　Vitadye makeup by E.
Elder classification
Eldopaque
　　E. Forte
　　E. Forte cream
Eldoquin Forte
EleCare medical food
elective
　　e. culture
　　e. low-risk recipient
Electra 1000C coagulation analyzer
electrical
electroacupuncture
Electro-Acuscope
electrocautery
electrocoagulated
electrocoagulation
　　e. biterminal device
　　pinpoint e.
electrode
　　Clarke-type e.
　　indifferent e.
　　e. siccation
electrodermal
　　e. diagnosis
　　e. testing
electrodermatome
electrodesiccation
electrofulguration
electroimmunodiffusion
electrolysis
electromagnetic
　　e. field
　　e. radiation
electromyographic feature
electromyography (EMG)
electron
　　e. beam
　　e. microscopy
electronic filter
electrooculogram
electrophilic ethylene episulfonium
electrophoresis
　　immunodeficiency e.
　　immunofixation e. (IFE)
　　polyacrylamide gel e. (PAGE)
　　pulsed field gel e. (PFGE)
　　SDS-polyacrylamide gel e.
　　serum immunofixation e. (SIFE)
　　serum protein e. (SPEP)
　　sodium dodecyl sulfate-
　　　polyacrylamide gel e. (SDS-
　　　PAGE)
　　temperature-controlled e.
　　urinary e.

　　urine immunofixation e. (UIFE)
　　urine protein e. (UPEP)
electrophoretic mobility shift assay
　(EMSA)
electrophoretogram
　　serum protein e. (SPE)
electrophototherapy
electrosection
electrosurgery
　　bipolar e.
electrosurgical epilation
electrotransfer test
element
　　kappa-deleting e.
　　promotor e.
　　Rev-responsive e. (RRE)
　　trace e.
elemental
　　e. diet
　　e. disorder
elementary lesion
element-binding
　　cAMP response e.-b. (CREB)
elephant
　　e. leg
　　e. skin
elephantiac
elephantiasic
elephantiasis
　　e. arabicum
　　e. arabum
　　e. asturiensis
　　congenital e.
　　filarial e.
　　e. graecorum
　　lymphangiectatic e.
　　e. neurofibromatosis
　　e. neuromatosa
　　neuromatosis e.
　　nevoid e.
　　nostras e.
　　e. nostras
　　e. nostra verrucosa
　　e. telangiectodes
　　e. tropica
elephantoid fever
Elestat eyedrops
elevation
　　blanched cutaneous e.
　　rest, ice, compresses, e. (RICE)
elevator
　　Freer septum e.
　　e. grain dust mite
elevatum
ELF
　　epithelial lining fluid
ELFD
　　epithelial lining fluid desensitization
Elgiloy

elicitation
Elidel
    E. cream
    E. tablet
elimination
    e. diet
    food e.
    immune e.
    e. procedure
    sweat chloride e.
Elimite Cream
ELISA
    enzyme-linked immunosorbent assay
    double-sandwich IgM ELISA
    ELISA test
    ELISA unit (EI.U)
ELISA-Light Chemiluminescent Detection system
ELISPOT
    enzyme-linked immunospot assay
    ELISPOT test
Elixicon
Elixir
    Allergy E.
    Brofed E.
    Bromaline E.
    Bromanate E.
    Bromphen E.
    Cold & Allergy E.
    Dimaphen E.
    Dimetane Decongestant E.
    Genatap E.
Elixophyllin
elizabethan
    Bartonella e.
Elliot sign
Ellipse compact spacer
elliptical
    e. biopsy
    e. incision
elliptocyte
Ellis-van Creveld syndrome
Ellman Surgitron
ELM
    epiluminescence light microscopy
elm
    American e.
    Chinese e.
    fall e.
    slippery e.
    e. tree
    e. tree pollen

Elocon topical
elongin
Elset long stretch bandage
Elta
    E. Dermal
    E. Dermal hydrogel dressing
    E. Dermal impregnated gauze
    E. Dermal wound cleanser
Eltor
eluate
    glomerular e.
EluSu
EM
    erythema multiforme
emaculation
ematode
embedded stinger
emboli (*pl. of* embolus)
embolia cutis medicamentosa
embolic
    e. gangrene
    e. nodule
embolism
    plasmodium e.
    pulmonary e.
embolization
    bronchial artery e.
    renal cholesterol e. (RCE)
embolus, pl. emboli
    atheromatous e.
    cholesterol e.
    septal e.
    septic e.
embryogenesis
embryology
EMC
    encephalomyocarditis
    EMC virus
emergency treatment
emerging virus
Emery-Dreifuss dystrophy
emetine
EMG
    electromyography
Emgel topical
EMIT
    enzyme-multiplied immunoassay technique
EMLA
    eutectic mixture of local anesthetics
    EMLA anesthetic disc

E

NOTES

EMLA *(continued)*
    EMLA cream
    EMLA topical
EMM
    erythema multiforme majus
EMMPRIN
Emo-Cort
emollient
    topical e.
7E3 monoclonal antiplatelet antibody
emotional
    e. dysfunction
    e. flushing
    e. hyperhidrosis
    e. stress
emperipolesis
emphlysis
emphractic
emphraxis
emphysema
    subcutaneous e.
empiric therapy
Empirin
Emplasterium urea **paste**
empty sella syndrome
empyema
empyesis
EMS
    eosinophilia-myalgia syndrome
EMSA
    electrophoretic mobility shift assay
emulsifiable ointment
emulsifier
emulsifying agent
emulsion
    Pusey e.
    radiodermatitis e. (RE)
    wound dressing e. (WDE)
E-Mycin-E
E-Mycin Oral
EN
    erythema nodosum
en
    e. bloc transplant
    e. bloc transplantation
    e. coup de sabre
    e. coup de sabre scalp lesion
    e. passant
ENA
    extractable nuclear antigen
    ENA antigen
enamel
    e. paint skin
    e. paint spot appearance
enanthem
enanthema
enanthematous
enanthesis
Enbrel plus ATG

Encap
    Novo-Rythro E.
encapsulated
    e. neuroma
    e. organism
encephalitide
encephalitis
    acute necrotizing e.
    Australian X e.
    Baló concentric e.
    bunyavirus e.
    California e. (CE)
    Coxsackie e.
    Dawson e.
    eastern equine e. (EEE)
    epidemic e.
    equine e.
    Far East Russian e.
    fox e.
    herpes simplex e.
    HHV6 e.
    hyperergic e.
    Ilhéus e.
    inclusion body e.
    Japanese B e.
    e. japonica
    e. lethargica
    Mengo e.
    Murray Valley e. (MVE)
    postvaccinal e.
    Powassan e.
    Russian autumn e.
    Russian spring-summer e.
    Russian tick-borne e.
    Saint Louis e.
    secondary e.
    subacute inclusion body e.
    varicella e.
    vernal e.
    e. virus
    von Economo e.
    woodcutter's e.
encephalitogen
encephalitogenic
Encephalitozoon cuniculi
encephalocele
encephalocraniocutaneous lipomatosis (ECCL)
encephalomyelitis
    allergic e.
    autoimmune e.
    avian infectious e.
    disseminated e.
    enzootic e.
    equine e.
    herpes B e.
    infectious porcine e.
    Kelly e.
    mouse e.

Venezuelan equine e. (VEE)
viral e.
virus e.
western equine e. (WEE)
zoster e.
encephalomyocarditis (EMC)
e. virus
encephalopathy
bovine spongiform e.
HIV e.
subacute spongiform e.
transmissible mink e.
transmissible spongiform e. (TSE)
encoding
naked DNA e.
end
e. cell
E. Lice
E. Lice Liquid
endemia
endemic
e. fogo selvagem
e. fungal infection
e. index
e. nonbacterial infantile
gastroenteritis
e. pemphigus foliaceus
e. syphilis
e. typhus
e. urticaria
endemica
urticaria multiformis e.
endemicum
Treponema e.
endemium
erythema e.
granuloma e.
endemoepidemic
Endep
endermic
endermism
end-inspiratory crackle
endobronchial brachytherapy
endocardial fibroproliferative
endocarditis
bacteria-free stage of bacterial e.
bacterial e.
enterococcal e.
infectious e.
Libman-Sacks e.
subacute bacterial e. (SBE)

endocrine
e. amyloidosis
e. disease
e. hormone imbalance
e. rhinitis
endocrinopathy
endocytosis
reverse e.
endoderm
Endodermophyton
endogenote
endogenous
e. antigen
e. antitumor immunity
e. dermatitis
e. factor
e. immune response
e. infection
e. ochronosis
e. pyrogen
endoluminal
endomophilous
endomysial mononuclear cell
endonuclease
endoparasitism
Endopearl bioabsorbable device
endopeptidase
Zn-dependent e.
endoperoxide synthase
endophthalmitis
endoplasmic reticulum
endoprotease
endosclerosis
endoscopy
intragastral provocation under e.
(IPEC)
zoom e.
EndoSheath
endosomal
e. acidification
e. localization motif
endosteal
endothelial
e. cell
e. cell proliferation
e. leukocyte adhesion molecule-1
(ELAM-1)
e. lysis
endothelial-derived nitric oxide
endothelial-relaxing factor
endothelin-1 (ET-1)
endothelioid

E

NOTES

endothelioma
  e. capitis
  e. cutis
endothelium-derived relaxation factor
endothelium vascular
endothrix infection
endotoxemia
endotoxicosis
endotoxic reaction
endotoxin
  e. shock
  e. signaling pathway
endovascular papillary angioendothelioma
end-product
end-stage organ disease
end-tidal cardiac disease (ETCO$_2$)
engagement
  immune e.
Engerix-B
English
  E. ivy
  E. plantain
  E. plantain weed pollen
  E. walnut tree pollen
englobe
englobement
Engman
  E. dermatitis
  E. disease
engrafted
engraftment
enhancement
  immunological e.
enhancer
  SEPA dermal absorption e.
enhancing antibody
enisoprost
ENL
  erythema nodosum leprosum
enolase
  neuron-specific e. (NSE)
Enomine
Enovil
enoxacin
enoxaparin
enrichment
  e. culture
  density gradient bone marrow progenitor e.
enseals
  potassium iodide e.
EN-tabs
  Azulfidine E.-t.
entactin
Entamoeba histolytica
ENTec Coblator plasma system
Entemopoxvirus

enteric
  e. coated acetylsalicylic acid (ECASA)
  e. coated aspirin
  e. cytopathogenic bovine orphan (ECBO)
  e. cytopathogenic bovine orphan virus
  e. cytopathogenic human orphan (ECHO)
  e. cytopathogenic human orphan virus
  e. cytopathogenic monkey orphan (ECMO)
  e. cytopathogenic monkey orphan virus
  e. cytopathogenic swine orphan (ECSO)
  e. cytopathogenic swine orphan virus
  e. fever
  e. infection
  e. pancreatic drainage
  portal (venous and) e. (P-E)
enteritidis
  Salmonella e.
enteritis
  e. anaphylactica
  Campylobacter fetus e.
  feline infectious e.
  e. of mink
  transmissible e.
enteroadherent
enteroaggregative
Enterobacter
  E. cloacae
  E. liquefaciens
  E. sakazakii
Enterobacteriaceae
enterobiasis
Enterobius vermicularis
enterochromaffin cell
enterococcal endocarditis
Enterococcus
  Enterococcus faecalis
  Enterococcus faecium
  vancomycin-resistant *Enterococcus* (VRE)
enterocolitica
  Yersinia e.
enterocolitis
  antibiotic e.
  dietary protein e.
  dietary protein-induced e.
  gold-induced e.
  necrotizing e. (NEC)
Enterocytozoon bieneusi
enterogenic reactive arthritis
enterohemorrhagic

enteroinvasive
enteropathic
    e. arthritis
    e. arthropathy
enteropathica
    acrodermatitis e. (AE)
enteropathy
    cow's mild-sensitive e.
    food protein-induced e.
    gluten e.
    gluten-sensitive e. (GSE)
    protein-losing e.
enterosepsis
enterotoxigenic
enterotoxin
    Escherichia coli e.
    staphylococcal e.
enteroviral
    e. exanthema
    e. infection
Enterovirus
enterovirus (EV)
    myelitic e.
    nonpolio e.
Entex
    E. LA
    E. PSE
entheseal ossification
enthesis
enthesitis
enthesitis-related arthritis
enthesopathy
    ankylosing e.
    metabolic e.
enthesophyte
enthetic
entire body imaging agent
Entocort
entomophthoramycosis basidiobolae
entrapment
    dorsal scapular nerve e.
    genitofemoral nerve e.
    ilioinguinal nerve e.
    interdigital nerve e.
    lateral femoral cutaneous nerve e.
    long thoracic nerve e.
    musculocutaneous nerve e.
    nerve e.
    e. neuropathy
    obturator nerve e.
    peroneal nerve e.
    radial nerve e.

    saphenous nerve e.
    sciatic nerve e.
    superficial peroneal nerve e.
    superficial radial nerve e.
    suprascapular nerve e.
    sural nerve e.
Entrophen
ENTsol
    E. adaptor
    E. Mist
    E. Packets
    E. Refillable Bottle
enucleation
Envacor test
envelope
    cornified cell e.
    viral e.
envenomation
env gene
environmental
    e. allergen
    e. change
    e. exposure unit (EEU)
    e. factor
    e. illness
    e. medicine
    e. mite infestation
    e. mycobacterial infection
    e. mycobacteriosis
    e. scabies
    e. scleroderma
    e. survey
    e. tobacco smoke (ETS)
environment progressive symptom sclerosis
envoplakin
enzootic
    e. bovine leukosis
    e. encephalomyelitis
    e. encephalomyelitis virus
enzymatic
    e. debriding agent
    e. saliva
enzyme
    angiotensin-converting e. (ACE)
    biotinidase e.
    CAT e.
    chloramphenicol acetyltransferase e.
    collagenolytic e.
    COX e.
    COX-1 e.
    cyclooxygenase e.

NOTES

183

enzyme *(continued)*
    dual-function e.
    epoxide hydrolase e.
    fyn kinase e.
    e. heme oxygenase
    immunoglobulin-complexed e. (ICE)
    lysosomal e.
    lytic e.
    matrix-degrading e.
    phospholipase e.
    prostanoid biosynthetic e.
    proteolytic e.
    e. replacement
    secretory PLA$_2$ e.
    steroidogenic e.
    ubiquitin-conjugating e.
    upstream e.
    e. worker's lung
enzyme-linked
    e.-l. immunoassay (EIA)
    e.-l. immunosorbent assay (ELISA)
    e.-l. immunosorbent assay test
    e.-l. immunospot assay (ELISPOT)
enzyme-multiplied immunoassay technique (EMIT)
enzyme-related panniculitis
EOA
    erosive osteoarthritis
eosin
    hematoxylin and e. (HE, H&E)
    e. stain
eosinophil
    e. chemotactic factor
    e. chemotactic factor of anaphylaxis (ECF-A)
    e. granule cationic protein
    e. peroxidase
    e. protein X
eosinophil-derived neurotoxin
eosinophilia
    airway e.
    blood e.
    peripheral blood e.
    prolonged pulmonary e.
    pulmonary infiltrate with e. (PIE)
    simple pulmonary e.
    tropical e.
eosinophilia-myalgia syndrome (EMS)
eosinophilic
    e. abscess
    e. arteritis
    e. bronchopneumonia
    e. cellulitis
    e. chemotaxis
    e. dermatitis
    e. fasciitis (EF)
    e. fasciitis syndrome
    e. gastroenteritis
    e. granuloma

    e. granulomatosis
    e. myalgia
    e. myalgia syndrome
    e. myositis
    e. panniculitis
    e. pneumonia
    e., polymorphic, and pruritic eruption associated with radiotherapy (EPPER)
    e. pulmonary syndrome
    e. pustular folliculitis
    e. spongiosis
    e. syndrome overlap
    e. synovitis
eosinophilopoiesis
eosinophiluria
eotaxin
ephedra
ephedrine
    aminophylline, amobarbital, and e.
    e. sulfate
Ephedsol
ephelis, pl. **ephelides**
    nevi, atrial myxoma, myxoid neurofibromas, and ephelides (NAME)
    nevi, atrial myxomas, myxomas of skin and mammary glands, and ephelides (NAME)
ephemeral
    e. fever of cattle
    e. fever virus
ephidrosis cruenta
epicanthus
Epicauta
    E. fabricii
    E. fabricii sting
    E. vitlata
    E. vitlata sting
Epicel
    E. autologous skin cell
    E. skin graft material
Epicoccum purpurascens
epicondylitis
Epics Elite flow cytometer
epicutaneous
    e. reaction
    e. test
epicuticle
epidemic
    e. acne
    e. arthritic erythema
    e. benign dry pleurisy
    e. cerebrospinal meningitis
    e. curve
    e. diaphragmatic pleurisy
    e. dropsy
    e. encephalitis
    e. exanthema

e. gastroenteritis virus
e. hemorrhagic fever
e. hepatitis
e. keratoconjunctivitis
e. keratoconjunctivitis virus
e. myalgia
e. myalgia virus
e. myositis
e. nausea
e. nonbacterial gastroenteritis
e. parotiditis
e. parotitis virus
e. pleurodynia
e. pleurodynia virus
e. polyarthritis
e. roseola
e. transient diaphragmatic spasm
e. tremor
e. typhus
e. vomiting
epidemica
    dermatitis exfoliativa e.
    nephropathia c.
    urticaria e.
epidemicity
epidemicum
    erythema arthriticum e.
epidemiography
epidemiologic
epidemiology
    The E. and Natural History of
    Asthma: Outcome and Treatment
    Regimens (TENOR)
epidermal
    e. allergen
    e. appendage
    e. cyst
    e. filaggrin
    e. growth factor (EGF)
    e. Langerhans cell
    e. necrolysis
    e. nevus
    e. stacking
    e. testing
    e. transit time
epidermal-dermal separation
epidermal-melanin unit
epidermatoplasty
epidermic-dermic nevus
epidermidalization
epidermides (*pl. of* epidermis)

epidermidis
    Staphylococcus e.
    stratum corneum e.
epidermidosis
epidermis, pl. **epidermides**
    a collarette of e.
    hyperkeratotic e.
    hyperplastic e.
epidermitis
epidermization
epidermodysplasia
    e. verruciformis (EV)
    e. verruciformis of Lewandowski-
    Lutz
epidermoid
    e. cancer
    e. carcinoma
    e. cyst
epidermolysis
    e. bullosa acquisita antigen
    e. bullosa atrophicans
    e. bullosa, dermal type
    e. bullosa dystrophica
    e. bullosa, epidermal type
    e. bullosa, Gravis type
    e. bullosa, inverse
    e. bullosa, junctional type
    e. bullosa, localized
    e. bullosa, Mitis type
    e. bullosa simplex
    e. bullosa simplex, generalized
    e. bullosa simplex herpetiformis
    e. bullosa simplex, localized
    e. bullosa simplex with mottled
    pigmentation
    e. bullosa with muscular dystrophy
    polydysplastic e.
    toxic bullous e.
epidermolytic
    e. acanthoma
    e. hyperkeratosis
    e. keratosis palmaris et plantaris
    e. palmoplantar keratoderma
epidermophytid
Epidermophyton
    E. floccosum
    E. inguinale
epidermophytosis
    e. cruris
    e. interdigitale
epidermosis

E

NOTES

epidermotropic
>   e. cutaneous toxoplasmosis
>   e. reticulosis

epidermotropism

EpiEZPen

Epifoam

Epifrin

epigenetic

epiglottiditis

epiglottitis
>   acute e.

epilans
>   eczema e.

EpiLaser laser-based hair removal system

epilate

epilation
>   electrosurgical e.
>   photo e.
>   wax e.

epilator
>   galvanic e.

epilatory

epilepticus
>   status e.

EpiLeukin

EpiLight
>   E. flashlamp
>   E. hair removal system

Epi-lock wound dressing

epiloia

epiluminescence light microscopy (ELM)

epiluminescent skin surface microscope

Epilyt

epimastical fever

epimerization

epinastine HCl

epinephrine
>   aqueous e.
>   e. hydrochloride
>   lidocaine and e.
>   self-injecting e.
>   subcutaneous e.
>   Xylocaine with e.

EpiPen Jr.

epiphenomenal

epiphora

epiphysial, epiphyseal

epiphysiodesis

epiphysiolysis

epiphysitis

Epiquick

episclera

episcleritis
>   nodular e.
>   nonrheumatoid e.
>   rheumatoid e.

episode
>   acute rejection e.

episodic
>   e. angioedema
>   e. bronchial obstruction
>   e. malnutrition

episomal DNA

episome
>   resistance-transferring e.

epispastic

EpiStar diode laser system

epistaxis

episulfonium
>   electrophilic ethylene e.

epithelial
>   e. cyst
>   e. degeneration
>   e. injury
>   e. keratitis
>   e. keratopathy
>   e. lining fluid (ELF)
>   e. lining fluid desensitization (ELFD)
>   e. nevus
>   e. tumor

epitheliale
>   molluscum e.

epithelialization

epithelial-mesenchymal

epitheliitis

epithelioid
>   e. blue nevus
>   e. cell
>   e. cell nevus
>   e. combined nevi Carney complex (ECN-CC)
>   e. granuloma
>   e. sarcoma

epithelioma
>   e. adenoides cysticum
>   apocrine e.
>   Borst-Jadassohn type intraepidermal e.
>   calcifying e.
>   e. capitis
>   e. contagiosum
>   e. cuniculatum
>   eccrine e.
>   Ferguson-Smith e.
>   Ferguson-Smith-type e.
>   Jadassohn e.
>   e. of Malherbe
>   Malherbe calcifying e.
>   multiple benign cystic e.
>   prickle-cell e.
>   sebaceous e.
>   squamous cell e.
>   superficial basal cell e.

epitheliomatocylindromatosus
>   nevus e.

epitheliomatosis

epitheliomatous
epitheliopathy
acute multifocal placoid pigment e.
epithelioserosa
zona e.
epitheliotropic
epithelite
epithelium
autologous cultured e.
bronchial e.
cat e.
columnar e.
cultured thymic e.
dog e.
ferret e.
goat e.
monkey e.
mouse e.
rabbit e.
sheep e.
sloughed bronchial e.
swine e.
tegumentary e.
epithelization
epithelize
Epitol
epitope
allergenic e.
alpha-Gal e.
B-cell e.
e. contraction
cryptic e.
3Gal e.
Gal-alpha-1 e.
e. homozygosity
J serovar-specific e.
e. mapping
ovalbumin-derived e.
shared e.
e. spreading
epitope-spreading phenomenon
EpiTouch laser
epitoxoid
epitrichium
Epivir
Epivir-HBV
epizootica
eczema e.
epizootic cellulitis
Epogen
eponychia
eponychium

epoprostenol
epoxide hydrolase enzyme
epoxy
e. resin
e. resin dermatitis
e. resin lung
EPP
erythropoietic porphyria
Eppendorf tube
EPPER
eosinophilic, polymorphic, and pruritic
eruption associated with radiotherapy
EPR
early-phase reaction
epsilometric test
epsilon-aminocaproic agent
Epsom salts
Epstein
E. disease
E. pearls
Epstein-Barr (EB)
E.-B. exanthema
E.-B. glycoprotein gp110
E.-B. nuclear antigen (EBNA)
E.-B. nuclear antigen test
E.-B. simplex
E.-B. virus (EBV)
E.-B. virus-associated malignancy
E.-B. virus-induced early antibody
E.-B. virus infection
E.-B. virus test
Epstein-Barr-specific immunoglobulin M test
ePTFE
expanded polytetrafluoroethylene
ePTFE implant
epulis
denture e.
e. fissuratum
giant cell e.
EQ-5D EuroQol questionnaire
Equagesic
equation
Chiou e.
equestrian panniculitis
equi
Babesia e.
Demodex e.
Rhodococcus e.
equilibrium
e. dialysis
Hardy-Weinberg e.

NOTES

equine
- e. abortion virus
- e. arteritis virus
- e. coital exanthema virus
- e. encephalitis
- e. encephalomyelitis
- e. infectious anemia
- e. infectious anemia virus
- e. influenza
- e. influenza virus
- e. *Morbillivirus*
- e. rhinopneumonitis
- e. rhinopneumonitis virus
- e. rhinovirus
- e. serum hepatitis
- e. viral arteritis

equinia
equivalence zone
equivalent
- human skin e. (HSE)
- living skin e. (LSE)

equuli
- *Actinobacillus e.*

ER
- Metadate ER

E-R
- Betachron E-R

eradicate
ErbB-2 protein
ERBE
- ERBE electrical coagulation instrument
- ERBE electrical cutting instrument

erbium
- e. laser
- 2040 e. SilkLaser

erbium:yttrium-aluminum-garnet (Er:YAG)
Ercaf
erectile
- e. dysfunction
- e. nevus

Ergamisol
ergocalciferol
Ergomar
Ergostat
ergosterole
ergotamine
- e. derivative
- Medihaler-Epi E.

ergotism
erinacei
- *Archeaopsylla e.*
- *Trichophyton e.*

eriparatide
erisipela de la costa
erosio interdigitalis blastomycetica
erosion
- bone e.
- bony e.
- glenoid e.
- punched-out e.
- radiographic e.
- subchondral e.
- e. volume

erosiva
erosive
- e. arthritis
- e. *Candida* balanitis
- e. chancre
- e. lichen planus
- e. osteoarthritis (EOA)
- e. polyarthritis

EROTIC
- European Organization for Research and Treatment of Cancer

error
- coefficient of e. (CE)

ERT
- estrogen replacement therapy

Ertaczo
ertapenem sodium
erubescence
erubescent
eruption
- acneform e.
- bullous pemphigoid-like e.
- butterfly e.
- creeping e.
- crustaceous e.
- cutaneous drug e.
- drug e.
- eczematous polymorphous light e.
- erythematous psoriasiform e.
- evanescent e.
- e. evolution
- familial polymorphous light e.
- feigned e.
- fixed drug e. (FDE)
- hypopigmented macular e.
- iodine e.
- juvenile spring e.
- Kaposi varicelliform e.
- lichenoid e.
- light e.
- medicinal e.
- morbilliform e.
- noneczematous persistent papular gold e.
- papulonecrotic e.
- papulosquamous e.
- pemphigus-like e.
- petechial e.
- pityriasis rosea-like e.
- polymorphic light e.
- polymorphous light e. (PMLE)
- posttraumatic pustular e.
- psoriasiform e.

purpuric phototherapy-induced e.
pustular e.
Rosen papular e.
scarlatiniform e.
scleroderma-like e.
seabather's e.
serum e.
skin e.
summer e.
tubercular e.
vesicopustular e.
vesicular e.

eruptione
variola sine e.

eruptive
e. fever
e. keratoacanthoma
e. pseudoangiomatosis
e. syringoma
e. vellus hair cyst
e. xanthoma

Erwinia
Er:YAG
erbium:yttrium-aluminum-garnet
Erybid
Erycette topical
Eryc Oral
EryDerm Topical
Erygel Topical
Erymax topical
EryPed Oral
erysipelas
ambulant e.
coast e.
e. de la costa
e. grave intemum
e. internum
e. migrans
migrant e.
e. perstans
e. perstans faciei
phlegmonous e.
e. pustulosum
surgical e.
e. verrucosum
e. vesiculosum
wandering e.
zoonotic e.

erysipelas-like
e.-l. dermatophytid
e.-l. erythema
e.-l. skin lesion

erysipelatous
erysipeloid
Rosenbach e.
e. of Rosenbach
erysipelothrix
Erysipelothrix dermatitis
Erysipelothrix rhusiopathiae
erysipelotoxin
Ery-Tab Oral
erythema
acral e.
acrodynic e.
e. annulare
e. annulare rheumaticum
anular e.
e. arthriticum
e. arthriticum epidemicum
bright e.
e. brucellum
e. caloricum
chilblain-like e.
e. chronicum
e. chronicum figuratum
melanodermicum
e. chronicum migrans (ECM)
circinate syphilitic e.
e. circinatum
congenital telangiectatic e.
e. congestivum
e. contagiosum
e. contusiforme
e. contusiformis
e. craquelé
e. desquamativum
diffuse e.
e. dose
drug-induced e.
e. dyschromicum perstans
e. endemium
epidemic arthritic e.
erysipelas-like e.
e. exfoliativa
facial e.
e. figuratum
e. figuratum perstans
e. fugax
e. gyratum
e. gyratum perstans
e. gyratum repens
hemorrhagic exudative e.
e. induratum
e. intertrigo

NOTES

E

189

erythema *(continued)*
  e. iris
  Jacquet e.
  e. keratodes
  linear extensor e.
  macular e.
  malar e.
  e. marginatum
  Milian e.
  morbilliform e.
  e. multiforme (EM)
  e. multiforme bullosum
  e. multiforme exudativum
  e. multiforme major
  e. multiforme majus (EMM)
  e. multiforme minor
  necrolytic migratory e.
  e. necroticans
  e. neonatorum toxicum
  ninth-day e.
  e. nodosum (EN)
  e. nodosum leprosum (ENL)
  e. nodosum migrans
  e. nodosum syphiliticum
  e. nuchae
  nummular e.
  palmar e.
  e. palmare
  e. palmare hereditarium
  e. papulatum
  papuloerosive e.
  e. papulosum
  e. paratrimma
  pellagroid e.
  periorbital violaceous e.
  periungual e.
  e. pernio
  e. polymorphe
  e. pudicitiae
  e. a pudore
  e. pudoris
  e. punctate
  e. punctatum
  radiation e.
  retiform e.
  rheumatic e.
  scarlatiniform e.
  e. scarlatiniforme
  e. simplex
  e. solare
  e. streptogenes
  symptomatic e.
  telangiectatic e.
  e. threshold
  toxic e.
  e. toxicum neonatorum
  e. traumaticum
  e. tuberculatum
  e. urticans

  e. venenatum
  violet-blue e.
erythematic
erythematosa
  acne e.
  dermatitis e.
erythematosquamous plaque
erythematosum
  eczema e.
erythematosus
  ACR diagnostic criteria for
    systemic lupus e.
  bullous systemic lupus e. (BSLE)
  chilblain lupus e.
  chronic cutaneous e. (CCE)
  chronic discoid lupus e.
  cutaneous lupus e.
  disseminated lupus e.
  drug-induced systemic lupus e.
  neonatal lupus e. (NLE)
  neuropsychiatric syndrome of
    systemic lupus e. (NPSLE)
  neuropsychiatric systemic lupus e.
    (NPSLE)
  pemphigus e.
  subacute cutaneous lupus e.
    (SCLE)
  systemic lupus e. (SLE)
  transient neonatal systemic lupus e.
  tumid lupus e.
erythematous
  e. macular dermatitis
  e. mark
  e. psoriasiform eruption
  e. syphilid
  e. vulvitis en plaque
  e. wheal
erythematovesicular
erythemogenic
erythermalgia
erythralgia
erythrasma
  Barensprung e.
erythredema
erythrism
erythristic
Erythro-Base
erythroblastosis
  fetal e.
  e. fetalis
erythroblastotic
erythrocatalysis
Erythrocin Oral
erythrocyanosis
  e. crurum
  e. crurum puellaris
  e. frigida
  e. frigida crurum puellarum
  e. supramalleolaris

erythrocyte
  e. adherence phenomenon
  e. adherence test
  e. cast
  C3-coated e.
  IgG-coated e.
  e. sedimentation rate (ESR)
  e. sheet rosette cell marker
erythrocytolysin
erythrocytolysis
erythrocytosis
  posttransplant e.
erythroderma, erythrodermia
  atypical ichthyosiform e.
  bullous congenital ichthyosiform e.
  e. desquamativum
  e. exfoliativa
  exfoliative e.
  ichthyosiform e.
  e. ichthyosiformis congenitalis
  lamellar congenital ichthyosiform e.
  lymphomatous e.
  nonbullous congenital
    ichthyosiform e.
  e. psoriaticum
  Sézary e.
  e. squamosum
  T-cell e.
  Wilson-Brocq e.
erythrodermatitis
erythrodermic
  e. psoriasis (PsoE)
  e. sarcoidosis
erythrodysesthesia syndrome
erythrogenic toxin
erythrokeratoderma variabilis (EKV)
erythrokeratodermia
  e. figurata variabilis
  progressive symmetric e. (PSEK)
  e. progressive symmetrica
  progressive symmetrical
    verrucous e.
erythrokeratolysis hiemalis
erythroleukemia cell line
erythrolysin
erythrolysis
erythromelalgia
erythromelanin
erythromelanosis
  e. follicularis faciei
  e. follicularis faciei et colli
erythromelia

erythromycin
  e. and benzoyl peroxide
  e., benzoyl peroxide topical gel
  e. and sulfisoxazole
  e. topical
erythromycin-sulfisoxazole
erythrophagia
erythrophagocytosis
erythroplakia
erythroplasia
  e. of Queyrat
  Zoon e.
erythropoietic
  e. coproporphyria (ECP)
  e. porphyria (EPP)
  e. protoporphyria
erythropoietin
erythropolis
  Rhodococcus e.
erythroprosopalgia
erythrose
  e. péribuccale pigmentaire of Brocq
  e. pigmentaire péribuccale
Eryzole Oral
ES
  excretory-secretory
eschar
  black e.
  burn e.
  e. separation
escharotic
escharotica
  dermatitis e.
  rupia e.
Escherichia
  E. coli
  E. coli enterotoxin
  E. coli polysaccharide antibody
E-selectin
ESF
  Painaid ESF
E-Solve-2 topical
esomeprazole magnesium
esophageal
  e. carcinoma
  e. dysfunction
  e. hypomotility
esophagitis dissecans superficialis
esophagomycosis
esophagram
Esoterica
  E. Facial

E

NOTES

Esoterica *(continued)*
    E. Regular
    E. Sensitive Skin Formula
    E. Sunscreen
espundia
ESR
    erythrocyte sedimentation rate
ESS
    excited skin syndrome
essential
    e. fatty acid (EFA)
    e. fatty acid deficiency
    e. fever
    e. mixed cryoglobulinemia
    e. oil
    e. pruritus
    e. telangiectasia
    e. thrombocytopenic purpura
established cell line
Estar Gel
Esteem synergy
EsteLux
    Palomar E.
    E. system
ester
    aminobenzoate e.
    fumaric acid e.
    isopropyl e.
    PABA e.
    phorbol e.
esterase
    C1 e.
    lymphocyte serine e.
    nonspecific e. (NSE)
    serine e.
esterified PABA
esthetics
esthiomene
estivae
estival, aestival
    e. vacciniform
estivale, aestivale
    hydroa e.
estivalis, aestivalis
    acne e.
    acne e.
    dermatitis e.
    protoporphyria e.
    prurigo e.
    pruritus e.
estradiol
estrogen
    conjugated e.
    e. replacement therapy (ERT)
estrone
Estroven
ET
    edema toxin

ET-1
    endothelin-1
et
    keratoderma palmaris e.
etanercept monotherapy
ETCO$_2$
    end-tidal cardiac disease
E-test
ethambutol hydrochloride
ethanol
    alkyl phenoxyl polyethoxy e.
ethanolamine
    amino ethyl e.
ether
    alkyl aryl e.
Ethezyme Papain-Urea Debriding ointment
Ethicon
    E. P and PS needle
    E. suture
ethidium bromide
Ethilon suture
ethinylestradiol
ethionamide
ethmoidectomy
ethmoid sinusitis
ethnicity factor
ethyl
    e. alcohol
    e. aminobenzoate
    e. chloride
    e. chloride and dichlorotetrafluoroethane
    e. hexanediol
    e. methacrylate
    tin e. (SnET2)
ethyl-2,3-dihydroxybenzoate
ethylenediamine dermatitis
ethylene oxide
ethyleneurea melamine formaldehyde resin
ethylnorepinephrine hydrochloride
ethylsuccinate
    oral erythromycin e.
Etibi
etidocaine hydrochloride
etidronate
    e. and calcium
    sodium e.
etidronate/calcium
etiolation
etiologic
etiology
    monoarticular arthritis of unknown e.
etiopathogenesis
etiopathogenic
etodolac
ETOPOPHOS infusion

etoposide phosphate infusion
etoricoxib
ETO Sleuth
E-Toxa-Clean Concentrate
Etretin
etretinate treatment
ETS
  environmental tobacco smoke
ETS-2% topical
Eubacterium aerofaciens
Eucalyptamint 2000
eucalyptus
  e. oil
  e. saligna
  e. tree
  e. tree pollen
Eucerin
  E. cream
  E. itch-relief moisturizing dry skin
    therapy spray
  E. Plus moisturizer
euchromatic
Eucommia ulmoides
Eudal-SR
eudiaphoresis
EULAR
  European League Against Rheumatism
Eulexin
eumelanin
eumycetoma
eumycotic mycetoma
eupatoria
  Agrimonia e.
eupeptic
euphoria
Euproctis
  E. chrysorrhoea
  E. chrysorrhoea sting
Eurax topical
Euro-Collins (EC)
  Euro-Collins solution
Euroglyphus maynei
europa
  Olea e.
europaeus
  Ulex e.
European
  E. Anti-ICAM Renal Transplant
    Study (EARTS)
  E. blastomycosis
  E. blister beetle sting
  E. cholera

  E. Confederation for Laboratory
    Medicine (ECLM)
  E. Consensus Lupus Activity
    Measure (ECLAM)
  E. Group for Bone Marrow
    Transplantation (EBMT)
  E. League Against Rheumatism
    (EULAR)
  E. Organization for Research and
    Treatment of Cancer (EROTIC)
European-American Lymphoma
  classification
Euro-Transplant Group
eustachian tube
eutectic mixture of local anesthetics
  (EMLA)
euthyroid
  sick e.
  e. sick syndrome
eutrichosis
Euxyl K 400
EV
  enterovirus
  epidermodysplasia verruciformis
evaluation
  acute physiology and chronic
    health e.
evanescent
  e. eruption
  e. macule
Evans blue stain
evening
  e. primrose
  e. primrose oil
everolimus
evisceration
  total abdominal e. (TAE)
E-Vista
E-Vitamin
evolution
  eruption e.
  lesion e.
Evoxac
evulsion
Ewart sign
ewengii
  Ehrlichia e.
Ewing tumor
ex
  e. vivo adenoviral transfection
  e. vivo cell expansion
  e. vivo organ storage

NOTES

E

exacerbation
exact
    E. Cream
    E. skin product
exaggerated bronchoconstrictor response
examination
    bone marrow e.
    full-body cutaneous e.
    full-body skin e. (FBSE)
    immunofluorescent e.
    KOH e.
    Neurobehavioral Cognitive Status e.
    retinal e.
    Wood light e.
exanthem
    unilateral laterothoracic e. (ULE)
    vesicular e.
exanthema, pl. exanthemas, exanthemata
    Boston e.
    echoviral e.
    enteroviral e.
    epidemic e.
    Epstein-Barr e.
    keratoid e.
    ordinal designation of the
      exanthemata
    polymorphous e.
    e. subitum
    vesicular e.
    viral e.
exanthematic typhus of São Paulo
exanthematicus
    ichthyismus e.
exanthematique
    typhus e.
exanthematous
    e. disease
    e. fever
    e. typhus
exanthesis arthrosia
excavatum
    pectus e.
Excedrin
    E. IB
    E. P.M.
excel
    Simplastin E.
excentrica
    hyperkeratosis e.
excess
    antibody e.
    antigen e.
    e. incidence (IDD)
excessive
    e. dryness
    e. hairiness
    e. secretion
    e. sweating
    e. water immersion

exchange
    donor-recipient plug e.
    e. plasmapheresis
    e. transfusion
exchanger
    heat/moisture e. (HME)
excimer
    E. laser therapy
    e. lasing medium
excision
    fusiform e.
    surgical e. (SE)
    tangential e.
    tangent-to-circle e.
    wide e.
excisional
    e. biopsy
    e. removal
excitation
    2-Photon E.
excited
    e. skin syndrome (ESS)
    e. state
exclamation point hair
exclusion
    allelic e.
excoriate
excoriated
    e. acne
    e. folliculitis
excoriation
    crusted e.
    necrotic e.
    neurotic e.
excrescence
    wart-like e.
excretion
    xanthine stone e.
excretory-secretory (ES)
excursion
Exelderm topical
exercise
    aquatic e.'s
    e. challenge testing
    isometric e.
    passive range of motion e.
    weight-bearing e.
exercise-induced
    e.-i. cholinergic urticaria
    e.-i. refractoriness
exertion
exfoliant
exfoliate
exfoliatio areata lingua
exfoliation
exfoliativa
    cheilitis e.
    dermatitis e.
    erythema e.

erythroderma e.
glossitis areata e.
keratolysis e.
exfoliative
e. dermatitis
e. erythroderma
e. psoriasis
Exgest
exhaust
exhaustion
nervous e.
obvious physical e.
Exidine
E. Scrub
E. solution
exilicauda
Centruroides e.
exine
Exirel
exoantigen
exocrine
exocrinopathic process
exocrinopathy
autoimmune e.
exocytosis
exogenetic
exogenote
exogenous
e. antigen
e. factor
e. hyperthyroidism
e. interleukin-12
e. ochronosis
e. pigmentation
e. polyunsaturated fatty acid
e. substance
exon 5
exonuclease
Exophiala
E. jeanselmei
E. werneckii
exophytic
exopolysaccharide
mucoid e. (MEP)
Exorex
exoserosis
exostosis, pl. **exostoses**
subungual e.
exotoxic
exotoxin
bacterial e.

botulinum A e.
streptococcal pyrogenic e. (SPE)
expanded
e. disability status scale (EDSS)
e. polytetrafluoroethylene (ePTFE)
e. polytetrafluoroethylene implant
expander
BioSpan tissue e.
Miami STAR tissue e.
expansion
clonal e.
ex vivo cell e.
pre-B cell e.
expectorant
Fedahist E.
Genamin E.
Myminic E.
Silaminic E.
Theramin E.
Triaminic E.
Tri-Clear E.
Triphenyl E.
expectorate
experimentally induced Köbner phenomenon (KP-e)
expiration
prolongation of e.
expiratory prolongation
explant
explantation
explosive-onset fever
explosive vomiting
exposure
aerosolized pollutant e.
allergen e.
cold e.
heat e.
light e.
limitation of e.
narrowband UVB therapeutic
light e.
occupational e.
prior drug e.
repeated e.
silica dust e.
sun e.
vinyl chloride e.
expression
cell surface e.
differential gene e.
human tyrosinase e.

E

NOTES

195

expressor
Heilen e.
Saalfield e.
Schamberg e.
Unna e.
Walton e.
Zimmerman-Walton e.
exsanguinous metabolic support perfusion
Exsel Shampoo
Exserohilum
E. jeanselmei
E. rostratum
exsiccation eczematid
extended criteria donor (ECD)
extender
Frechet e.
Extendryl
extensor surface
extensum
hemangioma planum e.
Extentabs
Dimetane E.
Dimetapp E.
exteriorization
externa
otitis e.
external
e. absorption
e. auditory canal (EAC)
e. meningitis
e. otitis
extra
e. articular harvest
Claritin e.
E. Strength Balm
E. Strength Bayer Enteric 500 Aspirin
E. Strength Doan's
extraarticular tissue
extracellular
e. cholesterolosis
e. crystalloid solution
e. matrix-degrading proteinase
e. matrix remodeling
e. signal-regulated kinase
e. toxin
extrachromosomal
extracorporeal
e. assist device
e. liver assist device (ELAD)
e. photochemotherapy
e. photophoresis (ECP)
extract
allergenic e.
allergic e.
alum-precipitated pyridine-extracted pollen e.
aqueous pollen e. (APE)

buffered charcoal yeast e. (BCYE)
dilute lyophilized allergen e.
glutaraldehyde-modified-tyrosine-absorbed e.
glycerinated e.
e. of henna
horse chestnut seed e.
inhalant allergen e.
liver e.
lyophilized e.
phenol-preserved e.
pollen e.
tobacco leaf e.
venom e.
whole-body e.
whole ragweed e. (WRE)
extractable nuclear antigen (ENA)
extraction
comedo e.
extractor
Amico e.
comedones e.
Schamberg comedo e.
Unna comedo e.
Walton e.
extraintestinal protozoa
extralobar
extraocular sarcoidosis
extrapulmonary
e. pneumocystosis
e. sarcoidosis
e. tuberculosis
extrauterine environmental stimulus
extravasation potential
extravascular granulomatous feature
extravillous
e. cytotrophoblast cell
e. trophoblastic damage
extrinsic
e. allergic alveolitis
e. asthma
e. compression of trachea
extrusion
exuberant
e. cicatrization
e. infectious
exudate
retinal e.
exudation
exudative
e. discoid
e. discoid and lichenoid
e. discoid and lichenoid dermatitis
e. neurodermatitis
e. papulosquamous disease
exudativum
erythema multiforme e.
exude

ExuDerm
  E. hydrocolloid
  E. hydrocolloid dressing
  E. hydrocolloid dressing material
Exu-Dry absorptive dressing
exulceratio simplex
ex-vivo liver perfusion
eye
  black e.
  e. folliculitis
  raccoon e.'s
  red e.
  vision, right e. (VOD)

eyebrow loss
eyedrops
  Elestat e.
eyeglass frame dermatitis
eyelash
  e. cosmetic
  e. loss
  e. pediculosis
eyelid
  e. cosmetic
  e. dermatitis
eyeline tattoo
Eye-Lube-A solution

NOTES

E

F
    F agent
    F genote
    F pilus
    F plasmid
F2
    prostaglandin F2 (PGF$_2$)
F12-MABP fusion protein
FA
    frequent episodic asthma
    FA virus
FAB
    French-American-British
    FAB classification
Fab
    Fab fragment
    Fab piece
FAB-1 cell marker
Faba vulgaris
Fab/c fragment
fabism
fabrication
    laser-assisted internal f. (LIFT)
fabricii
    Epicauta f.
Fabry
    F. angiokeratoma
    F. disease
    F. syndrome
Fabry-Anderson disease
faccinia
face
    Hippocratic f.
    F.'s Only
    f. peel
    ringworm of the f.
face-lift
facet
    f. joint arthropathy
    f. joint hypertrophy
    f. joint osteoarthritis
facetal joint
facial
    f. actinic keratosis
    f. angioedema
    f. erythema
    Esoterica F.
    f. foundation
    f. moisturizer
    f. nerve palsy
    f. pain
    f. powder
    f. resurfacing
    f. undercover cream
    f. vitiligo

faciale
    granuloma f.
    pyoderma f.
facialis
    herpes f.
    pyodermia f.
    zona f.
faciei
    atrophoderma reticulatum
      symmetricum f.
    chloasma f.
    erysipelas perstans f.
    erythromelanosis follicularis f.
    keratosis pilaris atrophicans f.
    lupus miliaris disseminatus f.
    pityriasis simplex f.
    pyoderma chancriforme f.
    seborrhea f.
    symmetricum f.
    tinea f.
facies
    adenoidal f.
    allergic f.
    coarse f.
    cushingoid f.
    dengue f.
    f. hepatica
    f. Hippocratica
    hound-dog f.
    leonine f.
    monkey f.
    moon f.
    myxedematous f.
    round f.
    tabetic f.
facility
    long-term-care f. (LTCF)
FACS
    fluorescent-activated cell sorting
FACSCalibur flow cytometer
FACScan flow cytometer
F-actin
    subplasmalemmal F-a.
factitia
    dermatitis f.
    urticaria f.
factitial
    f. dermatitis
    f. panniculitis
factitious
    f. dermatitis
    f. purpura
    f. urticaria
facto
    de f.

F

factor
    f. A, B, C, D, E, H, I
    activated vitamin K-dependent f.
    albumin-autoagglutinating f.
    alloantigen-independent risk f.
    allogenic effect f.
    angiogenesis f.
    anticomplementary f.
    antiperinuclear f. (APF)
    bacteriocin f.
    basic fibroblast growth f. (bFGF)
    B-cell differentiation/growth f.
    Bittner milk f.
    chemokinetic f.
    chemotactic f.
    ciliary neurotrophic f.
    complement chemotactic f.
    control of emotional f.
    cytokine synthesis inhibitory f.
    D deficiency f.
    f. (D, H, I) deficiency
    endogenous f.
    endothelial-relaxing f.
    endothelium-derived relaxation f.
    environmental f.
    eosinophil chemotactic f.
    epidermal growth f. (EGF)
    ethnicity f.
    exogenous f.
    fertility f.
    f f. I, II, IIa, III
    gender f.
    genetic f.
    f. Gm
    granulocyte colony-stimulating f.
      (G-CSF)
    growth f. (GF)
    Hageman f.
    H deficiency f.
    hemopoietic f.
    heparin-binding epidermal growth
      factor-like growth f. (HB-EGF)
    heparin-binding growth f. (HBGF)
    hepatocyte growth f. (HGF)
    histamine-releasing f. (HRF)
    I deficiency f.
    IgG rheumatoid f. (IgG RF)
    IgM rheumatoid f.
    f. I, II, VII, VIII, IX, X, XI, XII
    immunoglobulin G rheumatoid f.
    immunoglobulin M rheumatoid f.
      (IgM RF)
    inhibition f.
    kappa-binding nuclear f.
    latent transforming growth f.
    LE f.
    leucine zipper transcription f.
    leukocytosis-promoting f.
    leukopenic f.

    macrophage-activating f. (MAF)
    macrophage colony-stimulating f.
      (M-CSF)
    macrophage-derived tumor
      necrosis f.
    migration-inhibitory f. (MIF)
    milk f.
    monocyte chemotactic f. (MCF)
    monocyte-derived neutrophil
      chemotactic f.
    multilineage colony-stimulating f.
    myeloma growth f.
    natural killer cell-stimulating f.
      (NKSF)
    nephritic f.
    nerve growth f. (NGF)
    neutrophil-activating f. (NAF)
    neutrophil chemotactant f.
    nuclear f.
    osteoclast-activating f. (OAF)
    osteoclast differentiation f.
    platelet f. 4 (PF4)
    platelet-activating f. (PAF)
    platelet activating/aggregating f.
      (PAF)
    platelet-aggregating f. (PAF)
    platelet-derived angiogenesis f.
      (PDAF)
    platelet-derived epidermal growth f.
      (PDEGF)
    platelet-derived growth f. A
      (PDGF-A)
    platelet-derived growth f. B
      (PDGF-B)
    positive rheumatoid f.
    prepro-von Willebrand f.
    progesterone-induced blocking f.
      (PIBF)
    properdin f. A, B, D, E
    psychogenic f.
    R f.
    recognition f.
    recombinant platelet-derived
      growth f.
    releasing f. (RF)
    f. replacement therapy
    resistance f.
    resistance-inducing f.
    resistance-transfer f.
    Rh f.
    rhesus f.
    Rheumatex test for rheumatoid f.
    rheumatoid f. (RF)
    Rheumaton test for rheumatoid f.
    rubber elongation f. (Hev b1)
    secretor f.
    sex f.
    soluble co-stimulatory f.
    steel f.

stem cell f. (SCF)
stimulating f. (SF)
streaking leukocyte f.
sun protection f. (SPF)
T-cell growth f. (TCGF)
T-cell replacing f.
thymic lymphopoietic f.
thymus-replacing f.
thyrotoxic complement-fixation f.
tissue f. (TF)
transcription f.
transfer f.
transforming growth f. (TGF)
trigger f.
trypanosome growth f. (TGF)
tumor lysis f.
tumor necrosis f. (TNF)
vascular endothelial growth f.
    (VEGF)
vascular endothelial growth f.-2
vascular permeability factor/vascular
    endothelial cell growth f.
    (VPF/VEGF)
f. VIII:C inhibitor
f. V Leiden
f. V Leiden mutation
von Willebrand f. (vWF)
Willebrand f.
work-setting f.
X f.
f. XIII

factor-1
B-cell growth f.-1
heparin-binding growth f.-1 (HBGF-
    1)
insulin-like growth f.-1 (IGF-1)
stromal-cell-derived f.-1 (SDF-1)
T-cell growth f.-1

factor-2
B-cell growth f.-2
keratinocyte growth f.-2 (KGF-2)
T-cell growth f.-2

factor-3
leukocyte antigen f.-3 (LAF-3)

factor-4

factor-alpha
transforming growth f.-a. (TGF-
    alpha)
tumor necrosis f.-a. (TNF-alpha)

factor-beta
tumor necrosis f.-b. (TNF-beta)

factor-beta
transforming growth f.-b. (TGF-B)

factor-inducing monocytopoiesis

factor-kappa B
nuclear f.-k. B (NF-κB)

facultative
f. anaerobe
f. bacterium
f. myiasis
f. skin color

FADD
Fas-associating protein with death
    domain

faecalis
Alcaligenes f.
Enterococcus f.
Streptococcus f.

faecium
Enterococcus f.
vancomycin-resistant *Enterococcus f.*
    (VREF)

faeni
Micropolyspora f.

Faget sign

fagopyrism

failure
adrenocortical f.
graft f.
impending respiratory f.
late-onset renal f.
multiple organ system f. (MOSF)
ovarian f.
premature ovarian f. (POF)
primary adrenocortical f.
renal f.
respiratory f.
secondary adrenocortical f.
severe respiratory f.
f. to thrive
ventilatory f.

failure-free survival (FFS)

Fairbanks arthritis phenotype

falciparum
Plasmodium f.

fall
f. dermatosis
f. elm
f. elm tree
hair f.

fall-and-rise phenomenon

false
f. agglutination

F

NOTES

false *(continued)*
    f. cyst
    f. diphtheria
    f. membrane
    f. ragweed
    f. ragweed weed pollen
false-negative
    f.-n. patch test
    f.-n. reaction
false-positive
    f.-p. patch test
    f.-p. reaction
    f.-p. syphilis test
famciclovir
familial
    f. acanthosis nigricans
    f. aggregation
    f. alpha-lipoprotein deficiency
    f. amyloidosis
    f. amyloidotic polyneuropathy
        (FAP)
    f. amyloidotic polyneuropathy
        syndrome
    f. apoprotein CII deficiency
    f. articular hypermobility syndrome
    f. benign chronic pemphigus
    f. benign pemphigus of Hailey-
        Hailey
    f. cholestasis syndrome
    f. cold urticaria
    f. combined hyperlipidemia
    f. confluent and reticulated
        papillomatosis
    f. continuous skin peel
    f. cryoglobulinemia
    f. dysautonomia
    f. dysbetalipoproteinemia
    f. dysplastic nevus syndrome
    f. erythrophagocytic
        lymphohistiocytosis
    f. granulomatous arthritis
    f. Hibernian fever (FHF)
    f. hypercholesterolemia
    f. hypermobility syndrome
    f. hypertriglyceridemia
    f. hypocalciuric hypercalcemia
    f. juvenile hyperuricemic
        nephropathy
    f. Mediterranean fever
    f. multiple mucocutaneous venous
        malformation
    f. myovascular fibroma
    f. nephropathic amyloidosis
        syndrome
    f. pancytopenia
    f. panmyelophthisis
    f. paroxysmal polyserositis
    f. PMLE
    f. polymorphous light eruption

    f. pulmonary fibroproliferative
    f. recurrent arthritis
    f. recurrent polyserositis
    f. reticuloendotheliosis
    f. rosacea-like dermatitis
    f. spondyloepiphyseal dysplasia
        tarda
    f. thrombocytopenia
    f. urticaria pigmentosa
    f. white folded mucosal dysplasia
family
    immunoglobulin supergene f.
    pentraxin protein f.
famotidine
Famvir
fan-beam collimator
Fanconi
    F. anemia
    F. syndrome
Fansimef
FAO
    Food Agricultural Organization
FAP
    familial amyloidotic polyneuropathy
Farber
    F. body
    F. disease
farcinica
    Nocardia f.
farcy bud
Far East Russian encephalitis
farinae
    Dermatophagoides f.
farinosus
    herpes f.
farmer's
    f. lung
    f. neck
    f. skin
farmyard pox
Farr
    F. assay
    F. law
    F. test
Fas
    Fas antigen
    Fas ligand gene
    soluble Fas (sFas)
**Fas-associating protein with death
    domain (FADD)**
Fas-based killing pathway
fascia
    f. lata
    palmar f.
    plantar f.
fasciatus
    Nosopsyllus f.
fascicular lymphosarcoma

fasciculata
    zona f.
fasciitis
    eosinophilic f. (EF)
    necrotizing f.
    nodular pseudosarcomatous f.
    plantar f.
    proliferative f.
    pseudosarcomatous f.
fasciitis-panniculitis syndrome
fascioliasis
Fasciolopsis buski
fascioscapulohumeral dystrophy
Fas-Fas
    F.-F. ligand
    F.-F. ligand molecule
fashion
    clear cells scattered in a
      buckshot f.
    ying-yang f.
Fasject
FasL
    FasL gene
    FasL molecule
fastidious
fastigium
Fastmelt
    Benadryl Allergy/Cold F.
    Benadryl Children's Allergy F.
fast-twitch morphology of muscle fiber
fat
    atrophy of f.
    hydrous wool f.
    f. malabsorption
    f. necrosis
fatal asthma
fat-replacement atrophy
fatty
    f. degeneration
    f. nevus
faucium
    Mycoplasma f.
faun tail nevus
favic alopecia
favid
    f. alopecia
    f. Favre-Racouchot syndrome
favism
favosa
    mycosis f.
    porrigo f.

    tinea f.
    trichomycosis f.
Favre-Racouchot
    F.-R. cyst
    F.-R. disease
    F.-R. skin
    F.-R. syndrome
favus
    f. circinatus
    f. herpeticus
    f. herpetiformis
    f. pilaris
Fb fragment
FBSE
    full-body skin examination
5-FC
    5-fluorocytosine
Fc
    Fc fragment
    Fc gamma receptor III
    Fc piece
    Fc receptor
FCXM
    flow cytometry cross-match
    FCXM assay
FDE
    fixed drug eruption
feather
    Australian parrot f.
    canary f.
    chicken f.
    cockatiel f.
    duck f.
    goose f.
    f. hydroid
    f. hydroid dermatitis
    mixed f.
    parakeet f.
    parrot f.
    pigeon f.
    turkey f.
FeatherTouch CO2 laser
feature
    electromyographic f.
    extravascular granulomatous f.
    immunologic f.
    pathologic f.
    sicca f.
febricitans
    pes f.
febricula

F

NOTES

febrile
  f. agglutinin
  aphtha f.'s
  hydroa f.
  f. urticaria
febrilis
  herpes f.
  urticaria f.
febrility
fecal fat determination
Fedahist
  F. Expectorant
  F. Expectorant pediatric
  F. Tablet
feeleii
  Legionella f.
feet (*pl. of* foot)
FEF$_{25-75\%}$
  mean forced expiratory flow during the
  middle of FVC
Fegan technique
Fegeler syndrome
feigned eruption
Feingold diet
Fekeeh
Feldene
feline
  f. agranulocytosis
  f. infectious enteritis
  f. infectious peritonitis
  f. leukemia
  f. leukemia-sarcoma virus complex
  f. rhinotracheitis virus
  f. viral rhinotracheitis
felineum
  Microsporum f.
felis
  Afipia f.
  Babesia f.
  Ctenocephalides f.
felon
  bone f.
  deep f.
  subcutaneous f.
  subcuticular f.
  subperiosteal f.
  thecal f.
Felty syndrome
female
  f. pattern alopecia
  f. pattern baldness
  f. pseudo-Turner syndrome
Femizol-M
femoral
  f. anteversion
  f. nerve
Femstat
femtomolar concentration
fenbufen

Fen-fan-ji
fennel
  dog f.
fenoprofen calcium
fenoterol
fentanyl
fenugreek
Fer antigen
Ferguson-Smith
  F.-S. epithelioma
  F.-S. keratoacanthoma
Ferguson-Smith-type epithelioma
fermentans
  Acidaminococcus f.
fermentation
  abnormal gut f.
fermented food
Fernandez reaction
ferox
  protoporphyria f.
  prurigo f.
Ferreira-Marques lipoatrophy
ferret epithelium
ferric
  f. chloride
  f. subsulfate
ferrugineum
  Microsporum f.
fertility
  f. agent
  f. factor
fescue
  meadow f.
fester
festoon
festooning
fetal
  f. alcohol syndrome
  f. death
  f. erythroblastosis
  f. hydantoin syndrome
  f. liver transplantation
  f. pig cell transplantation
  f. thymus transplantation
  f. ventral mesencephalic tissue
    transplantation
fetalis
  erythroblastosis f.
  hydrops f.
  ichthyosis f.
  keratosis diffusa f.
fetid sweat
fetoprotein
  alpha f.
fetor oris
fetus
  harlequin f.
Feuerstein
  ringhook method of F.

fever

Aden f.
African endemic relapsing f.
African hemorrhagic f.
African swine f.
Argentinean hemorrhagic f.
Argentine hemorrhagic f.
black f.
f. blister
Bolivian hemorrhagic f.
bouquet f.
boutonneuse f.
bovine ephemeral f.
breakbone f.
bullous f.
Bunyamwera f.
Bwamba f.
camp f.
cerebrospinal f.
childbed f.
Colorado tick f. (CTF)
Congo-Crimean hemorrhagic f.
  (CCHF)
continued f.
Crimean-Congo hemorrhagic f.
dandy f.
date f.
3-day f.
deer fly f.
dengue hemorrhagic f.
diphasic milk f.
dumdum f.
Dutton relapsing f.
Ebola hemorrhagic f.
elephantoid f.
enteric f.
epidemic hemorrhagic f.
epimastical f.
eruptive f.
essential f.
exanthematous f.
explosive-onset f.
familial Hibernian f. (FHF)
familial Mediterranean f.
flood f.
food f.
Fort Bragg f.
glandular f.
grain f.
Haverhill f.
hemoglobinuric f.
hemorrhagic f.

herpetic f.
hospital f.
humidifier f.
Ilhéus f.
inundation f.
island f.
jail f.
Japanese river f.
jungle yellow f.
Katayama f.
kedani f.
Korean hemorrhagic f.
Lassa hemorrhagic f.
laurel f.
louse-borne relapsing f.
low-grade f.
malignant catarrhal f.
Malta f.
Manchurian hemorrhagic f.
Marseilles f.
Mediterranean erythematous f.
Mediterranean exanthematous f.
Mediterranean spotted f.
metal fume f.
miliary f.
mill f.
miniature scarlet f.
monoleptic f.
mud f.
nodal f.
Omsk hemorrhagic f.
o'nyong-nyong f.
Oroya f.
Pahvant Valley f.
pappataci f.
papular f.
paratyphoid f.
pharyngoconjunctival f.
Phlebotomus f.
polka f.
polyleptic f.
preicteric f.
pretibial f.
protein f.
puerperal f.
Pym f.
pyogenic f.
Q f.
quinine f.
Quotidian f.
rat-bite f.
recrudescent typhus f.

F

NOTES

fever *(continued)*
  relapsing f.
  rheumatic f.
  Rift Valley f.
  Rocky Mountain spotted f.
  rose f.
  Ross River f.
  saddleback f.
  sandfly f.
  San Joaquin Valley f.
  scarlet f.
  Schamberg f.
  ship f.
  shipping f.
  Sindbis f.
  slow f.
  solar f.
  f. sore
  South African hemorrhagic f.
  South African tick f.
  Southeast Asian f.
  spotted f.
  steroid f.
  streptobacillary f.
  swamp f.
  swine f.
  symptomatic f.
  syphilitic f.
  f. therapy
  tick f.
  tickborne relapsing f.
  traumatic f.
  trench f.
  tsutsugamushi f.
  typhoid f.
  undifferentiated type f.
  undulant f.
  f. of unknown origin (FUO)
  viral hemorrhagic f. (VHF)
  viral sandfly f.
  Wesselsbron f.
  West African f.
  West Nile f.
  Whitmore f.
  wound f.
  yellow f.
  Zika f.
Feverall
few-foods diet
fexofenadine
  f. HCl/pseudoephedrine HCl
  f. and pseudoephedrine
FF
  fibrofolliculoma
f factor I, II, IIa, III
FFS
  failure-free survival
FHF
  familial Hibernian fever

FI
  fungal infection
  fusion inhibitor
FIA
  Freund incomplete adjuvant
fiber
  A-alpha nerve f.
  afferent nerve f.
  alpha nerve f.
  blocking vagal afferent f.
  blocking vagal efferent f.
  elastic f.
  fast-twitch morphology of
    muscle f.
  Gomori silver impregnation for
    reticulin f.
  Herxheimer f.
  lattice f.
  parasympathetic nerve f.
  preelastic f.
  reticulin f.
  reticulum f.
  slow-twitch morphology of
    muscle f.
fiberglass dermatitis
fiber-knob
  Ad f.-k.
fiberoptic
  f. bronchoscope
  f. bronchoscopy
Fibracol
  F. collagen
  F. collagen-alginate dressing
Fibrel gel
fibric acid
fibril
  amyloid f.
  collagen f.
  f. structure
fibrillar collagen
fibrillarin
fibrillation
fibrillin
fibrillin-containing microfibril
fibrillogenesis
  in vitro f.
fibrillogenic *N*-terminal fragment
fibrin
  f. deposition
  f. glue
  f. matrix
  f. sealant
fibrinogen level
fibrinoid
  f. change
  f. necrosis
fibrinolysin and deoxyribonuclease
fibrinolysis
fibrinolytic purpura

fibrinopeptide
fibrinous degeneration
fibroblast
    B cell f.
    human embryonic lung f.
    f. interferon
    f. lineage synoviocyte
    macrophage f.
    f. mediation
    rheumatoid synovial f.
    Swiss 3T3 f.
    synovial f.
    T cell f.
    tissue-activated f.
    type B f.
fibroblastic tissue
fibroblast-like spindle cell
fibroblast-shaped synoviocyte
fibrocartilage
    meniscal f.
fibrocartilage-cell lacunae
fibrocytic dysmucopolysaccharidosis
fibrodysplasia ossification progressiva
fibroepithelial polyp
fibroepithelioma
    f. basal cell carcinoma
    f. of Pinkus
fibrofog
fibrofolliculoma (FF)
fibrogen-associated amyloidosis
fibrogenesis imperfecta ossium
fibrokeratoma
    acquired digital f.
    acral f.
    digital f.
fibroma
    aponeurotic f.
    collagenous f.
    f. durum
    familial myovascular f.
    infantile digital f.
    irritation f.
    juvenile aponeurotic f.
    f. lipomatodes
    f. molle
    f. molle gravidarum
    pedunculated f.
    f. pendulum
    perifollicular f. (PFF)
    peripheral ossifying f.
    periungual f.
    rabbit f.

    senile f.
    Shope f.
fibromatogenic
fibromatosis
    aggressive infantile f.
    f. colli
    congenital generalized f.
    diffuse infantile f.
    digital f.
    gingival f.
    juvenile hyaline f.
    juvenile palmoplantar f.
    palmoplantar f.
    plantar f.
    subcutaneous pseudosarcomatous f.
    f. virus of rabbit
fibromatous
fibromectomy
fibromodulin CS/DS
fibromucinoidosus
    lichen f.
fibromyalgia trigger point
fibronectin
    plasma f.
    f. receptor
fibronectin-deficient type Ehlers-Danlos syndrome
fibroplasia
    papular f.
fibroplasias
    papillary dermal f.
fibroproliferative
    endocardial f.
    familial pulmonary f.
fibrosa
    osteitis f.
fibrosarcoma
    Earle L f.
fibrosing
    f. alveolitis
    f. basal cell carcinoma
    f. disease
    f. syndrome
fibrosis
    apical lobe f.
    glomerular f.
    idiopathic pulmonary f. (IPF)
    interstitial f.
    mediastinal f.
    nodular subepidermal f.
    obliterative granulomatous f.
    parenchymal f.

F

NOTES

fibrosis *(continued)*
    perifollicular f.
    periglandular f.
    perineural f.
    peripheral f.
    portal tract f.
    progressive interstitial f.
    pulmonary f.
    retroperitoneal f.
    serosal f.
    subepidermal nodular f.
    subepithelial f.
    Symmers pipe-stem f.
fibrositis
fibrosum
    molluscum f.
fibrosus
    anulus f.
    lupus f.
    nevus f.
fibrothorax
fibrotic arteriosclerosis
fibrous
    f. arcade
    f. bacterial virus
    f. dysplasia
    f. hamartoma of infancy
    f. histiocytoma
    f. hyperplasia
    f. pannus
    f. papule
    f. papule fibroxanthoma
    f. sheath
    f. xanthoma
fibroxanthoma
    fibrous papule f.
FICH
    food ingestion challenge
Ficoll cushion
Ficoll-Hypaque
ficosis
fiddle-back
    f.-b. spider
    f.-b. spider bite
fiddler neck
field
    electromagnetic f.
Fiessinger-Leroy-Reiter syndrome
Fiessinger-Leroy syndrome
Fiessinger-Rendu syndrome
fifth disease
fig
    f. wart
    weeping f.
figurata
    keratosis rubra f.
    psoriasis f.
figurate psoriasis

figuratum
    erythema f.
figuratus
figure
    flame f.
filaggrin
    epidermal f.
    protein f.
filament
    intermediate f.
filamentary keratitis
filamentous
    f. actin
    f. bacterial virus
    f. bacteriophage
Filaria
    F. bancrofti
    F. loa
filaria, pl. **filariae**
filarial
    f. abscess
    f. elephantiasis
    f. nematode
filariasis
    Bancroft f.
    Bancroftian f.
    brugian f.
    Loiasis f.
    timorian f.
filaricidal
Filatov-Dukes disease
Filatov spot
filgrastim
filiform
    f. tumor
    f. wart
filiformis
    verruca f.
Filipovitch sign
filler
    AcryDerm Strands f.
    Cutinova Cavity f.
    DermAssist f.
    Humatrix Microclysmic Gel f.
    Multidex f.
    PolyWic f.
filles
    acne excoriée des jeunes f.
film
    Bioclusive MVP transparent f.
    BlisterFilm transparent f.
    CarraFilm transparent f.
    Centurion SiteGuard MVP
      transparent f.
    DermAssist transparent f.
    No Sting barrier f.
    NUVO barrier f.
    Omniderm transparent f.
    OpSite Flexigrid transparent f.

Polyskin II transparent f.
Polyskin M.R. transparent f.
polyurethane f. (PUF)
Pro-Clude transparent f.
ProCyte transparent f.
SureSite transparent f.
Tegaderm HP transparent f.
Transeal transparent f.

Filmtab

Biaxin F.
Rondec F.

Filoviridae virus
Filovirus
filter

ARI Group I–IV f.
electronic f.
HEPA f.
high-efficiency particulate air f.
membrane f.
Nucleopore f.

filtrable virus
fimbriatum

Gliocladium f.

Finacea
finding

immunofluorescence f.
serum protein electrophoretic f.
x-ray f.

Fine Line wrinkle treatment
fine-needle aspiration biopsy (FNAB)
Finevin cream
finger

blubber f.
bolster f.
bowed f.
clubbed f.
dead f.
Hippocratic f.
F. Phantom pulse oximeter testing
    system
sausage f.
seal f.
snapping f.
spade f.
speck f.
trigger f.
vibration-induced white f. (VWF)
waxy f.
whale f.
white f.

finger-in-glove appearance

fingernail

half-and-half f.

finger-packing doughy cemented
fingerprint

Galton system of classification
    of f.'s

fingertip

f. fissure
f. unit (FTU)

finish

antipill f.
textile f.

Finkelstein

F. disease
F. test

Finn chamber
FIO₂

fraction of inspired oxygen

fir

Douglas f.

fire

f. ant
f. ant anaphylaxis
f. ant sting
f. coral
f. coral dermatitis
f. coral sting
Saint Anthony f.
Saint Anthony's f.
f. sponge dermatitis

firebush
fireweed
firm lesion
first

F. Check rapid diagnostic test
f. degree frostbite
f. disease

first-degree burn
first-pass drug effect
first-set rejection
fir-tree-like pattern
Fischer stripper
FISH

fluorescence in situ hybridization
    FISH protocol in bone marrow
        transplantation

fish

f. oil
scorpion f.
f. skin
f. tapeworm anemia
tuna f.

F

NOTES

Fisher
    F. method
    F. syndrome
    F. two-tailed exact test
Fisher-Race theory
fish-mouth
    f.-m. healing
    f.-m. wound
fish-tank granuloma
Fisoneb ultrasonic nebulizer
fissuratum
    acanthoma f.
    epulis f.
    granuloma f.
fissure
    anal f.
    fingertip f.
    interpalpebral f.
fissured tongue
fissuring
fistula, pl. **fistulae, fistulas**
    f. in ano
    arteriovenous f.
    aural f.
    bronchopleural f.
    coronary f.
    dental f.
    pilonidal f.
    postbiopsy f.
Fite stain
Fitz-Hugh and Curtis syndrome
Fitzpatrick
    F. classification of skin type
    F. wrinkle score
fixation
    f. forceps
    Ilizarov external f.
    open reduction and internal f.
    (ORIF)
    f. reaction
fixed
    f. airflow obstruction
    f. charge density
    f. cutaneous sporotrichosis
    f. drug eruption (FDE)
    f. drug reaction
    f. pulmonary infiltrate
    f. virus
FK506
    tacrolimus
**FL3095 fluorescence spectrometer
system**
flaccid
flagellar
    f. agglutinin
    f. antigen
flagellate hyperpigmentation
flag sign
Flagyl Oral

flake
    sulfur f.
flaky paint dermatosis
Flamazine
flame
    f. figure
    f. nevus
flammeus
    nevus f.
    f. nevus
    osteohypertrophic nevus f.
Flantadin
flap
    advancement f.
    Brandy f.
    cheek-based 2-stage f.
    interpolation f.
    island pedicle f.
    Juri f.
    Karapandzic f.
    Marzola f.
    oblique advancement f.
    O to T f.
    O to Z f.
    pedicled f.
    rhombic f.
    rotation f.
    sliding-bucket mucosal f.
    transposition f.
flare
    premenstrual f.
    wheal and f.
Flarex Ophthalmic
flashlamp
    EpiLight f.
    f. photoepilation
Flash portable spirometer
flashscanner-enhanced CO_2 laser
flask
    Dewar f.
flat
    f. condyloma
    f. feet
    f. papular syphilid
    f. wart
flatworm
flavedo
flavicollis
    Apodemus f.
Flavimonas orzihabitans
Flaviviridae
Flavivirus
Flavobacterium meningosepticum
flavus
    Aspergillus f.
flax
flaxseed
FLB
    4-layer bandage

flea
> cat f.
> chigger f.
> dog f.
> northern rat f.
> Oriental rat f.
> sand f.
> f. venom

flea-borne typhus
flea-collar dermatitis
fleckeri
> *Chironex f.*

Flegel disease
Fleischner syndrome
flesh
> goosebump f.
> proud f.

flesh-colored
fleshfly
Flexderm hydrogel sheet
flexed tenosynovitis
Flexercell Strain Unit
flexible
> f. collodion
> f. silicone implant

Flexigrid
flexion
> f. contracture
> f. deformity

Flexi-Trak skin anchoring device
flexneri
> *Shigella f.*

flexor
> f. hallucis longus tendinitis
> f. surface

Flex-Power Performance Sports cream
flexural
> f. area
> f. eczema
> f. psoriasis

flexure
Flexzan foam wound dressing
flight
> matrix-assisted laser desorption
> ionization-time of f. (MALDI-
> TOF)

floating-tooth sign
floccosum
> *Epidermophyton f.*
> limit of *f.*

flocculation
> f. reaction
> f. test

Flolan
Flonase
flood fever
floor-sit maneuver
flop
> dory f.

flora
> gut microbial f.
> saprophytic f.

Florey unit
florid
> f. dermatitis
> f. oral papillomatosis

Florida seaweed dermatitis
Florinef Acetate
floristic zone
Florone
> F. cream
> F. E
> F. E topical

flour
> soybean f.
> wheat f.

Flovent Rotadisk powder
flow
> f. cytometry
> f. cytometry cross-match (FCXM)
> peak expiratory f. (PEFR)
> peak nasal inspiratory f. (PNIF)
> sinusoidal blood f.

flow-cytometry cross match assay
flower
> pansy f.

flowmeter
> Personal Best Peak F.

flowmetry
> laser Doppler f. (LDF)

FlowPRA beads assay
Floxin
> F. injection
> F. oral

FLPD
> vascular FLPD

FLS
> fibroblast-like synoviocyte

flu
> Connaught f.

flucatisone propionate/salmeterol
(FP/Salm Combo)

F

NOTES

fluconazole
fluctuance
fluctuant
fluctuating
fluctuation
5-flucytosine
fludrocortisone acetate
fluence
flufenamic acid
fluffy alveolar infiltrate
fluid
    basal transalveolar f.
    cutting f.
    epithelial lining f. (ELF)
    intravenous f.
    middle ear f. (MEF)
    simulated gastric f. (SGF)
    simulated intestinal f. (SIF)
    synovial f. (SF)
    tetanus toxoid, f.
    f. therapy
fluid-filled pressure transducer
fluid-phase C1q-binding assay
Flu-Imune
fluke
    blood f.
    intestinal f.
    tissue f.
Flumadine oral
flunisolide nasal solution
fluocinolone
    f. acetonide, hydroquinone, tretoin hydroquinone, tretinoin, and f.
    f. ointment
fluocinonide
Fluoderm
Fluogen
Fluonex topical
Fluonid topical
fluoresce
fluorescein-conjugated monoclonal antibody immunofluorescent test
fluorescein-tagged monoclonal antibody immunofluorescent test
fluorescence
    f. overlay antigen mapping (FOAM)
    f. polarization immunoassay (FPIA)
    f. quenching
    f. in situ hybridization (FISH)
    f. in situ hybridization protocol in bone marrow transplantation
fluorescent
    f. antibody technique
    f. microscopy
    f. sun lamp
    f. treponemal antibody absorption doublestaining (FTA-ABS)

    f. treponemal antibody-absorption test
fluorescent-activated cell sorting (FACS)
fluorescentiae
    stadium f.
Fluorethyl
fluoride
    sodium f.
Fluori-Methane Topical Spray
fluorinated
    f. corticosteroid
    f. corticosteroid-occlusive therapy
    f. pyrimidine
fluorochrome
fluorochroming
5-fluorocytosine (5-FC)
fluorometholone
    sodium sulfacetamide and f.
fluorometric procedure
Fluoroplex topical
Fluor-Op Ophthalmic
fluoroquinolone antibiotic
fluoroscopy
5-fluorouracil (5-FU)
fluorouracil cream
fluoxetine
    f. HCl
    f. hydrochloride
fluphenazine hydrochloride
flurandrenolide
flurazepam
flurbiprofen
Fluro-Ethyl Aerosol
Flurosyn topical
Flury
    F. strain rabies virus
    F. strain vaccine
flush
    f. area
    autonomic epilepsy f.
    carcinoid f.
    chlorpropamide f.
    dry f.
    histamine f.
    idiopathic f.
    medullary carcinoma f.
    wet f.
flushing
    emotional f.
    menopausal f.
    neural-mediated f.
    paroxysmal f.
    pulmonary f.
    thermal f.
flutamide
Flutex topical
fluticasone propionate aqueous nasal spray (FPANS)
Flutide Diskhaler

flutter device
flux
 f. allergen
 soldering f.
Fluzone
fly
 f. bite
 black f.
 f. blister
 buffalo f.
 caddis f.
 deer f.
 sarcophagi f.
 screw-worm f.
 sewer f.
 Spanish f.
 stable f.
 tsetse f.
 tumbu f.
fly-borne disease
flying blister
Flynn-Aird syndrome
FMD
 foot-and-mouth disease
 FMD virus
FML Forte Ophthalmic
FML-S Ophthalmic suspension
FNAB
 fine-needle aspiration biopsy
FOAM
 fluorescence overlay antigen mapping
foam
 CarraSmart f.
 f. cell
 clobetasol propionate f.
 f. dressing
 Luxiq ViaFoam betamethasone
  valerate f.
 Olux f.
 Reston f.
foamy
 f. agent
 f. histiocyte
 f. virus
focal
 f. acantholytic dyskeratoma
 f. acantholytic dyskeratosis
 f. acral hyperkeratosis
 f. amyloidosis
 f. anoxia
 f. dermal hypoplasia
 f. embolic glomerulonephritis

 f. histiocytosis
 f. infection
 f. inflammation
 f. reaction
 f. rupture of basement membrane
focus, pl. foci
 granulomatous f.
focusing
 isoelectric f. (IEF)
foenum-gaecum
 Trigonella f.-g.
Foerster forceps
FOII powder inhaler
foil
 f. bath pulsed ultraviolet
  actinotherapy
 f. bath PUVA
fold
 aryepiglottic f.
 crural f.
 Dennie infraorbital f.
 Dennie-Morgan infraorbital f.
 immunoglobulin f.
 lateral nail f.
 Morgan f.
 nail f.
 nasolabial f. (NLF)
 villous f.
folding
 protein f.
Folex PFS
foliacée
 lame f.
foliaceous pemphigus
foliaceus
 endemic pemphigus f.
 pemphigus f. (PF)
folic
 f. acid
 f. acid deficiency
folinic acid
follicle
 agminated f.
 hair f.
 hypertrophic lymphoid f.
 pilosebaceous f.
 tertiary f.
follicle-stimulating hormone (FSH)
follicular
 f. abscess
 f. accentuation
 f. alopecia

F

NOTES

213

follicular *(continued)*
    f. atrophoderma
    f. degeneration syndrome
    f. hyperkeratosis
    f. ichthyosis
    f. impetigo
    f. infundibular cyst
    f. isthmus cyst
    f. keratosis
    f. lichen planus
    f. mange
    f. melanin unit
    f. mucinosis
    f. mycosis fungoides
    f. nummular dermatitis
    f. nummular eczema
    f. occlusion triad
    f. orifice
    f. papule
    f. plug
    f. poroma
    f. pustule
    f. syphilid
    f. vulvitis
follicularis
    alopecia f.
    ichthyosis f.
    isolated dyskeratosis f.
    keratosis f.
    lichen planus f.
folliculis
folliculitis
    agminate f.
    f. barbae
    Bockhart f.
    Candida f.
    f. cheloidalis
    f. cruris atrophicans
    f. decalvans
    f. decalvans cryptococcica
    f. decalvans et lichen spinulosus
    eosinophilic pustular f.
    f. et perifolliculitis abscedens et
      suffodiens
    excoriated f.
    eye f.
    f. gonorrhoeica
    gram-negative f.
    hot tub f.
    industrial f.
    keloidal f.
    f. keloidalis
    f. nares perforans
    oil f.
    perforating f.
    Pityrosporum f.
    pustular f.
    scalp f.
    superficial f.

    f. ulerythema reticulata
    f. ulerythematosa reticulata
    f. varioliformis
folliculorum
    Acarus f.
    Demodex f.
    pityriasis f.
folliculosis
    traumatic anserine f.
folliculotropism
folliculus
Follmann balanitis
fomes
fomite
Fong syndrome
Fonsecaea
    F. compactum
    F. pedrosoi
food
    f. additive
    F. Agricultural Organization (FAO)
    f. allergy
    f. antigen
    antigenemically cross-reacting f.
    f. asthma
    f. dye
    EleCare medical f.
    f. elimination
    fermented f.
    f. fever
    f. hypersensitivity
    f. ingestion challenge (FICH)
    f. intolerance
    f. protein-induced enterocolitis
      syndrome (FPIES)
    f. protein-induced enteropathy
    Tetramune fish f.
**food-associated exercise-induced
   anaphylaxis**
food-borne
    f.-b. botulism
    f.-b. disease
food-induced respiratory disease
foot, pl. **feet**
    athlete's f.
    claw f.
    Dr. Scholl's Athlete's F.
    edema of feet
    flat feet
    fungous f.
    Hong Kong f.
    immersion f.
    Madura f.
    moccasin f.
    mossy f.
    neuropathic f.
    perforating ulcer of f.
    reddening of sole of f.
    ringworm of f.

sea boot f.
shelter f.
tennis shoe f.
f. tetter
trench f.
tropical immersion f.
tropic immersion f. (TIF)
warm water immersion f. (WWIF)
f. yaw
foot-and-mouth
f.-a.-m. disease (FMD)
f.-a.-m. disease virus
f.-a.-m. disease virus vaccine
for
f. skin (FS)
f. skin reverse cutting needle
Foradil dry powder inhaler
foramen of Monro
foramina
neural f.
forbidden-clone theory
force
f. transducer
van der Waals f.
forced air system disease
forceps
Adson toothed f.
Allis f.
Barraquer f.
Bergh f.
Bishop-Harmon ophthalmic f.
Brown-Adson f.
Carmalt f.
Castroviejo f.
Desjardins f.
Dyonics basket f.
fixation f.
Foerster f.
Frankel-Adson f.
Graefe f.
Hartmann ear f.
IM Jaws alligator f.
iris f.
Jacobson f.
jeweler's f.
Lalonde hook f.
Mixter f.
mosquito f.
Semken f.
splinter f.
suction loose body f.

thumb f.
Walter splinter f.
Forchheimer
F. sign
F. spot
Fordyce
angiokeratoma of F.
F. angiokeratoma
F. condition
F. disease
F. granule
F. spot
forearm ischemic exercise test
forefoot
f. valgus
f. varus
foreign
f. body giant cell
f. body granuloma
f. body radiation
f. body rhinitis
f. protein
f. protein therapy
f. serum
foreign-body reaction
forelock
occipital f.
white frontal f.
Forestier disease
forest yaw
fork
tuning f.
form
hyphal f.
IKDC Subjective Knee F.
involution f.
pentamidine in aerosol f.
replicative f. (RF)
yeast f.
formaldehyde resin
formalin
formalinize
formans
dermopanniculosis f.
formation
anterior synechia f.
antigenic antibody lattice f.
keloid f.
lamellipodia f.
mesangial complex f.
posterior synechia f.
scar f.

F

NOTES

formation *(continued)*
    spike f.
    syndesmophyte f.
    web f.
formication
formoterol
    f. fumarate dry powder inhaler
Formo-Test test
formula
    Alimentum f.
    amino acid-based low fat
      proprietary f.
    Anti-Acne Control F.
    Bayer Select Pain Relief F.
    Berkow f.
    Castellani Natural F.
    f. change
    Contac Allergy F.
    Esoterica Sensitive Skin F.
    Friedewald f.
    Grecian F.
    Neocate f.
    Nursoy f.
    Nutramigen f.
    Parkland burn resuscitation f.
    Poisson-Pearson f.
    Triaminic AM Decongestant F.
    Vivonex f.
formulary
formulation
    amphotericin B liposomal f.
fornix, pl. **fornices**
    inferior f.
Forsius-Eriksson-type ocular albinism
Forssman
    F. antibody
    F. antigen
    F. antigen-antibody reaction
FortaDerm wound dressing
Fortaz
Fort Bragg fever
Forte
    Aristocort F.
    Citanest F.
    Eldopaque F.
    Eldoquin F.
    Robinul F.
    Solaquin F.
    Stieva-A F.
    Triam F.
Forteo
Fortical
Fortovase
fortuitum
    Mycobacterium f.
Fosamax
foscarnet sodium
Foscavir injection
fosfomycin tromethamine

Foshay test
Fos protooncogene
fossa, pl. **fossae**
    antecubital f.
    coronoid f.
    glenoid f.
    olecranon f.
    popliteal f.
Foster needle holder
Fostex
    F. Bar
    F. BPO Gel
    F. Medicated Cleansing
    F. Wash
Fostril lotion
Fothergill disease
FotoFacial treatment
FotoFinder Derma
Fototar
foundation
    anhydrous facial f.
    facial f.
    National Psoriasis F.
    oil-based facial f.
    water-based facial f.
    water-free facial f.
fountain-spray splatter
Fournier
    F. disease
    F. gangrene
    F. syphiloma
fourth disease
foveation
foveolate
fowl
    f. diphtheria
    f. erythroblastosis virus
    leukemia of f.'s
    f. leukosis
    f. lymphomatosis
    f. lymphomatosis virus
    f. myeloblastosis virus
    f. neurolymphomatosis virus
    f. paralysis
    f. pest
    f. plague
    f. plague virus
fowleri
    Naegleria f.
Fowler solution
fowlpox virus
fox
    F. curette
    F. disease
    f. encephalitis
    f. encephalitis virus
    F. impetigo
Fox-Fordyce disease

foxtail
    meadow f.
FPANS
    fluticasone propionate aqueous nasal
    spray
FPIA
    fluorescence polarization immunoassay
FPIES
    food protein-induced enterocolitis
    syndrome
FPNS
    flocculus projecting neurons
FP/Salm Combo
fractional sterilization
fraction of inspired oxygen (FIO$_2$)
fracture
    Colles f.
    f. fusi
    F. Intervention Trial
    intraarticular f.
    march f.
    Segond f.
    stress f.
    subchondral f.
    transchondral f.
fragarius
    nevus f.
fragilis
    Bacteroides f.
fragilitas
    f. crinium
    f. unguium
fragility
    bone f.
fragment
    Fab f.
    Fab/c f.
    Fb f.
    Fc f.
    fibrillogenic *N*-terminal f.
    Fv f.
    Klenow f.
    Spengler f.
fragmentation
    elastic-fiber f.
fraise
    diamond f.
frambesia tropica
frambesiformis
    sycosis f.
frambesiform syphilid
frambesioma

framboesia
    sycosis f.
framboesiaeformis
    sycosis f.
framboesianus
    lichen f.
framboesioides
    mycosis f.
frame-shift
    f.-s. mutagen
    f.-s. mutation
Framingham risk score
Franceschetti-Jadassohn syndrome
Franceschetti-Klein syndrome
Francis disease
Francisella tularensis
Frankel-Adson forceps
Frankfort horizontal plane
frank virilization
Franschetti-Klein syndrome
fraterna
    Hymenolepis f.
Frazier-Shepherd skin hook
Frazier skin hook
FRC
    functional residual capacity
FreAmine
Frechet
    F. extender
    F. 3-flap slot correction
freckle
    f. of Hutchinson
    Hutchinson f.
    melanotic f.
freckling
    axillary f.
Frederickson type IIa, IIb
  hyperlipidemia
free
    f. cartilage graft
    f. margin
    f. radical
    f. salicylate level
freeborni
    Anopheles f.
freehand technique
Freeman-Sheldon syndrome
Freer septum elevator
free-tissue xenograft
freeze-dried
    f.-d. protein
    f.-d. skin

F

NOTES

freezing
    surface f.
Frei
    F. antigen
    F. bubo
    F. test
Freiberg disease
Frei-Hoffmann reaction
French-American-British (FAB)
    F.-A.-B. classification
French measles
Freon
frequency
    f. of allergy symptom
    ciliary beat f.
    f. doubled neodymium:yttrium-
      aluminum-garnet laser
frequent episodic asthma (FA)
freshening peel
fresh frozen plasma
Freund
    F. complete adjuvant test
    F. incomplete adjuvant (FIA)
freundii
    Citrobacter f.
Frey
    F. hair
    F. syndrome
friction
    adhesional and glide f.
    f. blister
    f. bulla
Friedewald formula
Friedländer pneumonia
Friend
    F. disease
    F. erythroleukemia cell
    F. leukemia virus
frigida
    erythrocyanosis f.
Frigiderm
frigoris
    stadium f.
fringe
    costal f.
Frish bacillus
Froben
FrogWear sunscreen clothing
frond
    villous f.
frontal bossing
frontalis
    acne f.
    alopecia liminaris f.
frost
    f. itch
    urea f.
frostbite
    first degree f.

frostnip
frozen
    f. plasma
    f. shoulder
frozen-thawed red cell
fruit
    F. of the Earth Moisturizing Aloe
    F. of the Earth Moisturizing Aloe
      Sport
frustrated
    f. phagocyte
    f. phagocytosis
frutescens
    Capsicum f.
FS
    for skin
    FS reverse cutting needle
    FS Shampoo topical
FSH
    follicle-stimulating hormone
FSL
    Actin FSL
FTA-ABS
    fluorescent treponemal antibody
      absorption doublestaining
    FTA-ABS test
FTU
    fingertip unit
5-FU
    5-fluorouracil
fuchsin
    acid f.
    f. body
fucosidosis
fugax
    erythema f.
fugitive
    f. swelling
    f. wart
fulguration
full-body
    f.-b. cutaneous examination
    f.-b. skin examination (FBSE)
full-coverage facial powder
full-thickness
    f.-t. burn
    f.-t. graft
fulminans
    acne f.
    purpura f.
fulminating smallpox
Fulvicin P/G
Fulvicin-U/F
fulvum
    Microsporum f.
fumagillin
fumarate
    clemastine f.
fumaric acid ester

fumes
    soldering f.
fumigation
fumigatus
    Aspergillus f.
Fun-boi
function
    barrier f.
    circadian f.
    decreased renal f.
    delayed graft f. (DGF)
    gene f.
    International Index of Erectile F.
      (IIEF)
    phagocytic f.
    poor marrow f.
    pulmonary f. (PF)
    secretory vesicle f.
functional
    f. abnormality in asthma
    f. affinity
    f. C1 esterase inhibitor
    f. class II–IV
    f. impairment
    f. polymorphism
    f. residual capacity (FRC)
funestus
    Anopheles f.
fungal
    f. arthritis
    f. bursitis
    f. culture
    f. disease
    f. id reaction
    f. infection (FI)
    f. scraping
fungate
fungating
    f. chancre
    f. sore
fungemia
fungi (*pl. of* fungus)
fungicidal
fungicide
fungiform
Fungi Imperfecti
Fungi-Nail
fungistasis
fungistat
fungistatic
fungitoxic
Fungizone intravenous

Fungoid
    F. AF Topical solution
    F. HC creme
    F. tincture
fungoides
    Alibert-Bazin type mycosis f.
    follicular mycosis f.
    granuloma f.
    microabscess of mycosis f.
    mycosis f. (MF)
fungosity
fungosus
    nevus vascularis f.
fungous
    f. foot
    f. gonitis
    f. infection
fungus, pl. **fungi**
    Alternaria alternata f.
    f. ball
    beefsteak f.
    bracket f.
    Cladosporium herbarum f.
    dematiaceous f.
    dimorphic fungi
    mosaic f.
    nonpathogenic f.
    opportunistic f.
    Phoma f.
    sac f.
    saprophytic fungi
    subcutaneous f.
    Trichophyton tonsurans f.
    umbilical f.
    zoophilic f.
funicular node
FUO
    fever of unknown origin
Furacin topical
Furadantin
Furalan
Furan
Furanite
furazolidone
furfur, pl. *furfures*
    Malassezia f.
    Microsporum f.
furfuracea
    alopecia f.
    dermatomycosis f.
    dermatophytosis f.
    impetigo f.

NOTES

F

furfuracea *(continued)*
    pityriasis f.
    seborrhea f.
    tinea f.
furfuraceous
    f. desquamation
    f. impetigo
furfurans
    porrigo f.
furfures (*pl. of furfur*)
furin convertase
furoate
    diloxanide f.
    mometasone f.
Furoxone
furrow
    Jadelot f.
    parallel f.
    transverse f.
furrowed tongue
furuncle
furuncular disease
furunculitis
    hospital f.
furunculoid
furunculosis orientalis
furunculous
furunculus
Fusarium
    F. chlamydosporum
    F. moniliforme
    F. oxysporum
    F. sacchari
    F. solani
fusca
    lamina f.

fuscoceruleus
    nevus f.
fusi (*pl. of* fusus)
fusidic acid
fusiform
    f. bacillus
    f. excision
fusin molecule
fusion
    f. inhibitor (FI)
    f. protein
    protoplast f.
    f. toxin
Fusobacterium nucleatum
fusospirochetal
    f. balanitis
    f. disease
    f. stomatitis
fusus, pl. **fusi**
    cortical fusi
    fracture fusi
Futcher line
fuzz
    peach f.
FVC
    mean forced expiratory flow during
      the middle of FVC ($FEF_{25-75\%}$)
Fv fragment
Fy antigen
FyBron
    F. alginate wound cover
    F. alginate wound dressing
fyn kinase enzyme

γ (*var. of* gamma)
G
    G antigen
    G protein
    G unit of streptomycin
G5 massage and percussion machine
GABA
    GABA inhibitory neurotransmitter
GABAergic neuron
gabapentin
Gabbromicina
GABHS
    group A beta-hemolytic *Streptococcus*
Gaboon ulcer
GAD
    glutamic acid decarboxylase
GAD65
gadolinium
GAG
    glycosaminoglycan
gag
    g. gene
    viral protein g.
gait
    g. analysis
    antalgic g.
    g. cycle
GAL
    gallus adeno-like
        GAL virus
            gallus adeno-like virus
Gal
    G. antibody
galactidrosis
galactophlysis
Gal-alpha-1 epitope
galantamine hydrobromide
galea
3Gal epitope
gallinae
    Dermanyssus g.
gallinarum
    neurolymphomatosis g.
    osteopetrosis g.
Gallipoli sore
gallium-aluminum-arsenide 904-nm laser
gallus
    g. adeno-like (GAL)
    g. adeno-like virus (GAL virus)
GALT
    gut-associated lymphoid tissue
Galton
    G. delta
    G. system of classification of
      fingerprints

galvanic epilator
Gamasidae
gamasoidosis
Gamastan
Gambel
    G. oak
    G. oak tree
gambiae
    Anopheles g.
gamekeeper's thumb
gametocytemia
gametophyte
Gamimune N
gamma, γ
    g. globulin
    g. hemolysis
    interferon g. (IFN-gamma)
gamma-1b
    interferon g.-1b
Gammabulin Immuno
gamma-camera
Gammagard S/D
gamma-glutamyltranspeptidase
gamma-heavy-chain disease
gamma-herpesvirus
gamma-linolenic acid
Gammar
Gammar-P I.V.
gammopathy
    benign monoclonal g.
    biclonal g.
    monoclonal g.
    polyclonal g.
ganciclovir
ganglion, pl. **ganglia**
    sensory g.
    trigeminal g.
ganglionectomy
    lumbar g.
ganglioneuroma
gangosa
gangraenescens
    granuloma g.
gangrene
    arteriosclerotic g.
    bacterial synergistic g.
    cold g.
    cutaneous g.
    decubital g.
    diabetic g.
    disseminated cutaneous g.
    dry g.
    embolic g.
    Fournier g.
    gas g.

G

gangrene *(continued)*
> hemorrhagic g.
> hospital g.
> hot g.
> infected vascular g.
> Meleney g.
> moist g.
> nosocomial g.
> peripheral g.
> Pott g.
> presenile spontaneous g.
> pressure g.
> progressive bacterial synergistic g.
> senile g.
> static g.
> symmetrical g.
> synergistic g.
> thrombotic g.
> venous g.
> wet g.
> white g.

gangrenosa
> dermatitis g.
> phagedena g.
> pyodermia g.
> vaccinia g.
> varicella g.

gangrenosum
> bullous hemorrhagic pyoderma g.
> ecthyma g.
> hemorrhagic pyoderma g.
> pyoderma g. (PG)

gangrenosus
> pemphigus g.

gangrenous stomatitis
Gantanol
Gantrisin oral
gap
> allergic g.

gaping mouth
Garamycin
> G. injection
> G. Ophthalmic
> G. Topical

Gardner-Diamond
> G.-D. purpura
> G.-D. syndrome

Gardnerella **vaginitis**
Gardner syndrome
gargoylism
garinii
> *Borrelia* g.

garlic
garment
> Marena compression g.
> g. nevus

garnet
> neodymium:yttrium-aluminum-g.
> (Nd:YAG)

GART
> genotypic antiretroviral resistance testing

GAS
> group A *Streptococcus*

gas
> g. abscess
> blood g.
> g. cautery
> g. chromatography
> g. gangrene
> g. gangrene antitoxin
> irritant g.

gaseous cellulitis
gasping disease
Gasterophilus
gastritis
> autoimmune atrophic g.

Gastrocrom oral
gastroenteritis
> acute infectious nonbacterial g.
> allergic eosinophilic g.
> endemic nonbacterial infantile g.
> eosinophilic g.
> epidemic nonbacterial g.
> infantile g.
> porcine transmissible g.
> rotavirus g.
> viral g.
> g. virus type A, B

gastroenterocolitis
> allergic eosinophilic g.

gastroenteropathy
> protein-losing g.

gastrointestinal
> g. hypersensitivity
> g. symptom
> g. ulceration

gastropathy
> NSAID g.

gastroprotective agent
gastroschisis
gastrotoxin
gatifloxacin
gating
Gaucher disease
gauge
> adjustable-depth g. (ADG)

Gaussian beam
gauze
> Aquaphor g.
> Biolex impregnated g.
> CarraGauze impregnated g.
> ClearSite impregnated g.
> Cover-Roll g.
> Curafil impregnated g.
> Curasol impregnated g.
> Dermagran impregnated g.
> DermAssist impregnated g.
> Elta Dermal impregnated g.

Gentell impregnated g.
Iodoform g.
MPM GelPad impregnated g.
nonstick g.
N-Terface g.
PanoGauze hydrogel-impregnated g.
PanoGauze impregnated g.
Restore impregnated g.
SkinTegrity impregnated g.
TransiGel impregnated g.

Gaviscon Prevent
GBS
group B *Streptococcus*
GC
glucocorticoid
G-CSF
granulocyte colony-stimulating factor
Ge
G. antigen
G. Jie Anti-asthma Pill
Gebauer ethyl chloride
Geiger electrocautery unit
gel
AccuSite injectable g.
adapalene g.
Advanced Formula Oxy
Sensitive G.
agarose g.
Anti-Itch g.
Avosil scar g.
Benzac AC G.
BenzaClin g.
Benzac W G.
bexarotene g.
Brevoxyl G.
Cann-Ease moisturizing nasal g.
Carmol 40 g.
Clear By Design G.
Clinac BPO g.
Clindagel topical g.
clindamycin/benzoyl peroxide g.
clindamycin phosphate topical g.
dapsone topical g.
Del Aqua-5 G.
Del Aqua-10 G.
Dermaflex G.
Desquam-E g.
Desquam-X g.
DiaB G.
diclofenac sodium g.
Differin g.
g. diffusion

g. diffusion precipitin test
g. diffusion precipitin test in one
dimension
g. diffusion reaction
Dryox G.
Duac topical g.
erythromycin, benzoyl peroxide
topical g.
Estar G.
Fibrel g.
Fostex BPO G.
H.P. Acthar G.
Humatrix Microclysmic g.
IntraSite g.
ionic polymer matrix wound g.
IPM wound g.
Ivy Stat g.
Kelo-cote topical g.
Keralyt G.
LAM IPM wound g.
MetroGel topical g.
metronidazole topical g.
NeoStrata Skin Lightening g.
NuSieve agarose g.
Panretin topical g.
Perfectoderm G.
g. phenomenon
precipitate in g.
PreSun lotion and g.
Retin-A Micro g.
Rosula aqueous g.
silicone g.
sodium dodecyl sulfate-
polyacrylamide gradient slab g.
Solaraze g.
SoloSite wound g.
T g.
tazarotene topical g.
Tisit Blue G.
tretinoin g.
Triaz g.
Vergogel G.
g. wound dressing
Zoderm g.

gelatin
g. allergy
g. compression boot
g. zymography
gelatinase
72-kD g.
92-kD g.

G

NOTES

gelcap
  Compoz g.
Gelfoam
Gell
  G. and Coombs classification
  G. and Coombs classification
    system
  G. and Coombs reaction
gelling phenomenon
Gelocast
  G. bandage
  G. Unna boot leg compression
    dressing
gelsolin amyloidosis
gem
  Ampliwax PCR G.
gemcitabine HCl
gemellus
  Paederus g.
geminata
  Solenopsis g.
Gemini automated centrifugal analyzer
Genac Tablet
Genahist oral
Genamin Expectorant
Gen-Amoxicillin
Genant method
Genapap
Genasense
Genaspor
Genatap Elixir
Gen-Beclo
Gen-Cyproterone
gender factor
gene
  g. array technique
  art/trs g.
  g. bank
  bax g.
  bcl-2, -6 g.
  Bruton tyrosine kinase g.
  CD40 ligand g.
  cell interaction g.
  CI g.
  c-myc g.
  COL1A1 g.
  COL2A1 type II procollagen g.
  g. complex
  CTNS g.
  g. defect
  g. disruption
  env g.
  FasL g.
  Fas ligand g.
  g. function
  gag g.
  germline V g.
  herpes thymidine kinase g.
  HLA-B60 g.

HLA-DR3 g.
hormone-related g.
housekeeping g.
IL-2 receptor alpha chain g.
immune response g.
immune suppressor g.
immunoglobulin g.
Ir g.
Is g.
J chain g.
JH g.
jun g.
luciferase reporter g.
manganese superoxide dismutase g.
g. manipulation
marker g.
master regulator g.
melanoma-associated g. (MAGE)
3'orf g.
g. overexpression
Patched g. (PTC)
pol g.
proapoptotic g.
P53 tumor suppressor g.
R g.
RAG1, RAG2 g.
recombinase-activating g.
recombination activationg.
sor g.
stealthing g.
sTNFR g.
g. structure
suicide g.
tat g.
g. therapy
TNF receptor II g.
g. transcription
transfer g.
transforming g.
tumor suppressor g.
V g.
vanA, vanH, vanS g.
V-D-J g.
VH g.
von Hippel-Lindau g. (VHL)
wt g.
X-encoded immune system g.
gene-based
  g.-b. vaccine
  g.-b. vector
gene-knockout technology
general
  g. immunity
  g. transduction
generalis
  acne g.
  seborrhea g.
generalisata
  alopecia g.

generalisatus
    herpes zoster g.
generalized
    g. anaphylaxis
    g. desquamation
    g. elastolysis
    g. epidermolysis bullosa simplex
    epidermolysis bullosa simplex, g.
    g. epidermolytic hyperkeratosis
    g. eruptive histiocytoma
    g. granuloma annulare
    g. heat urticaria
    g. hives
    g. hyperhidrosis
    g. lentiginosis
    g. maculopapular rash
    g. melanosis
    g. morphea
    g. morphea variant
    g. myxedema
    g. plane xanthoma
    g. plane xanthomatosis
    g. pruritus
    g. pustular psoriasis
    g. Shwartzman phenomenon
    g. vaccinia
    g. vitiligo
    g. weakness
    g. xanthelasma
generation time
genetic
    g. C2 deficiency
    g. depression of immune system
    g. determinant
    g. disease
    g. disorder
    g. factor
    g. marker
    microbial g.'s
    g. predisposition
    g. recombination
    g. therapy
Gengou phenomenon
Gengraf
geniposidic acid
Gen-Ipratropium
genistein
genistein-inhibited movement
genital
    g. aphthous ulcer
    g. atopic dermatitis
    g. erosive lichen planus

    g. hair
    g. herpes
    g. herpes simplex virus
    g. hidradenitis suppurativa
    g. lentigo
    g. leukoderma
    g. lichen sclerosus
    g. lichen simplex chronicus
    g. neurodermatitis
    g. papulosquamous lesion
    g. plasma cell mucositis
    g. pruritus
    g. psoriasis
    g. Reiter syndrome
    g. squamous cell carcinoma
    g. tumor
    g. wart
genitalis
    herpes g.
genitalium
    Mycoplasma g.
genitofemoral nerve entrapment
genitourinary lesion
Gennerich treatment
genodermatology
genodermatosis
    neurologic g.
genome
    viral g.
genome-side linkage analysis
genomic
    g. analysis
    g. glucocorticoid mechanism
Genoptic S.O.P. Ophthalmic
genospecies
genote
    F g.
genotoxic
genotype
    XXYY g.
genotypic antiretroviral resistance testing (GART)
genotyping
Genpril
Gen-Probe rapid tuberculosis test
Gensan
Gentab-LA
Gentacidin Ophthalmic
Gentak Ophthalmic
gentamicin
    prednisolone and g.
    g. sulfate

G

NOTES

Gentell
- G. alginate wound cover
- G. alginate wound dressing
- G. foam wound dressing
- G. hydrogel dressing
- G. impregnated gauze
- G. wound cleanser

gentian violet
GentleLASE
- G. laser
- G. Plus laser system

GentlePeel skin exfoliation system
genu valgum
Geocillin
geode
geographic
- g. difference
- g. pattern
- g. stippling of nail
- g. tongue

geographica
- lingua g.
- psoriasis g.

geophilic
geotrichosis
Geotrichum
gerbil
Geref
Gerhardt
- G. disease
- G. phenomenon
- G. reaction
- G. test

Gerhardt-Mitchell disease
geriatric
- g. dermogram
- g. psoriasis

Gerimal II
germ
- hair g.
- primary epithelial g.
- g. theory

German
- G. chamomile
- G. cockroach
- G. measles
- G. measles virus

germander
germicidal
germicide
germinal
germinative
- g. cell
- g. time

germinativum
- stratum g.

Germiston virus

germline
- g. transcription
- g. V gene

geroderma
gerontine
gerstaeckeri
- *Triatoma g.*

Gerstmann-Straussler-Scheinker syndrome
GESICA
- Argentinian Study Group for Prevention of Cardiac Insufficiency
- GESICA trial

gestationis
- hydroa g.
- impetigo g.
- pemphigoid g.
- protoporphyria g.
- prurigo g.

GF
- growth factor

GFD
- gluten-free diet

GFN
- G. 1000/DM50 sustained release
- G. 550/PSE 60/DM30 sustained release

GG
- Slo-Phyllin GG

ggELISA
GH
- growth hormone

Ghon complex
ghoul hand
GI 198745
Gianotti-Crosti
- G.-C. disease
- G.-C. syndrome

giant
- g. cell
- g. cell arteritis syndrome
- g. cell epulis
- g. cell granuloma
- g. cell myocarditis
- g. cell myositis
- g. cell tumor
- g. condyloma
- g. congenital pigmented nevus
- g. desert centipede
- g. desert centipede bite
- g. eccrine acrospiroma
- g. hives
- g. lichenification
- g. ragweed
- g. urticaria

giantism
Giardia lamblia
Gibbs-Gradle scissors

Gibert
>G. disease
>G. pityriasis

Giemsa stain
gift spot
gigantea
>lichenificatio g.
>urticaria g.

giganteum
>molluscum g.

Gila
>G. monster
>G. monster bite

Gilbert syndrome
Gilchrist
>G. disease
>G. mycosis

Gilead
>balm of G.

Gillette Blue Blade
Gillies needle holder
ginger
ginger-based product
gingiva
gingival
>g. fibromatosis
>g. hyperplasia
>g. lymphoma

gingivitis
>acute necrotizing ulcerative g.
>(ANUG)
>desquamative g.
>gonococcal g.
>ulcerative g.

gingivostomatitis
>acute herpetic g.
>herpetic g.

ginkgo
Ginkgo biloba
ginseng
>red g.

gio
>cao g.

girdle
>shoulder g.

Girdlestone pseudarthrosis
Giroux-Barbeau syndrome
GIVIO
>Interdisciplinary Group for Cancer Care
>Evaluation in Italy

GL-701
glabella

glabra
>*Glycyrrhiza* g.
>verruca g.

glabrata
>*Candida* g.
>*Torulopsis* g.

glabrate
glabrosa
>tinea g.

glabrous skin
gladiatorum
>herpes g.

gland
>apocrine sweat g.
>axillary venom g.
>Boerhaave sweat g.
>Brunner g.
>ceruminous g.
>cirrhotic lacrimal g.
>coil g.
>eccrine sweat g.
>ectopic sebaceous g.
>holocrine g.
>hyperplasia of sebaceous g.
>Krause g.
>lymph g.
>meibomian g.
>merocrine g.
>Moll g.
>oil g.
>paired venom g.
>parotid g.
>Philip g.
>salivary g.
>sebaceous g. (SG)
>stink g.
>sweat g.
>thyroid g.
>Zeis g.

glanders
glandular fever
glandularis
>cheilitis g.

glans penis
Glanzmann thrombasthenia
glass
>g. body
>Wood g.

Glaucon
glebae
>*Acanthamoeba* g.

G

NOTES

227

glenohumeral
- g. arthritis
- g. degeneration
- g. joint
- g. ligament
- g. osteoarthritis
- g. synovitis

glenoid
- g. component
- g. erosion
- g. fossa
- g. labrum

glenoidplasty

glenoplasty

gliadin
- deamidated g.

glial nodule

Gliocladium fimbriatum

glioma
- nasal g.
- optic g.

gliomatous proliferation

global rating of pain

globi (*pl. of* globus)

globosa
- *Malassezia g.*

globosum
- *Chaetomium g.*

globulin
- alpha$_2$ g.
- antihuman g.
- antithymocyte g. (ATG, ATGAM, Atgam)
- beta-$_{1F}$ g.
- beta-$_{1E}$ g.
- beta-$_{1C}$ g.
- gamma g.
- hepatitis B immune g. (H-BIG)
- human gamma g.
- immune serum g.
- intravenous gamma g. (IVGG)
- intravenous immune serum g. (IVIG)
- lymphocyte immune g.
- Minnesota antilymphoblast g.
- pertussis immune g.
- placenta-eluted gamma g.
- rabbit antithymocyte g. (RATG)
- respiratory syncytial virus IV immune g.
- RH$_o$(D) g.
- tetanus immune g.
- vaccinia immune g.
- varicella-zoster immune g.
- zoster immune g.

globus, pl. **globi**

glomangioma

glomangiomatosis

glomera (*pl. of* glomus)

glomerata
- *Dactylis g.*

glomerular
- g. eluate
- g. fibrosis
- g. hyperfiltration

glomeruli (*pl. of* glomerulus)

glomerulitis

glomeruloid hemangioma

glomerulonephritis
- acute crescentic g.
- acute hemorrhagic g.
- crescentic g.
- diffuse proliferative g.
- focal embolic g.
- hypocomplementemic g.
- immune complex g.
- lupus g.
- membranoproliferative g.
- membranous g.
- mesangiocapillary g. (MCGN)
- pauciimmune g.
- postinfectious g.
- postpyodermal acute g.
- poststreptococcal g. (PSGN)
- primary pauciimmune necrotizing g.
- proliferative g.
- rapidly progressive necrotizing g. (RPNG)

glomerulosa
- zona g.

glomerulosclerosis

glomerulus, pl. **glomeruli**

glomus, pl. **glomera**
- g. body
- neuromyoarterial g.
- g. tumor

glomuvenous malformation

Glossina **bite**

glossitis, pl. **glossitides**
- g. areata exfoliativa
- atrophic g.
- benign migratory g.
- *Candida* g.
- g. dissecans
- Hunter g.
- median rhomboid g. (MRG)
- migratory g.
- Moeller g.
- g. parasitica
- parenchymatous g.
- g. of pellagra
- g. rhombica mediana
- rhomboid g.
- g. rhomboidea mediana

glossodynia
- *Candida* g.

glossopyrosis

glossy
> g. skin
> g. tongue

glove
> Biobrane g.
> Bluettes cotton knit-lined g.
> cotton g.
> Dermapor g.
> g. dermatitis
> invisible g.
> Nimble Fingers g.
> vinyl g.'s

glove-powder inhalation test
glove-use test
glow
> sunset g.

glowing red lip
glucagon
> gut g.

glucagonoma syndrome
Glucantime
glucocerebrosidase
glucocorticoid (GC)
> intraarticular g.
> g. withdrawal syndrome

glucocorticoid-induced osteoporosis
glucocorticoid-inducible protein
glucocorticoid-mediated stress-induced immune alteration
glucocorticosteroid
gluconate
> calcium g.
> chlorhexidine g.

gluconic acid
gluconolactone
Glucoprime
glucosamine sulfate
glucose
glucose-6-phosphatase deficiency
glucuronate
> trimetrexate g.

glucuronic acid
glucuronidase
glucuronidation salicylate
glue
> bee g.
> fibrin g.
> Loctite 15494 ethyl cyanoacrylate g.

GLUS
> granulomatous lesions of unknown significance
> GLUS syndrome

glutamate
> monosodium g. (MSG)

glutamic acid decarboxylase (GAD)
glutamine-rich polypeptide
glutaraldchyde
glutaraldehyde-modified-tyrosine-absorbed extract
glutathione-dependent, cytosolic isozyme
glutathione-S-transferase (GST)
gluten
> g. enteropathy
> g. intolerance
> g. shock

gluten-free diet (GFD)
gluten-sensitive enteropathy (GSE)
glutinosa
> *Alnus* g.
> *Rehmannia* g.

GLY
> glycerol

glycation
> nonenzymatic g. (NEG)

glycerin
> DermAssist G.

glycerinated extract
glycerol (GLY)
> g. guaiacolate

Glycerol-T
glyceryl monostearate
glycine
glycine-rich
> g.-r. beta-glycoprotein
> g.-r. beta-glycoproteinase

glycobiology
glycocalyx
Glycofed
glycogenolysis
glycogen storage disease
glycol
> Diprolene G.
> propylene g.
> salicylic acid and propylene g.

glycolic acid
glycolipid lipidosis
glycolysis
glycophorin antigen
glycophosphatidylinositol anchor

G

NOTES

glycoprotein
    beta$_2$-g. II
    homopentameric g.
    human cartilage g. 39
    g. IIa (GPIIa)
    g. IIb (GPIIb)
    g. IIb-IIIa (GPIIb-IIIa)
    lysosomal g.
    multifunctional extracellular g.
    myelin-oligodendrocyte g. (MOG)
    pregnancy alpha-2 g. (PAG)
    pregnancy-associated g.
glycoproteinosis
glycopyrrolate
glycosaminoglycan (GAG)
    g. chain
glycoside
    cardiac g.
glycosphingolipid
    g. deposit
    g. metabolism
glycosphingolipidosis
glycosylation
glycosylphosphatidylinositol (GPI)
**glycosylphosphatidylinositol-anchored
  protein**
glycyl-transfer
    g.-t. ribonucleic acid
    g.-t. ribonucleic acid synthetase
glycyl-tRNA synthetase
Glycyphagus domesticus
Glycyrrhiza
    G. glabra
    G. uralensis
Glydant
Gly Derm skin care product
Glyquin cream
Gm
    Gm allotype
    Gm antigen
    factor Gm
GMP
    guanosine monophosphate
GMS
    Grocott methenamine silver
G-myticin topical
gnat bite
Gnathostoma spinigerum
gnathostomiasis
GNB
    gram-negative bacillus
    gram-negative bacteremia
gnotobiology
gnotobiota
gnotobiote
gnotobiotic
goat epithelium
goatpox virus
goat-serum-derived

goat's milk
goblet
    g. cell
    g. cell degranulation
    g. cell hyperplasia
    g. cell metaplasia
Goeckerman
    G. regimen
    G. treatment
Goggia sign
gold
    African G.
    g. allergy
    g. 4-amino-2-mercaptobenzoic acid
    g. dermatitis
    parenteral g.
    g. retinoid
    g. salts
    G. Schnapps syndrome
    Selsun G.
    g. therapy
    g. thiopropanolsulphonate
    g. thiosulphate
goldenrod pollen
gold-induced
    g.-i. aplasia
    g.-i. enterocolitis
golfer's
    g. elbow
    g. skin
golf tee hair
Golgi
    G. apparatus
    G. complex
Goltz-Gorlin syndrome
Goltz syndrome
**Gomori silver impregnation for
  reticulin fiber**
gonadal dysgenesis
gonadotropin
    chorionic human recombinant g.
gonarthrosis
gondii
    Toxoplasma g.
gonitis
    fungous g.
gonococcal
    g. arthritis
    g. arthropathy
    g. conjunctivitis
    g. gingivitis
    g. ophthalmia
    g. septicemia
    g. stomatitis
gonococcemia
gonococcic tenosynovitis
gono-opsonin
gonophage

gonorrhea
    oropharyngeal g.
    pharyngeal g.
    rectal g.
gonorrheal
    g. bubo
    g. dermatosis
    g. keratosis
    g. tenosynovitis
    g. urethritis
gonorrhoeae
    Neisseria g.
    tetracycline-resistant *Neisseria* g.
     (TRNG)
gonorrhoeica
    folliculitis g.
gonorrhoica
    macula g.
gonotoxemia
gonotoxin
Good antigen
goodness-of-fit chi-square test
Goodpasture syndrome
goose
    g. bump
    g. feather
gooseberry
goosebump flesh
gooseflesh
goosefoot weed pollen
Gopalan syndrome
Gordofilm Liquid
gordonae
    Mycobacterium g.
Gordon phenomenon
Gorham disease
Gorlin-Chaudhry-Moss syndrome
Gorlin-Goltz syndrome
Gorlin syndrome
Gorman syndrome
Gormel creme
Gorney-Freeman straight facelift scissors
Gorney straight facelift scissors
Göthlin test
Gottron
    G. papule
    G. sign
    G. syndrome
Gott shunt
Gougerot
    G. and Blum disease

    pigmented purpuric lichenoid
     dermatitis of G.
    G. syndrome
    G. triad
Gougerot-Blum
    G.-B. dermatosis
    G.-B. disease
    G.-B. syndrome
Gougerot-Carteaud
    papillomatosis of G.-C.
    G.-C. syndrome
Gougerot-Sjögren disease
goundou
gout
    chronic tophaceous g.
    clinical g.
    intercritical g.
    juvenile g.
    saturnine g.
    tophaceous g.
    underexcretion-type g.
gouttes
    parapsoriasis en g.
gouty
    g. arthritis
    g. panniculitis
Gower
    G. maneuver
    panatrophy of G.
gp110
    EBV glycoprotein g.
    Epstein-Barr glycoprotein g.
GP47 protein
GP67 protein
gp91^{phox} level
GPB
    gram-positive bacillus
    gram-positive bacteremia
GPI
    glycosylphosphatidylinositol
GPI-anchored protein
GP ib-IX complex
GPIIa
    glycoprotein IIa
GPIIb
    glycoprotein IIb
GPIIb-IIIa
    glycoprotein IIb-IIIa
GPL unit
GPMT
    guinea pig maximization test
G-protein-coupled receptor

G

NOTES

gracile
 Lophatherum g.
grade
 International Society for Heart and Lung Transplant g.
 ISHLT g.
gradient
 alveolar-arterial oxygen g.
grading
 wound g. 1-6
Gradle scissors
graecorum
 elephantiasis g.
 lepra g.
Graefe forceps
Graffi virus
graft
 AlloDerm processed tissue g.
 AlloDerm universal dermal tissue g.
 allogenic g.
 autogeneic g.
 autologous g.
 autoplastic g.
 composite g.
 g. failure
 free cartilage g.
 full-thickness g.
 H g.
 heterologous g.
 heteroplastic g.
 heterospecific g.
 homologous g.
 homoplastic g.
 g. injury
 interspecific g.
 intrahepatic islet g.
 islet composite g.
 isogeneic g.
 isologous g.
 isoplastic g.
 osteochondral g.
 Papineau g.
 pinch g.
 g. reinfection
 g. rejection
 g. septoplasty
 split-thickness skin g. (STSG)
 g. survival rate
 syngeneic g.
 Thiersch g.
 g. thrombosis
 g. vessel disease (GVD)
 white g.
 XenoDerm g.
 xenogeneic g.
GraftCyte gauze wound dressing
grafting
 bone g.

 CDR g.
 hair g.
Graftskin
graft-versus-host reaction
graft-versus-leukemia (GVL)
 g.-v.-l. effect
Graham-Little-Piccardi-Lasseur syndrome
Graham Little syndrome
grain
 g. dust
 g. fever
 g. itch
grama grass
gramicidin
 neomycin, polymyxin b, and g.
gram-negative
 g.-n. bacilli arthritis
 g.-n. bacillus (GNB)
 g.-n. bacteremia (GNB)
 g.-n. cocci
 g.-n. folliculitis
 g.-n. organism
 g.-n. rod
gram-positive
 g.-p. bacillus (GPB)
 g.-p. bacteremia (GPB)
 g.-p. cocci
 g.-p. organism
 g.-p. rod
Gram stain
Gr antigen
granular
 g. cell
 g. cell layer
 g. cell myoblastoma
 g. cell schwannoma
 g. cell tumor
 g. degeneration
 g. papulation
 g. vaginitis
granulate
granulation
 red g.
 g. tissue
granule
 azurophil g.
 Birbeck g.
 bismuth g.
 Bollinger g.
 cytoplasmic g.
 dextranomer g.
 Fordyce g.
 keratohyaline g.
 lamellar g.
 Langerhans cell g.
 membrane-coating g.
 Much g.
 Paneth cell g.
 Snaplets-FR G.

sulfur g.
tertiary g.
Granulex
granulocyte
    g. colony-stimulating factor (G-CSF)
    g. transfusion
granulocytic leukemia
granulocytopenia
granuloma
    actinic g.
    amebic g.
    anular elastolytic giant cell g.
    aquarium g.
    beryllium g.
    bilharzial g.
    Candida g.
    caseating g.
    clear-cut g.
    coccidioidal g.
    coli g.
    diaper g.
    elastolytic giant cell g.
    g. endemium
    eosinophilic g.
    epithelioid g.
    g. faciale
    fish-tank g.
    g. fissuratum
    foreign body g.
    g. fungoides
    g. gangraenescens
    giant cell g.
    g. gluteale infantum
    histiocytic g.
    Hodgkin g.
    infectious g.
    g. inguinale
    g. inguinale tropicum
    interstitial g.
    lethal midline g.
    lipoid g.
    lipophagic g.
    g. lycopodium
    Majocchi g.
    g. malignum
    mercury g.
    metastatic g.
    midline lethal g.
    Miescher actinic g.
    mixed inflammatory g.
    mixed interstitial and palisaded g.

monilial g.
g. multiforme
necrobiotic g.
necrotizing g.
noncaseating g.
O'Brien actinic g.
oily g.
orbital g.
palisaded g.
palisading g.
paracoccidioidal g.
parasitic g.
perifollicular g.
peripheral giant cell g.
g. pudendi
pyogenic g.
g. pyogenicum
reticulohistiocytic g.
sarcoid g.
schistosome g.
sea urchin g.
silica g.
swimming pool g.
g. telangiectaticum
trichophytic g.
g. trichophyticum
g. venereum
zirconium g.
granulomatis
    Calymmatobacterium g.
    Donovania g.
granulomatosa
    cheilitis g.
    Miescher cheilitis g.
granulomatosis
    allergic g.
    Churg-Strauss g.
    g. disciformis et progressiva
    eosinophilic g.
    lethal midline g.
    limited Wegener g.
    lipid g.
    lipophagia g.
    lymphomatoid g.
    midline g.
    Miescher-Leder g.
    necrobiosis g.
    g. rhinitis
    Wegener g. (WG)
granulomatous
    g. angiitis
    g. arteritis

G

NOTES

233

granulomatous *(continued)*
    g. bacterial infection
    g. cheilitis
    g. cutaneous T-cell lymphoma
    g. dermal infiltrate
    g. disease
    g. focus
    g. hepatitis
    g. idiopathic arthritis
    g. inflammatory reaction
    g. lesions of unknown significance
      (GLUS)
    g. pyoderma
    g. rosacea
    g. slack skin
    g. vasculitis
granulosis rubra nasi
granulosity
granulosum
    stratum g. (SG)
granulosus
    Echinococcus g.
granzyme
    g. B (GrB)
    g. B-mediated cleavage
grape cell
grapefruit
grapeseed
grasper
    nonsuction g.
grass
    alfalfa g.
    Bahia g.
    Bermuda g.
    blue g.
    brome g.
    Canada blue g.
    canary g.
    common reed g.
    crab g.
    cultivated barley g.
    cultivated corn g.
    cultivated oat g.
    cultivated rye g.
    cultivated wheat g.
    grama g.
    Johnson g.
    June g.
    meadow fescue g.
    meadow foxtail g.
    orchard g.
    perennial rye g.
    g. pollen
    g. pollen concentration
    redtop A g.
    salt g.
    sorghum g.
    sweet vernal g.
    timothy g.

    velvet g.
    vernal g.
    wild rye g.
Graves disease
Gravicon VC25
gravidarum
    chloasma g.
    fibroma molle g.
    hydroa g.
    melasma g.
    prurigo g.
    striae g.
gravimetric
    g. assessment
    g. device
gravis
    icterus g.
    junctional epidermolysis bullosa
      atrophicans generalisata g.
    myasthenia g. (MG)
gravis-type Ehlers-Danlos syndrome
gravitational
    g. particle collection
    g. sampler
    g. ulcer
Gravol
gray-patch
    g.-p. ringworm
    g.-p. tinea capitis
gray-scale intensity
GrB
    granzyme B
grease
    silicone g.
greasewood
greasy
    g. scaly lesion
    g. surface
Grecian Formula
5G1.1 recombinant C5 complement inhibitor
green
    g. amaranth
    g. ash
    g. ash tree
    g. coffee bean
    Guignet g.
    g. hair
    indocyanine g. (ICG)
    malachite g.
    g. monkey virus
    g. nail
    g. nail syndrome
    Paris g.
    g. pepper
    G. soap tincture
    g. tea polyphenol (GTP)
Greenblatt
    groove sign of G.

Greenhow disease
Greenspan scale
green-striped nail
Greither syndrome
grenz
  g. ray
  g. ray therapy
  g. ray treatment
Griesinger disease
Griess
  G. analysis
  G. reaction
Grifulvin V
grinder
  Kontes Pellet Pestle disposable microtissue g.
grind test
grip, grippe
  devil g.
Grisactin Ultra
Griscelli syndrome (GS)
grisea
  Madurella g.
griseofulvin
  ultramicrosize g.
Grisolle sign
Grisovin-FP
Gris-PEG
grocer's itch
Grocott methenamine silver (GMS)
groin
  ringworm of the g.
  g. ulcer
Grönblad-Strandberg syndrome
groove
  ectodermal g.
  Harrison g.
  nail g.
  g. sign
  g. sign of Greenblatt
  transverse nasal g.
grooved tongue
gross
  g. lesion
  G. leukemia virus
Grossan nasal irrigator
Grotthus-Draper law
ground
  g. itch
  g. substance
ground-glass
  g.-g. appearance

g.-g. opacification
g.-g. pattern
grounding pad
groundsel tree
group
  g. A beta-hemolytic streptococcal infection
  g. A beta-hemolytic *Streptococcus* (GABHS)
  g. A carbohydrate antibody
  g. agglutination
  g. agglutinin
  g. antigens
  g. A *Streptococcus* (GAS)
  g. A *Streptococcus* infection
  blood g.
  g. B *Streptococcus* (GBS)
  Contact Dermatitis Research G.
  cross-reactive antigen g. (CREG)
  g. C rotavirus
  cytophil g.
  Dermatology Teachers Exchange G. (DTEG)
  determinant g.
  Duffy blood g.
  Euro-Transplant G.
  g. immunity
  International Contact Dermatitis Research G. (ICDRG)
  g. JK *Corynebacterium* sepsis
  g. JK organism
  Kell-Cellano blood g.
  Kidd blood g.
  Lewis blood g.
  Lutheran blood g.
  MNS blood g.
  North American Contact Dermatitis G. (NACDG)
  Pigmented Lesion Study G. (PLSG)
  g. reaction
  retrovirus g.
  support g.
  syntenic g.
  g. 5 topical steroid
grouping
  blood g.
  chemical g.
Grover disease
growing season
growth
  g. factor (GF)

G

NOTES

growth *(continued)*
> g. hormone (GH)
> g. hormone deficiency
> g. phase
> g. retardation

Gruber reaction
Gruber-Widal reaction
gryphosis
gryphotic
gryposis unguium
GS
> Griscelli syndrome

GSE
> gluten-sensitive enteropathy

GST
> glutathione-S-transferase

GTP
> green tea polyphenol
> guanosine triphosphate

guaiacolate
> glycerol g.

Guaifed-PD
guaifenesin
> g. and phenylpropanolamine
> g., phenylpropanolamine, and
>   phenylephrine
> g. and pseudoephedrine
> theophylline and g.

Guaifenex
> G. DM
> G. LA
> G. PPA 75
> G. PSE

GuaiMAX-D
Guaipax
Guaitab
Guaivent PD capsule
Guaivent/PSE
Guama virus
guanethidine
guanine
guanosine
> g. monophosphate (GMP)
> g. triphosphate (GTP)

guanylic acid
Guard
> Aspirin Plus Stomach G.

guar gum
Guarnieri body
Guaroa virus
Gubler-Robin typhus
Guiatex
Guiatuss PE
guideline
> National Asthma Education and
>   Prevention Program G.'s (NAEPP)

Guignet green
Guillain-Barré syndrome

guillermondii
> *Candida* g.

guinea
> g. corn yaw
> g. pig
> g. pig maximization test (GPMT)
> g. worm
> g. worm infection

Gulf War syndrome (GWS)
gum
> guar g.
> karaya g.
> g. rash
> G. tragacanth
> vegetable g.

Gumboro disease
gumma of tertiary syphilis
gummatous
> g. meningitis
> g. syphilid
> g. syphilis
> g. ulcer

gummosa
> scrofuloderma g.

gummy
Günther
> G. disease
> G. syndrome

gustatory
> g. hyperhidrosis
> g. rhinitis

gut
> g. glucagon
> g. homeostasis
> g. microbial flora

gut-associated
> g.-a. lymphoid disease
> g.-a. lymphoid tissue (GALT)

Guthrie skin hook
gutless adenovirus
guttata
> morphea g.
> parapsoriasis g.
> psoriasis g.

guttate
> g. hypomelanosis
> g. parapsoriasis
> g. psoriasis

guttering
> limbal g.

Guyon
> tunnel of G.

GV
> Healon GV

GVD
> graft vessel disease

GVH
> GVH disease

GVL
graft-versus-leukemia
G-well
G-w. Lotion
G-w. Shampoo
GWS
Gulf War syndrome
gymnosperm
Gynecort topical
Gyne-Lotrimin
gypseum
Microsporum g.
Trichophyton g.

gypsy
g. moth larva
g. moth larva sting
gyrase
DNA g.
gyrata
cutis verticis g.
psoriasis g.
gyrate psoriasis
gyratum
erythema g.
gyrose

NOTES

H

H agglutinin
H antigen
H deficiency factor
H F Antidote
H graft

1H

Campath 1H

H-2

H-2 antigen
H-2 complex

H2

H2 blocker
prostaglandin H2 (PGH$_2$)

H5N1 virus

HA

hepatitis A
hydroxyapatite

Ha-1A monoclonal antibody

HA1, HA2 virus

HAA

hepatitis A antigen
hepatitis-associated antigen

Haake rheometer

haarscheibe tumor

HAART

highly active antiretroviral therapy

Habermann disease

Haber syndrome

Haber-Weiss reaction

habit

h. tic deformity
wolf-biter h.

habitus

marfanoid h.

habumatone

hackberry tree

HAE

hereditary angioneurotic edema

HAEM

herpes-associated erythema multiforme
herpes simplex-associated erythema
multiforme

haematobium

Schistosoma h.

Haemonchus contortus

haemophilum

Mycobacterium h.

Haemophilus

H. ducreyi
H. influenzae meningitis
H. influenzae type b (HIB)
H. parahaemolyticus
H. parainfluenzae
H. suis

haemorrhagica

Haenel symptom

Haffkine vaccine

Hafnia alvei

Hagedorn needle

Hageman factor

Hailey-Hailey

H.-H. disease (HHD)
familial benign pemphigus of H.-H.

Haines directory

hair

acquired progressive kinking of
the h. (APKH)
animal h.
axillary h.
bamboo h.
bayonet h.
beaded h.
black dot h.
bubble h.
h. bulb
burrowing h.
h. cast
club h.
h. collar sign
corkscrew h.
cortex of h.
crackled h.
cuticle of h.
h. cyst
deer h.
h. disc
H. dressing screening tray test
exclamation point h.
h. fall
h. follicle
h. follicle mite
h. follicle mite scabies
h. follicle nevus
Frey h.
genital h.
h. germ
golf tee h.
h. grafting
green h.
horse h.
ingrowing h.
ingrown h.
kinky h.
knotted h.
lanugo h.
h. loss
h. matrix
h. melanin
moniliform h.

H

239

hair *(continued)*
    nettling h.
    nonvellus h.
    h. removal efficiency (HRE)
    ringed h.
    h. rudiment
    h. and scalp
    Schridde cancer h.
    h. shaft
    spun-glass h.
    stellate h.
    telogen h.
    terminal h.
    h. transplant
    tuft of h.
    twisted h.
    vellus h.
    whisker h.
    woolly h.
HAIR-AN
    hyperandrogenism, insulin resistance, and acanthosis nigricans
    HAIR-AN syndrome
hairdressing solution
hairiness
    excessive h.
hair-like structure
hair-matrix carcinoma
hair-on-end appearance
hair-standing-on-end appearance
hairy
    h. cell (HC)
    h. cell leukemia (HCL)
    h. hamartoma
    h. leukoplakia
    h. mole
    h. nevus
Halberstaedter-Prowazek body
halcinonide
Halcion
Haldrone
Halfan
half-and-half
    h.-a.-h. fingernail
    h.-a.-h. nail
half-buried mattress stitch
half-moon
    red h.-m.
Halfprin
halitosis
Hallermann-Streiff syndrome
Hallopeau
    H. acrodermatitis
    acrodermatitis continua of H.
    H. disease
Hallopeau-Siemens
    H.-S. epidermolysis bullosa
    H.-S. syndrome

hallux
    h. rigidus
    h. valgus
    h. varus
halo
    anemic h.
    h. melanoma
    h. nevus
    purpuric h.
    red h.
    h. vest
halobetasol propionate
haloderma, halodermia
halodes
    Helminthosporium h.
halofantrine hydrochloride
halofuginone
halogen acne
halogenated salicylanilides
halogenoderma
halogenosis
    vegetating h.
Halog-E topical
Halog topical
haloprogin
Halotex topical
Halothane
Halotussin PE
HALS
    Health and Activity Limitation Survey
Halsey needle holder
Halsted
    H. law
    H. mosquito hemostat
Haltone
Haltran
Hamamelis virginiana
hamartoma, pl. **hamartomata**
    Becker hairy h.
    eccrine angiomatous h.
    hairy h.
    neurocristic h.
    pilar neurocristic h.
    smooth muscle h.
Hamilton
    H. bandage
    H. pseudophlegmon
    H. test
Hamman-Rich syndrome
Hamman sign
hammer toe
hamster
Ham test
HAM/TSP
    HTLV-1-associated myelopathy or tropical spastic paraparesis
Hanalux Oslo light
hand
    accordion h.

Breuerton view of the h.
chrome holes on the h.
crab h.
h. dermatosis
h. eczema
edema of h.
ghoul h.
Hunstad h.
Marinesco succulent h.
mechanic h.
neutrophilic dermatosis of the
 dorsal h. (NDDH)
pulling boat h.
ringworm of the h.
trench h.
Handages dressing
hand-and-foot syndrome
hand-foot-and-mouth
 h.-f.-a.-m. disease
 h.-f.-a.-m. disease virus
1-hand 2-foot syndrome
handheld dermatoscope
Handisol phototherapy device
handlebar palsy
Hand-Schüller-Christian disease
HANE
 hereditary angioneurotic edema
hanging skin
hangnail
Hanks balanced salt solution (HBSS)
Hansamed strip
Hansen
 H. bacillus
 H. disease
Hantaan virus
Hantavirus **infection**
hapalonychia
haploidentical
haplotype
haplotype-shared transfusion
Happle syndrome
HappySkin Acne Light
hapten
 conjugated h.
 h. inhibition of precipitation
 h. mechanism of hemolytic anemia
haptenated protein
haptene
Hapten-type reaction
haptoglobin
HAQ
 Health Assessment Questionnaire

Stanford Health Assessment
 Questionnaire
 HAQ DI
Harada syndrome
hard
 h. chancre
 h. corn
 h. keratin
 h. nevus
 h. pad disease
 h. pad virus
 h. palate
 h. papilloma
 h. sore
 h. tick
 h. ulcer
harderoporphyrin
hard-milled soap
Hardonk criteria
Hardy-Weinberg equilibrium
harlequin
 h. fetus
 h. ichthyosis
 ichthyosis h.
Harrison groove
Harris pressure mat
Harter syndrome
Hartmann
 H. ear forceps
 H. hemostat
Hartnup disease
harvest
 extra articular h.
 h. mite
 h. mite bite
Harvey murine sarcoma virus
harzianum
 Trichoderma h.
Hashimoto
 H. disease
 H. thyroiditis
Hashimoto-Pritzker disease
Hassall corpuscle
HAT
 hypoxanthine, aminopterin and thymidine
 HAT medium
Hata phenomenon
Hatchcock sign
hatchetti
 Acanthamoeba h.
Hauch
 ohne H.

NOTES

H

HAV
  hepatitis A virus
    HAV RNA
Haverhill fever
Haversian system
Havrix vaccine
Hawaiian Tropic Herbal
Hawes-Pallister-Landor syndrome
hay asthma
Hayek oscillator
Hayem corpuscle
Hayfebrol Liquid
hayfever
Hay-Wells syndrome
hazard
  univariate Cox proportional h.
hazel
  witch h.
hazelnut
  h. tree
  h. tree pollen
HB
  hepatitis B
    Recombivax HB
HB$_s$
  hepatitis B surface
HB$_s$Ab, HBsAb
  antibody to hepatitis B surface antigen
HB$_s$Ag, HBsAg
  hepatitis B surface antigen
HB$_c$
  hepatitis B$_c$
HB$_c$Ab, HBcAb
  antibody to hepatitis B core antigen
HB$_c$Ag, HBcAg
  hepatitis B core antigen
HbCO
  carboxyhemoglobin
HBD
  heart-beating donor
HBDT
  human basophil degranulation test
HB$_e$, HBe
  hepatitis B$_e$
HB$_e$Ab, HBeAb
  antibody to hepatitis Be antigen
HB-EGF
  heparin-binding epidermal growth factor-
  like growth factor
HBGF
  heparin-binding growth factor
HBGF-1
  heparin-binding growth factor-1
H-BIG
  hepatitis B immune globulin
  hepatitis B immunoglobulin
HBO
  hyperbaric oxygen

HbO$_2$
  oxyhemoglobin
HbOC/DTP vaccine
HbOC vaccine
HBsAb (*var. of* HB$_s$Ab)
HBsAg (*var. of* HB$_s$Ag)
HBSS
  Hanks balanced salt solution
HBT
  home-based telemetry
    HBT Sleuth
HBV
  hepatitis B virus
    HBV bDNA signal amplification
    HBV DNA
    HBV DNA probe test
HC
  hairy cell
  hepatitis C
    Dermaflex HC
    Prevex HC
    Sarna HC
    Ti-U-Lac HC
HCA
  hybrid capture assay
    Orabase HCA
HCB
  hexachlorobenzene
HCD
  heavy-chain disease
HCH
  hexachlorocyclohexane
HCL
  hairy cell leukemia
HCl
  hydrochloride
    aminolevulinic acid HCl
    amiprilose HCl
    butenafine HCl
    cevimeline HCl
    doxepin HCl
    epinastine HCl
    fexofenadine HCl/pseudoephedrine
      HCl
    fluoxetine HCl
    gemcitabine HCl
    hydroxyzine HCl
    moxifloxacin HCl
    paroxetine HCl
    pioglitazone HCl
    pramoxine HCl
    promethazine HCl
    pseudoephedrine HCl
    sertraline HCl
    valacyclovir HCl
HCO$_3$
  bicarbonate

HCP
> hereditary coproporphyria
> histiocytic cytophagic panniculitis

HCQ
> hydroxychloroquine

HCT
> hematopoietic stem cell transplantation

HCV
> hepatitis C virus
>> RIBA HCV
>> HCV by RIBA
>> HCV RNA

HCV-related cirrhosis

HD
> hemodialysis
> hepatitis D

HDCV
> human diploid cell rabies vaccine

HDI
> isocyanate HDI

HDIT
> high-dose immunosuppressive therapy

IIDM
> house dust mite

HDMFP
> house dust mite fecal pellet

HDV
> hepatitis D virus

HE
> hematoxylin and eosin
> hepatitis E

H&E
> hematoxylin and eosin
> hematoxylin and eosin stain

head
> cobalt-chrome h.
> h. compression test
> h. distraction test
> h. louse
> H. & Shoulders Shampoo
> H. zone

headache tablet

headlight sign

Heaf test

healed ulcer

healing
> fish-mouth h.
> Pressure Ulcer Scale for H. (PUSH)
> wound h.

Healon GV

health
> H. and Activity Limitation Survey (HALS)
> H. Assessment Questionnaire (HAQ)
> H. Assessment Questionnaire Disability Index
> h. maintenance organization (HMO)
> National Institutes of H. (NIH)

health-related quality of life

healthy
> h. carrier
> h. years of life lost (HYLL)

He antigen

hearing
> h. aid dermatitis
> h. loss

heart
> AbioCor implantable replacement h.
> h. allograft
> h. antigen
> h. rate reserve (HRR)
> h. transplantation (HTX)

heart-beating donor (HBD)

heart-lung
> h.-l. circuit
> h.-l. transplantation (HLT)

heartseases

heartworm

heat
> h. exposure
> h. lamp
> prickly h.
> h. rash
> h. therapy
> h. urticaria

Heath curette

heat-induced urticaria

heat/moisture exchanger (HME)

heat-phenol inactivated vaccine

heat-shock
> h.-s. protein (HSP)
> h.-s. protein 70 (HSP-70)

heavy chain

heavy-chain disease (HCD)

Heberden node

Hebra
> H. disease
> H. erythema multiforme
> melanotic prurigo of H.
> H. ointment
> H. pityriasis

NOTES

H

Hebra *(continued)*
    protoporphyria of H.
    H. prurigo
hebraeum
    Amblyomma h.
Hecht
    H. phenomenon
    H. pneumonia
Heck syndrome
HED
    hypohidrotic ectodermal dysplasia
heel
    black h.
    cracked h.
    h. pain
    h. spur
Heelbo decubitus protector
Heerfordt syndrome
height loss
Heilen expressor
Heine Optotechnik
Heiner syndrome
Heinz body
Hektoen phenomenon
HEL
    hen egg lysozyme
    HEL protein
HeLa cell
Helanthus
helical
helicis
    chondrodermatitis nodularis
      chronica h.
Helicobacter
    H. mustelae
    H. pylori
heliopathy
Helioseal
heliotherapy
heliotrope rash
Helisal rapid blood test
Helistat collagen matrix sponge
helix
    triple h.
HELLP
    hemolysis, elevated liver enzymes, low
    platelet
    HELLP syndrome
helminth
    multicellular h.
helminthiasis elastica
helminthic parasitic disease
Helminthosporium
    H. halodes
    H. savitum
Heloderma
    H. suspectum
    H. suspectum bite

heloma
    h. durum
    h. molle
helosis
helotomy
helper
    h. T cell
    h. virus
helper-suppressor cell ratio
helplessness
    learned h.
Helweg-Larssen syndrome
hemacytometer
hemadsorption
    h. virus test
    h. virus type 1, 2
hemagglutinating
    h. antibody
    h. cold autoantibody
hemagglutination
    h. inhibition
    passive h. (PHA)
    reverse passive h.
    h. test
    viral h.
hemagglutinin
    influenza virus h.
hemalum
    Mayer h.
hemangioendothelioma
    kaposiform h. (KHE)
    malignant h.
    retiform h.
    spindle cell h.
hemangioma, pl. **hemangiomata**
    h. birthmark
    capillary h.
    cavernous h.
    cherry h.
    h. congenitale
    deep h.
    DeMorgan h.
    dyschondroplasia with h.
    glomeruloid h.
    h. hypertrophicum cutis
    involuting flat h.
    microvenular h.
    mixed h.
    nuchal h.
    h. planum extensum
    port-wine h.
    sclerosing h.
    senile h.
    spider h.
    strawberry h.
    superficial h.
    synovial h.
    targetoid hemosiderotic h. (THH)

ulcerated h.
verrucous h.
hemangiomata
hemangioma-thrombocytopenia syndrome
hemangiomatosis
Osler h.
Parkes-Weber h.
pulmonary capillary h.
thrombocytopenic h.
unilateral h.
visceral h.
hemangiomatous tissue
hemangiopericytoma (HPC)
benign h.
borderline malignant h.
malignant h.
hemarthritic disability
hemarthrosis
hemarthrotic disability
hematid
hematidrosis
hematogenous metastasis
hematoidin crystal
hematologic
h. disorder
h. lupus
h. reaction
hematolysis
hematoma
paroxysmal hand h.
spontaneous spinal epidural h.
(SSEH)
subungual h.
hematopoiesis
hematopoietic
h. chimerism
h. failure syndrome
h. PGD$_2$ synthase
h. progenitor cell (HPC)
h. progenitor cell transplantation
h. progenitor transplantation
h. reconstitution
h. stem cell
h. stem cell transplant
h. stem cell transplantation (HCT,
HSCT)
h. system
hematotoxin
hematotropic
hematoxin

hematoxylin
h. and eosin (HE, H&E)
h. and eosin stain (H&E)
hematoxylin-eosin
h.-e. staining
hematoxyphilic inclusion
hematuria
hemiarthroplasty
McKeever and MacIntosh h.
hemiatrophy
progressive facial h.
Romberg h.
hemiballismus
hemicallotasis procedure
hemichannel
connexin h.
hemidesmosome
hemidiaphoresis
hemidiaphragm
hemidrosis
hemidysplasia
congenital h.
unilateral h.
hemihepatectomy
hemihidrosis
hemihyperhidrosis
hemihypertrophy
hemijoint
Hemiptera
hemipterus
Cimex h.
hemithorax
hemoagglutination
hemoagglutinin
hemoantitoxin
hemochromatosis
hemochromatotic arthritis
hemocyanin
keyhole limpet h.
hemocytoblast
hemocytometer
hemoderma
hemodialysis (HD)
perforating disease of h.
hemodialysis-associated amyloidosis
hemoglobin
h. crystal
h. C, S disease
hemoglobinopathy
hemoglobinophilic
hemoglobinuria
nocturnal h.

NOTES

H

hemoglobinuria *(continued)*
  paroxysmal cold h.
  paroxysmal nocturnal h. (PNH)
hemoglobinuric
  h. fever
  h. nephrosis
hemolysate
hemolysin
  alpha h.
  bacterial h.
  beta h.
  cold h.
  heterophil h.
  immune h.
  natural h.
  specific h.
  h. unit
  warm-cold h.
hemolysinogen
hemolysis
  acute intravascular h.
  autoimmune h.
  beta h.
  biologic h.
  conditioned h.
  h., elevated liver enzymes, low
    platelet (HELLP)
  h., elevated liver enzymes, low
    platelet count
  gamma h.
  immune h.
  venom h.
  viridans h.
hemolytic
  h. anemia of newborn
  h. chain
  h. disease of newborn
  h. plaque assay
  h. sickle cell disease
  h. streptococcus
  h. uremic syndrome (HUS)
hemolyzation
hemolyze
hemopexin
hemophagocytic syndrome
hemophagocytosis
hemophil
hemophilia
  acquired h.
hemophiliac patient
hemophilic arthropathy
hemopoietic factor
hemoprecipitin
hemoptysis
  Manson h.
hemorrhage
  iliopsoas h.
  intraalveolar h.
  intraosseous h.

  intraventricular h.
  petechial h.
  pulmonary h.
  punctate h.
  retinal h.
  splinter h.
  subaponeurotic h.
hemorrhagic
  h. arthritis
  h. bulla
  h. cystitis
  h. dengue
  h. diathesis
  h. edema
  h. exudative erythema
  h. fever
  h. fever with renal syndrome
    (HFRS)
  h. gangrene
  h. lesion
  h. pian
  h. pyoderma gangrenosum
  h. rash
  h. smallpox
  h. telangiectasia
hemorrhagica
  purpura h.
  scarlatina h.
  urticaria h.
  variola h.
hemorrhagicus
  lichen h.
  pemphigus h.
hemorrhagin
hemosiderin
  h. deposition
  h. hyperpigmentation
hemosiderin-laden macrophage
hemosiderosis
  idiopathic pulmonary h.
  pulmonary h.
  synovial h.
hemostasis
  chemical h.
hemostat
  Halsted mosquito h.
  Hartmann h.
hemostatic
  h. agent
  h. collodion
  h. disorder
hemostatica
  dermatitis h.
hemothorax, pl. **hemothoraces**
  catamenial h.
hemotoxic
hemotoxin
  cobra h.
hemotropic

hemp
 western water h.
Hemril-HC Uniserts
hen
 h. egg lysozyme (HEL)
 h. egg lysozyme protein
Henderson-Paterson body
Hendersonula toruloidea
Hendra virus
He-Ne lasing medium
Henle-Koch pustulate
Henle layer
henna
 extract of h.
Henoch purpura
Henoch-Schönlein
 H.-S. purpura (HSP)
 H.-S. syndrome (HSS)
 H.-S. vasculitis
henselae
 Bartonella h.
 Rochalimaea h.
HEP
 hepatoerythrocytic porphyria
HEPA
 high-efficiency particulate air
 high-efficiency particulate arresting
 HEPA filter
Hepadnaviridae
hepadnavirus
Hepandrin
heparinase 2
heparin-binding
 h.-b. epidermal growth factor-like
  growth factor (HB-EGF)
 h.-b. growth factor (HBGF)
 h.-b. growth factor-1 (HBGF-1)
heparinization
heparinoid therapy
heparin sulfate
hepatic
 h. ischemia and reperfusion (HIR)
 h. ischemia and reperfusion injury
 h. nevus
 h. porphyria
 h. portoenterostomy
 h. sickling
 h. sinusoid
hepatica
 facies h.
hepaticojejunostomy
 Roux-en-Y h.

hepaticum
 chloasma h.
hepatitic
hepatitis
 h. A (HA)
 h. A antigen (HAA)
 aggressive h.
 anicteric virus h.
 autoimmune chronic h.
 h. A vaccine
 h. A virus (HAV)
 h. B (HB)
 h. B_e (HB_e, HBe)
 h. B_c (HB_c)
 h. B core antigen (HB_cAg, HBcAg)
 h. B DNA detection
 h. Be antigen
 h. B immune globulin (H-BIG)
 h. B immunoglobulin (H-BIG)
 h. B surface (HB_s)
 h. B surface antigen (HB_sAg, HBsAg)
 h. B vaccine
 h. B viral DNA assay
 h. B virus (HBV)
 h. B virus branched chain deoxyribonucleic acid signal amplification
 h. C (HC)
 cholangiolitic h.
 cholestatic h.
 h. contagiosa canis
 h. C RNA detection
 h. C virus (HCV)
 h. C virus antibody detection
 h. C virus-related cirrhosis
 h. D (HD)
 delta antigen h.
 h. D virus (HDV)
 h. E (HE)
 epidemic h.
 equine serum h.
 h. E virus (HEV)
 h. G
 granulomatous h.
 h. G virus (HGV)
 infectious h.
 infectious canine h.
 isoniazid-induced h.
 long incubation h.
 lupoid h.

NOTES

H

hepatitis *(continued)*
 mouse h.
 murine h.
 NANB h.
 non-A-E h.
 non-A non-B h.
 peliosis h.
 posttransfusion h. (PTH)
 serum h. (SH)
 short incubation h.
 transfusion h.
 viral h. (VH)
 h. virus
 virus A h.
hepatitis-associated
 h.-a. antigen (HAA)
 h.-a. lichen planus
hepatobiliary disease
hepatocellular chimerism
hepatocyte
 h. growth factor (HGF)
 immortalized human h.
hepatoerythrocytic porphyria (HEP)
hepatoerythropoietic porphyria
hepatolenticular degeneration
hepatolysin
hepatomegaly
hepatopulmonary syndrome (HPS)
hepatosplenic
 h. schistosomiasis
 h. tuberculosis
hepatosplenomegaly
hepatotoxic
hepatotoxicity
hepatotoxin
hepatotrophic
Hep-B-Gammagee
HEPES buffer
heptacarboxylporphyrin III
Heptavax immunization
Heptovir
herald patch
herb
 mucilage-containing h.
herbal
 H. Answer
 Hawaiian Tropic H.
 h. therapy
herbimycin-inhibited movement
Herbogesic
herd immunity
hereditaria
 alopecia h.
hereditarium
 erythema palmare h.
hereditary
 h. allergy
 h. angioneurotic edema (HAE, HANE)

 h. arthroophthalmopathy
 h. cardiopathic amyloidosis
 h. coproporphyria (HCP)
 h. disease
 h. hemorrhagic angioma
 h. hemorrhagic telangiectasia (HHT)
 h. hemorrhagic telangiectasis
 h. hypomelanosis
 h. lymphedema
 h. multiple trichoepithelioma
 h. osteoonychodysplasia (HOOD)
 h. periodic fever syndrome
 h. sclerosing poikiloderma (HSP)
 h. sensory radicular neuropathy
 h. spherocytosis
 h. vascular disorder
 h. vibratory angioedema
heredofamilial
 h. amyloidosis
 h. urticaria
heredolues
heredoluetic
heredopathia atactica polyneuritiformis
heredosyphilis
heredosyphilitic
heres
 Scolopendra h.
Herisan
heritable
 h. connective tissue disease
 h. disorder
Herlitz
 H. disease
 H. epidermolysis bullosa
 H. syndrome
Hermal kit
Hermansky-Pudlak syndrome type IV, VI
hernia
 diaphragmatic h.
herniated
 h. nucleus pulposus (HNP)
 h. presacral fat pad
herniation
 disc h.
herpangina pharyngitis
Herpasil
Herp-Check
herpes
 h. B encephalomyelitis
 h. catarrhalis
 h. circinatus bullosus
 h. cornea
 h. desquamans
 h. digitalis
 h. facialis
 h. farinosus
 h. febrilis
 genital h.

h. genitalis
h. gladiatorum
inoculation h.
h. iridis
h. iris
h. labialis
h. menstrualis
h. mentalis
nasal h.
neonatal h.
h. neonatalis
h. odeus
orolabial h.
h. pharyngitis
h. phlyctaenodes
h. praepuffalis
h. progenitalis
h. simplex
h. simplex-associated erythema
multiforme (HAEM)
h. simplex conjunctivitis
h. simplex encephalitis
h. simplex infection
h. simplex recurrens
h. simplex virus (HSV)
h. simplex virus arthritis
h. simplex virus thymidine kinase
(HSVTK)
h. simplex virus type I, II
h. thymidine kinase gene
h. tonsurans
h. tonsurans maculosus
toxoplasmosis, other, rubella,
cytomegalovirus, and h.
traumatic h.
h. vegetans
h. whitlow
wrestler h.
h. zoster (HZ)
h. zoster generalisatus
h. zoster infection
h. zoster ophthalmicus
h. zoster oticus
h. zoster varicellosus
h. zoster virus
herpes-associated erythema multiforme
(HAEM)
Herpesviridae
herpesvirus
h. 8
canine h.
caprine h.

h. hominis
human h. 1–7
human h. 6 (HHV6)
human h. 6A
human h. 6B
Kaposi sarcoma h. (KSHV)
McKrae strain of h.
h. saimiri (HVS)
h. simiae
suid h.
h. type 1
herpesvirus-8
Herpesvirus saimiri
herpetic
h. angina
h. fever
h. gingivostomatitis
h. infection
h. keratoconjunctivitis
h. meningoencephalitis
h. paronychia
h. stromal keratitis (HSK)
h. sycosis
h. ulcer
h. vulvovaginitis
h. whitlow
zoster sine h.
herpeticum
eczema h.
herpeticus
favus h.
herpetiform
h. aphtha
h. aphthous stomatitis
h. distribution of lesion
h. pemphigus (HP)
herpetiforme
hydroa h.
herpetiformis
epidermolysis bullosa simplex h.
favus h.
impetigo h.
morphea h.
herpetoid
Herpetoviridae
herpetovirus
canine h.
caprine h.
Herplex
H. Liquifilm
H. Ophthalmic

NOTES

H

herringbone
    h. nail
    h. pattern
Hertoghe sign
Herxheimer
    H. fiber
    H. reaction
    H. spiral
HES
    hypereosinophilic syndrome
Hess test
HETE
    hydroxyeicosatetraenoic acid
heteroagglutinin
heteroantibody
heteroantiserum
heterochromia iris
heteroclitic, heteroclytic
    h. antibody
heterocyclic antidepressant
heterocytotropic
    h. anaphylaxis
    h. antibody
heterodermic
heterodimer
heterodimeric complex
heterodimerization
heteroduplex analysis
heteroduplexing method
heterogenetic
    h. antibody
    h. antigen
heterogenic, heterogeneic
    h. enterobacterial antigen
heterogenote
heterogenous vaccine
heterograft
heterokeratoplasty
heterologous
    h. antiserum
    h. desensitization
    h. graft
    h. protein
    h. serotype
    h. serum
heterology
heterolysin
heterolysis
heterolytic
heteromerization
heterooligomeric complex
heteroosteoplasty
heteropathy
heterophil
    h. antibody
    h. antigen
    h. hemolysin

heterophile
    h. antibody
    h. antigen
heteroplasia
    osseous h.
heteroplastic graft
heteroplastid
heteroplasty
heterospecific graft
heterotopia
    cephalic brainlike h.
heterotopic
    h. heart transplantation (HHT)
    h. plate count bacteria
heterotransplantation
heterotrichosis superciliorum
heterotrimer
heterotrimeric cell-membrane-bound molecule
heterovaccine therapy
heterozygosity
    loss of h. (LOH)
heterozygous
heuristic
HEV
    hepatitis E virus
    high endothelial venule
Hev
    Hev b1
    Hev b6
Hevea
    H. brasiliensis
    H. brasiliensis latex
hevein (Hev b6)
HEVI
    hibernal epidemic viral infection
hexacetonide
    triamcinolone h.
hexachloride
hexachlorobenzene (HCB)
hexachlorocyclohexane (HCH)
hexachlorophene
Hexadenovirus
Hexadrol
    Decadron and H.
    H. phosphate
hexagonus
    Ixodes h.
hexahydrate
    aluminum chloride h.
hexamer
hexamethylmelamine
hexamethyl violet
hexanediol
    ethyl h.
hexasaccharide
    hyaluronan h.
Hexascan Mark (I, II) model robotic scanning device

Hexit
hexon antigen
hexosaminidase
hexose monophosphate shunt (HMS)
HFA
    Proventil HFA
HFRS
    hemorrhagic fever with renal syndrome
HGA
    homogentisic acid
HGF
    hepatocyte growth factor
HGH
    human growth hormone
HGP-30W vaccine
HGPRT
    hypoxanthine-guanine
        phosphoribosyltransferase
        HGPRT deficiency
HGV
    hepatitis G virus
H$_1$, H$_2$ antihistamine
HHD
    Hailey-Hailey disease
HHT
    hereditary hemorrhagic telangiectasia
    heterotopic heart transplantation
HHV-1–7
HHV6
    human herpesvirus 6
        HHV6 encephalitis
HIB
    Haemophilus influenzae type b
hibernal epidemic viral infection (HEVI)
hibernoma
Hibiclens topical
Hibiscus sabdariffa
Hibistat topical
Hibitane
HibTITER
Hib-TT vaccine
hiccup, hiccough
hickey
    stingray h.
hickory
    shagbark h.
    h. tree
Hi-Cor topical
HID
    hyperimmunoglobulinemia syndrome

hidden
    h. margin
    h. nail skin
hidebound
    h. appearance
    h. disease
hidradenitis
    h. axillaris
    h. axillaris of Verneuil
    eccrine h.
    idiopathic recurrent palmoplantar h.
    neutrophilic eccrine h. (NEH)
    palmoplantar eccrine h. (PEH)
    recurrent palmoplantar h.
    h. suppurativa
hidradenoma
    clear cell h.
    cystic h.
    malignant nodular h.
    nodular h.
    papillary h.
    h. papilliferum
    poroid h.
    solid h.
hidroa
hidroacanthoma simplex
hidrocystoma
    apocrine h.
    eccrine h.
hidromeiosis
hidropoiesis
hidropoietic
hidrorrhea
hidrosadenitis
hidroschesis
hidrosis
hidrotic ectodermal dysplasia
HIE
    hyper-IgE
hiemalis
    acrodermatitis h.
    dermatitis h.
    erythrokeratolysis h.
    prurigo h.
    pruritus h.
hierarchical clustering discrimination logic
high
    h. avidity
    h. cyclosporine
    h. dose tolerance
    h. endothelial venule (HEV)

NOTES

high *(continued)*
  h. endothelial venule cell
  h. frequency oscillation
  h. frequency oscillatory ventilator
  h. frequency of recombination
  h. frequency transduction
  h. inflammatory response
  h. liquid content
  h. lung volume
  h. mole count
  h. molecular weight (HMW)
  h. molecular weight-melanoma-
    associated antigen (HMW-MAA)
high-arched palate
high-dose immunosuppressive therapy
  (HDIT)
high-efficiency
  h.-e. particulate air (HEPA)
  h.-e. particulate air filter
  h.-e. particulate arresting (HEPA)
high-egg-passage vaccine
high-energy, pulse-doublet waveform
high-frequency
  h.-f. jet ventilation
  h.-f. microsatellite instability
  h.-f. positive pressure ventilation
high-grade small noncleaved cell
  malignant lymphoma
highly
  h. active antiretroviral therapy
    (HAART)
  h. polymorphic microsatellite
    marker
high-performance liquid chromatography
  (HPLC)
high-resolution
  h.-r. computed tomography (HRCT)
  h.-r. computed tomography scan
high-risk recipient (HRR)
Higouménaki sign
hilar
  h. adenopathy
  h. lymphadenopathy
Hildenbrand typhus
hilus tuberculosis
HIM
  hyper-IgM syndrome
hindfoot
  h. problem
  h. splint
  h. varus
Hind III polymorphism
hinge region
Hinton test
hip
  h. deflexion
  snapping h.
Hippocratic
  H. countenance

  H. face
  H. finger
  H. look
  H. nail
  H. visage
  H. wreath
Hippocratica
  facies H.
HIR
  hepatic ischemia and reperfusion
  HIR injury
hirci
  barbula h.
Hirsch mucosal clamp
Hirschowitz syndrome
Hirschsprung disease
Hirst spore trap
hirsute
hirsuties
hirsutism
  Apert h.
  constitutional h.
  idiopathic h.
hirtellous
hirudiniasis
Hirudin-sensitive protease
Hismanal
HISS
  human immune status survey
Histadyl
Histaject injection
Histalet
  H. Forte Tablet
  H. Syrup
  H. X
Histalon
histaminase
histamine
  h. challenge
  h. dihydrochloride
  h. flush
  h. H_1 agonist
  h. liberator
  h. phosphate
  h. shock
histamine-releasing
  h.-r. factor (HRF)
  h.-r. factor deficiency
histaminergic
Histantil
Histatab
Histatrol
Hista-Vadrin Tablet
Histenol-Forte
histidinemia
histidyl-tRNA synthetase
histiocyte
  alveolar infiltration by h.
  foamy h.

interstitial infiltration by h.
palisading h.
histiocytic
h. cytophagic panniculitis (HCP)
h. granuloma
h. lymphoma
h. medullary reticulosis
h. response
histiocytoma
h. cutis
fibrous h.
generalized eruptive h.
malignant fibrous h. (MFH)
histiocytosis
acute disseminated h.
atypical h.
Blackfan-Diamond Langerhans
cell h.
cephalic h.
chronic h.
focal h.
indeterminate cell h.
juvenile xanthogranuloma h.
Langerhans cell h. (LCH)
malignant h.
multifocal h.
nodular non-X h.
regressing atypical h.
sea-blue h.
sinus h. (SH)
skin-limited h.
h. X
h. Y
histoblot method
histochemical
histocompatibility
h. antigen
h. antigen class I
h. locus (HL)
major h.
h. testing
Histofreezer
H. cryosurgical wart remover
H. cryosurgical wart treatment
histoid leprosy
histoincompatibility
histoincompatible
histologic
h. architecture
h. change
h. lesion
histological

histology
joint h.
Histolyn-CYL
histolytica
Ameba h.
Entamoeba h.
Torula h.
histone antibody
histone-DNA antibody
Histopaque
Histoplasma
H. capsulatum
H. duboisii
histoplasmin
histoplasmin-latex test
histoplasmosis
African h.
cutaneous h.
primary pulmonary h.
progressive disseminated h.
history
Köbner phenomenon by h. (KP-h)
relevant sting h.
histotope
histotoxic
His-Werner disease
Hitzelberger sign
Hitzig syndrome
HIV
human immunodeficiency virus
HIV DNA amplification assay
HIV DNA PCR test
HIV encephalopathy
HIV neutralizing antibody
HIV protease inhibitor
HIV-1
human immunodeficiency virus-1
HIV-2
human immunodeficiency virus-2
HIV-1E virus
HIV-associated
hive
bullous h.'s
generalized h.'s
giant h.'s
Hivid
HIVIG
human immunodeficiency virus
immunoglobulin
HL
histocompatibility locus

NOTES

H

HLA
    human leukocyte antibody
    human leukocyte antigen
        HLA allele
        HLA antigen
        HLA B60
        HLA class 1
        HLA class 1 associated disease
        HLA complex
        HLA Cw6
        HLA intercellular interaction
        HLA typing
HLA-129
HLA-A
HLA-A11
HLA-B
HLA-B8
HLA-B13
HLA-B17
HLA-B60 gene
HLA-B27 gene product
HLA-C
HLA-Cw6
HLA-DP
HLA-DQ
HLA-DQ1
    human leukocyte class II antigen
HLA-DR
HLA-DR2
HLA-DR4
    allele H.-D.
HLA-DR7
    allele H.-D.
HLA-DR3 gene
HLA-DRB1 allele
HLA-DRB and HLA-DRQ DNA typing
HLA-DRw4
HLA-DRw52
HLA-E
HLA-F
HLA-G DNA
HLT
    heart-lung transplantation
HM-175
HME
    heat/moisture exchanger
        Tracheolife HME
HMG-CoA
    3-hydroxy-3-methylglutaryl coenzyme A
        HMG-CoA reductase inhibitor
HMO
    health maintenance organization
HMPAO-SPECT
    technetium-99m hexamethylpropylene
    amine oxime-single-photon-emission
    computed tomography
HMR-3480
HMS
    hexose monophosphate shunt

    hypothetical mean strain
    HMS Liquifilm
    HMS Liquifilm Ophthalmic
HMW
    high molecular weight
HMW-MAA
    high molecular weight-melanoma-
    associated antigen
HNP
    herniated nucleus pulposus
Ho antigen
hobnail tongue
Hodgkin
    H. disease
    H. granuloma
    H. lymphoma
Hoechst staining
Hof area
Hoffman-Clayton procedure
Hoffman sign
Hofmann violet
hog
    h. cholera
    h. cholera vaccine
    h. cholera virus
holder
    Baumgartner needle h.
    Carb-N-Sert needle h.
    Castroviejo blade h.
    Castroviejo needle h.
    Collier needle h.
    Crile-Wood needle h.
    Diamond Jaw needle h.
    Foster needle h.
    Gillies needle h.
    Halsey needle h.
    Neuro-smooth needle h.
    neurosurgery needle h.
    Olsen-Hegar needle h.
    smooth jawed needle h.
    Webster needle h.
Hollister medial adhesive bandage
Hollister-Stier Laboratory
Holmes-Adie syndrome
holmium ethylenediamine tetramethylene
    phosphonic acid
holocrine gland
holoenzyme
Hologic
holothurin
Holt-Oram syndrome
homatropine hydrobromide
home
    h. cleaning product
    h. remedy
home-based telemetry (HBT)
homeobox protein
homeopathy
homeoplasia, homoioplasia

homeoplastic
homeostasis
  gut h.
homeostasis-driven proliferation
homeotherapy
homing receptor
hominis
  Actinobacillus h.
  Actinomyces h.
  Dermatobia h.
  herpesvirus h.
  Mycoplasma h.
  Pentatrichomonas h.
  poliovirus h.
  Sarcoptes h.
  Staphylococcus h.
homme rouge
homocystinuria
homocytotropic
  h. anaphylaxis
  h. antibody
  h. reaction
homodimer
homodimeric
homodimerization
homogenate
homogeneous
homogenous
homogentisic acid (HGA)
homograft reaction
homoioplasia (*var. of* homeoplasia)
homolog
  C-terminal h.
  murine h.
homologous
  h. antigen
  h. antiserum
  h. desensitization
  h. graft
  h. to lymphotoxin, shows inducible
  expression and competes with
  herpes simplex virus glycoprotein
  D for herpes virus entry
  mediator, a receptor expressed by
  T lymphocyte (LIGHT)
  h. serotype
  h. serum
  h. serum jaundice
homology
  h. of chain
  DNA h.
  h. of strand

homolysin
homolysis
homopentameric glycoprotein
homophil
homophilic cell-cell adhesion
homoplastic graft
homotransplantation
homotrimeric
homozygosity
  epitope h.
homozygous
  h. autosomal recessive deletion
  h. typing cell
homunculus
honeybee
  African h.
  h. sting
honeycomb
  h. atrophy
  h. hyperkeratosis
  h. lung
  h. nevus
  h. plaque
  h. ringworm
  h. staining pattern
  h. tetter
honeymoon period
Hong
  H. Kong foot
  H. Kong influenza
  H. Kong toe
HOOD
  hereditary osteoonychodysplasia
hoof-and-mouth disease
hook
  Dortu phlebectomy h.
  double-hook Tyrell skin h.
  dura twist skin h.
  Frazier-Shepherd skin h.
  Frazier skin h.
  Guthrie skin h.
  Joseph skin h.
  Millet phlebectomy h.
  Muller phlebectomy h.
  Oesch phlebectomy h.
  Ramelet phlebectomy h.
  single-hook Frazier skin h.
  skin h.
  Tyrell skin h.
  Varady phlebectomy h.
hookworm
  cat h.

NOTES

H

Hoover sign
Hopf
    acrokeratosis verruciformis of H.
Hopkins lupus cohort
hops
hordeolum
Horder spot
horizontal
    h. growth phase
    h. mattress stitch
    h. section
    h. transmission
Hormodendron, Hormodendrum
    H. compactum
    H. pedrosoi
hormonal change
hormone
    adrenocorticotropic h. (ACTH)
    alpha-melanocyte-stimulating h.
      (alpha-MSH)
    autocrine h.
    beta-melanocyte-stimulating h.
    follicle-stimulating h. (FSH)
    growth h. (GH)
    human growth h. (HGH)
    immunoreactive h.
    melanocyte-stimulating h. (MSH)
    polypeptide h.
    syndrome of inappropriate excretion
      of antidiuretic h. (SIADH)
    thymic h.
    thyroid-stimulating h. (TSH)
hormone-related gene
horn
    cicatricial h.
    cutaneous h.
    nail h.
    sebaceous h.
    warty h.
hornbeam
Horner syndrome
hornet
    h. sting
    white-faced h.
    yellow h.
hornification
horny
    h. cell
    h. cell layer
    h. spine
horripilation
horror
    h. autotoxicans
    h. autotoxicus
horse
    h. chestnut seed extract
    h. hair
    infectious arteritis virus of h.'s
    h. serum

horsefly bite
horsepox virus
hortae
    Piedraia h.
Horton disease
hose
    Medi-Strumpf support h.
hospital
    h. fever
    h. furunculitis
    h. gangrene
hospital-acquired infection
host
    accidental h.
    amplifier h.
    dead-end h.
    h. defect
    humoral h.
    h. immunity
    immunocompromised h.
    reservoir h.
    h. response
host-cell lysis
host-generated neutrophils recruitment
host-immune process
hot
    h. comb alopecia
    h. gangrene
    h. quartz vapor lamp
    h. tub folliculitis
Hotchkiss-McManus
    H.-M. stain
    H.-M. technique
hot-cross-bun skull
hotfoot
hound-dog facies
Houpt
    DIDMOS syndrome of Sontheimer
      and H.
    drug-induced delayed multiorgan
      hypersensitivity syndrome of
      Sontheimer and H.
24-Hour
    Claritin-D 24-H.
hour
    Actifed 12 H.
    Sudafed 12 H.
hourglass
house
    h. dust
    h. dust mite (HDM)
    h. dust mite fecal pellet (HDMFP)
    h. dust mite F, P
housefly
housekeeping gene
housemaid's knee
housewives'
    h. dermatitis
    h. eczema

Houssay animal
Howell-Evans
    H.-E. keratoderma
    H.-E. syndrome
Howell-Jolly body
H2Oxyl
Hoyne sign
HP
    herpetiform pemphigus
    hypersensitivity pneumonitis
        Bensal HP
        Tegaderm HP
HPA
    hypothalamic-pituitary-adrenal
        HPA axis
H.P. Acthar Gel
HPC
    hemangiopericytoma
    hematopoietic progenitor cell
        HPC bacteria
        HPC cell
HPLC
    high-performance liquid chromatography
HPS
    hepatopulmonary syndrome
HPV
    human papillomavirus
    human parvovirus
HQ
    NeoStrata HQ
HRCT
    high-resolution computed tomography
        HRCT scan
HRE
    hair removal efficiency
HRF
    histamine-releasing factor
        HRF deficiency
HRR
    heart rate reserve
    high-risk recipient
HS
    hyperplastic synovium
HSCT
    hematopoietic stem cell transplantation
        nonmyeloablative HSCT
HSE
    human skin equivalent
HSK
    herpetic stromal keratitis

H-SLAP
    human stromelysin aggregated
    proteoglycan
        H-SLAP test
HSNC
    human skin nurse cell
hSOSI
    human son of sevenless
HSP
    heat-shock protein
    Henoch-Schönlein purpura
    hereditary sclerosing poikiloderma
        mycobacteria HSP
HSP-70
    heat-shock protein 70
HSS
    Henoch-Schönlein syndrome
0157-H7 strain
HSV
    herpes simplex virus
        Mollaret HSV
HSV-thymidine kinase ex-vivo cell therapy
HSVTK
    herpes simplex virus thymidine kinase
H-tetanase
HTLV-1-associated myelopathy or tropical spastic paraparesis (HAM/TSP)
HTLV-1 retinovirus
HTLV-I
    human T-cell leukemia virus I
    human T-cell lymphotrophic virus type I
HTLV-II
    human T-cell lymphotrophic virus type II
HTLV-III
    human T-cell leukemia virus III
HTX
    heart transplantation
Hu-901
hu1124
Hu antigen
huff cough
Huile Solaire Bronzage
human
    h. alpha-1-proteinase inhibitor
    h. androgen receptor assay (HUMARA)
    h. anti-CMV antibody
    h. anticytomegalovirus antibody
    h. basophil degranulation test (HBDT)

NOTES

H

human *(continued)*
    h. bite
    h. cartilage glycoprotein 39
    CD4, immunoglobulin G,
      recombinant h.
    chickenpox immune globulin (h.)
    h. cloned DNA
    h. cutaneous leishmaniasis
    cytomegalovirus immune globulin
      intravenous, h.
    h. dermatosparaxis type Ehlers-
      Danlos syndrome
    h. diploid cell rabies vaccine
      (HDCV)
    h. embryonic lung fibroblast
    h. gamma globulin
    h. granulocytic ehrlichiosis
    h. growth hormone (HGH)
    h. herpesvirus 1–7
    h. herpesvirus 6 (HHV6)
    h. herpesvirus 6A
    h. herpesvirus 6B
    h. host defense defect
    h. immune status survey (HISS)
    h. immunodeficiency virus (HIV)
    h. immunodeficiency virus-1 (HIV-
      1)
    h. immunodeficiency virus-2 (HIV-
      2)
    h. immunodeficiency virus antigen
      testing
    h. immunodeficiency virus
      deoxyribonucleic acid amplification
      assay
    h. immunodeficiency virus DNA
      amplification
    h. immunodeficiency virus
      immunoglobulin (HIVIG)
    h. leukemia-associated antigen
    h. leukocyte antibody (HLA)
    h. leukocyte antigen (HLA)
    h. leukocyte antigen allele
    h. leukocyte class II antigen
      (HLA-DQ1)
    h. lymphocyte antigen
    h. mammary tumor virus
    measles immune globulin h.
    h. measles immune serum
    h. monocyte chemoattractant
      protein-1
    h. normal immunoglobulin
    h. nude defect
    h. papillomavirus (HPV)
    h. papillomavirus infection
    h. parvovirus (HPV)
    h. parvovirus B19
    h. pertussis immune serum
    poliomyelitis immune globulin (h.)
    rabies immune globulin, h.

    h. RD
    h. recombinant deoxyribonuclease
    h. retrovirus
    h. rhabdomyosarcoma
    h. scarlet fever immune serum
    h. skin equivalent (HSE)
    h. skin nurse cell (HSNC)
    h. small intestinal allograft
    h. son of sevenless (hSOS1)
    specific immune globulin (h.)
    h. stromelysin aggregated
      proteoglycan (H-SLAP)
    h. stromelysin aggregated
      proteoglycan test
    h. T-cell leukemia/lymphoma virus
    h. T-cell leukemia virus
    h. T-cell leukemia virus I (HTLV-
      I)
    h. T-cell leukemia virus III
      (HTLV-III)
    h. T-cell lymphotrophic virus
    h. T-cell lymphotrophic virus type
      I (HTLV-I)
    h. T-cell lymphotrophic virus type
      II (HTLV-II)
    h. T-cell lymphotrophic virus type
      III
    tetanus immune globulin, h.
    h. thymus lymphocyte antigen
    h. tyrosinase expression
    h. umbilical vein endothelial cell
      (HUVEC)
Human-CFSE Flow Kit
humanized
    h. anti-CD3 monoclonal antibody
    h. BTI-322
humanus
    Pediculus h.
HUMARA
    human androgen receptor assay
Humatin
Humatrix
    H. Microclysmic gel
    H. Microclysmic Gel filler
Humatrope
HuMax-CD4
humectant
Humibid LA
humidified oxygen
humidifier
    h. fever
    h. lung
humidity
humid tetter
Humira
humoral
    h. abnormality
    h. antibody
    h. defect

h. host
h. immune response
h. immunity
h. immunity status panel
hump
buffalo h.
dowager h.
Hunermann disease
Hunstad
H. hand
H. tumescent liposuction system
Hunter
H. glossitis
H. mucopolysaccharidosis
H. robe
H. syndrome
hunterian chancre
Hunter-Thompson syndrome
hunting
h. phenomenon
h. reaction
Hunt syndrome
Huriez syndrome
Hurler
H. disease
H. syndrome
Hurler-Scheie
H.-S. mucopolysaccharidosis
H.-S. syndrome
Hurst disease
HUS
hemolytic uremic syndrome
Hutchinson
chilblain lupus erythematosus of H.
freckle of H.
H. freckle
H. mask
melanotic freckle of H.
H. sign
H. summer protoporphyria
H. summer prurigo
H. teeth
H. triad
Hutchinson-Gilford
H.-G. progeria
H.-G. syndrome
HUVEC
human umbilical vein endothelial cell
HUVS
hypocomplementemic urticarial vasculitis
syndrome
Huxley layer

HVD
hypoxic ventilatory drive
HVPT
hyperventilation provocation test
HVS
herpesvirus saimiri
hyperventilation syndrome
Hyalase
Hyalgan
hyaline
h. articular cartilage
h. basement membrane
h. degeneration
hyalinosis
h. cutis et mucosa
systemic h.
hyalinum
Scytalidium h.
hyalohyphomycosis
Hyalomma variegatum
hyaluran
hyaluronan
h. hexasaccharide
h. injection
h. oligosaccharide
hyaluronate
h. injection
sodium h.
hyaluronate-polylysine complex
hyaluronic
h. acid
h. acid injection
hyaluronidase
h. activity
h. deficiency
hybrid
h. antibody
h. capture assay (HCA)
H. Capture II DNA-based test for
human papillomavirus
h. cell
SV40-adenovirus h.
h. total arthroplasty
hybridization
h. buffer
clonospecific oligoprobe h.
comparative genomic h.
deoxyribonucleic acid h.
DNA h.
fluorescence in situ h. (FISH)
sequence-specific oligonucleotide
probe h. (SSOP)

NOTES

H

hybridization *(continued)*
in situ h. (ISH)
h. test
hybridoma antibody
hyCARE G
Hycodan
Hycomine
Hycor rheumatoid factor IgA ELISA autoimmune test
Hycort
H. Topical
H. topical
Hycotuss
Hy-C trial
hyCure
h. collagen
h. collagen hemostatic wound dressing
hydantoin
h. anticonvulsant
DMDM h.
hydantoin/EDTA
hydatid rash
Hyde disease
Hydeltrasol injection
Hydeltra-TBA injection
Hyderm
hydradenitis
hydradenoma
hydralazine-associated lupus-like syndrome
hydralazine syndrome
Hydramyn Syrup
hydrarthrosis
intermittent h.
Hydrasorb foam wound dressing
hydrate
chloral h.
H. Injection
tacrolimus h.
hydrated petrolatum
hydration
adequate h.
DuoDerm hydroactive gel for wound h.
skin h.
vigorous h.
hydrazine
isonicotine h. (INH)
Hydrea
Hydrisinol
hydro
Cutinova H.
hydroa
h. estivale
h. febrile
h. gestationis
h. gravidarum
h. herpetiforme

h. puerorum
h. vacciniforme
h. vesiculosum
HydroBrader irrigating/aspirating dermabrader
hydrobromide
galantamine h.
homatropine h.
hydrocarbon
aliphatic h.
aromatic h.
hydrocephalus
hydrochloride (HCl)
amantadine h.
amiprilose h.
amitriptyline h.
amprolium h.
aneurin h.
bacampicillin h.
benzphetamine h.
bupivacaine h.
butenafine h.
chloroguanide h.
chloroprocaine h.
chlorpromazine h.
chlortetracycline h.
ciprofloxacin h.
Cleocin h.
clonidine h.
cyclizine h.
cyproheptadine h.
cytarabine h.
daunorubicin h.
demeclocycline h.
diphenhydramine h.
diphenidol h.
dyclonine h.
eflornithine h.
epinephrine h.
ethambutol h.
ethylnorepinephrine h.
etidocaine h.
fluoxetine h.
fluphenazine h.
halofantrine h.
hydroxyzine h.
isoxsuprine h.
levocabastine h.
lidocaine h.
lomefloxacin h.
mechlorethamine h.
meclizine h.
mefloquine h.
mepivacaine h.
methapyrilene h.
minocycline h.
Mustargen H.
naftifine h.
naloxone h.

olopatadine h.
oxymetazoline h.
oxytetracycline h.
pararosaniline h.
paroxetine h.
phenoxybenzamine h.
phenylephrine h.
phenylpropanolamine h.
piperazine h.
pramoxine h.
prazosin h.
procaine h.
promethazine h.
propranolol h.
ranitidine h.
rimantadine h.
sertraline h.
spectinomycin h.
terbinafine h.
tetracaine h.
tetrahydrozoline h.
vancomycin h.
ziprasidone h.
hydrochlorothiazide (HCTZ)
hydrocodone bitartrate
Hydrocol
H. hydrocolloid dressing
H. Sacral
H. Thin
hydrocolloid
BGC Matrix h.
CombiDERM ACD h.
Comfeel h.
Curaderm h.
Cutinova Thin h.
DermAssist h.
Dermatell h.
h. dressing
ExuDerm h.
Nu-Derm h.
RepliCare h.
Restore h.
SignaDress sterile h.
Tegasorb h.
Tegasorb Thin h.
Triad h.
Ultec h.
hydrocortisone
h. acetate
h. acetate cream
acetic acid, propanediol diacetate,
and h.

bacitracin, neomycin, polymyxin b,
and h.
Bactine H.
benzoyl peroxide and h.
h. butyrate
chloramphenicol, polymyxin b,
and h.
clioquinol and h.
colistin, neomycin, and h.
iodoquinol and h.
lidocaine and h.
neomycin and h.
neomycin, polymyxin b, and h.
oxytetracycline and h.
polymyxin b and h.
h. sodium succinate
urea and h.
h. valerate
Hydrocortone
H. Acetate
H. Phosphate
Hydrocort topical
hydrocystoma
hydrofiber dressing
hydrofluoroalkane
hydrofluoroalkane-134a
hydrogel
Carrasyn h.
h. dressing
h. sheet
Tegagel h.
hydrogen
h. breath test
h. peroxide
hydroid
feather h.
hydrolase
LTA$_4$ h.
hydrolysis of surfactant
hydrolyze
HydroMed wound dressing
Hydron Burn Bandage
Hydropel
hydroperoxyeicosatetraenoic acid
Hydrophen
Hydrophiinae
hydrophila
Aeromonas h.
hydrophilic
h. petrolatum
h. polymer dressing
hydrophobia

NOTES

H

hydrophobic ascorbic acid
hydropic change in pneumocyte
hydrops fetalis
hydroquinone
    h. cream
    monobenzyl ether of h.
    h., tretinoin, and fluocinolone
    h. USP and glycolic acid
HydroSkin
    H. cream
    H. lotion
    H. ointment
Hydrosone
Hydro-Tex topical
hydrotherapy
hydrous wool fat
hydroxide
    dysprosium ferric h.
    lactic acid with ammonium h.
    methylmercury h.
    potassium h. (KOH)
    sodium h.
hydroxyacid
hydroxyapatite (HA)
    h. chondrocalcinosis
    h. crystal deposition
hydroxychloroquine (HCQ)
    h. sulfate
    h. therapy
hydroxyeicosatetraenoic acid (HETE)
5-hydroxyindoleacetic acid
hydroxyl
16-hydroxylated metabolite
hydroxylation
5-hydroxy-L-tryptophan
hydroxylysine content of collagen
hydroxylysylpyridinoline
    cross-link h.
3-hydroxy-3-methylglutaryl
    3-h.-3-m. coenzyme A (HMG-CoA)
    3-h.-3-m. coenzyme A reductase
      inhibitor
hydroxyprogesterone caproate
hydroxyproline
hydroxypropyl cellulose
hydroxyquinoline sulfate
hydroxyurea
hydroxyzine
    h. HCl
    h. hydrochloride
    theophylline, ephedrine, and h.
      (TEH)
HyFil hydrogel dressing
hyfrecator
    Birtcher h.
Hy-Gestrone injection
hygiene
    bronchial h.

hygroma
    cystic h.
hygroscopicity
Hylaform Plus wrinkle treatment
hylan G-F 20
HYLL
    healthy years of life lost
Hylutin injection
Hymenolepis
    H. fraterna
    H. nana
Hymenoptera
    Hymenoptera sting
    Hymenoptera venom
    Hymenoptera venom anaphylaxis
hymenopterous vespid
hyomagnesemia
hyoscyamine sulfate oral
Hypafix
Hy-Pam oral
Hyperab
hyperabduction
hyperacanthosis
hyperacute organ rejection
hyperaldosteronism
    primary h.
hyperalgesia
    zone of h.
hyperalgia
    thermal h.
hyperalimentation
hyperandrogenism, insulin resistance,
    and acanthosis nigricans (HAIR-AN)
hyperbaric
    h. oxygen (HBO)
    h. oxygen therapy
hyperbilirubinemia
hypercalcemia
    familial hypocalciuric h.
hypercalciuria
hypercapnia
    permissive h.
hypercarbia
hypercarotenemia
hypercholesteremic xanthoma
hypercholesterolemia
    familial h.
hypercoagulable state
hypercortisolism
hyperekplexia
hyperelastica
    cutis h.
hyperemia
    zone of h.
hypereosinophilia
hypereosinophilic syndrome (HES)
hyperephidrosis
hyperergia
hyperergic encephalitis

hyperesthesia
hyperesthetic zone
hyperextensibility
hyperextensible skin type I–VIII
hyperextension
hyperfiltration
    glomerular h.
hypergammaglobulinemia
    M-component h.
    polyclonal h.
    h. of Waldenström
hypergammaglobulinemic purpura
Hypergel hydrogel dressing
hypergia
hypergic
hyperglobulinemia
hyperglobulinemic purpura
hypergranulosis
hypergranulotic dyscornification
HyperHep
hyperhidrosis
    axillary h.
    emotional h.
    generalized h.
    gustatory h.
    h. lateralis
    h. oleosa
    primary h.
    unilateral h.
hyperhistidinemia
hyperhistidinuria
hyperhomocystinemia
hyperhydration
hypericin
Hypericum montana
hyperidrosis
hyper-IgE (HIE)
    h.-IgE syndrome
hyper-IgM
    immunodeficiency with h.-IgM
    h.-IgM syndrome (HIM)
hyperimmune
    h. bovine colostrum IgC
      concentrate
    h. gamma globulin preparation
    h. serum
    h. state
hyperimmunization
hyperimmunoglobulin E
hyperimmunoglobulinemia
    h. D, E syndrome
    h. syndrome (HID)

hyperinfection
hyperinflation
Hyperion
    H. Advanced alginate dressing
    H. bordered hydrocolloid dressing
    H. hydrophilic wound gel hydrogel
      dressing
    H. thin hydrocolloid dressing
    H. wound cleanser
hyperirritability
hyperirritable skin
hyperkalemia
hyperkeratinization
hyperkeratomycosis
hyperkeratosis, pl. **hyperkeratoses**
    dystrophic palmoplantar h.
    h. eccentrica
    epidermolytic h.
    h. excentrica
    h. figurata centrifuga atrophica
    focal acral h.
    follicular h.
    h. follicularis et parafollicularis
    h. follicularis et parafollicularis in
      cutem penetrans
    h. follicularis vegetans
    generalized epidermolytic h.
    honeycomb h.
    h. lenticularis perstans
    h. lingua
    multiple minute digitate h.
    subungual h.
    h. subungualis
    h. universalis congenita
hyperkeratotic
    h. epidermis
    h. scabies
    h. spicule
hyperleukocytosis
hyperlinearity
    palmar h.
    plantar h.
hyperlinear palm
hyperlipemic xanthoma
hyperlipidemia
    familial combined h.
    Frederickson type IIa, IIb h.
hyperlipoproteinemia
    medication-induced h.
    multiple-type h.
    primary h.
    secondary h.

NOTES

H

hyperliposis
hypermelanization
hypermelanosis
    linear and whorled nevoid h.
    nevoid h.
hypermelanotic
**hypermobile-type Ehlers-Danlos
  syndrome**
hypermobility syndrome
hypermutation
    somatic h.
hyperneocytosis
hyperonychia
hyperorthocytosis
hyperostosis
    ankylosing h.
    h. cranialis
    diffuse idiopathic skeletal h.
      (DISH)
    idiopathic skeletal h.
    sternoclavicular h.
    sternocostoclavicular h.
hyperostotica
    spondylosis h.
hyperostotic syndrome
hyperoxaluria
hyperparathyroidism
    secondary h.
hyperperistalsis
hyperpermeability
    dermal venular h.
hyperphenylalaninemia
hyperpigmentation
    bronze h.
    cutaneous h.
    flagellate h.
    hemosiderin h.
    industrial h.
    longitudinal nail h.
    marble cake h.
    mercury h.
    metal h.
    minocycline h.
    oral postinflammatory h.
    periorbital h.
    postinflammatory h.
    reticulate h.
    zebra-like h.
hyperplasia
    angiolymphoid h.
    basaloid folliculolymphoid h.
    benign h.
    congenital sebaceous gland h.
    crypt h.
    fibrous h.
    gingival h.
    goblet cell h.
    inflammatory fibrous h.
    intravascular papillary endothelial h.

    pseudoepitheliomatous h.
    psoriasiform epidermal h.
    rete ridge h.
    reticuloendothelial h.
    h. of sebaceous gland
    sebaceous senile h.
    senile sebaceous h.
    synovial h.
hyperplastic
    h. epidermis
    h. mucus-secreting goblet cell
    h. synovium (HS)
hyperprebetalipoproteinemia
hyperreactivity
    bronchial h.
    nonspecific bronchial h.
hyperresponsiveness
    airway h. (AHR)
hypersecretion
    mucus h.
hypersensitiveness
hypersensitivity
    h. angiitis
    atopic h.
    cell-mediated h.
    contact h.
    delayed h. (DH)
    delayed-type h. (DTH)
    drug h.
    food h.
    gastrointestinal h.
    immediate h.
    immediate gastrointestinal h.
    latex h.
    h. pneumonitis (HP)
    h. pneumonitis panel
    h. reaction
    reaginic h.
    h. skin testing
    tuberculin-type h.
    h. vasculitis
hypersensitization
hypersomnia
hypersplenism
hypersteatosis
hypersusceptibility
hypertelorism
    ocular h.
hypertension
    benign intracranial h.
    mild h.
    portopulmonary h. (PPHTN)
    primary pulmonary h. (PPH)
    pulmonary h.
Hyper-Tet
hyperthyroidism
    clinical h.
    exogenous h.
    overt h.

hypertonia
hypertrichiasis
hypertrichophrydia
hypertrichosis
    h. lanuginosa
    nevoid h.
    h. partialis
    h. universalis
hypertriglyceridemia
    familial h.
hypertrophic
    h. cervical pachymeningitis
    h. cicatrix
    h. lichen planus
    h. lymphoid follicle
    h. osteoarthropathy
    h. ringworm
    h. rosacea
    h. scar
    h. smooth muscle layer
    h. tonsil
hypertrophica
    acne h.
hypertrophicum
    h. cutis
    eczema h.
    h. simplex
    strawberry h.
    verrucous h.
hypertrophicus
    corneus h.
    lichen corneus h.
    lichen planus h.
    lupus erythematosus h.
hypertrophy
    facet joint h.
    left ventricular h.
    papillary h.
    progressive synovial h.
    submucosal gland h.
    h. of tongue papilla
hypertylosis
hyperuricemia
hyperuricuria
hypervaccination
hypervariable region
hyperventilation
    isocapnic h. (ISH)
    h. provocation test (HVPT)
    h. syndrome (HVS)
hyperviscosity syndrome
hypervitaminosis A, C, D, E

hyperzincuria
hypha, pl. **hyphae**
    spaghetti and meatballs appearance
      of spores and hyphae
hyphal form
hyphomycotic sycosis
hypoadrenalism
hypoallergenic
    h. diet
    h. product
hypoallergenicity
hypobaric hypoxia
hypocapnia
hypochondriasis
    monosymptomatic h.
hypochondrogenesis
hypochromic normocytic anemia
hypocomplementemia
hypocomplementemic
    h. glomerulonephritis
    h. urticarial vasculitis
    h. urticarial vasculitis syndrome
      (HUVS)
    h. vasculitis urticarial syndrome
hypoderm
hypodermatic
hypodermiasis
hypodermic needle separation
hypodermitis sclerodermiformis
hypodermolithiasis
hypodontia
hypoergia
hypoergic
hypofibrinogenemia
hypofibrinolytic
hypogammaglobulinemia,
  hypogammaglobinemia
    acquired h.
    primary h.
    secondary h.
    X-linked h.
hypogammaglobulinemic
hypoglycemia
hypogonadism
hypohidrosis
    h., ephelides and enteropathy, and
      respiratory tract infection
    postmiliarial h.
hypohidrotic ectodermal dysplasia
  (HED)
hypolymphemia
hypomelanism

NOTES

H

hypomelanosis
congenital circumscribed h.
guttate h.
hereditary h.
idiopathic guttate h.
h. of Ito
hypometabolism brain lesion
hypomotility
esophageal h.
hyponychial
hyponychium
hyponychon
hypoparathyroidism
immunodeficiency with h.
hypophosphatasia
hypophosphatemia
hypophysitis
lymphocytic h.
lymphoid h.
hypopigmentation
postinflammatory h.
reticulate h.
hypopigmented
h. macular eruption
h. macule
hypopigmenter
hypopituitarism
hypoplasia
cartilage-hair h.
dermal h.
focal dermal h.
thymic h.
hypoprothrombinemia
hypopyon iritis
hyposensitivity
hyposensitization
oral h.
hypostatica
dermatitis h.
hypostaticum
ulcus h.
hypostome
barbed h.
hyposulfite
sodium h.
HypoTears PF solution
hypotension
orthostatic h.
hypothalamic-pituitary-adrenal (HPA)
h.-p.-a. system
hypothalamic-pituitary adrenal axis
hypothalamo-pituitary adrenal
hypothermic
h. injury
h. perfusion
hypothesis, pl. **hypotheses**

cotriggering h.
missing self h.
Saunders-Zwilling h.
unitarian h.
hypothetical
h. mean organism
h. mean strain (HMS)
hypothyroidism
idiopathic h.
hypotonia
hypotonicity
hypotonic solution
hypotrichiasis
hypotrichosis
hypoventilation
hypovitaminosis A, B
hypovolemic shock
hypoxanthine, aminopterin and thymidine (HAT)
hypoxanthine-guanine
h.-g. phosphoribosyltransferase (HGPRT)
h.-g. phosphoribosyltransferase deficiency
hypoxemia
arterial h.
rapid eye movement sleep-related h.
REM sleep-related h.
rest h.
hypoxia
hypobaric h.
neonatal h.
synovial h.
hypoxic
h. vasoconstriction
h. ventilatory drive (HVD)
Hyprogest
H. 250
H. injection
Hyrexin-50 Injection
Hysone topical
hysterical
h. edema
h. reaction
hystriciasis
hystrix
ichthyismus h.
ichthyosis h.
Hy-Tape
HY-TEC automated allergy diagnostic system
Hytone topical
Hyzine-50 Injection
HZ
herpes zoster

I

    I antigen
    I cell
    I deficiency factor
    I invariant
    I pilus
    I region

I3

    prostacyclin I3

IA

    infrequent episodic asthma
    intraarticular

Ia

    Ia antigen
    Ia cell marker

Ia+

    immune-associated antigen-positive
    macrophage

IA-A-F

    idiopathic anaphylaxis-angioedema-
    frequent

IA-A-I

IAET

    International Association of Enterostomal
    Therapy
      IAET stages

IA-G-F

    idiopathic anaphylaxis-generalized-
    frequent

IA-G-I

    idiopathic anaphylaxis-generalized-
    infrequent
    idiopathic anyaphylaxis-generalized-
    infrequent

IAHIA

    immune adherence immunosorbent assay

Iamin

    I. Gel wound dressing
    I. hydrogel dressing
    I. wound cleanser

IAPP

    islet amyloid polypeptide
    IAPP amylin

IA-Q

    idiopathic anaphylaxis-questionable

IAS

    illness attitude scale

iatrogenic

    i. calcinosis
    i. Cushing syndrome
    i. immunosuppression
    i. infection
    i. pneumothorax
    i. polymorphism

IA-V

    idiopathic anaphylaxis-variant

IB

    Excedrin IB
    Midol IB
    Motrin IB
    Pamprin IB
    Sine-Aid IB

I-B1 radiolabeled antibody

ibandronate

Ibaraki virus

IBD

    inflammatory bowel disease

IBIDS

    ichthyosis plus BIDS
    ichthyosis plus brittle hair, intellectual
    impairment, decreased fertility, short
    stature
      IBIDS syndrome

IBR

    infectious bovine rhinotracheitis
      IBR virus

IBS

    ichthyosis bullosa of Siemens
    inflammatory bowel syndrome
    irritable bowel syndrome

Ibuprin

ibuprofen

    Arthritis Foundation i.
    pseudoephedrine and i.

Ibuprohm

Ibu-Tab

IBV

    infectious bronchitis virus

IC

    immune complex
    inspiratory capacity

ICA

    islet cell antibody

ICAM

    intercellular adhesion module

ICAM-1

    intercellular adhesion molecule-1

ICC

    immunocytochemistry
    intraclass correlation coefficient

iccosome

ICD

    irritant contact dermatitis

ICDRG

    International Contact Dermatitis Research
    Group

ICE

    immunoglobulin-complexed enzyme
      ICE disorder

ice
    i. compress
    i. cube test
    dry i.
    i. pack
ice-pick type scar
ICG
    indocyanine green
ichthammol
ichthyismus
    i. exanthematicus
    i. hystrix
Ichthyol
ichthyosiform
    i. dermatosis
    i. erythroderma
    i. sarcoidosis
ichthyosis
    acquired i.
    autosomal dominant lamellar i.
    autosomal recessive i.
    i. bullosa of Siemens (IBS)
    i. congenita neonatorum
    i. fetalis
    follicular i.
    i. follicularis
    harlequin i.
    i. harlequin
    i. hystrix
    i. intrauterina
    lamellar i.
    i. lethalis
    i. linearis circumflexa (ILC)
    i. lingua
    nacreous i.
    nonbullous congenital
      erythrodermic i.
    i. palmaris et plantaris
    i. plus BIDS (IBIDS)
    i. plus brittle hair, intellectual
      impairment, decreased fertility,
      short stature (IBIDS)
    i. plus brittle hair, intellectual
      impairment, decreased fertility,
      short stature syndrome
    recessive X-linked i.
    i. sauroderma
    i. scutulata
    i. sebacea
    i. sebacea corneae
    senile i.
    i. serpentina
    i. simplex
    i. spinosa
    i. thysanotrichica
    i. uteri
    i. vulgaris
    i. vulgaris ichthyotic
    X-linked i.

ichthyotic
    ichthyosis vulgaris i.
ICM-3
ICOS
    inducible costimulatory
icosahedral
ICOS molecule
ICP
    intracranial pressure
ICS
    inhaled corticosteroid
icteric
icteroid
icterus
    acquired hemolytic i.
    i. gravis
    i. melas
    i. neonatorum
    i. praecox
ICU
    immunological contact urticaria
    immunologic contact unit
ID
    immune deficiency
    immunodiffusion
    infecting dose
    infectious disease
IDA
    idiopathic destructive arthritis
idarubicin
IDD
    excess incidence
IDDM
    insulin-dependent diabetes mellitus
IDEC-114, -131
identical twin donor
identification
    i. bracelet
    i. tag
identity
    reaction of partial i.
idioagglutinin
idioheteroagglutinin
idioheterolysin
idioisoagglutinin
idioisolysin
idiolysin
idiopathic
    i. acute eosinophilic pneumonia
    i. anaphylaxis-angioedema-frequent
      (IA-A-F)
    i. anaphylaxis-generalized-frequent
      (IA-G-F)
    i. anaphylaxis-generalized-infrequent
      (IA-G-I)
    i. anaphylaxis-questionable (IA-Q)
    i. anaphylaxis-variant (IA-V)
    i. anaphylaxis-generalized-infrequent
      (IA-G-I)

i. aortitis
i. atrophoderma
i. atrophoderma of Pasini and Pierini
i. calcinosis cutis
i. clubbing
i. cold agglutinin disease
i. cold urticaria
i. destructive arthritis (IDA)
i. eczematous disease
i. environmental intolerance (IEI)
i. flush
i. giant esophageal ulcer
i. guttate hypomelanosis
i. hirsutism
i. hypereosinophilic syndrome (IHES)
i. hypertrophic osteoarthritis
i. hypothyroidism
i. inflammatory myopathy (IIM)
i. late-onset eczema
i. livedo reticularis
i. lobular panniculitis
i. nephrotic syndrome
i. panhypopituitarism
i. panuveitis
i. periostosis
i. polyserositis
i. posterior uveitis
i. pulmonary fibrosis (IPF)
i. pulmonary hemosiderosis
i. recurrent palmoplantar hidradenitis
i. rhinitis (IR)
i. roseola
i. skeletal hyperostosis
i. solar urticaria
i. thrombocytopenic purpura (ITP)

idiopathica
livedo reticularis i.

idiopeptide
idiosyncrasy
idiosyncratic
i. drug reaction
i. sensitivity

idiotope
set of i.'s

idiotype
i. antibody
i. autoantibody
cross-reactive i.

idiotypic
i. antigen
i. antigenic determinant

IDM
infant of diabetic mother

idoxuridine (IDUR)
id reaction
idrosis
IDSA
Infectious Disease Society of America

IDU
injecting-drug use

IDUR
idoxuridine

iduronic acid
IEC
intestinal epithelial cell

IEF
isoelectric focusing

IEI
idiopathic environmental intolerance

IEM
immune electron microscopy

I:E ratio
inspiratory to expiratory ratio

IF
immunofluorescence

IF-A
inflammatory factor of anaphylaxis

IFE
immunofixation electrophoresis

Ifex
IFN
interferon

IFN-alpha
interferon alpha

IFN-beta
interferon beta

IFN-gamma
interferon gamma

ifosfamide
Ig
immunoglobulin
Ig class

IgA
immunoglobulin A
IgA antiendomysial antibody
IgA antigliadin antibody
IgA deficiency
IgA dermatosis
IgA nephropathy
serum IgA

NOTES

IgD
  immunoglobulin D
IGDR
  interstitial granulomatous drug reaction
IgE
  immunoglobulin E
    IgE antibody
    latex-specific IgE
    IgE radioallergosorbent test
    total serum IgE
IgE-dependent immunologic drug reaction
IgE-mediated
    IgE-m. food allergy
    IgE-m. response
IgE-sensitized cell
IGF-1
  insulin-like growth factor-1
IgG
  immunoglobulin G
    aggregated human IgG
    IgG antibody
    IgG avidity test
    biotinylated antihuman IgG
    Candida albicans IgG
    circulating antiepidermal BMZ IgG
    IgG complex
    IgG heavy chain
    IgG RF
    IgG rheumatoid factor (IgG RF)
    IgG subclass determination
    IgG subclass level
    IgG titer
IgG1
  immunoglobulin G1
IgG4
  immunoglobulin G4
IgG-coated erythrocyte
IgG-RF complement aggregate
IGIV
  immunoglobulin, intravenous
    Nordimmun IGIV
IgM
  immunoglobulin M
    IgM anticardiolipin antibody
    indirect enzyme immunoassay for
      anti-*Mycoplasma pneumoniae* IgM
    IgM nephropathy
    IgM RF
    IgM rheumatoid factor
    serum IgM
    X-linked immunodeficiency with
      hyper IgM
IgM-coated cell
ignea
    zona i.
ignis
    sacer i.

ignorance
    clonal i.
IGT
  impaired glucose tolerance
IHC
  immunohistochemistry
IHES
  idiopathic hypereosinophilic syndrome
IIa
    glycoprotein IIa (GPIIa)
IIb
    glycoprotein IIb (GPIIb)
IIb-IIIa
    glycoprotein IIb-IIIa (GPIIb-IIIa)
IIEF
  International Index of Erectile Function
IIF
  indirect immunofluorescence
IIM
  idiopathic inflammatory myopathy
IKDC
  International Knee Documentation
    Committee
  international Knee Documentation
    Committee
    IKDC Subjective Knee Form
IL
  interleukin
IL-1
    IL-1 interleukin
    IL-1 receptor
IL-1–15
  interleukin-1–15
IL-2
  interleukin-2
    IL-2 cytokine
    IL-2 receptor alpha chain (CD25)
      deficiency
    IL-2 receptor alpha chain gene
    IL-2 receptor-b and cytotoxic
      activity
IL-10
  IL-10 gene promoter
  recombinant human IL-10
IL-12p40 deficiency
IL-12 receptor beta-1 mutation
IL-1-alpha
  interleukin-1-alpha
ILC
  ichthyosis linearis circumflexa
IL-1, -2, -3, -4, -10, -13 cytokine
ILD
  interstitial lung disease
Ilhéus
    I. encephalitis
    I. fever
    I. virus
iliacus

ilii
  osteitis condensans i.
ilioinguinal nerve entrapment
iliopectineal
  i. bursitis
  i. ligament
iliopsoas
  i. bursitis
  i. hemorrhage
iliotibial band syndrome
Ilizarov external fixation
ill
  louping i.
ill-defined border
illinition
illness
  i. attitude scale (IAS)
  environmental i.
  opportunistic i. (OI)
  roseola-like i.
Illouz cannula
illuminator
  BLU-U blue light photodynamic
    therapy i.
ILO
  International Labor Organization
  ILO pneumoconiosis classification
iloprost
Ilosone
  I. oral
  I. Pulvules
Ilotycin Ophthalmic
IL-1ra
  interleukin-1 receptor antagonist
ILSI
  International Life Science Institute
ILVEN
  inflamed linear verrucous epidermal
    nevus
  inflammatory linear verrucous epidermal
    nevus
IM
  infectious mononucleosis
  IM Jaws alligator forceps
image
  store and forward i.'s
imaging
  ImmuRAID antibody i.
  laser Doppler perfusion i.
  magnetic resonance i. (MRI)
  magnetization transfer i. (MTI)

  videomicroscopic i.
  volumetric magnetization transfer i.
imbalance
  endocrine hormone i.
  protease-antiprotease i.
imbricata
  tinea i.
IMC
  index of marrow conversion
I-Methasone
imglucerase
imidazole
  i. carboxamide
  pyrindinyl i.
imidazolidinyl urea
imipenem/cilastatin
imipenem and cilastatin
imipramine
imiquimod
Imitrex
  I. injection
  I. oral
immediate
  i. active cutaneous anaphylaxis
  i. allergy
  i. antigen release
  i. contact urticaria
  i. contagion
  i. gastrointestinal hypersensitivity
  i. hypersensitivity
  i. hypersensitivity reaction
  i. nasal response (INR)
  i. phase reaction (IPR)
  i. skin reactivity
  i. skin response (ISR)
  i. tanning
  i. telogen release
  i. transfusion reaction
  i. wheal reaction
immersion
  excessive water i.
  i. foot
  oil i.
immitis
  Coccidioides i.
  Dirofilaria i.
immobilization
  Treponema pallidum i. (TPI)
immobilizing antibody
immortalization
immortalized human hepatocyte
ImmTher

NOTES

immune
    i. activation
    i. adherence
    i. adherence immunosorbent assay
      (IAHIA)
    i. adherence phenomenon
    i. adhesion test
    i. adsorption
    i. agglutination
    i. agglutinin
    i. bacteriolysis
    i. complex (IC)
    i. complex assay
    i. complex clearance
    i. complex disease
    i. complex disorder
    i. complex glomerulonephritis
    i. complex immunologic drug
      reaction
    i. complex-mediated drug reaction
    i. complex nephritis
    i. complex vasculitis
    i. deficiency (ID)
    i. deposit
    i. deviation
    i. dysregulation
    i. dysregulation, polyendocrinopathy,
      enteropathy, X-linked (IPEX)
    i. electron microscopy (IEM)
    i. elimination
    i. engagement
    i. globulin, intramuscular
    i. globulin, intravenous
    i. hemolysin
    i. hemolysis
    i. inflammation
    i. interferon
    i. memory
    i. modulator
    i. neutropenia
    i. opsonin
    i. paralysis
    i. precipitation
    i. privileged site
    i. protein
    i. response (Ir)
    i. response gene
    i. serum (IS)
    i. serum globulin
    i. suppressor (Is)
    i. suppressor gene
    i. surveillance
    i. system
    i. system modulator
    i. theory
    i. thrombocytopenia
    i. tolerance
immune-associated antigen-positive
  macrophage (Ia+)

immune-derived amyloidosis
immune-mediated
    i.-m. coagulation disorder
    i.-m. disease
    i.-m. membranous nephritis
    i.-m. thyroiditis
Immunex
immunifacient
immunity
    acquired i.
    active i.
    adoptive i.
    antiviral i.
    artificial active i.
    artificial passive i.
    bacteriophage i.
    cell-mediated i. (CMI)
    concomitant i.
    i. deficiency
    endogenous antitumor i.
    general i.
    group i.
    herd i.
    host i.
    humoral i.
    infection i.
    innate i.
    local i.
    maternal i.
    natural i.
    passive i.
    relative i.
    specific active i.
    specific passive i.
immunization
    active i.
    Heptavax i.
    passive i.
    i. requirement
    Standards for Pediatric I. (SPI)
    viral i.
immunize
Immuno
    Gammabulin I.
immunoadjuvant
immunoagglutination
immunoassay
    antinuclear antibody screening by
      enzyme i.
    double antibody i.
    enzyme-linked i. (EIA)
    fluorescence polarization i. (FPIA)
    ImmunoCard i.
    solid phase i. (SPIA)
    thin-layer i.
    urine myoglobin i.
immunobead assay
immunoblast
immunoblastic sarcoma of B, T cell

immunoblot
immunoblotting
immunobullous disease
Immuno-C
ImmunoCAP
ImmunoCard
    I. immunoassay
    I. STAT! Rotavirus test
    I. used for diagnosis of
      Helicobacter pylori
immunochemical
    i. abnormality
    i. assay
    i. relative
immunochemistry
immunocompetence
immunocompetent
    i. cell
    i. tissue therapy
immunocomplex
immunocompromised host
immunoconglutinin
immunocyte
immunocyte-derived amyloidosis
immunocytochemical
immunocytochemistry (ICC)
immunodeficiency
    acquired i.
    common variable unclassifiable i.
    i. disease
    i. disorder
    i. electrophoresis
    partial albinism with i.
    phagocytic dysfunction disorders i.
    secondary i.
    severe combined i. (SCID)
    i. syndrome
    i. with hyper-IgM
    i. with hypoparathyroidism
    X-linked severe combined i.
      (XSCID)
immunodeficient
immunodepressant
immunodepressor
immunodeterminant
immunodiagnosis
immunodiffusion (ID)
    antinuclear antibody i.
    i. assay
    double i.
    radial i. (RID)

    single radial i. (SRID)
    i. technique
immunodominant
immunoelectrophoresis
    2-dimensional i.
    quantitative i. (QIE)
    rocket i. (RIE)
immunoenhancement
immunoenhancer
immunoferritin
immunofixation electrophoresis (IFE)
immunofluorescence (IF)
    i. analysis
    antinuclear antibody i.
    i. assay
    cytometric indirect i.
    direct i.
    i. finding
    indirect i. (IIF)
    i. method
    i. microscopy
    i. technique
immunofluorescent
    i. examination
    i. stain
immunogen
immunogenetics
immunogenetic wild-type adenovirus
immunogenic
    i. peptide
    i. protein
immunogenicity
immunoglobulin (Ig)
    i. A (IgA)
    anti-D i.
    antihuman parvovirus i. G
    chickenpox i.
    i. class
    i. class switching
    i. D (IgD)
    i. delta chain
    DiffGAM bovine anti-*Clostridium*
      difficile i.
    i. domain
    i. E (IgE)
    i. E-mediated food allergy
    i. epsilon chain
    i. E-sensitized cell
    i. fold
    i. G (IgG)
    i. G1 (IgG1)
    i. G4 (IgG4)

NOTES

immunoglobulin *(continued)*
    i. gene
    i. gene rearrangement
    i. G heavy chain
    i. G rheumatoid factor
    i. G rheumatoid factor complement
      aggregate
    i. heavy chain
    hepatitis B i. (H-BIG)
    human immunodeficiency virus i.
      (HIVIG)
    human normal i.
    intravenous i.
    i. IV
    i. light chain-origin amyloid
      deposit
    lyophilized i. G
    i. M-coated cell
    measles i.
    i. membrane
    monoclonal i.
    i. M rheumatoid factor (IgM RF)
    i. mu chain
    nephropathic i.
    pertussis i.
    poliomyelitis i.
    rabies i.
    i. replacement therapy
    RH$_0$(D) i.
    secretory i.
    i. subclass
    subcutaneous i. (SCIG)
    i. superfamily
    i. supergene family
    tetanus i.
    thyroid-binding inhibitory i. (TBII)
    thyrotropin-binding inhibitory i.
      (TBII)
    varicella-zoster i. (VZIG)
immunoglobulin-complexed
    i.-c. enzyme (ICE)
    i.-c. enzyme disorder
immunoglobulin, intravenous (IGIV)
immunoglobulin M (IgM)
immunoglobulin-secreting cell
immunogold electron microscopy
immunohematology
immunohistochemical
immunohistochemistry (IHC)
    Ki-67 i.
immunoisolating microreactor
immunolocalization
immunologic
    i. adjuvant
    i. complication
    i. contact unit (ICU)
    i. contact urticaria
    i. disorder
    i. drug reaction

    i. dysfunction
    i. feature
    i. high dose tolerance
    i. inflammatory disease
    i. memory
    i. organ damage
    i. pregnancy test
    i. response
immunological
    i. competence
    i. contact urticaria (ICU)
    i. defense
    i. deficiency
    i. enhancement
    i. mechanism
    i. paralysis
    i. surveillance
    i. tolerance
immunologically
    i. activated cell
    i. competent cell
    i. privileged site
immunologist
immunology
    cancer i.
    i. laboratory technique
    therapeutic i.
immunometric technique
immunomodulating drug regimen
immunomodulation
immunomodulator
    topical i. (TIM)
immunomodulatory
immunopathology
immunoperoxidase
immunophenotype
immunophilin-binding drug
immunophilin isomerase activity
immunopotentiation
immunopotentiator
immunoprecipitation
    i. assay
    chromatin i. (ChIP)
immunoproliferative
    i. disorder
    i. small intestinal disease (IPSID)
immunoprophylaxis
    passive i.
immunoproteasome
immunopurging
    complement-mediated tumor cell i.
immunoradiometric assay (IRMA)
immunoreactant
    proinflammatory i.
immunoreaction
immunoreactive
    i. hormone
    i. insulin (IRI)

immunoreceptor tyrosine-based activation motif (ITAM)
immunoregulation
immunoregulatory
    i. circuit
    i. defect
immunoselection
immunosenescence
immunosorbent
ImmunoSpot
    in-house I. (IS)
immunostimulatory
    i. DNA sequence (ISS)
    i. oligodeoxynucleotide (ISS-ODN)
immunosuppressant cocktail
immunosuppression
    iatrogenic i.
    postgrafting i.
    tacrolimus-based i.
    TGF-induced i.
    transforming growth factor-induced i.
immunosuppression-associated leukoencephalopathy
immunosuppressive
    i. agent
    i. drug
    i. therapy (IST)
immunosurveillance
immunosympathectomy
immunotherapy
    adoptive i.
    allergen i.
    antiimmunoglobulin E i.
    biological i.
    cancer i.
    cellular adoptive i.
    passive i.
    rush i. (RIT)
    short-term i. (STI)
    specific i. (SIT)
    specific injection i. (SIT)
    sublingual i. (SLIT)
    sublingual-swallow i.
    venom i. (VIT)
immunotolerance
immunotoxin
immunotransfusion
Immupath
ImmuRAID antibody imaging
ImmuRAIT-LL2 monoclonal antibody
Immuthiol

Imogam
Imovax
    I. Rabies intradermal vaccine
    I. Rabies intramuscular vaccine
impaction sampler
impactor
    Anderson cascade i.
    Cascade i.
    rotating air i.
    rotating arm i.
impaired
    i. glucose tolerance (IGT)
    i. neutrophil chemotaxis
impairment
    chronic phase shoulder i.
    functional i.
    restrictive functional i.
    subacute phase shoulder i.
Impatiens biflora
impending respiratory failure
imperfecta
    dentinogenesis i.
    lethal osteogenesis i.
    osteogenesis i.
    severe deforming osteogenesis i.
    Sillence type II–IV osteogenesis i.
Imperfecti
    Fungi I.
impermeable
impermeant solution additive
impetigines (*pl. of* impetigo)
impetiginization
    secondary i.
impetiginize
impetiginized
impetiginous
    i. cheilitis
    cheilitis granulomatosa i.
    i. syphilid
impetigo, pl. impetigines
    Bockhart i.
    bullous i.
    bullous staphylococcal i.
    i. circinata
    i. contagiosa
    i. contagiosa bullosa
    i. eczematodes
    follicular i.
    Fox i.
    i. furfuracea
    furfuraceous i.
    i. gestationis

NOTES

impetigo *(continued)*
    i. herpetiformis
    i. neonatorum
    nonbullous i.
    i. simplex
    i. staphylogenes
    i. syphilitica
    i. variolosa
    i. vulgaris
impingement
    i. sign
    i. syndrome
implant
    Avanta i.
    bovine collagen dermal i.
    cartilage i.
    collagen i.
    ePTFE i.
    expanded polytetrafluoroethylene i.
    flexible silicone i.
    Medpor surgical i.
    Neer II i.
    osteochondral i.
    perichondrial i.
    periosteal i.
    SoftForm facial i.
    Spectrum Designs facial i.
    Zyderm collagen i.
    Zyplast collagen i.
implantation
    collagen i.
    i. cyst
importance
    allergic i.
impregnated pad
impregnation
    silver i.
improper repair of DNA
ImuLyme vaccine
Imuran
IMX
    whole-body antibody technique
in
    in noma ulcer
    in situ
    in situ hybridization (ISH)
    in situ squamous cell carcinoma
    in toto
    in vitro
    in vitro anergy
    in vitro cytotoxic assay
    in vitro fibrillogenesis
    in vitro mechanical compression
    in vitro proliferative lymphocyte
     response
    in vitro purging
    in vitro test
    in vivo
    in vivo reaction

inactivate
inactivated
    Japanese encephalitis virus
     vaccine, i.
    i. poliovirus vaccine (IPV)
    poliovirus vaccine, i.
    i. serum
inactivation
    nonrandom X chromosome i.
inactivator
    anaphylatoxin i.
inadvertent trauma
inaperturate
Inc.
    Jacobson Resonance Enterprises, I.
    Laser Photonics, I.
    Ligand Pharmaceuticals, I.
incarnati
incarnatus
    pilus i.
    unguis i.
incentive spirometry
incidence
    excess i. (IDD)
incision
    elliptical i.
    Mercedes Benz i.
    Risdon i.
incisional biopsy
incisor
    overriding maxillary i.
inclusion
    i. body
    i. body disease
    i. body encephalitis
    i. body myositis
    i. cell
    i. conjunctivitis virus
    i. cyst
    cytoplasmic i.
    i. dermoid
    hematoxyphilic i.
    Rocha-Lima i.
incognito
    scabies i.
    tinea i.
incognitus
    Mycoplasma i.
incompatibility
    ABO i.
incompatible blood transfusion reaction
incomplete
    i. agglutinin
    i. antibody
    i. antigen
    i. neurofibromatosis
inconspicua
    Candida i.
incontinence of pigment

incontinentia
    i. pigmenti
    i. pigmenti achromians
increased sympathoadrenal activity
incrementi
    stadium i.
incrustation
incubation period (IP)
incubative stage
incubatory carrier
Indanyl carbenicillin
Inderal LA
Indermil
    I. tissue adhesive
    I. topical adhesive
indeterminate
    i. cell histiocytosis
    i. leprosy
index, pl. **indices, indexes**
    algofunctional Lequesne i.
    apoptotic i.
    Asthma Symptom Utility I.
    Atopic Dermatitis Area and
      Severity I. (ADASI)
    Atopic Dermatitis Severity I.
      (ADSI)
    Bath AS Functional I.
    chemotherapeutic i.
    cutaneous tolerance i. (CTI)
    Eczema Area and Severity I.
      (EASI)
    endemic i.
    Health Assessment Questionnaire
      Disability I.
    International Prognostic I.
    Lansbury articular i.
    Lequesne algofunctional i.
    Lequesne functional i.
    leukopenic i.
    i. of marrow conversion (IMC)
    metacarpal i.
    organ system failure i. (OSFI)
    phagocytic i.
    plaque i.
    Psoriasis Area and Severity I.
      (PASI)
    Psoriasis Area Severity I. (PASI)
    Reliable Change I.
    Ritchie articular i.
    SASSAD severity i.
    SCORAD i.

    self-administered Psoriasis Area and
      Severity I. (SAPASI)
    semiquantitative disease extent i.
    Singh i.
    SLE Disease Activity I. (SLEDAI)
    splenic i.
    stimulation i. (SI)
    tension-time i.
    tumor burden i. (TBI)
    ultraviolet light i.
    volume thickness i. (VTI)
    Western Ontario and McMaster
      Universities Osteoarthritis I.
      (WOMAC)
Indian tick typhus
India rubber skin
indica
    Azadirachta i.
indicanidrosis
indication
indicator system
indices (*pl. of* index)
indifferent electrode
indigenous
indinavir sulfate
indirect
    i. agglutination
    i. agglutination test
    i. assay
    i. coelenterate dermatitis
    i. Coombs test
    i. Coombs titer
    i. enzyme immunoassay for anti-
      Mycoplasma pneumoniae IgM
    i. fluorescent antibody
    i. fluorescent antibody test
    i. hemagglutination test
    i. immunofluorescence (IIF)
indium chloride scan
indium-labeled scanning
Indocid PDA
Indocin
    I. IV injection
    I. SR oral
Indocollyre
indocyanine green (ICG)
indolent
    i. bubo
    i. nonpitting edema
    i. papule
    i. ulcer
indomethacin

NOTES

Indotec
induced
    i. phagocytosis
    i. sensitivity
inducer cell
inducible
    i. costimulatory (ICOS)
    i. nitric oxide synthase
    i. skin color
induction
    antilymphocyte i.
    lysogenic i.
    ovulation i.
    i. period
indurata
    acne i.
    tuberculosis cutis i.
indurated
    i. border
    i. chancre
    i. lymphangitis
    i. papule
    i. plantar keratoma (IPK)
    i. welt
induration
    brawny i.
    scaling, erythema, and i. (SEI)
induratio penis plastica
indurativa
    tuberculosis cutis i.
induratum
    erythema i.
industrial
    i. dermatitis
    i. dermatosis
    i. folliculitis
    i. hyperpigmentation
    i. smog
Inerpan dressing
inertial suction sampler
infancy
    acropustulosis of i.
    capillary hemangioma of i.
    fibrous hamartoma of i.
    transient erythroporphyria of i.
    transient hypogammaglobulinemia
      of i.
Infanrix vaccine
infant
    i. of diabetic mother (IDM)
    sudden unexpected death in i.'s
      (SUDI)
    sudden unexplained death in i.'s
      (SUDI)
infantile
    i. acne
    i. acropustulosis
    i. acute hemorrhagic edema of the
      skin

    i. colic
    i. digital fibroma
    i. digital myofibroblastoma
    i. eczema
    i. gastroenteritis
    i. gastroenteritis virus
    i. myofibromatosis
    i. neuroblastoma
    i. perianal pyramidal protrusion
    i. purulent conjunctivitis
infantilis
    lipodystrophia centrifugalis
      abdominalis i.
    prurigo i.
    roseola i.
infantum
    acrodermatitis papulosa i.
    cholera i.
    dermatitis excoriativa i.
    dermatitis exfoliativa i.
    dermatitis gangrenosa i.
    granuloma gluteale i.
    lichen i.
    roseola i.
infarction
    diabetic muscle i. (DMI)
infarctive
    i. inflammatory disease
    i. lesion
Infazinc
infected vascular gangrene
infecting dose (ID)
infection
    alopecia, nail dystrophy, ophthalmic
      complication, thyroid dysfunction,
      hypohidrosis, ephelides and
      enteropathy, and respiratory
      tract i. (ANOTHER)
    anorectal herpes simplex virus i.
    atrium of i.
    atypical mycobacterial i.
    bacterial i.
    banal bacterial i.
    beta-hemolytic streptococcus i.
    Candida i.
    candidal i.
    chlamydial i.
    chronic Epstein-Barr virus i.
    chronic parvovirus B19 i.
    closed-space i.
    congenital HIV i.
    congenital human immunodeficiency
      virus i.
    cross i.
    cryptogenic i.
    dermatophyte i.
    dermatophyte fungal i.
    disc space i.
    disseminated gonococcal i.

documented bacterial i. (DBI)
documented viral i. (DVI)
droplet i.
EBV i.
ectothrix i.
endemic fungal i.
endogenous i.
endothrix i.
enteric i.
enteroviral i.
environmental mycobacterial i.
Epstein-Barr virus i.
focal i.
fungal i. (FI)
fungous i.
granulomatous bacterial i.
group A beta-hemolytic
   streptococcal i.
group A *Streptococcus* i.
guinea worm i.
Hantavirus i.
herpes simplex i.
herpes zoster i.
herpetic i.
hibernal epidemic viral i. (HEVI)
hospital-acquired i.
human papillomavirus i.
hypohidrosis, ephelides and
   enteropathy, and respiratory
   tract i.
iatrogenic i.
i. immunity
laryngeal i.
latent i.
loa loa i.
mass i.
metazoan i.
mixed nail i.
multiplicity of i. (MOI)
mycobacterial i.
natural focus of i.
necrotizing i.
nondermatophyte fungal i.
nontuberculous mycobacterial i.
nosocomial i.
ocular herpes simplex virus i.
ocular herpes zoster virus i.
opportunistic systemic fungal i.
overwhelming postsplenectomy i.
   (OPSI)
paravaccinia virus i.
phycomycotic i.

pneumococcal i.
primary herpes simplex i.
protozoan i.
pyodermatous i.
pyogenic i.
recurrent i.
repeated respiratory i.
reservoir of i.
rhinocerebral i.
rickettsial i.
scalp i.
seatworm i.
secondary i.
sexually acquired i.
Shigella i.
spirochete i.
Streptococcus i.
subcutaneous fungal i.
subcutaneous necrotizing i.
superficial i.
sycosiform fungous i.
systemic fungal i.
tinca i.
transcervical i.
transforming i.
transplacental i.
unusual opportunistic i.
upper respiratory tract i. (URTI)
urinary tract i. (UTI)
vaccinia i.
varicella-zoster i.
vesicular viral i.
Vincent i.
viral respiratory i.
Western blot i.
yeast i.
zoonotic i.
infection-immunity
infectiosity
infectiosum
   ecthyma i.
infectious
   i. angioma
   i. arteritis virus of horses
   i. arthritis
   i. avian bronchitis
   i. bovine rhinotracheitis (IBR)
   i. bovine rhinotracheitis virus
   i. bronchitis virus (IBV)
   i. bulbar paralysis
   i. canine hepatitis
   i. disease (ID)

NOTES

infectious *(continued)*
    I. Disease Society of America (IDSA)
    i. ectromelia virus
    i. eczematoid dermatitis
    i. eczematous dermatitis
    i. endocarditis
    exuberant i.
    i. granuloma
    i. hepatitis
    i. hepatitis virus
    i. labial dermatitis
    i. mononucleosis (IM)
    i. nucleic acid
    i. papilloma of cattle
    i. papilloma virus
    i. perichondritis
    i. plasmid
    i. polyneuritis
    i. porcine encephalomyelitis
    i. porcine encephalomyelitis virus
    i. rhinitis
    i. wart
infectiousness
infectiva
    polioencephalitis i.
infective
infectivity
inferior fornix
infest
infestans
    Phytophathoria i.
infestation
    Cheyletiella i.
    environmental mite i.
    louse i.
    mite i.
    Pediculus humanus capitis i.
    ping-pong i.
    Pthirus pubis i.
infiltrate
    Assmann tuberculous i.
    diffuse pulmonary i.
    fixed pulmonary i.
    fluffy alveolar i.
    granulomatous dermal i.
    lymphoid i.
    patchy i.
    perivascular i.
    transient migratory i.
    transient pulmonary i.
infiltration
    adipose i.
    inflammatory i.
    lymphocytic i.
    peribronchiolar lymphocyte i.
infiltrative basal cell carcinoma
infiltrator
    showerhead i.

Infinity sensor
Inflamase
    I. Forte Ophthalmic
    I. Mild Ophthalmic
inflame
inflamed
    i. linear verrucous epidermal nevus (ILVEN)
    i. ulcer
inflammation
    allergic i.
    chronic jejunal i.
    cutaneous neurogenic i.
    diffuse i.
    focal i.
    immune i.
    interstitial i.
    intraocular i.
    mucosal i.
    necrotizing scleritis with adjacent i.
    necrotizing scleritis without adjacent i.
    neutrophilic i.
    neutrophil-mediated joint i.
    occult bowel i.
    i. reaction
    urate-associated i.
inflammatory
    i. arthritis
    i. bowel disease (IBD)
    i. bowel syndrome (IBS)
    i. cascade
    i. cell
    i. dermatosis
    i. edema
    i. factor of anaphylaxis (IF-A)
    i. fibrous hyperplasia
    i. infiltration
    i. linear verrucous epidermal nevus (ILVEN)
    i. lung disease
    i. macrophage
    i. plaque
    i. tinea capitis
    i. ulcer
inflation
inflatum
    Scopulariopsis i.
infliximab monoclonal antibody
inflorescence
influenza, pl. **influenzae**
    i. A
    A/Texas/36/91-like i.
    avian i.
    A-Wuhan/359/95-like i.
    i. B
    B/Beijing/184/93-like i.
    i. C
    equine i.

Haemophilus influenzae type b (HIB)
Hong Kong i.
sequela of i.
Spanish i.
swine i.
i. virus
i. virus hemagglutinin
i. virus vaccine
influenzal meningitis
infolded
infranate
infrapatellar bursitis
infrequent episodic asthma (IA)
infriction
infundibulocystic basal cell carcinoma
infundibulofolliculitis
disseminated recurrent i.
recurrent i.
infundibulum
tumor of the follicular i. (TFI)
infusion
allogenic bone marrow cell i.
donor lymphocyte i. (DLI)
ETOPOPHOS i.
etoposide phosphate i.
ingestion
L-tryptophan i.
ingestive
Ingram
I. regimen for psoriasis
I. technique
ingress
neutrophil i.
ingrowing hair
ingrown
i. hair
i. nail
inguinale
acanthoma i.
Epidermophyton i.
granuloma i.
lymphogranuloma i.
inguinalis
tinea i.
inguinal ligament
INH
isonicotine hydrazine
Inhal-Aid bronchodilator
inhalant
i. allergen

i. allergen extract
toxic i.
inhalation
Atrovent Aerosol I.
i. breath unit
NebuPent I.
smoke i.
inhaled
i. corticosteroid (ICS)
i. dander
inhaler
AeroBid-M Oral Aerosol I.
AeroBid Oral Aerosol I.
Beclovent Oral I.
Beconase AQ Nasal I.
Chiesi powder i.
Diskhaler i.
Diskus i.
dry power i. (DPI)
FOII powder i.
Foradil dry powder i.
formoterol fumarate dry powder i.
Inhalet i.
InspirEase i.
Intal Oral I.
metered-dose i. (MDI)
Nebuhaler i.
nebulized i.
Orion i.
pressurized metered-dose i. (pMDI)
Rondo i.
Rotahaler i.
Spinhaler i.
Turbuhaler i.
Vancenase AQ I.
Vancenase Nasal I.
Vanceril Oral I.
Inhalet inhaler
inheritance
pattern of i.
X-linked recessive i.
inherited
i. complement deficiency syndrome
i. epidermolysis bullosa
i. patterned lentiginosis
inhibin
inhibiting antibody
inhibition
allogenic i.
eicosanoid i.
i. factor
i. fluorescent antibody

NOTES

inhibition *(continued)*
> hemagglutination i.
> leukotriene i.
> prostaglandin synthesis i.
> xanthine i.

inhibitor
> 5-alpha-reductase i.
> alpha$_1$-trypsin i.
> angiogenesis i.
> caspase i.
> C1 esterase i.
> collagenase i.
> COX-1 i.
> COX-2 i.
> COX/LO i.
> cysteine proteinase i.
> decarboxylase i.
> factor VIII:C i.
> functional C1 esterase i.
> fusion i. (FI)
> 5G1.1 recombinant C5
> complement i.
> HIV protease i.
> HMG-CoA reductase i.
> human alpha-1-proteinase i.
> 3-hydroxy-3-methylglutaryl coenzyme
> A reductase i.
> MAO i.
> mast cell i.
> myosin ATPase i.
> nonnucleoside reverse
> transcriptase i. (NNRTI)
> nucleoside analog RT i. (NRTI)
> nucleoside reverse transcriptase i.
> phosphodiesterase isoenzyme i.
> polypeptide i.
> protein C1 esterase i.
> recombinant human tissue factor
> pathway i. (r-hT-FPI)
> secretory leukoprotease i.
> soybean trypsin i. (STI)
> surface-targeted plasmin i.
> synthesis i.
> target of rapamycin i.
> tissue factor pathway i. (TFPI)
> TNF i.
> TOR i.
> transcriptase i.
> tumor necrosis factor i.
> tyrosinase i.
> tyrosine kinase i.

inhibitor
> calcineurin i. (CNI)

in-house ImmunoSpot (IS)
injectable
> i. collagen
> i. dye
> tinzaparin sodium i.

injecting-drug use (IDU)

injection
> Adlone I.
> Adrucil i.
> Aloprim I.
> Amcort I.
> A-methaPred i.
> Amikin i.
> amphotericin B lipid complex i.
> AquaMEPHYTON i.
> Aristocort Forte i.
> Aristocort Intralesional i.
> Aristospan Intra-articular i.
> Aristospan Intralesional i.
> Articulose-50 i.
> Bactocill i.
> Bena-D i.
> Benadryl I.
> Benahist i.
> Ben-Allergin-50 I.
> Benoject i.
> Bicillin C-R 900/300 i.
> Bicillin L-A i.
> Brethine i.
> Bricanyl i.
> Bronkephrine i.
> Calciferol i.
> Carbocaine i.
> Celestone Phosphate I.
> Cel-U-Jec I.
> Ceredase i.
> Chlor-Trimeton I.
> Cipro i.
> Cleocin Phosphate I.
> collagen i.
> conjunctival i.
> Cophene-B i.
> Cortone Acetate i.
> Crysticillin A.S. i.
> Cytoxan i.
> Decadron I.
> Dehist i.
> depMedalone I.
> Depoject I.
> Depo-Medrol I.
> Depopred I.
> D.H.E. 45 i.
> Diflucan i.
> Dihyrex I.
> Dinate I.
> Diphenacen-50 I.
> Dizac i.
> D-Med I.
> Doxychel i.
> Dramilin I.
> Duralone I.
> Duralutin i.
> Duranest i.
> Dymenate I.
> Floxin i.

I

Foscavir i.
Garamycin i.
Histaject i.
hyaluronan i.
hyaluronate i.
hyaluronic acid i.
Hydeltrasol i.
Hydeltra-TBA i.
Hydrate I.
Hy-Gestrone i.
Hylutin i.
Hyprogest i.
Hyrexin-50 I.
Hyzine-50 I.
Imitrex i.
Indocin IV i.
intraarticular i.
intralesional i.
intratendinous i.
Isocaine HCl i.
Jenamicin i.
Kantrex i.
Keflin i.
Kefurox i.
Kenaject I.
Kenalog I.
Key-Pred I.
Key-Pred-SP I.
Konakion i.
Levophed i.
Lyphocin i.
Marmine I.
Medralone I.
meropenem for i.
Metro IV I.
Minocin IV i.
Monistat IV I.
M-Prednisol I.
Nafcil i.
Nallpen i.
Nasahist B i.
ND-Stat i.
Nebcin i.
Neosar i.
Netromycin i.
Neucalm-50 I.
Neupogen i.
Neut i.
Nordryl i.
Novocain i.
Nydrazid i.
Octocaine i.

Oraminic II i.
Ornidyl i.
Osmitrol i.
Pentacarinat i.
Pentam-300 I.
Permapen i.
Pfizerpen i.
Pfizerpen-AS i.
Phenazine I.
Phenergan I.
Polocaine i.
Pontocaine i.
Predaject i.
Predalone i.
Predcor i.
Predicort-50 i.
Prednisol TBA i.
Pro-Depo i.
Prodrox i.
Prograf i.
Prometh i.
Prorex I.
Prostaphlin i.
Prothazine i.
Retrovir i.
Rifadin I.
Sandimmune i.
sensitizing i.
soft-tissue i.
Solu-Medrol I.
Spectam i.
subcutaneous i.
Supartz i.
Tac-3, -40 I.
tacrolimus i.
Terramycin IM i.
Toposar i.
Toradol i.
Triam-A I.
Triam Forte I.
Triamonide I.
Tri-Kort I.
Trilog I.
Trilone I.
Trisoject I.
Trobicin i.
Unipen i.
Ureaphil I.
Valium i.
Vancocin i.
Vancoled i.
VePesid i.

NOTES

injection *(continued)*
    V-Gan i.
    Vibramycin i.
    Vistaril I.
    Vistazine I.
    Vumon i.
    Wellcovorin i.
    Wycillin i.
    Zantac i.
    Zetran i.
    Zinacef i.
    zoledronic acid for i.
    Zovirax i.
injury
    cold-induced cell i.
    epithelial i.
    graft i.
    hepatic ischemia and reperfusion i.
    HIR i.
    hypothermic i.
    I/R i.
    ischemia-reperfusion i.
    oligodendrocyte i.
    photoacoustic i.
    preservation perfusion i.
    preservation reperfusion i.
    reperfusion i.
    sesamoid i.
    sinusoidal lining cell i.
    transfusion-related acute lung i.
      (TRALI)
    whiplash i.
ink-spot lentigo
innate immunity
inner
    i. canthus
    i. root sheath
innocent bystander cell
inoculability
inoculable
inoculate
inoculating
inoculation herpes
inoculum
    plantar i.
inosinic
    i. acid
    i. acid dehydrogenase
Inosiplex
inositol
    i. phospholipid turnover
    i. triphosphate
    i. triphosphate pathway
Inoviridae
INR
    immediate nasal response
    International Normalization Ratio
    INR clotting test
INRO surgical prosthetic nail

insect
    i. allergen
    i. allergy
    i. bite
    biting i.
    i. dermatitis
    i. sting
    i. sting kit
    i. virus
insecticide
insensible perspiration
insensitive sweat
inserta
    variola i.
insidious onset
insipidus
    nephrogenic diabetes i.
insolation
Insomnal
inspiratory
    i. capacity (IC)
    i. to expiratory ratio (I:E ratio)
    i. positive airway pressure (IPAP)
    i. "Velcro" crackle
InspirEase inhaler
Inspiron
instability
    high-frequency microsatellite i.
    low-frequency microsatellite i.
    microsatellite i. (MSI)
InstaGene Matrix resin
Instat collagen matrix sponge
institute
    International Life Science I. (ILSI)
institutional review board (IRB)
instructive theory
instrument
    Derma I.'s
    diamond fraise dermabrasion i.
    ERBE electrical coagulation i.
    ERBE electrical cutting i.
    IOS immunodiagnostic testing i.
    nail fold capillaroscopic i.
    ProLine endoscopic i.
insufficiency
    adrenal i.
    adrenocortical i.
    Argentinian Study Group for
      Prevention of Cardiac I.
      (GESICA)
insula
insulin
    i. allergy
    i. antagonist
    immunoreactive i. (IRI)
    i. lipoatrophy
    lispro i.
    i. reaction
    i. resistance

single-peak pork i.
i. skin test
i. tumor
insulin-dependent diabetes mellitus (IDDM)
insulin-like
i.-l. growth factor-1 (IGF-1)
i.-l. growth factor BP3 complex
insusceptibility
intake
caloric i.
reference nutrient i. (RNI)
Intal
I. Nebulizer solution
I. Oral Inhaler
Integra artificial skin
Integrated Wound Manager
integrin
integrin-mediated adhesion
integrity
Braden score for skin i.
integument
integumentary system
integumentum commune
Intelligent dressing
intemum
erysipelas grave i.
intense
i. pulsed light (IPL)
i. pulsed light source (IPLS)
intensity
gray-scale i.
interaction
adhesin-receptor i.
B7:counterreceptor i.
cell-cell i.
cognate i.
drug i.
HLA intercellular i.
receptor-ligand i.
T-cell counter-receptor i.
tumor/stromal i.
intercellular
i. adhesion module (ICAM)
i. adhesion molecule-1 (ICAM-1)
i. bridge
i. edema
i. machinery
i. space
intercensal
intercritical gout

interdigital
i. clavus
i. dermatitis
i. maceration
i. nerve entrapment
interdigitale
epidermophytosis i.
interdigitalis
mycosis i.
Interdisciplinary Group for Cancer Care Evaluation in Italy (GIVIO)
interface
alveolar-lung parenchymal i.
dermoepidermal i.
Monarch Mini Mask nasal i.
interference
bacterial i.
interfering
defective i. (DI)
interferon (IFN)
i. alfa-2a
i. alfa-2b
i. alfa-2b and ribavirin combination pack
i. alfa-n3
i. alpha (IFN-alpha)
antigen i.
i. B-1b
i. beta (IFN-bcta)
fibroblast i.
i. gamma (IFN-gamma)
i. gamma-1b
i. gamma receptor deficiency
immune i.
leukocyte i.
pegylated i.
recombinant gamma i.
therapeutic i.
i. therapy
interferon-alpha
interferon-independent mechanism
interleukin (IL)
IL-1 i.
interleukin-1–15 (IL-1–15)
interleukin-2 (IL-2)
i.-2 adjunctive chemotherapy
interleukin-12
exogenous i.-12
interleukin-1-alpha (IL-1-alpha)
interleukin-1 receptor antagonist (IL-1ra)

NOTES

interlobular
- i. artery
- i. septa

intermedia
- beta-thalassemia i.

intermediate
- i. carcinoma
- i. cyclosporine
- i. filament
- i. leprosy
- reactive oxygen i. (ROI)

intermedius
- *Streptococcus i.*

intermetacarpal

intermittent
- i. carrier
- i. hair-follicle dystrophy
- i. hydrarthrosis
- i. mandatory ventilation
- i. positive pressure breathing (IPPB)
- i. sterilization

internal
- i. hair apparatus
- i. meningitis

international
- I. Association of Enterostomal Therapy (IAET)
- I. Contact Dermatitis Research Group (ICDRG)
- I. Index of Erectile Function (IIEF)
- i. Knee Documentation Committee (IKDC)
- I. Labor Organization (ILO)
- I. Life Science Institute (ILSI)
- I. Normalization Ratio (INR)
- i. normalized ratio clotting test
- I. Pancreas Transplant Registry (IPTR)
- I. Prognostic Index
- I. Society for Heart and Lung Transplant (ISHLT)
- I. Society of Heart and Lung Transplantation (ISHLT)
- I. Society for Heart and Lung Transplant biopsy
- I. Society for Heart and Lung Transplant grade

internum
- erysipelas i.

interpalpebral fissure

interpapillary ridge

Interpersonal Support Evaluation List (ISEL)

interphalangeal
- distal i. (DIP)
- i. joint
- proximal i. (PIP)

interplant

interplanting

interpolation flap

interpretation
- patch test i.

interquartile range (IQR)

interrogans
- *Leptospira i.*

interspecific graft

interstitial
- i. fibrosis
- i. granuloma
- i. granulomatous drug reaction (IGDR)
- i. infiltration by histiocyte
- i. inflammation
- i. lung disease (ILD)
- i. nephritis
- i. pressure

interstitium
- lung i.

intertinctus
- strophulus i.

intertriginous
- i. area
- i. psoriasis
- i. region

intertrigo
- bacterial i.
- *Candida* i.
- diaper rash i.
- eczema i.
- i. eczema
- erythema i.
- monilial i.
- i. with ulceration

intertrochanteric
- varus i.

interval
- anterior atlantodental i. (AADI)
- confidence i. (CI)
- i. mapping technique
- posterior atlantodental i. (PADI)

intervention
- avocational i.
- psychosocial i.
- vocational i.

interzone

intestinal
- i. biopsy
- i. bypass arthritis
- i. epithelial cell (IEC)
- i. fluke
- i. lipodystrophy
- i. mucosal dysfunction
- i. nematode
- i. polyp
- i. protozoa

i. transplantation
i. ulceration
intestinalis
pneumatosis i.
intestinotoxin
intimal
i. arteritis
i. collagen
intimitis
proliferative i.
intine
intolerance
carbohydrate i.
cow-milk protein i.
disaccharide i.
drug i.
food i.
gluten i.
idiopathic environmental i. (IEI)
lactose i.
intoxication
anaphylactic i.
bromide i.
metal i.
intraalveolar hemorrhage
Intra-articular
Aristospan I.-a.
intraarticular (IA)
i. depocorticosteroids
i. fracture
i. glucocorticoid
i. injection
i. ossicle
i. osteoid osteoma
i. therapy
i. tophus
intrabursal
intracellular
i. calcium chelator
i. crystalloid solution
i. digestion
i. edema
i. toxin
intraclass correlation coefficient (ICC)
intracranial pressure (ICP)
intractable
i. plantar keratosis
i. pyoderma
i. wheezing
intracutaneous
i. nevus

i. reaction
i. test
intracytoplasmic inclusion cell
intradermal
i. anesthetic
i. melanocyte
i. nevus
i. reaction
i. skin test
i. test concentration
IntraDop probe
intraepidermal
i. abscess
i. acanthoma
i. blistering disease
i. bulla
i. carcinoma
i. microabscess
i. microabscess of psoriasis
i. neutrophilic IgA dermatosis
i. nevus
i. vesiculation
intraepithelial mast cell
intragastral provocation under endoscopy (IPEC)
intragraft pressure
intrahepatic
i. cholestasis of pregnancy
i. islet graft
intralesional
Aristospan I.
i. corticosteroid therapy
i. injection
intralysosomal
intramural thrombus
intramuscular
immune globulin, i.
in-transit metastasis
intraocular inflammation
intraosseous hemorrhage
intraperitoneal glucose tolerance test (IPGTT)
intrapsychic stress
IntraSite
I. gel
I. hydrogel dressing
intrasplenic transplantation (isp-Tx)
intrasynovial complement level
intratendinous injection
intrathoracic blood volume (ITBV)
intrauterina
ichthyosis i.

NOTES

intravascular
    i. endothelial proliferation
    i. endothelial proliferative lesion
    i. papillary endothelial hyperplasia
    i. ultrasound (IVUS)
disseminated intravascular coagulation (DIC)
intravenous
    i. fluid
    Fungizone i.
    i. gamma globulin (IVGG)
    i. glucose tolerance test (IVGTT)
    immune globulin, i.
    i. immune serum globulin (IVIG)
    i. immunoglobulin
    immunoglobulin, i. (IGIV)
    respiratory syncytial virus immune globulin i. (RSV-IGIV)
    Rh immune globulin i. (RhIGIV)
    Rous sarcoma virus immune globulin i. (RSV-IGIV)
intraventricular hemorrhage
intravesical
    i. oxychlorosene sodium
    i. silver nitrate
intrinsic
    i. affinity
    i. allergy
    i. association constant
    i. asthma
    i. muscle atrophy
Intron A
intron-exon boundary
Intropin
intrusion
    alpha wave i.
intubation
intussusception
inunct
inunction
inundation fever
InV
    InV allotype
    InV group antigen
invaccination
invadens
    aegleria i.
invaginata
    trichorrhexis i.
invagination
Invanz
invariant
    i. chain
    i. chain CS
    I i.
invasion
    angiolymphatic i.
    pagetic petrous bony i.
    stage of i.

invasionis
    stadium i.
invasive
    i. aspergillosis
    i. candidiasis
    i. squamous cell carcinoma
invecta
    Solenopsis i.
inventory
    Children's Depression I.
    Psoriasis Life Stress I. (PLSI)
inversa
    acne i.
    junctional epidermolysis bullosa atrophicans i.
inverse
    i. anaphylaxis
    epidermolysis bullosa, i.
    i. pityriasis rosea
    i. psoriasis
    i. ratio ventilation (IRV)
inversus
    situs i.
inverted follicular keratosis
inveterata
    psoriasis i.
Invirase
invisible glove
involuting flat hemangioma
involution form
involvement
    axial i.
    cardiovascular i.
    juvenile rheumatoid arthritis with spinal i.
    kidney i.
    lung i.
    20-nail i.
    20-nail i.
    nervous system i.
    palm-sole i.
    peripheral nerve i.
    predominant DIP joint i.
    predominant distal interphalangeal joint i.
    psoriatic arthritis with spinal i.
    renal i.
    skin i.
    subaxial i.
    T-cell i.
INVOS Cerebral Oximeter
Io
    Io caterpillar
    Io moth larva
    Io moth larva sting
Iobid DM
ioderma
Iodex Regular

iodica
> purpura i.

iodide
> i. acne
> potassium i.
> propidium i.
> saturated solution of potassium i.
> (SSKI)

iodine
> i. bush
> i. eruption
> radiolabeled i.

iodized collodion
iodochlorhydroxyquin
iododerma
Iodoflex absorptive dressing
Iodoform gauze
iodophor
iodoquinol and hydrocortisone
Iodosorb absorptive dressing
Iofed PD
Iohist DM
ionic polymer matrix wound gel
Ionil
Ionil-T plus
ionizing radiation
iontophoresis
iontophoretic unit
**IOS immunodiagnostic testing
  instrument**
IP
> incubation period

IPAP
> inspiratory positive airway pressure

IPEC
> intragastral provocation under endoscopy

IPEX
> immune dysregulation,
> polyendocrinopathy, enteropathy, X-
> linked
>>   IPEX syndrome

IPF
> idiopathic pulmonary fibrosis

IPGTT
> intraperitoneal glucose tolerance test

I-Phrine Ophthalmic solution
IPITx
> isolated pancreatic islet transplantation

IPK
> indurated plantar keratoma

IPL
> intense pulsed light

IPLS
> intense pulsed light source

IPM wound gel
IPPB
> intermittent positive pressure breathing

IPR
> immediate phase reaction

ipratropium
> i. bromide
> i. bromide aerosol

IPSID
> immunoproliferative small intestinal
> disease

IPTR
> International Pancreas Transplant
> Registry

IPV
> inactivated poliovirus vaccine

IQR
> interquartile range

IR
> idiopathic rhinitis

I/R
> ischemia and reperfusion

Ir
> immune response
> Ir gene

IR502 psoriasis vaccine
IRB
> institutional review board

Irgasan
IRI
> immunoreactive insulin

irides (*pl. of* iris)
iridescent virus
iridis
> herpes i.

iridocyclitis
Iridoviridae
Iridovirus
I/R injury
iris, pl. **irides**
> erythema i.
> i. forceps
> herpes i.
> heterochromia i.
> i. lesion
> lichen i.
> syphilis of i.

iritis
> hypopyon i.
> plastic i.

NOTES

IRMA
  immunoradiometric assay
iron
  i. deficiency
  i. deficiency anemia
  i. oxide pigment
  i. storage disease
irradiance
irradiate
irradiation
  allograft i.
  therapeutic i.
  thoracoabdominal i. (TAI)
  thymic i. (TI)
  total body i. (TBI)
  total-lymphoid i.
  total lymphoid i. (TLI)
  whole-body i. (WBI)
irregular border
irrigation
  joint i.
  tidal i.
irrigator
  Grossan nasal i.
irritable bowel syndrome (IBS)
irritans
  Pulex i.
  Trombicula i.
irritant
  i. contactant
  i. contact dermatitis (ICD)
  i. contact urticaria
  contributory i.
  i. gas
  i. hand dermatitis
  mild i.
  i. patch-test reaction
  i. patch-test response
  primary i.
irritate
irritation
  crab larvae i.
  i. fibroma
IRV
  inverse ratio ventilation
IS
  immune serum
  in-house ImmunoSpot
Is
  immune suppressor
  Is gene
Isaacs syndrome
Isambert disease
ISAtx247 immunosuppressive drug
ischemia
  cold i.
  digital i.
  donor-related warm i.

  i. and reperfusion (I/R)
  transient cerebral i.
ischemia-reperfusion injury
ischemic
  i. bone necrosis
  i. bone pain
  i. ulcer
ischial bursitis
ischidrosis
ischiogluteal bursitis
Iscove modified Dulbecco medium
ISEL
  Interpersonal Support Evaluation List
isethionate
  pentamidine i.
  piritrexim i.
ISH
  isocapnic hyperventilation
  in situ hybridization
ISHLT
  International Society for Heart and Lung
    Transplant
  International Society of Heart and Lung
    Transplantation
  ISHLT biopsy
  ISHLT grade
island
  i. disease
  i. fever
  i. pedicle flap
  i. of sparing
  i. wound dressing
islet
  i. allograft rejection
  i. alpha cell
  i. amyloid polypeptide (IAPP)
  i. cell antibody (ICA)
  i. cell transplant
  i. composite graft
  i. transplantation
isoagglutination
isoagglutinin
isoagglutinogen
isoallotypic determinant
isoantibody
isoantigen
  Rh i.
Isocaine HCl injection
isocapnic
  i. condition
  i. hyperventilation (ISH)
Isoclor
isocoproporphyrin
isocyanate
  i. disease
  i. HDI
  i. MDI
  i. TDI
isocytolysin

Isodine
Isoelast adhesive short stretch bandage
isoelectric focusing (IEF)
isoenzyme
    PLA$_2$ i. (type IIA, IV, V)
isoerythrolysis
isoetharine
    Arm-a-Med i.
    Dey-Lute i.
isoeugenol
isoflurane
isoform
    catabolin i.
    i. PDGF-A
    i. PDGF-B
isogeneic graft
isograft
isohemagglutination
isohemagglutinin
    saline i.
isohemolysin
isohemolysis
isoimmune
    i. neonatal neutropenia
    i. neonatal thrombocytopenia
isoimmunization
isokinetic collection
Isolage
isolate
    spirochetal i.
isolated
    i. dyskeratosis follicularis
    i. limb perfusion
    i. pancreatic islet transplantation
    (IPITx)
isoleucyl-tRNA synthetase
isoleukoagglutinin
isologous graft
isolysin
isolysis
isolytic
isomeric response
isometric exercise
isomorphic
    i. effect
    i. phenomenon
    i. response
isoniazid
    rifampin and i.
isoniazid-induced hepatitis
isonicotine hydrazine (INH)
isopathy

isophagy
isophil antibody
isophile antigen
Isoplast adhesive short stretch bandage
isoplastic graft
isoprecipitin
isoprenaline
Isoprinosine
isopropyl
    i. alcohol
    i. ester
    i. myristate
isoproterenol
    Arm-a-Med I.
    Dey-Dose I.
    Dispos-a-Med I.
    nebulized i.
    i. and phenylephrine
Isopto
    I. Atropine Ophthalmic
    I. Cetapred Ophthalmic
    I. Frin Ophthalmic solution
    I. Homatropine Ophthalmic
    I. Hyoscine Ophthalmic
    I. Plain solution
    I. Tears solution
isopyknic
isosensitize
isoserum treatment
Isospora belli
isosporiasis
isothiocyanate
    allyl i.
    rhodamine i.
isotransplantation
isotretinoin
Isotrex
isotype
isotypic
isoxsuprine hydrochloride
isozyme
    glutathione-dependent, cytosolic i.
    PLA$_2$ i.
Ispaghula
isp-Tx
    intrasplenic transplantation
ISR
    immediate skin response
isradipine
israelii
    Actinomyces i.

NOTES

ISS
immunostimulatory DNA sequence
ISS-ODN
immunostimulatory oligodeoxynucleotide
IST
immunosuppressive therapy
isthmic spondylolisthesis
isthmus
I-Sulfacet Ophthalmic
Isuprel
IT
ACE IT
AsthmaCare Education: Intensive
Training
Italian
I. cypress
I. cypress tree
Italy
Interdisciplinary Group for Cancer
Care Evaluation in I. (GIVIO)
ITAM
immunoreceptor tyrosine-based activation
motif
ITBV
intrathoracic blood volume
itch
Absorbine Jock I.
baker's i.
barber's i.
barn i.
bath i.
Boeck i.
clamdigger's i.
coolie i.
copper i.
copra i.
Cortef Feminine I.
Cuban i.
dew i.
dhobie i.
Dogger Bank i.
frost i.
grain i.
grocer's i.
ground i.
jock strap i.
kabure i.
ked i.
lumberman's i.
mad i.
Malabar i.
i. mite
Moeller i.
Norway i.
poultryman's i.
prairie i.
I. Relief Gel Spritz
rice i.
Saint Ignatius i.

straw i.
summer i.
swamp i.
swimmer's i.
toe i.
vulvar i.
warehouseman's i.
washerwoman's i.
water i.
winter i.
7-year i.
itching
nasal i.
i. purpura
itch-scratch-lichenification cycle
Itch-X
itchy
i. red bump disease
i. soft palate
i. throat
Ito
hypomelanosis of I.
nevus of I.
I. nevus
Ito-Reenstierna test
ITP
idiopathic thrombocytopenic purpura
chronic ITP
itraconazole
I-Tropine Ophthalmic
IV
Avelox IV
Cubicin powder for IV
Merrem IV
moxifloxacin HCl IV
Synercid IV
I.V.
Gammar-P I.V.
Ivarest cream
ivermectin
Iverson dermabrader
IVGG
intravenous gamma globulin
IVGTT
intravenous glucose tolerance test
IVIG
intravenous immune serum globulin
IVUS
intravascular ultrasound
ivy
I. Cleanse medicated wipe
English i.
poison i.
I. Soothe cream
I. Stat gel
I. Super Dry topical liquid
IvyBlock Lotion
IX
protoporphyrin IX (PPIX)

Ixodes
    I. cookei
    I. dammini
    I. dammini tick
    I. hexagonus
    I. pacificus
    I. pacificus tick
    I. persulcatus

    I. ricinus
    I. ricinus wood tick
    I. scapularis
    I. spinipalpis
ixodiasis
ixodic
Ixodidae

NOTES

J

J chain
J chain gene
J serovar-specific epitope
J5 lipopolysaccharide
Jaa

Jaa Amp
Jaa Pyral
jaagsiekte
Jaa-Prednisone
Jaccoud

J. arthritis
J. arthropathy
jacket

yellow j.
Jackson-Lawler syndrome
Jackson-Sertoli syndrome
Jackson-Weiss syndrome
Jacobi poikiloderma
Jacobsen syndrome
Jacobson

J. forceps
J. Resonance Enterprises, Inc.
J. resonator device
Jacob ulcer
Jacquet

J. erosive diaper dermatitis
J. erythema
Jadassohn

anetoderma of J.
J. anetoderma
J. disease
J. epithelioma
nevus sebaceus of J. (NSJ)
sebaceous nevus of J.
J. sebaceous nevus
J. testerma
Jadassohn-Bloch test
Jadassohn-Lewandowsky

J.-L. law
J.-L. syndrome
Jadassohn-Pellizzari anetoderma
Jadassohn-Tièche nevus
Jadelot

J. furrow
J. line
Jaeger plate
Jaffe-Campanacci syndrome
jail fever
JAK2

Janus kinase 2
Jak

Janus family tyrosine kinase
Jak kinase

Jak3 deficiency
Jakob-Creutzfeldt (JC)

J.-C. disease
JAM

joint alignment and motion
jambolan bark
James C. White tar ointment
Jamestown Canyon virus (JCV)
Janeway lesion
Janus

J. family tyrosine kinase (Jak)
J. kinase 2 (JAK2)
J. reaction
Japanese

J. B encephalitis
J. B encephalitis virus
J. cedar
J. cedar tree
J. encephalitis virus vaccine (JE-VAX)
J. encephalitis virus vaccine, inactivated
J. hot foot dermatitis
J. lacquer tree
J. river fever
J. sargassum
J. sargassum allergy
japonica

Cryptomeria j.
encephalitis j.
japonicum

Schistosoma j.
Jarisch-Herxheimer reaction
Jarisch ointment
JAS

juvenile ankylosing spondylitis
jasmine
jaundice

catarrhal j.
homologous serum j.
jaw

j. claudication
j. cyst
lumpy j.
phossy j.
pincer j.
JC

Jakob-Creutzfeldt
JC virus
JCV

Jamestown Canyon virus
JDMS

juvenile dermatomyositis
JDMS/PM

juvenile dermatomyositis/polymyositis

jeanselmei
> *Exophiala j.*
> *Exserohilum j.*

Jeanselme nodule

JEB
> junctional epidermolysis bullosa

JEB-PA
> junctional epidermolysis bullosa-pyloric atresia syndrome

jejuni
> *Campylobacter j.*

jelly
> petroleum j.
> Vaseline petroleum j.

jellyfish
> box j.
> Portuguese j.
> j. sting

Jenamicin injection

Jerne
> J. plaque assay
> J. technique

Jessner
> lymphocytic infiltrate of J.
> J. Peel
> J. syndrome

Jessner-Kanof
> benign lymphocytic infiltrate of J.-K.
> J.-K. disease

jet-bubble mechanism

jet nebulizer

JE-VAX
> Japanese encephalitis virus vaccine

jeweler's forceps

jewelweed

JH
> JH gene
> JH virus

JIA
> juvenile idiopathic arthritis

jigger

JKA cell

Jk antigen

Jo-1
> Jo-1 antibody
> Jo-1 antigen

Jobbins antigen

Job syndrome

jock strap itch

jodbasedow
> j. disease
> j. phenomenon

Joest body

jogger's
> j. nipples
> j. toe

John
> J. Bunn Mini-Mist nebulizer
> J. Dory fish prick testing

johnin

Johnson
> J. grass
> J. smut

joint
> acromioclavicular j.
> active j.
> j. alignment and motion (JAM)
> apophysial j.
> atlantoaxial j.
> carpometacarpal j.
> Charcot j.
> Clutton j.
> coding j.
> j. congruence
> costovertebral-girdle j.
> cricoarytenoid j.
> distal radicular j. (DRUJ)
> j. effusion
> facetal j.
> glenohumeral j.
> j. histology
> interphalangeal j.
> j. irrigation
> j. lavage
> Luschka j.
> manubriosternal j.
> metatarsophalangeal j.
> occipitoaxial j.
> patellofemoral j.
> peripheral j.
> prosthetic j.
> j. protection technique
> j. protection training
> pseudoneuropathic j.
> radiocarpal j.
> j. space narrowing
> sternoclavicular j.
> sternocostal j.
> subtalar j.
> j. swelling
> temporomandibular j. (TMJ)
> trochleo-ginglymoid j.
> zygapophysial j.

jointedness
> loose j.

jojoba oil

Jones criteria

Jones-Mote
> J.-M. radiation
> J.-M. reaction

Jonston
> J. alopecia
> J. area

Jopling classification

Jordan anomaly

jordanis
    Legionella j.
josamycin
Joseph skin hook
Jouvence
JPD
    juvenile plantar dermatitis
Jr.
    Aerolate Jr
    Congess Jr
    EpiPen Jr.
JRA
    juvenile rheumatoid arthritis
Js antigen
JTA
    juvenile temporal arteritis
juccuya
judacia
    Parietaria j.
judaica
judgment
    clinical j.
Juglans regia
jugulation
jun
    jun gene
    Jun protooncogene
junction
    craniocervical j.
    dermal-epidermal j. (DEJ)
    dermoepidermal j.
    j. nevus
    pannus-cartilage j.
junctional
    j. CD8+ cutaneous lymphoma
    j. epidermolysis bullosa (JEB)
    j. epidermolysis bullosa atrophicans generalisata gravis
    j. epidermolysis bullosa atrophicans generalisata mitis
    j. epidermolysis bullosa atrophicans inversa
    j. epidermolysis bullosa atrophicans localisata
    j. epidermolysis bullosa progressiva
    j. epidermolysis bullosa-pyloric atresia syndrome (JEB-PA)
    j. epidermolysis bullosa with pyloric atresia
    j. nevus
    j. variant

June
    J. grass
    J. grass pollen
jungle
    j. rot
    j. yellow fever
Jüngling disease
Junin virus
Junior Strength Motrin
juniper
    j. mix
    j. mix tree
    j. tar
    Western j.
Juquitiba virus
Juri flap
Jurkat
    J. cell
    J. cell migration
    J. T-cell line
Just Tears solution
jute
juvenile
    j. ankylosing spondylitis (JAS)
    j. aponeurotic fibroma
    j. biotin deficiency
    j. chronic arthritis
    j. chronic polyarthritis
    j. colloid milium
    j. dermatomyositis (JDMS)
    j. dermatomyositis/polymyositis (JDMS/PM)
    j. elastoma
    j. gout
    j. hyaline fibromatosis
    j. idiopathic arthritis (JIA)
    j. melanoma
    j. myositis
    j. palmoplantar fibromatosis
    j. papillomatosis
    j. pityriasis rubra pilaris
    j. plantar dermatitis (JPD)
    j. plantar dermatosis
    j. rheumatoid arthritis (JRA)
    j. rheumatoid arthritis rash
    j. rheumatoid arthritis with spinal involvement
    j. spring eruption
    j. temporal arteritis (JTA)
    j. xanthogranuloma (JXG)
    j. xanthogranuloma histiocytosis
    j. xanthoma

NOTES

juvenilis
 verruca plana j.
juxtaarticular
 j. node
 j. nodule

 j. osteopenia
 j. osteoporosis
juxtacrine stimulation
JXG
 juvenile xanthogranuloma

κ

K

K antigen
K cell
Euxyl K 400
K virus

k82 ImmunoCap test

KA

keratoacanthoma

Kabuki syndrome

kabure itch

Kaffir pox

kala azar

Kalcinate

kale

kaleidoscope phenomenon of autoimmunity

Kaletra

K. capsule
K. oral solution

Kalginate

K. alginate dressing
K. alginate wound cover

Kalischer disease

kallak

kallikrein

k. activity
basophil k.
plasma k.

Kaltostat alginate dressing

Kamisyoyo-san

kanamycin

k. sulfate
k. and vancomycin (KV)

Kandahar sore

kangri cancer

Kank-A

kansasii

Mycobacterium k.

Kantrex

K. injection
K. oral

Kanzaki disease

kaolin clotting time

Kaopectate

Kaplan

K. PenduLaser 115
K. PenduLaser 115 laser system

Kaplan-Meier method

Kaplan PenduLaser 115

kapok mattress

Kaposi

K. disease
K. sarcoma (KS)
K. sarcoma herpesvirus (KSHV)

K. varicelliform eruption
K. xeroderma

kaposiform hemangioendothelioma (KHE)

kappa, κ

k. light chain

kappa-binding nuclear factor

kappa-deleting element

Karapandzic flap

karaya

k. gum
k. gum dermatitis

Karnofsky score

Kartagener syndrome

Kasabach-Merritt

K.-M. phenomenon
K.-M. syndrome

Kashin-Beck disease

Kassowitz-Diday law

Katayama fever

Kathon

Kathon-CG

Kauffmann-White scheme

Kawasaki

K. disease (KD)
K. syndrome

Kaye scissors

Kayser-Fleischer ring

KD

Kawasaki disease

kD, kd, kdal

kilodalton

220-kD protein

kedani fever

ked itch

Keep Clear Anti-Dandruff Shampoo

Keflex

Keflin injection

Keftab

Kefurox injection

kefyr

Candida k.

Kefzol

Kelev strain rabies virus

Kell blood antibody type

Kell-Cellano blood group

Keller ultraviolet test

Kelley-Seegmiller syndrome

Kellgren

K. disease
K. score

Kellgren-Lawrence stage

kellicotti

Paragonimus k.

Kelly encephalomyelitis

K

Kelo-cote topical gel
keloid
    k. acne
    Addison k.
    Alibert k.
    k. formation
keloidal
    k. basal cell carcinoma
    k. blastomycosis
    k. folliculitis
    k. scarring
    k. type scar
keloidalis
    acne k. (AK)
    folliculitis k.
keloidosis
Kemstro
Kenacort
    K. oral
    K. Syrup
    K. Tablet
Kenaject-40
Kenaject Injection
Kenalog
    K. H
    K. Injection
    K. in Orabase
    K. topical
Kenalog-10, -40
Kendall correlation coefficient
Kenicef
Kenonel topical
Kentucky bluegrass
Kenya tick typhus
Keragen
Keralyt Gel
Kerastick
    Levulan K.
keratiasis
keratic
keratin
    k. 13
    k. 19
    hard k.
    nail k.
    soft k.
keratinase
keratin 6HF (K6HF)
keratinization
    ectopic k.
keratinize
keratinized cell
keratinocyte
keratinocyte
    apoptotic k.
    dyskeratotic k.
    k. growth factor-2 (KGF-2)
    subconfluent k.
keratinocytic adhesion

keratinous
    k. cyst
    k. material
    k. sheet
keratitis
    k. deafness
    epithelial k.
    filamentary k.
    herpetic stromal k. (HSK)
    k. rosacea
keratitis-deafness cornification disorder
keratitis-ichthyosis-deafness (KID)
    k.-i.-d. syndrome
keratoacanthoma (KA)
    k. centrifugum marginatum
    eruptive k.
    Ferguson-Smith k.
    multiple k.
    solitary k.
keratoangioma
keratoatrophoderma
keratoconjunctivitis
    atopic k.
    epidemic k.
    herpetic k.
    k. sicca
    vernal k.
    virus k.
keratoconus
keratocyte
keratoderma
    k. blennorrhagica
    k. blennorrhagicum
    carnauba-wax-like k.
    k. climacterica
    k. climactericum
    k. eccentrica
    epidermolytic palmoplantar k.
    Howell-Evans k.
    lymphedematous k.
    mutilating k.
    k. palmaris et
    k. palmaris et plantaris
    palmoplantar k. (PPK)
    k. plantare sulcatum
    punctate k.
    punctate porokeratotic k.
    k. punctatum
    Richner-Hanhart k.
    senile k.
    symmetric k.
    k. symmetrica
    Unna-Thost k.
    Vorner variant of Unna-Thost k.
keratodermatitis
keratodermia
keratodermic sandal
keratodes
    erythema k.

keratoelastoidosis marginalis
keratogenesis
keratogenetic
keratogenous zone
keratohyaline granule
keratoid exanthema
keratolysis
    k. exfoliativa
    k. exfoliativa areata manuum
    k. neonatorum
    pitted k.
    k. plantare sulcatum
keratolytic
    k. agent
    k. paint
keratoma
    k. diffusum
    k. disseminatum
    k. hereditaria mutilans
    k. hereditarium mutilans
    indurated plantar k. (IPK)
    k. malignum
    k. malignum congenitale
    k. palmare et plantare
    k. plantare sulcatum
    senile k.
keratomalacia
keratomycosis lingua
keratonosis
keratopachyderma
keratopathy
    band k.
    epithelial k.
keratoplastic
keratosa
    acne k.
keratose
keratosic cone
keratosis, pl. keratoses
    actinic k.
    arsenical k.
    aural k.
    k. blennorrhagica
    k. climactericum
    k. diffusa fetalis
    facial actinic k.
    follicular k.
    k. follicularis
    k. follicularis contagiosa
    k. follicularis spinulosa decalvans
    gonorrheal k.
    intractable plantar k.

    inverted follicular k.
    k. labialis
    lichenoid k.
    k. lichenoides chronica
    lichen planus-like k.
    nevoid k.
    nevus follicularis k.
    k. nigricans
    k. obliterans
    oral k.
    k. palmaris et plantaris
    k. palmaris et plantaris of the
      Meleda type
    k. palmaris et plantaris of Unna-
      Thost
    k. palmoplantaris punctata
    pedunculated seborrheic k.
    k. pilaris
    k. pilaris atrophicans
    k. pilaris atrophicans faciei
    k. pilaris rubra
    k. rubra figurata
    seborrheic k.
    senile k.
    k. senilis
    smoker k.
    solar k.
    stucco k.
    k. suprafollicularis
    suramin k.
    tar k.
    k. universalis congenita
    k. vegetans
keratotic
    k. angioma
    k. material
    k. papule
    k. plug
    k. scabies
    k. surface
keratouveitis
Keri moisturizer
kerion
    k. celsi
    Celsus k.
    tinea k.
kerionic
Kern determinant
kernicterus
keroid
kerosene
kerotherapy

K

NOTES

ketanserin
ketoconazole
ketone
    methyl ethyl k. (MEK)
ketoprofen
11-keto-reductase
ketorolac tromethamine
ketotifen
Ketotop
Ketron-Goodman disease
Kettle syndrome
Keutel syndrome
Kevadon
Keyes punch
keyhole limpet hemocyanin
Key-Pred Injection
Key-Pred-SP Injection
KF-1 antigen
KGF-2
    keratinocyte growth factor-2
KHE
    kaposiform hemangioendothelioma
khellin
    topical k.
K6HF
    keratin 6HF
Ki-67
    Ki-67 immunohistochemistry
    Ki-67 marker detection
KI antigen
KID
    keratitis-ichthyosis-deafness
    KID syndrome
Kidd
    K. blood antibody type
    K. blood group
Kidde apparatus
kidney
    k. allograft
    k. bean
    k. disease
    k. involvement
    Madin-Darby bovine k. (MDBK)
    k. transplantation (KTx)
Kienböck-Adamson point
Kienböck disease
Kiesselbach plexus
Kikuchi disease
Kilham rat virus
killed-virus vaccine
killer
    k. cell
    k. cell inhibitory receptor (KIR)
    k. inhibitor receptor-human
      leukocyte antigen (KIR-HLA)
    k. inhibitor receptor-human
      leukocyte antigen complex
    natural k. (NK)

killing test
kilodalton (kD, kd, kdal)
45-kilodalton protein
Kimura disease
kinase
    c-jun N-terminal k.
    creatinine k.
    extracellular signal-regulated k.
    herpes simplex virus thymidine k.
      (HSVTK)
    Jak k.
    Janus k. 2 (JAK2)
    Janus family tyrosine k. (Jak)
    mitogen-activated protein k.
      (MAPK)
    phosphoinositide 3 k.
    Polo-like k. (PLK)
    serine-threonine k.
    sphigosine k.
    Tec family of cytoplasmic protein
      tyrosine k.
    tyrosine k.
Kindler syndrome
kindling
    limbic k.
Kinerase
    K. cream
    K. lotion
    K. N6-furfuryladenine skin cream
Kineret
kinesiology
    applied k.
kinetics
    single-hit k.
Kinetin
kinetochore
kingae
    actinomycetemcomitans,
      Cardiobacterium hominis, Eikenella
      corrodens and Kingella k.
kininase
kinin system
kinky-hair
    k.-h. disease
    k.-h. syndrome
kinky hair
Kinyoun stain
KIR
    killer cell inhibitory receptor
Kirby-Bauer agar
KIR-HLA
    killer inhibitor receptor-human leukocyte
      antigen
    KIR-HLA complex
Kirsten-MSV Ras oncogene
Kisenyi sheep disease virus
kissing
    k. bug
    k. bug bite

kit
- AlaBLOT k.
- Alatest latex-specific IgE allergen test k.
- Arrow pneumothorax k.
- Carmol scalp treatment k.
- Cell Proliferation k.
- Circulon System Step 1, 2 venous ulcer k.
- Cleanmix DNA purification k.
- Dsg1/3 ELISA k.
- Hermal k.
- Human-CFSE Flow k.
- insect sting k.
- MarBlot test k.
- Murine-CFSE Flow k.
- Murine in vivo k.
- Persona ovulation predicting k.
- Pro-Vent arterial blood sampling k.
- Quantikine ELISA k.
- RNeasy Maxi k.
- RNeasy Mini k.
- Screening Patch Test K.

Kitamura
- acropigmentatio reticular of K.
- K. reticulate acropigmentation

Klaron lotion

Klauder syndrome

Klebsiella
- *K. oxytoca*
- *K. pneumoniae*
- *K. rhinoscleromatis*

Klein
- K. cannula
- K. pump

Klein-Waardenburg syndrome

Klenow fragment

Klerist-D Tablet

Kligman's ointment

Klinefelter syndrome

Klippel-Feil syndrome

Klippel-Trenaunay-Parkes-Weber syndrome

Klippel-Trenaunay syndrome

Klippel-Trenaunay-Weber syndrome

Klonopin

Klout

Km
- Km allotype
- Km allotypic determinant
- Km antigen

knee
- housemaid's k.
- knock k.
- mechanical disorder of k.

knemometry

Kniest dysplasia

knife
- chalazion k.

Knight-Taylor brace

knob
- adenovirus fiber k.

knobby skin

knock knee

knot
- surfer's k.

knotted hair

knottin scaffold

knuckle pad

Kobberling-Duncan disease

Kobberling-Dunnigan syndrome

Köbner
- K. disease
- K. effect
- K. epidermolysis bullosa
- K. phenomenon (KP)
- K. phenomenon by history (KP-h)

Koch
- K. bacillus
- K. law
- K. old tuberculin
- K. phenomenon
- K. postulate

kochia

Koebner
- K. effect
- K. phenomenon
- K. reaction

koebnerization

Koenen tumor

Koeppe nodule

Kogoj
- K. pustule
- spongiform pustule of K.

KOH
- potassium chloride stain
- potassium hydroxide
- KOH examination
- KOH preparation
- KOH scraping

Köhler
- K. disease
- K. line

K

NOTES

Kohn pore
koilocytotic
koilonychia
occupational k.
kojic acid
Kolmer test
Kolmogorov-Smirnov test
Komed lotion
Konakion injection
Kondon's Nasal
Kontes Pellet Pestle disposable
microtissue grinder
Koongol virus
Koplik spot
Korean
K. hemorrhagic fever
K. hemorrhagic fever virus
K. yellow moth dermatitis
Kostmann syndrome
Kotonkan virus
Kozak sequence
KP
Köbner phenomenon
KP-e
experimentally induced Köbner
phenomenon
KP-h
Köbner phenomenon by history
Krabbe disease
kra-kra (*var. of* craw-craw)
Kramer-Collins Spore trap
kraurosis
k. penis
k. vulvae
Krause gland
kringle 4 domain of plasminogen
Krisovski sign
Kromayer lamp
Kronofed
krusei
Candida k.
Kruskal-Wallis test

krypton lasing medium
Krysolgan
KS
Kaposi sarcoma
KSHV
Kaposi sarcoma herpesvirus
KT
Orudis KT
KTP
potassium titanyl phosphate
KTP laser
KTx
kidney transplantation
Kulchitsky cell
Kupffer cell
kurtosis
Kurunegala ulcer
Kuru syndrome
Küstner fish allergy
KV
kanamycin and vancomycin
Kveim
K. antigen
K. test
Kveim-Stilzbach antigen
kwashiorkor
marasmic k.
Kwell
K. Cream
K. Lotion
K. Shampoo
Kwellada
Kyasanur
K. Forest disease
K. Forest disease virus
kyphoscoliosis type Ehlers-Danlos
syndrome
kyphoscoliotic type
kyphosis
cervicothoracic k.
Kyrle disease

L

L dose
L unit of streptomycin
L2 linker region
LA

Dexone LA
Entex LA
Guaifenex LA
Humibid LA
Inderal LA
Nolex LA
Partuss LA
PhenaVent LA
Solurex L.A.
Touro LA
Westrim LA
Zephrex LA
L.A.

Dalalone L.A.
Dexasone L.A.
Phenylfenesin L.A.
Theoclear L.A.
La

L. antigen
L. Crosse virus
LABD

linear IgA bullous dermatosis
labeling

affinity l.
T-cell antibody l.
Labello Active
labia (*pl. of* labium)
labial

l. herpes simplex virus
l. melanotic macule
labialis

herpes l.
keratosis l.
myxadenitis l.
labium, pl. **labia**
laboratory

Hollister-Stier L.
Medical Research Council L.'s
(MRCL)
Northern Research L.'s
Venereal Disease Research L.
(VDRL)
labrum

glenoid l.
lacerate
laceration
Lachman test
Lac-Hydrin V
lackluster skin

lacquer

Penlac nail l.
Lacril Ophthalmic solution
lacrimal
Lacrisert
lactalbumin

alpha l.
lactase
lactate

aluminum l.
ammonium l.
l. dehydrogenase
l. dehydrogenase virus
lactea

crusta l.
lactenin
lactic

l. acid
l. acidosis
l. acid and sodium-PCA
l. acid with ammonium hydroxide
l. dehydrogenase (LDH)
l. dehydrogenase agent
LactiCare-HC topical
lactiflora

Paeonia l.
Lactinol
lactobacillary milk
Lactobacillus

L. acidophilus
L. casei
lactobin
lactoferrin
lactoglobulin

beta l.
lactose

l. intolerance
l. malabsorption
lactovegetarian diet
lacuna, pl. **lacunae**

fibrocartilage-cell lacunae
osteocyte lacunae
lacunata

Moraxella l.
LAD

leukocyte adhesion deficiency
linear IgA disease
LAD1

leukocyte adhesion deficiency type 1
LAD2

leukocyte adhesion deficiency type 2
LAD3

leukocyte adhesion deficiency type 3
LAD4

leukocyte adhesion deficiency type 4

L

LAD-01 ER:YAG lightweight portable laser unit
LADA
   latent autoimmune diabetes of adults
ladder
   nucleosome l.
Laelaps echidninus
Laemmli sample buffer
laeta
   Loxosceles l.
LAF-3
   leukocyte antigen factor-3
Lafora disease
lag phase
LaGrange scissors
Laguna Negra virus
Lahey scissors
Lahore sore
laidlawii
   Acholeplasma l.
LAK
   lymphokine-activated killer
   LAK cell
lake
   venous l.
Lalonde hook forceps
la main en lorgnette
LAMB
   lentigines, atrial myxoma, mucocutaneous
   myxomas, and blue nevi
   LAMB syndrome
lambda
   l. bacteriophage
   l. light chain
Lambert-Eaton
   L.-E. myasthenic syndrome (LEMS)
   L.-E. syndrome
lamblia
   Giardia l.
lamb's
   l. quarters
   l. quarters weed pollen
lame foliacée
lamella
   cornoid l.
lamellar
   l. body (LB)
   l. congenital ichthyosiform
   erythroderma
   l. desquamation
   l. dominant
   l. dyshidrosis
   l. dystrophy
   l. exfoliation of the newborn
   l. granule
   l. ichthyosis
   l. plate
   l. scale
lamelliform

lamellipodia formation
lamina
   basal l.
   cell l.
   l. densa
   l. fusca
   l. lucida
   l. propria
   l. propria immune cell
   l. splendens
laminated epithelial plug
laminin
LAM IPM wound gel
Lamisil
   L. oral
   L. Tablet
   L. topical
   L. topical cream
Lamis PressureFuse automatic pressure control
lamivudine
   l. triphosphate (3TC)
   zidovudine and l.
lamotrigine
lamp
   black light fluorescent l.
   black ray l.
   carbon arc l.
   cold quartz l.
   CureLight l.
   fluorescent sun l.
   heat l.
   hot quartz vapor l.
   Kromayer l.
   narrowband UVB l.
   24, 50 Philips 100W TL-01 l.
   quartz l.
   quartz-iodine l.
   sun l.
   ultraviolet A l.
   ultraviolet B l.
   UVA l.
   UVB l.
   uviol l.
   Wood l.
   xenon arc l.
Lamprene
Lamprey cannula
Lanacort
Lan antigen
Lanaphilic Topical
Lancefield classification
lanceolata
   Plantago l.
lance-ovate macule
Lancereaux-Mathieu disease
lancet
   Pharmacia l.
   Phazet l.

Lander Dandruff Control
Landouzy
    L. disease
    L. purpura
Landry-Guillain-Barré syndrome
Landry syndrome
Landschutz tumor
Lane disease
Langenbeck retractor
Langer-Giedion syndrome
Langerhans
    L. cell
    L. cell granule
    L. cell histiocytosis (LCH)
Langer line
Langhans cell
langue au chat
Laniazid oral
lanolin
    anhydrous l.
    l., cetyl alcohol, glycerin, and
    petrolatum
Lanophyllin-GG
lanosum
    Microsporum l.
Lansbury articular index
lansingensis
    Legionella l.
Lantiseptic skin care product
lanuginosa
    acquired hypertrichosis l.
    hypertrichosis l.
lanuginous
lanugo hair
Lanvisone topical
laparoscopic
    l. donor nephrectomy (LDN)
    l. live donor nephrectomy (LLDN)
lapinization
lapinized
LAR
    late asthmatic response
larbish
large
    l. artery disease
    l. cell lymphoma
    l. external transformation-sensitive
    (LETS)
    l. granular lymphocyte (LGL)
    l. vessel vasculitis
large-joint inflammatory arthritis
large-molecular-weight drug

large-plaque
    parapsoriasis l.-p.
    l.-p. parapsoriasis
Lariam
Larrey-Weil disease
Larsen
    L. grading system
    L. syndrome
larva, pl. **larvae**
    brown-tail moth l.
    l. currens
    gypsy moth l.
    Io moth l.
    l. migrans
    l. migrans profundus
larvalis
    porrigo l.
laryngeal
    l. edema
    l. infection
    l. papillomatosis
laryngomalacia
laryngotracheitis
    avian infectious l.
laryngotracheobronchitis
    acute l.
Lasgue sign
Lasan
    L. cream
    L. Unguent
Laschal scissors
L-ascorbic acid
LaseAway
    Polytec PI L.
Lasègue sign
laser
    alexandrite l.
    ALEXlazr l.
    argon l.
    argon-pumped tunable-dye l.
    Athos l.
    Aura L.
    Candela l.
    carbon dioxide l.
    CO_2 l.
    Coherent UltraPulse CO_2 l.
    continuous-wave l.
    copper bromide l.
    copper vapor l.
    CW dye l.
    Derma K l.
    diode l.

L

NOTES

laser *(continued)*
- l. Doppler flowmetry (LDF)
- l. Doppler perfusion imaging
- l. Doppler velocimetry
- dye l.
- EpiTouch l.
- erbium l.
- FeatherTouch CO2 l.
- flashscanner-enhanced CO_2 l.
- frequency doubled neodymium:yttrium-aluminum-garnet l.
- gallium-aluminum-arsenide 904-nm l.
- GentleLASE l.
- l. hair removal
- KTP l.
  - potassium titanyl phosphate laser
- LightSheer l.
- long-pulsed dye l.
- long-pulsed potassium-titanyl-phosphate l.
- low-dose Excimer 308-nm l.
- Luxar NovaPulse l.
- LX 20 l.
- medical free electron l. (MFEL)
- Nd:YAG l.
- neodymium:yttrium-aluminum-garnet l.
- New Star model 130 l.
- NLite l.
- 308-nm Excimer l.
- normal-mode ruby l. (NMRL)
- PhotoDerm l.
- Photogenica l.
- L. Photonics, Inc.
- l. plume
- potassium titanyl phosphate l. (KTP laser)
- pulsed-dye l. (PDL)
- Q-switched alexandrite l.
- Q-switched Nd:YAG l.
- Q-switched neodymium:YAG l. (QSYAG)
- Q-switched ruby l. (QSRL)
- quasicontinuous-wave l.
- ruby l.
- ScleroPlus flashlamp-pumped pulsed tunable dye l.
- Sharplan SilkTouch flashscan surgical l.
- Silk L.
- SilkTouch l.
- Skinlight erbium:YAG l.
- l. skin resurfacing (LSR)
- solid-state dye l.
- Spectrum ruby l.
- l. surgery
- SurgiPulse XJ l.
- l. therapy
- titanium:sapphire l.
- TruPulse l.
- UltraPulse CO_2 l.
- VersaLight l.
- VersaPulse l.
- Viridis pulsed l.
- Xanar 20 Ambulase CO_2 l.
- XeCl excimer l.
- YAG l.
- yttrium-aluminum-garnet l.

laser-assisted
- l.-a. internal fabrication (LIFT)
- l.-a. internal fabrication technique

"Laser bra" procedure
Laserflo laser Doppler
Lasertrolysis hair removal
Lasix
lasofoxifene
Lassa
- L. hemorrhagic fever
- L. virus

Lassar
- L. betanaphthol paste
- L. plain zinc paste

lata
- condyloma l.
- condylomata l.
- fascia l.
- perianal condylomata l.

late
- l. asthmatic response (LAR)
- l. benign syphilis
- l. cardiovascular syphilis
- l. centrilobar necrosis
- l. congenital syphilis
- l. latent syphilis
- l. onset neurofibromatosis
- l. osseous syphilis
- l. pulmonary response (LPR)
- l. respiratory systemic syndrome (LRSS)
- l. yaw

latency
latens
- scarlatina l.

latent
- l. allergy
- l. allotype
- l. autoimmune diabetes of adults (LADA)
- l. class analysis
- l. infection
- l. microbism
- l. period
- l. rat virus
- l. stage
- l. syphilis
- l. transforming growth factor

late-onset
  l.-o. renal failure
  l.-o. spondyloepiphyseal dysplasia
late-phase
  l.-p. allergic reaction (LPAR)
  l.-p. cutaneous reaction (LPCR)
  l.-p. response
lateral
  l. collateral ligament (LCL)
  l. femoral cutaneous nerve
    entrapment
  l. nail fold
  l. rotation mattress
lateralis
  hyperhidrosis l.
  nevus unius l.
  onychia l.
lateris
  nevus unius l.
laterosporus
  Bacillus l.
latex
  l. agglutination assay
  l. agglutination test
  l. allergy
  l. allergy test
  l. ELISA for antigen protein
    (LEAP)
  l. fixation reaction
  l. fixation test
  Hevea brasiliensis l.
  l. hypersensitivity
  l. particle agglutination
  polystyrene l.
  l. product
  l. RIA panel
latex-fruit syndrome
latex-specific IgE
Laticaudinae
Latranal
latrodectism
Latrodectus
  L. mactans
  L. mactans antivenom
  L. mactans bite
LATS
  long-acting thyroid stimulator
lattice fiber
latticelike
latticework

latum
  condyloma l.
  Diphyllobothrium l.
Laugier-Hunziger syndrome
laurel fever
Laurin angle
Lauth violet
LAV
  lymphadenopathy-associated virus
lava bean
lavage
  bronchoalveolar l. (BAL)
  joint l.
law
  Behring l.
  Farr l.
  Grotthus-Draper l.
  Halsted l.
  Jadassohn-Lewandowsky l.
  Kassowitz-Diday l.
  Koch l.
  Marfan l.
  Planck l.
  l. of priority
  Profeta l.
  von Behring l.
Lawrence-Seip syndrome
laxa
  cutis l.
laxity
  ligament l.
lax skin
layer
  adherent mucus gel l.
  barrier l.
  basal cell l.
  Bowman l.
  cornified l.
  granular cell l.
  Henle l.
  horny cell l.
  Huxley l.
  hypertrophic smooth muscle l.
  lucid l.
  malpighian l.
  mushroom-hook l.
  palisade l.
  prickle cell l.
  Profore wound contact l.
  spinous l.
  squamous cell l.
4-layer bandage (FLB)

NOTES

lazarine leprosy
Lazaro
    mal de San L.
lazaroid
Lazarus (LZRS)
LazerSporin-C Otic
lazy
    l. leukocyte syndrome (LLS)
    l. NK cell
lazy-S closure
LB
    lamellar body
LBL
    lymphoblastic lymphoma
    lymphoblastic leukemia
L-canavaline
LCH
    Langerhans cell histiocytosis
LCL
    lateral collateral ligament
LCM
    lymphocytic choriomeningitis
        LCM virus
LCP
    leukocytapheresis
LCR-based HLA typing
LCV
    leukocytoclastic vasculitis
LD
    lethal dose
    living donor
LDA-1 antigen
LDF
    laser Doppler flowmetry
LDH
    lactic dehydrogenase
        LDH agent
LDL-C
    low-density lipoprotein cholesterol
LDLT
    living donor liver transplantation
LDN
    laparoscopic donor nephrectomy
L-DOPA
    levodopa
L+ dose
LDP-02 humanized monoclonal antibody
LE
    LE cell
    LE cell phenomenon
    discoid LE
    LE factor
lead
    l. poisoning
    l. stomatitis
    l. time
leaflet
    mitral l.
    tricuspid valvular l.

leaf litter
leak
    proton l.
Le antigen
LEAP
    latex ELISA for antigen protein
learned helplessness
leather
lectin
    mannan-binding l. (MBL)
    mannose-binding l. (MBL)
    l. pathway
lectularius
    Cimex l.
LED
    light-emitting diode
    lupus erythematosus disseminatus
Ledderhose syndrome
Ledebouriella saseloides
Ledercillin VK oral
leech
Leede-Rumpel phenomenon
leek
leflunomide
left
    l. side down-head up position
    l. ventricular hypertrophy
leg
    Barbados l.
    elephant l.
Legg-Calvé-Perthes disease
Legionella
    L. anisa
    L. birminghamensis
    L. bozemanii
    L. cincinnatiensis
    L. dumoffii
    L. feeleii
    L. jordanis
    L. lansingensis
    L. longbeachae
    L. maceachernii
    L. micdadei
    L. oakridgensis
    L. pneumophila
legionellosis
Legionnaires disease
leg-raise maneuver
legume
Leicester
    L. disease
    L. score
Leichtenstern phenomenon
Leiden
    factor V L.
Leiner
    L. dermatitis
    L. disease
leiodermia

leiomyoma
l. cutis
uterine l.
leiomyosarcoma
leiotrichous
Leishman-Donovan body
Leishmania
L. *donovani*
L. *major*
L. *orientalis*
L. *tropica*
leishmaniasis
acute cutaneous l.
American l.
l. americana
anergic l.
anthroponotic cutaneous l.
antimonial drug therapy for l.
chronic cutaneous l.
diffuse cutaneous l.
disseminated cutaneous l. (DCL)
dry cutaneous l.
human cutaneous l.
lupoid l.
mucocutaneous l. (MCL)
nasopharyngeal l.
New World l.
Old World l.
pseudolepromatous l.
l. recidivans
recidivans l. (RL)
rural cutaneous l.
l. tegumentaria diffusa
l. tropica
urban cutaneous l.
visceral l. (VL)
viscerotropic l. (VTL)
wet cutaneous l.
zoonotic cutaneous l.
leishmania test
leishmanid
leishmanin test
leishmaniosis
**Leishman-Montenegro-Donovan
  intradermal test**
leishmanoid
dermal l.
post-kala-azar dermal l.
Leitz periplan photomicroscope
Leloir disease
lemic
Lemierre disease

lemon
LEMS
Lambert-Eaton myasthenic syndrome
lenercept
length
restriction fragment l.
Lennert lymphoma
Lennhoff sign
lens
lenscale
lens-induced uveitis
lenticula
lenticularis
dermatofibrosis l.
lenticular syphilid
lenticulopapular
lentigines (*pl. of* lentigo)
lentiginosis
agminated l.
centrofacial l.
generalized l.
inherited patterned l.
periorificial l.
l. profusa
lentiginous
lentigo, pl. **lentigines**
lentigines, atrial myxoma,
  mucocutaneous myxomas, and
  blue nevi (LAMB)
lentigines, electrocardiographic
  defects, ocular hypertelorism,
  pulmonary stenosis, abnormalities
  of genitalia, retardation of
  growth, deafness (LEOPARD)
genital l.
ink-spot l.
l. maligna
l. maligna melanoma (LMM)
l. melanoma (LM)
nevoid l.
nevus spilus l.
PUVA-induced l.
reticulated black solar l.
senile l.
l. senilis
simple l.
l. simplex
solar lentigines
solar ink-spot l.
Touraine centrofacial l.
lentil
Lentivirinae

L

NOTES

lentivirus
lentogenic
Lenz-Majewski syndrome
leonine facies
leontiasis
LEOPARD
    lentigines, electrocardiographic defects,
      ocular hypertelorism, pulmonary
      stenosis, abnormalities of genitalia,
      retardation of growth, deafness
      LEOPARD syndrome
leopard skin
leper
Lepidoglyphus destructor
Lepidoptera
lepidosis
Lépine-Froin syndrome
Leporipoxvirus
lepothrix
lepra
    l. alba
    l. alphoides
    l. alphos
    l. anaesthetica
    l. arabum
    l. bacillus
    l. cell
    l. conjunctivae
    l. graecorum
    l. maculosa
    l. mutilans
    l. nervorum
    l. nervosa
    l. tuberculoides
    Willan l.
leprae
    Mycobacterium l.
leprechaunism
leprid
leprologist
leprology
leproma
lepromatous
    l. leprosy
    l. nodule
    polar l.
    l. reaction
lepromin
    l. reaction
    l. test
leprosarium
leprose
leprosery
leprostatic
leprosum
    erythema nodosum l. (ENL)
leprosus
    lichen l.
    pemphigus l.

leprosy
    anesthetic l.
    articular l.
    Asturian l.
    borderline lepromatous l.
    borderline tuberculoid l.
    diffuse lepromatous l.
    dimorphous l.
    dry l.
    histoid l.
    indeterminate l.
    intermediate l.
    lazarine l.
    lepromatous l.
    Lombardy l.
    Lucio l.
    macular l.
    maculoanesthetic l.
    Malabar l.
    mixed l.
    mutilating l.
    neural l.
    nodular l.
    paucibacillary l.
    polar lepromatous l.
    pure neural l.
    reactional l.
    smooth l.
    spotted l.
    subclinical l.
    subpolar lepromatous l.
    trophoneurotic l.
    tuberculoid l.
    uncharacteristic l.
    virchowian l.
    water-buffalo l.
leprotic
leprotica
    alopecia l.
leprous
leptochroa
leptodermic
Leptospira interrogans
leptospirosis
Leptothrix
Leptotrombidium akamushi
Lequesne
    L. algofunctional index
    L. functional index
Leredde syndrome
Leri-Weill syndrome
Leroy I cell
Lesch-Nyhan syndrome
Lescol fluvastatin sodium
Leser-Trélat sign
lesion
    acneform l.
    Andersson l.
    angel kisses l.

angioinvasive l.
angioproliferative l.
anular distribution of l.
arciform distribution of l.
l. arrangement
atrophic hyperkeratotic l.
atrophie blanche l.
blanchable red l.
blistering l.
blueberry muffin l.
blue-gray l.
brown-black l.
bullous skin l.
bull's eye l.
Bywaters l.
coin-sized l.
l. color
l. configuration
l. consistency
cutaneous pustular l.
dermal l.
devil's bite l.
discoid l.
l. distribution
division (I–IV) l.
eczematous l.
elementary l.
en coup de sabre scalp l.
erysipelas-like skin l.
l. evolution
firm l.
genital papulosquamous l.
genitourinary l.
greasy scaly l.
gross l.
hemorrhagic l.
herpetiform distribution of l.
histologic l.
hypometabolism brain l.
infarctive l.
intravascular endothelial
  proliferative l.
iris l.
Janeway l.
lichenified l.
linear distribution of l.
low-grade squamous
  intraepithelial l. (LSIL)
l. margination
medium l.
metachronous tissue l.
l. morphology

mother l.
nickel and dime l.
nonblanchable, abnormally
  colored l.
nummular l.
ocular l.
oil drop l.
osseous l.
osteolytic bone l.
papulopustular l.
papulosquamous l.
papulovesicular l.
pigmented skin l. (PSL)
polycyclic distribution of l.
polypoid l.
precancerous l.
primary l.
proliferative l.
pruritic l.
psoriasiform l.
pulmonary l.
purpuric l.
pustular l.
pyodermatous skin l.
raspberry l.
reticular l.
ripe l.
rolled shoulder l.
Romanus l.
salt and pepper l.
satellite l.
scaling skin-colored l.
secondary l.
silvery scaly l.
l. size
skin l.
skin-colored l.
slope-shouldered l.
smooth skin-colored l.
soft l.
space-occupying l.
special l.
squamous intraepithelial l. (SIL)
square-shouldered l.
stork-bite l.
l. surface characteristic
synchronous tissue l.
traumatic l.
ulcer l.
ulceronecrotic l.
varicelliform l.
vasculitic l.

L

NOTES

313

lesion *(continued)*
  Vaughn-Jackson l.
  venular l.
  vesicobullous l.
  vesiculopustular l.
  vulvar l.
  weeping l.
  white l.
  wire-loop l.
  yellow l.
  zosteriform distribution of l.

LET
  leukocyte esterase test

lethal
  l. chondrodysplasia
  l. dose (LD)
  l. midline granuloma
  l. midline granulomatosis
  l. osteogenesis imperfecta
  l. toxin (LT)

lethalis
  ichthyosis l.

lethargica
  encephalitis l.

LETS
  large external transformation-sensitive

Letterer-Siwe disease

Leu-3+ helper T cell

leu-CAM
  leukocyte cell adhesion molecule

leucin

leucine
  l. zipper motif
  l. zipper transcription factor

leucine-zipper
  basic-region l.-z. (bZIP)

Leucomax

Leucotropin

leucovorin calcium

leukapheresis cycle

leukapheresis-induced amelioration

leukaphersis-based immunomodulatory therapy

leukasmus

leukemia
  African Burkitt l.
  aleukemic l.
  angiocentric l.
  angiodestructive l.
  B-cell l.
  B-cell chronic lymphocytic l. (B-CLL)
  B-cell lymphocytic l.
  blastic NK-cell l.
  body cavity-based B-cell l.
  Burkitt l.
  CD56+ l.
  CD30+ cutaneous l.
  chronic myeloid l. (CML)

chronic T-cell l.
cutaneous B-cell l.
cutaneous B-cell lymphocytic l.
l. cutis
donor-transmitted l.
feline l.
l. of fowls
gingival l.
granulocytic l.
granulomatous cutaneous T-cell l.
hairy cell l. (HCL)
high-grade small noncleaved cell malignant l.
histiocytic l.
Hodgkin l.
junctional CD8+ cutaneous l.
large cell l.
Lennert l.
lymphoblastic l. (LBL)
lymphocytic l.
lymphoepithelioid l.
lymphoid l.
malignant l.
MALT l.
mantle cell l.
marginal zone B-cell l. (MZBL)
Mediterranean l.
monocytic l.
mucosa-associated lymphoid tissue l.
murine l.
myeloid l.
myelomonocytic l.
natural killer cell l.
NK/T-cell l.
non-Hodgkin l. (NHL)
null cell l.
null-type non-Hodgkin l.
peripheral T-cell l.
pleomorphic l.
primary cutaneous B-cell l.
primary cutaneous B-cell lymphocytic l.
primary cutaneous T-cell l.
primary effusion l.
prolymphocytic l. (PLL)
pseudomalignant l.
pulmonary l.
retrovirus-associated l.
Revised European-American L. (REAL)
secondary cutaneous B-cell l.
secondary cutaneous B-cell lymphocytic l.
signet ring l.
subcutaneous panniculitis-like T-cell l. (SPTL)
subcutaneous T-cell l.
T-cell l.

T-cell large granuloma
  lymphocyte l.
T-cell lymphocytic l.
thymus-derived l.
U-cell l.
undefined-cell l.
leukemia/lymphoma
  adult T-cell l./l. (ATLL)
leukemic
  l. arthritis
  l. reticuloendotheliosis
leukemid
Leukeran
leukin
Leukine
leukoagglutinin
leukocidin
leukoclastic
leukocytactic
leukocytapheresis (LCP)
leukocytaxia
leukocyte
  l. adhesion deficiency (LAD)
  l. adhesion deficiency type 1
    (LAD1)
  l. adhesion deficiency type 2
    (LAD2)
  l. adhesion deficiency type 3
    (LAD3)
  l. adhesion deficiency type 4
    (LAD4)
  l. antigen factor-3 (LAF-3)
  l. attachment assay
  l. cell adhesion molecule (leu-
    CAM)
  l. chemotaxis
  l. chimerism
  l. common antigen
  l. concentrate
  l. esterase test (LET)
  l. factor antigen-1 (LFA-1)
  l. function-associated antigen 1
    (LFA-1)
  l. histamine release
  l. histamine release test
  l. interferon
  l. migration
  passenger l.
  polymorphonuclear l. (PML)
leukocyte-poor preparation

leukocytoclastic
  l. angiitis
  l. vasculitis (LCV)
leukocytolysin
leukocytolysis
leukocytolytic
leukocytosis
leukocytosis-promoting factor
leukocytotactic
leukocytotaxia
leukocytotoxin
leukoderma
  acquired l.
  l. acquisitum centrifugum
  chemical l.
  l. colli
  contact l.
  genital l.
  occupational l.
  patterned l.
  syphilitic l.
leukodermatous
leukodermia
leukoencephalitis
  acute epidemic l.
  subacute sclerosing l.
leukoencephalopathy
  immunosuppression-associated l.
  progressive multifocal l. (PML)
  reversible posterior l. (RPLE)
leukokeratosis oris
leukolysin
leukolysis
leukolytic
leukonecrosis
leukonychia
  apparent l.
  partial l.
  l. striata
leukopathia
  acquired l.
  l. punctata reticularis symmetrica
  l. symmetrica progressiva
  l. unguis
leukopathy
  symmetric progressive l.
leukopenia
leukopenic
  l. factor
  l. index
leukoplakia
  acquired dyskeratotic l.

L

NOTES

leukoplakia *(continued)*
    Candida l.
    candidal l.
    hairy l.
    oral hairy l. (OHL)
    proliferative verrucous l.
    l. vulva
leukoplakic vulvitis
leukoplasia
leuko-poor
    l.-p. blood component
    l.-p. red blood cell
leukorrhea
LeukoScan diagnostic agent
leukosialin
leukosis
    avian l.
    enzootic bovine l.
    fowl l.
leukotactic
leukotaxia
leukotaxine
leukotaxis
leukotoxin
leukotrichia annularis
leukotrichous
leukotriene (LT)
    l. B4 (LTB4)
    l. C, E
    l. inhibition
    l. receptor antagonist (LTRA)
    l. reduction
    l. regulation
LeukoVAX
Leukovirus
leupeptin
leuprolide acetate
LeuTech radiolabeled antibody
Leutrol
levalbuterol
levamisole
Levaquin
levarterenol bitartrate
Levay antigen
level
    $beta_2$-microglobulin l.
    Clark l. (I–V)
    fibrinogen l.
    free salicylate l.
    gp91^{phox} l.
    IgG subclass l.
    intrasynovial complement l.
    liver transaminase l.
    no observed adverse effect l.
      (NOAEL)
    peak serum l.
    recommended exposure l. (REL)
    serum complement l.

    specific IgE antibody l.
    total serum IgE l.
Lever
    L. 2000
    L. 2000 moisture response soap
    L. and Schamberg-Lever
      classification
Leviviridae
levocabastine hydrochloride
levodopa (L-DOPA)
    l. stain
levofloxacin
levonorgestrel
Levophed injection
levothyroxine sodium
Levulan
    L. Kerastick
    L. photodynamic therapy
Levulin PDT system
Lewandowski
    nevus elasticus of L.
    rosacea-like tuberculid of L.
Lewandowski-Lutz
    L.-L. disease
    epidermodysplasia verruciformis
      of L.-L.
Lewandowsky nevus elasticus
Lewis
    L. blood antibody type
    L. blood group
    triple response of L.
    L. triple response
    L. X oligosaccharide
Lewis-Summer syndrome
Leyden disease
Leydig cell tumor
Lf
    Lf dose
    Lf unit
LFA
    lymphocyte function-associated antigen
LFA-1
    leukocyte factor antigen-1
    leukocyte function-associated antigen 1
LGDA
    lichenoid and granulomatous dermatitis
      of AIDS
LGL
    large granular lymphocyte
L-glutathione
LH 7:2 antigen
LHE apparatus
Lhermitte-Duclos disease
Lhermitte sign
L'Homme rouge
Liacopoulos phenomenon
liarozole
liasis
Liatest C4b-BP test

liberator
histamine l.
Libman-Sacks
L.-S. endocarditis
L.-S. syndrome
Librium
lice (*pl. of* louse)
Lice-Enz Shampoo
lichen
l. agrius
l. albus
l. amyloidosis
l. chronicus simplex
l. corneus hypertrophicus
l. fibromucinoidosus
l. framboesianus
l. hemorrhagicus
l. infantum
l. iris
l. leprosus
l. myxedematosus
myxedematous l.
l. nitidus
l. nuchae
l. obtusus
l. obtusus corneus
l. pilaris
l. pilaris seu spinulosus
l. planus actinicus
l. planus annularis
l. planus et acuminatus atrophicans
l. planus follicularis
l. planus hypertrophicus
l. planus-like keratosis
l. planus overlap syndrome
l. planus pemphigoid
l. planus pigmentosus
l. planus verrucosus
l. ruber
l. ruber acuminatus
l. ruber moniliformis
l. ruber planus
l. ruber verrucosus
sclerosus l.
l. sclerosus
l. sclerosus et atrophicans
l. sclerosus scleroatrophy
l. scrofulosorum
l. striatus
l. striatus epidermal nevus
l. strophulosus
l. syphiliticus

l. trichophyticus
tropical l.
l. tropicus
l. urticatus
Wilson l.
lichenificatio gigantea
lichenification
giant l.
lichenified
l. dermatitis
l. lesion
l. plaque
licheniformis
Bacillus l.
lichenization
lichenoid
l. acute pityriasis
l. amyloidosis
chronica parapsoriasis l.
l. chronic dermatosis
l. contact dermatitis
l. eczema
l. eruption
exudative discoid and l.
l. and granulomatous dermatitis of AIDS (LGDA)
l. keratosis
parapsoriasis l.
l. phase
pityriasis l.
tuberculosis cutis l.
lichenoides
melanodermatitis toxica l.
parapsoriasis l.
pityriasis l.
tuberculosis cutis l.
lichen-type scale
Lich-Gregoire
L.-G. repair
L.-G. ureteroneocystostomy
Lich technique
licorice
Lidakol cream
LidaMantle HC topical
Liddle syndrome
Lidemol
Lidex-E topical
Lidex topical
lidocaine
bacitracin, neomycin, polymyxin b, and l.
l. and epinephrine

NOTES

317

lidocaine *(continued)*
>l. hydrochloride
>l. and hydrocortisone
>l. and prilocaine

Lidoderm
LidoPen
life
>Dermatology-Specific Quality of L. (DSQL)
>health-related quality of l.
>quality of l. (QOL)
>l. root

life-year
>quality-adjusted l.-y. (QALY)

LIFT
>laser-assisted internal fabrication
>LIFT technique

lifting technique
ligament
>alar l.
>glenohumeral l.
>iliopectineal l.
>inguinal l.
>lateral collateral l. (LCL)
>l. laxity
>l. of Struthers
>transverse l.

ligamentosa
>spondylitis ossificans l.

ligamentous disorder
ligamentum nuchae
ligand
>addressing l.
>Fas-Fas l.
>nuclear factor-kappa B l.
>osteoprotegerin l.
>peptide l.
>L. Pharmaceuticals, Inc.
>P-selectin l.
>receptor activator of nuclear factor kappa B l. (RANKL)
>retinoid X receptor-selective l.
>tumor necrosis factor-related apoptosis-inducing l. (TRAIL)

ligase chain reaction
LIGHT
>homologous to lymphotoxin, shows inducible expression and competes with herpes simplex virus glycoprotein D for herpes virus entry mediator, a receptor expressed by T lymphocyte

light
>actinic l.
>Boyd surgical l.
>Castle examination l.
>l. chain
>CureLight Broadband red l.
>l. eruption
>l. exposure

>Hanalux Oslo l.
>HappySkin Acne L.
>intense pulsed l. (IPL)
>l. microscopy
>midrange spectrum ultraviolet l.
>midrange-wavelength ultraviolet l. (UVB)
>oral administration of psoralen and subsequent exposure to long wavelength ultraviolet l. (PUVA)
>persistent reactivity to l. (PLR)
>l. scatter technique
>l. treatment
>ultraviolet l.
>l. urticaria
>Wood l.

light-emitting diode (LED)
LightSheer
>L. diode laser system for permanent hair removal
>L. laser
>L. SC
>L. SC laser hair removal system

light-sparing effect
lignieresii
>*Actinobacillus l.*

lignocaine monoethylgylycine xylidine excretion test
Likert scale
lilacinus
>*Paecilomyces l.*

lilac tree
lima bean
limb
>l. defect
>l. pain

limbal
>l. guttering
>l. vernal conjunctivitis

limb-girdle dystrophy
limbi (*pl. of* limbus)
limbic kindling
limb-mammary syndrome
limbus, pl. **limbi**
>limbi conjunctiva
>limbi palpebrales anteriores
>limbi palpebrales posteriores

lime
liminal
liminaris
>alopecia l.

limit
>l. of *floccosum*
>permissible exposure l. (PEL)

limitation of exposure
limited
>l. cutaneous systemic sclerosis
>l. joint mobility syndrome
>l. progressive systemic sclerosis

l. scleroderma
l. Wegener granulomatosis
limnophilus
  Paederus l.
Limulus amebocyte lysate assay
lincomycin
lincosamide
lindane
Lindner body
line
  Beau l.
  l.'s of Blaschko
  Blaschko l.
  Borsieri l.
  Cantle l.
  cell l.
  cement l.
  l.'s of cleavage
  Dennie l.
  Dennie-Morgan l.
  erythroleukemia cell l.
  established cell l.
  Futcher l.
  Jadelot l.
  Jurkat T-cell l.
  Köhler l.
  Langer l.
  marionette l.
  Mees l.
  MOLT-18, human T cell l.
  Morgan l.
  Muehrcke l.
  Pastia l.
  pigmentary demarcation l.
  Ramos B-cell l.
  RA synoviocyte l.
  Relaxed Skin Tension L. (RSTL)
  Sergent white l.
  tram l.
  Voigt l.
  white l.
linea, pl. **lineae**
  l. alba
  l. albicans
  l. IgM dermatosis of pregnancy
  l. nigra
  lineae striae atrophicae
linear
  l. atrophoderma of Moulin
  l. atrophy
  l. distribution
  l. distribution of lesion

l. epidermal nevus
l. extensor erythema
l. focal elastosis
l. IgA bullous dermatosis (LABD)
l. IgA bullous dermatosis of
  childhood
l. IgA bullous disease in children
l. IgA disease (LAD)
l. lichen planus
l. petechia
l. porokeratosis
l. progressive systemic sclerosis
l. scleroderma
l. scleroderma variant
l. streaking
l. telangiectasis
l. and whorled nevoid
  hypermelanosis
linearis
  morphea l.
linearity
  Mantel-Haenszel test for l.
liner
  Ac'cents permanent lash l.
linezolid
lingua, pl. **linguae**
  exfoliatio areata l.
  l. geographica
  hyperkeratosis l.
  ichthyosis l.
  keratomycosis l.
  l. nigra
  nigrities l.
  pityriasis l.
  l. plicata
  psoriasis l.
  l. scrotalis
  tylosis l.
lingula, pl. **lingulae**
liniment
  Sloan l.
lining
  synovial l.
linkage disequilibrium
linked suppression
linker
  tonofilament-cytoplasmic plaque l.
  transmembrane l.
link-protein-stabilized aggregate
linnaean system of nomenclature
linoleic acid
Linomide

L

NOTES

linter
    cotton l.
Linton procedure for varicose veins
Linum usitatissimum
Lioresal
LIP
    lymphocytic interstitial pneumonitis
lip
    blubbery l.
    l. cosmetic
    cracked l.
    dry l.
    glowing red l.
    pseudocolloid of l.
lipedematous alopecia
lipid
    l. granulomatosis
    5-lipoxygenase-generated l.
    l. liquid crystal
    neutral l.
    l. peroxidation
    skin l.
    l. storage disease
lipid-free cleanser
lipidosis
    glycolipid l.
Lipkote
    Coppertone L.
Lipman-Pearson protein alignment
    program
lipoatrophia annularis
lipoatrophic diabetes
lipoatrophy
    anular l.
    centrifugal l.
    Ferreira-Marques l.
    insulin l.
    partial l.
    postinfection l.
    semicircular l.
lipoblastomatosis
    benign l.
lipochrome histiocytosis disease
lipocortin
lipodermatosclerosis
lipodystrophia centrifugalis abdominalis
    infantilis
lipodystrophy
    acquired generalized l.
    acquired partial face-sparing l.
    congenital total l.
    intestinal l.
    localized l.
    partial face-sparing l.
    progressive l.
    total l.
lipogranuloma
    sclerosing l.
lipogranulomatosis subcutanea

lipoid
    l. dermatoarthritis
    l. granuloma
    l. pneumonia
    l. proteinosis
lipoidica
    necrobiosis l.
lipolytica
    Candida l.
lipoma
    l. arborescens
    atypical l.
    pleomorphic l.
    spindle cell l.
    synovial l.
lipomatodes
    fibroma l.
    molluscum l.
    nevus l.
lipomatosis
    benign symmetric l.
    encephalocraniocutaneous l. (ECCL)
    mediastinal l.
    multiple symmetric l.
lipomatosus
    nevus l.
lipomelanic reticulosis
lipomelanotic
Lipomel melanoma vaccine
Liponyssus bacoti
lipophagia granulomatosis
lipophagic granuloma
lipophilic yeast
lipophosphoglycan (LPG)
lipopolysaccharide (LPS)
    J5 l.
    l. vaccine
lipopolysaccharide-induced arthritis
lipopolysaccharide-stimulated
lipoprotein
    l. lipase deficiency
    l. polymorphism
    very-low-density l. (VLDL)
liposarcoma
liposculpture
liposomal doxorubicin
liposome
    clodronate-containing l.
liposuction
    syringe-assisted l.
liposuction-assisted curettage
LipoTECA cream
lipoteichoic acid (LTA)
lipotrophy
    semicircular l.
lipovaccine
Lipovnik virus
lipoxin

lipoxygenase
>l. interaction product
>5-l.
>l. pathway

5-lipoxygenase-generated lipid
Lipschütz
>L. body
>L. cell
>L. ulcer

Lipsorex
lipstick
lip-switch
lip-tip vitiligo
liquefaciens
>*Enterobacter l.*
>*Serratia l.*

liquefaction
>l. degeneration
>l. necrosis

Liqui-Caps
>Vicks 44 Non-Drowsy Cold & Cough L.-C.

liquid
>l. air
>Anaplex L.
>Band-Aid L.
>Barc L.
>bland aerosolized l.
>Children's Motion Sickness l.
>Chlorafed L.
>End Lice L.
>l. ethyl chloride
>Gordofilm L.
>Hayfebrol L.
>l. human serum
>Ivy Super Dry topical l.
>Lortuss DM oral l.
>Lotrimin AF Spray L.
>Occlusal-HP L.
>L. paraffin
>L. petrolatum
>L. Pred
>L. Pred oral
>Pyrinyl II L.
>Rhinosyn L.
>Rhinosyn-PD L.
>Ryna L.
>Sudafed Plus L.
>Tisit L.
>Triple X L.

liquidambar

Liquifilm
>L. Forte solution
>Herplex L.
>HMS L.
>L. Tears
>L. Tears solution

Liqui-Gels
>Robitussin Severe Congestion L.-G.

Liquimat lotion
Liquiprin
LiquiShield-A Skin Protectant
LiquiVent
Lisch nodule
lisofylline
lispro insulin
lissotrichic
list
>Interpersonal Support Evaluation L. (ISEL)

Lister
>L. scissors
>L. tubercle

listerial
Listeria monocytogenes
listeriosis
listerism
listhesis
>subaxial l.

listing
>UNOS transplant l.

Lite
>TheraPress DUO L.

lithium succinate
litmus paper
Littauer scissors
litter
>leaf l.

Little League elbow
Litx system
live
>Bacillus Calmette-Guérin l.
>measles virus vaccine, l.
>l. oak
>l. oak tree
>l. oral polio vaccine
>l. oral poliovirus vaccine
>rubella virus vaccine, l.
>varicella virus vaccine l.

livedo
>l. annularis
>lupus l.
>l. pattern

NOTES

L

321

livedo *(continued)*
- l. racemosa
- l. reticularis
- l. reticularis idiopathica
- l. reticularis symptomatica
- l. telangiectatica
- l. vasculitis

livedoid
- l. dermatitis
- l. vasculitis
- l. vasculopathy

livedo-patterned disease

liver
- l. allograft
- l. allotransplantation
- bioartificial l. (BAL)
- l. disease
- ELAD artificial l.
- l. extract
- l. palm
- l. spot
- l. transaminase level

lividity

living
- activities of daily l.
- l. donor (LD)
- l. donor liver transplantation (LDLT)
- l. skin equivalent (LSE)

livor

Livostin Ophthalmic

lizard skin

LLDN
- laparoscopic live donor nephrectomy

LLS
- lazy leukocyte syndrome

LM
- lentigo melanoma

LMM
- lentigo maligna melanoma

LN
- lupus nephritis

Loa
- *L. loa*

loa
- *Filaria l.*
- *Loa l.*
- *L. loa* infection

5-LO-activating protein

loading
- mechanical l.

loaiasis

Lobana wound cleanser

lobar bronchus

lobenzarit disodium

loblolly
- l. pine
- l. pine tree

Lobo disease

lobomycosis

lobster

lobucavir

lobular panniculitis

local
- l. anaphylaxis
- l. anesthetic allergy
- l. immunity

localisata
- junctional epidermolysis bullosa atrophicans l.

localized
- l. acquired cutaneous pseudoxanthoma elasticum
- l. albinism
- l. angiokeratoma
- l. cutaneous amyloidosis
- epidermolysis bullosa, l.
- l. epidermolysis bullosa simplex
- epidermolysis bullosa simplex, l.
- l. granuloma annulare
- l. lipodystrophy
- l. mucocutaneous candidiasis
- l. neurodermatitis
- l. pagetoid reticulosis
- l. pemphigoid of Brunsting-Perry
- l. progressive systemic sclerosis
- l. pustular psoriasis
- l. scleroderma
- l. tuberculous meningitis
- l. vitiligo

loci (*pl. of* locus)

Locilex
- L. pexiganan acetate cream
- L. topical cream

Locoid topical

locomotor ataxia

Loctite 15494 ethyl cyanoacrylate glue

loculation

locus, pl. **loci**
- histocompatibility l. (HL)
- l. minoris resistentiae
- T l.

locust
- black l.
- l. tree pollen

lodgepole
- l. pine
- l. pine tree

Lodine

lodoxamide tromethamine

Loesche classification

Loewenthal reaction

Löffler syndrome

LOFFLEX
- low-fiber, fat-limited exclusion diet

Lofgren syndrome

Löfqvist tourniquet

logarithmic phase

logic
hierarchical clustering
discrimination l.
logit transformation
LogMAR visual acuity
LOH
loss of heterozygosity
loiasis
Loiasis filariasis
LoKara lotion
Lolium perenne **allergen**
Lol p allergen (I-III)
Lombardy leprosy
lomefloxacin hydrochloride
Lomir
lomustine
London
L. Drugs Sport
L. Drugs Sunblock
L. Drugs Sunscreen
lonestari
Borrelia l.
Lone Star tick
long
l. incubation hepatitis
l. thoracic nerve entrapment
l. thoracic nerve palsy
long-acting
Sinex L.-a.
l.-a. thyroid stimulator (LATS)
longbeachae
Legionella l.
long-distance running
long-handled dressing reacher
longibrachiatum
Trichoderma l.
longior
Tyroglyphus l.
longitudinal
l. hyperpigmented band
l. melanonychia
l. nail hyperpigmentation
long-pulse
super l.-p. (SLP)
long-pulsed
l.-p. dye laser
l.-p. potassium-titanyl-phosphate
laser
long-term-care facility (LTCF)
long-term repeat sequence (LTR)
Loniten oral

look
Hippocratic l.
loop
l. diuretic
Roux-Y l.
Loo punch
loose
l. anagen hair syndrome
l. body
l. jointedness
l. skin
loperamide
lophate
Lophatherum gracile
lopinavir/ritonavir
l. capsule
l. oral solution
lopinavir and ritonavir
Loprox
Lopurin
Lorabid
loracarbef
loratadine and pseudoephedrine
lordosis
lumbar l.
lorgnette
la main en l.
Loroxide
Lortat-Jacobs disease
Lortuss DM oral liquid
Losartan
loss
chronic blood l.
eyebrow l.
eyelash l.
hair l.
hearing l.
height l.
l. of heterozygosity (LOH)
powered air l.
transepidermal water l. (TEWL)
weight l.
lost
healthy years of life l. (HYLL)
Lotemax
loteprednol
lotion
Active Dry L.
alcoholic white shake l.
alpha hydroxy acid l.
Alpha Keri l.
Amerigel l.

NOTES

lotion *(continued)*
    Aqua Glycolic L.
    Aquanil l.
    A/T/S l.
    Aveeno skin replenishing cleansing l.
    Balneol l.
    BlemErase L.
    Caladryl l.
    calamine l.
    Carmol 10 body l.
    Carmol scalp treatment l.
    Clear Confident antifungal topical l.
    clobetasol propionate l.
    Clobex l.
    clotrimazole/betamethasone dipropionate l.
    colored alcoholic shake l.
    Complex 15 l.
    dihydroxyacetone self-tanning l.
    Fostril l.
    G-well L.
    HydroSkin l.
    IvyBlock L.
    Kinerase l.
    Klaron l.
    Komed l.
    Kwell L.
    Liquimat l.
    LoKara l.
    Lotrimin AF L.
    Lotrisone l.
    Lubriderm daily UV l.
    MetroLotion topical l.
    Neutrogena Healthy Skin face l.
    Neutrogena On-The-Spot Acne L.
    Neutrogena Sensitive Skin sunblock l.
    nonalcoholic white shake l.
    Nova Perfecting L.
    Ombrelle sunscreen l.
    Panscol L.
    Pen-Kera l.
    Pennsaid topical l.
    Reactive Skin Decontamination L.
    Scabene L.
    Sebasorb l.
    Shade UvaGuard sunscreen l.
    Skinvisible l.
    sodium sulfacetamide l.
    sulfacetamide sodium scalp treatment l.
    talc l.
    tanning l.
    Tecnu Outdoor Skin Cleanser l.
    Tinver L.
    T4N5 liposome l.
    triamcinolone l. (TAL)

Lotriderm
Lotrimin
    L. AF Cream
    L. AF Lotion
    L. AF Solution
    L. AF Spray Liquid
    L. AF Spray Powder
Lotrisone lotion
Lou Gehrig disease
Louis-Bar syndrome
louping
    l. ill
    l. ill virus
louse, pl. **lice**
    body l.
    clothes l.
    crab l.
    End Lice
    head l.
    l. infestation
    pubic l.
    scalp l.
    sucking l.
louse-borne
    l.-b. relapsing fever
    l.-b. typhus
lousiness
lousy
Lovibond
    L. angle
    L. profile sign
low
    l. absolute glomerular filtration rate
    l. air-loss bed
    l. avidity
    l. back pain
    l. cyclosporine
    l. flow rate
    l. frequency transduction
    l. inflammatory response
    l. plasma albumin
    l. urine pH
    l. virulence vaccine
low-density lipoprotein cholesterol (LDL-C)
low-dose Excimer 308-nm laser
low-egg-passage vaccine
Löwenstein-Jensen agar
lower respiratory tract symptoms (LRSx)
low-fiber, fat-limited exclusion diet (LOFFLEX)
low-frequency microsatellite instability
low-grade
    l.-g. fever
    l.-g. squamous intraepithelial lesion (LSIL)
low-phenylalanine diet
low-tyrosine diet

Loxosceles
>L. *laeta*
>L. *reclusa*
>L. *reclusa* bite

loxoscelism
>necrotic cutaneous l.
>viscerocutaneous l.

lozenge
>zinc gluconate l.

LP
>AstraZeneca LP

LPAR
>late-phase allergic reaction

LPCR
>late-phase cutaneous reaction

LPG
>lipophosphoglycan

l-phenylalanine mustard

LPI excimer laser system

LPR
>late pulmonary response

LPS
>lipopolysaccharide

LPS-induced arthritis

Lr dose

LRS
>lymphoreticular system

LRSS
>late respiratory systemic syndrome

LRSx
>lower respiratory tract symptoms

2-L rubber bag

LSE
>living skin equivalent

L-selectin

LSIL
>low-grade squamous intraepithelial lesion

LSR
>laser skin resurfacing

LT
>lethal toxin
>leukotriene

LTA
>lipoteichoic acid

LTA$_4$
>LTA$_4$ hydrolase
>LTA$_4$ hydrolase gene disruption

LTB4
>leukotriene B4
>dihydroxy leukotriene, LTB4

LTC4
>cysteinyl leukotriene, LTC$_4$
>LTC4 synthase

LTCF
>long-term-care facility

LTR
>long-term repeat sequence

LTRA
>leukotriene receptor antagonist

L-tryptophan
>L-t. ingestion

Lu antigen

Lubath oil

lubricant

lubricant/emollient
>Bag Balm l./e.
>Udder Butter l./e.

lubrication
>elastohydrodynamic l.
>skin l.

lubricin

Lubriderm
>L. daily UV lotion
>L. moisturizer

LubriTears solution

lucent cleft

lucida
>lamina l.

lucid layer

lucidum
>stratum l.

luciferase reporter gene

luciliae
>*Crithidia* l.

Lucio
>diffuse leprosy of L.
>L. leprosy
>L. leprosy phenomenon

Lucké
>L. adenocarcinoma
>L. carcinoma
>L. virus

lucotherapy

Ludiomil

Ludwig angina

Luer-Lok syringe

lues
>l. nervosa
>l. tarda
>l. venerea

luetic mask

Lufyllin

L

NOTES

325

lugdunensis
 Staphylococcus l.
Luikart dissector
Lukes-Collins non-Hodgkin lymphoma classification
lumbar
 l. corset
 l. ganglionectomy
 l. lordosis
 l. spinal stenosis
 l. spine
lumberman's itch
lumbosacral supporter
lumbricoides
 Ascaris l.
lumican
luminal antigen
lumiracoxib
Lumitene
lumpy
 l. jaw
 l. skin disease
Lunar bone density machine
lunata
 Curvularia l.
lunate
lunate-capitate
lunch-time peel
Lund-Browder
 L.-B. burn scale
 L.-B. classification
lung
 l. allograft
 bathtub refinisher's l.
 l. biopsy
 bird-breeder's l.
 bird-fancier's l. (BFL)
 butterfly l.
 cheese washer's l.
 diffuse interstitial fibrosis of the l.
 l. disease
 enzyme worker's l.
 epoxy resin l.
 farmer's l.
 honeycomb l.
 humidifier l.
 l. interstitium
 l. involvement
 malt-worker's l.
 mushroom-picker's l.
 mushroom-worker's l.
 paprika-splitter's l.
 pituitary snuff taker's l.
 plastic-worker's l.
 smallpox-handler's l.
 thresher's l.
lunula, pl. **lunulae**
 diffusion of the l.
 red l.

 spotted l.
 l. unguis
Lunyo virus
lupiform
lupinosa
 porrigo l.
lupoid
 l. acne
 l. hepatitis
 l. leishmaniasis
 l. sclerosis
 l. sycosis
 l. ulcer
luposa
 tuberculosis cutis l.
lupus
 l. alopecia
 l. arthritis
 cardiopulmonary l.
 Cazenave l.
 l. cerebritis
 chilblain l.
 cutaneous l.
 discoid l.
 drug-induced l.
 l. erythematosus cell
 l. erythematosus cell test
 l. erythematosus discoides
 l. erythematosus disseminatus (LED)
 l. erythematosus hypertrophicus
 l. erythematosus, neonatal
 l. erythematosus panniculitis
 l. erythematosus phenomenon
 l. erythematosus profundus
 l. erythematosus tumidus
 l. erythematous-like rash
 l. fibrosus
 l. glomerulonephritis
 hematologic l.
 l. livedo
 l. lymphaticus
 l. miliaris disseminatus faciei
 musculoskeletal l.
 l. mutilans
 neonatal l.
 l. nephritis (LN)
 neurologic l.
 l. papillomatosus
 l. pernio
 l. profundus/panniculitis
 renal l.
 l. sebaceous
 l. sebaceus
 l. serpiginosus
 l. superficialis
 l. syndrome
 l. thrombophilia
 l. tuberculosus

l. verrucosus
l. vorax
l. vulgaris
lupus-like syndrome
lupus-scleroderma overlap syndrome
Luschka joint
lusitaniae
    Candida l.
Lustra-AF
Lustra cream
Lutheran blood group
Lutz-Miescher disease
Lutzomyia
Lutz-Splendore-Almeida disease
Luxar NovaPulse laser
Luxiq ViaFoam betamethasone valerate foam
lwoffi
    Acinetobacter l.
LXA₄ R
LX 20 laser
Ly antigen
Lyb antigen
lycopenemia
lycopodium
    granuloma l.
Lyderm
Lyell
    L. disease
    L. syndrome
Lymantria
    L. dispar
    L. dispar sting
Lyme
    L. arthritis
    L. borreliosis
    L. disease DNA detection
    L. disease (stage 1–3)
Lymephobia
LYMErix
lymph
    l. cell
    l. gland
    l. node
    l. node biopsy
    l. nodule
    vaccine l.
    l. varix
lymphadenitis
    dermatopathic l.
    necrotizing l.

regional granulomatous l.
tuberculosis l.
lymphadenoma
lymphadenomatosis
lymphadenopathy
    angioblastic l.
    dermatopathic l.
    drug-induced l.
    hilar l.
    persistent generalized l. (PGL)
lymphadenopathy-associated virus (LAV)
lymphadenosis
    benign l.
    l. benigna cutis
    l. cutis benigna
lymphangiectasia
lymphangiectasis
lymphangiectatica
    pachyderma l.
lymphangiectatic elephantiasis
lymphangiectodes
lymphangioendothelioma
    benign l.
lymphangioleiomyomatosis
lymphangioma
    l. capillare varicosum
    l. cavernosum
    cavernous l.
    l. circumscriptum
    l. cysticum
    solitary simple l.
    l. superficium simplex
    l. tuberosum multiplex
    l. xanthelasmoideum
lymphangiomyomatosis
lymphangiosarcoma
    postmastectomy l.
lymphangitis
    ascending l.
    l. carcinomatosa
    indurated l.
    penile sclerosing l.
    sclerosing l.
lymphapheresis
lymphatic
    l. cisternae
    dermal l.'s
    l. malformation
    l. nevus
lymphaticus
    lupus l.

L

NOTES

lymphaticus *(continued)*
    nevus l.
    varix l.
lymphatolytic serum
Lymphazurin
lymphedema
    chronic hereditary l.
    hereditary l.
    l. praecox
    primary l.
    secondary l.
lymphedema-distichiasis syndrome
lymphedematous keratoderma
lymphoablative technique
lymphoblastic lymphoma (LBL)
lymphoblastoma
lymphocele
LymphoCide antibody
lymphocutaneous pattern
lymphocytapheresis
lymphocyte
    l. activation
    B l.
    l. chemoattractant activity
    l. function assay
    l. function-associated antigen (LFA)
    l. homing receptor
    homologous to lymphotoxin, shows
      inducible expression and competes
      with herpes simplex virus
      glycoprotein D for herpes virus
      entry mediator, a receptor
      expressed by T l. (LIGHT)
    l. immune globulin
    large granular l. (LGL)
    peripheral blood l. (PBL)
    l. recirculation
    sensitized l.
    l. serine esterase
    l. subset count
    T l.
    T-helper-2 l. (TH2)
    l. transformation
    transformed l.
    tumor-infiltrating l. (TIL)
lymphocytic
    l. apoptosis
    l. choriomeningitis (LCM)
    l. disease
    l. hypophysitis
    l. infiltrate of Jessner
    l. infiltration
    l. infiltration of the skin
    l. interstitial pneumonitis (LIP)
    l. leukemia
    l. vasculitis
lymphocytoma
    Borrelia l.
    l. cutis

lymphocytopenia
lymphocytosis
    diffuse infiltrative l.
    l. syndrome
lymphocytotoxic antibody
lymphoderma
lymphoepithelioid lymphoma
lymphogenous metastasis
lymphogranuloma
    l. benignum
    l. inguinale
    l. venereum antigen
    l. venereum conjunctivitis
    l. venereum virus
lymphogranulomatosis
    l. benigna
    l. maligna
    Schaumann benign l.
lymphohistiocytic
lymphohistiocytosis
    familial erythrophagocytic l.
lymphoid
    l. cell
    l. hypophysitis
    l. infiltrate
    l. leukemia
lymphokine
    production of l.
lymphokine-activated killer (LAK)
lympholeukocyte
lymphoma-associated follicular mucinosis
lymphomagenesis
lymphoma/leukemia
lymphomatoid granulomatosis
lymphomatosis
    avian l.
    fowl l.
    ocular l.
    visceral l.
lymphomatous erythroderma
lymphopathia venereum
lymphopenia
lymphopenic thymic dysplasia
lymphoplasmacytapheresis
lymphoplasmacytic
lymphoplasmacytoid lymphoma cell
Lymphoprep Tube
lymphoproliferative disease
lymphoreticular
    l. cell
    l. disorder
    l. system (LRS)
lymphoreticulosis
    benign inoculation l.
lymphosarcoma
    fascicular l.
    sclerosing l.
lymphosarcomatosis
lymphoscintigraphy

lymphostatic verrucosis
lymphotoxicity
lymphotoxin
lymphotrophism
lymphotropic retrovirus
Lynghya dermatitis
Lyofoam
    L. A, C, T foam dressing
    L. Extra foam dressing
Lyon effect
lyophilized
    l. extract
    l. immunoglobulin G
Lyphocin injection
Lyra laser system
lysate
lyse
lysin
lysine mutation
lysinogen
lysinogenic
lysis
    endothelial l.
    host-cell l.
    NK cell l.
    reactive l.
lysogen
lysogenesis

lysogenic
    l. bacterium
    l. induction
    l. strain
lysogenicity
lysogenization
lysogeny
lysosomal
    l. enzyme
    l. glycoprotein
    l. proteinase
lysosomotropic antimalarial drug
lysozyme
    hen egg l. (HEL)
lysozyme-associated amyloidosis
lyssa
Lyssavirus
lysyl oxidase
Lyt antigen
lytic
    l. enzyme
    l. Epstein-Barr virus
Lytta
    L. vesicata
    L. vesicata sting
lyze
LZRS
    Lazarus

L

NOTES

329

M

M antigen
Back-Ese M
CarraSorb M
M cell
oncostatin M (OSM)
M protein

M1

streptococcal M1

2M

A 2M

M3

streptococcal M3

MA

monoarthritis

Maalox H2 Acid Controller

MAb

MEDI-507 anti-CD2 Mab

MAb-170 monoclonal antibody

MABP

maltose-binding protein

MabThera monoclonal antibody

MAb therapy

MAC

membrane attack complex
membranolytic attack complex
microcystic adnexal carcinoma
Mycobacterium avium complex

maceachernii

Legionella m.

macerate

macerated

maceration

interdigital m.
plantar m.

machination

machine

CPM m.
G5 massage and percussion m.
Lunar bone density m.
Northland bone density m.
PhotoDerm m.
m. preservation (MP)
Respitrace m.
Sysmex SE-9500 m.

machinery

intercellular m.

machine-worker dermatitis

Machupo virus

MacIsaac disease

MacMARCKS protein

Macritonin

Macrobid

macrocheilia, macrochilia

macrocheiria, macrochiria

macrochimerism

multilineage m.
transient m.

macrocytase

macrodactylia

Macrodantin

macroglobulinemia

Waldenström m. (WM)

macroglossia

macrolabia

macrolide antimicrobial agent

macromelia

macromolecule

bacterial m.

macronychia

macrophage

activated m.
alveolar m.
armed m.
associated m.
m. colony-stimulating factor (M-CSF)
dendritic m.
m. fibroblast
hemosiderin-laden m.
immune-associated antigen-positive m. (Ia+)
inflammatory m.
m. inflammatory protein (MIP)
marginal metallophilic m.
marginal zone m.
m. migration inhibition test
scavenger m.
system of m.

macrophage-activating factor (MAF)

macrophage-derived

m.-d. chemokine (MDC)
m.-d. tumor necrosis factor

macrophage-like synoviocyte

macrophagic myofasciitis

macrophagocyte

macroscopic agglutination test

macrosteatosis

macrovascular

macrovesicular steatosis

mactans

Latrodectus m.

macula, pl. **maculae**

m. atrophica
cerebral m.
m. cerulea
m. gonorrhoica
mongolian m.
Saenger m.
m. solaris

M

macular
> m. amyloidosis
> m. atrophy
> m. erythema
> m. leprosy
> m. purpura
> m. rash
> m. syphilid

maculata
> parapsoriasis m.
> pityriasis m.

maculate

maculation

maculatum
> atrophoderma striatum et m.

macule
> ash-leaf m.
> atrophic m.
> cayenne pepper-like m.
> confetti m.
> congenital hypomelanotic m.
> darkly pigmented m.
> evanescent m.
> hypopigmented m.
> labial melanotic m.
> lance-ovate m.
> mongolian m.

maculoanesthetic leprosy

maculoerythematous

maculopapular rash

maculopapule

maculosa
> lepra m.
> purpura m.
> urticaria m.

maculosus
> herpes tonsurans m.
> nevus m.

Madajet XL local anesthesia

madarosis

Madelung disease

madescent

madidans
> eczema m.

Madin-Darby
> M.-D. bovine kidney (MDBK)
> M.-D. bovine kidney cell

mad itch

madre
> buba m.

Madura
> M. boil
> M. foot

madurae
> *Actinomadura m.*

Madurella
> *M. grisea*
> *M. mycetomi*

maduromycosis

mAECA
> monoclonal antiendothelial cell antibody

maedi virus

MAF
> macrophage-activating factor

mafenide acetate

Maffucci syndrome

mafosfamide

Magan

MAGE
> melanoma-associated gene

Magellan Monitor

maggot
> Congo floor m.
> m. therapy

magnesium
> esomeprazole m.
> m. salicylate
> m. sulfate

magnetic resonance imaging (MRI)

magnetic-resonance imaging-compatible hollow-fiber bioreactor

magnetization transfer imaging (MTI)

magnolia

magnus
> *Peptostreptococcus m.*

Magsal

MAI
> *Mycobacterium avium-intracellulare*
> MAI bacteremia

MAINA
> monoclonal antibody immobilization of neutrophil antigens

maintenance
> m. cyclosporine monotherapy (mCsA)
> m. dose

Majocchi
> M. disease
> M. granuloma
> M. purpura
> purpura annularis telangiectodes of M.

major
> m. agglutinin
> aphthae m.
> *Babesia m.*
> m. basic protein (MBP)
> erythema multiforme m.
> m. histocompatibility
> m. histocompatibility complex class II allele DRB1, DRB3, DRB4, DRB5, and DQB1
> m. histocompatibility complex class I, II
> m. histocompatibility complex restriction (MHC)
> *Leishmania m.*

m. outer membrane protein
  (MOMP)
thalassemia m.
variola m.
majus
  Chelidonium m.
  erythema multiforme m. (EMM)
  unclassified erythema multiforme m.
makeup
  Covermark corrective m.
  Dermablend m.
mal
  m. de Cayenne
  m. de los pintos
  m. del pinto
  m. de Meleda
  m. de San Lazaro
  m. morado
  m. perforans
  m. perforant
  m. perforant du pied
Malabar
  M. itch
  M. leprosy
  M. ulcer
malabarica
  phlegmasia m.
malabsorption
  fat m.
  lactose m.
malachite green
malacoplakia
maladie du sommeil
malady
  Mortimer m.
malaise
malakoplakia
malaleuca tree
malar
  m. butterfly rash
  m. erythema
malaria
  apocrine m.
  cerebral m.
  m. prophylaxis
  therapeutic m.
malariae
  Plasmodium m.
malarial therapy
Malassezia
  M. furfur
  M. furfur pustulosis

M. globosa
M. obtusa
M. ovalis
M. pachydermatis
M. restricta
M. slooffiae
M. sympodialis
malathion
malayi
  Brugia m.
MALDI-TOF
  matrix-assisted laser desorption
  ionization-time of flight
male
  m. pattern alopecia
  m. pattern baldness
maleate
  azatadine m.
  brompheniramine m.
  chlorpheniramine m.
  dexchlorpheniramine m.
  methysergide m.
malformation
  capillary m.
  cystic lymphatic m.
  familial multiple mucocutaneous
    venous m.
  glomuvenous m.
  lymphatic m.
  venous m.
Malherbe
  calcifying epithelioma of M.
  M. calcifying epithelioma
  epithelioma of M.
  M. tumor
malic acid
maligna
  lentigo m.
  lymphogranulomatosis m.
  onychia m.
  papulosis atrophicans m.
  pustula m.
  scarlatina m.
  variola m.
malignancy
  B-cell m.
  Epstein-Barr virus-associated m.
  myositis with m.
  nonmelanoma cutaneous m.
  systemic m.
malignant
  m. acanthosis nigricans

M

NOTES

333

malignant *(continued)*
 m. angioendotheliomatosis
 m. atrophic papulosis
 m. blue nevus
 m. bubo
 m. catarrhal fever
 m. catarrhal fever virus
 m. catarrh of cattle
 m. chondroid syringoma
 m. clear cell acrospiroma
 m. degeneration
 m. down
 m. dyskeratosis
 m. eccrine poroma
 m. eccrine spiradenoma
 m. fibrous histiocytoma (MFH)
 m. glomus tumor (MGT)
 m. hemangioendothelioma
 m. hemangiopericytoma
 m. histiocytosis
 m. lentigo melanoma
 m. lymphoma
 m. melanoma in situ
 m. mole syndrome
 m. neoplasia
 m. neoplastic disease
 m. neuroleptic syndrome
 m. nodular hidradenoma
 m. papillomatosis
 m. papillomatosis of Degos
 m. peripheral nerve sheath tumor
 m. porokeratosis
 m. potentially fatal asthma
 m. progression
 m. pustule
 m. pyoderma
 m. smallpox
 m. systemic mastocytosis
 m. transformation
maligne
 papulose atrophicante m.
malignum
 granuloma m.
 keratoma m.
malignus
 pemphigus m.
malingering
Malis scissors
Mallazine Eye drops
mallei
 Malleomyces m.
mallein
malleinization
Malleomyces
 M. mallei
 M. pseudomallei
mallet toe
malleus
Mallorca miliary actinic acne

malnutrition
 episodic m.
 protein-energy m. (PEM)
malodorous sweat
Maloney leukemia virus
malpighian layer
malpighii
 stratum m.
MALT
 mucosa-associated lymphoid tissue
 MALT lymphoma
malt
Malta fever
maltase
 acid m.
Maltese cross
maltodextrin
 Calgitrol calcium alginate wound
 dressing with m.
maltophilia
 Pseudomonas m.
 Stenotrophomonas m.
 Xanthomonas m.
maltose-binding protein (MABP, MBP)
malt-worker's lung
malum
 m. coxae senilis
 m. perforans
 m. perforans pedis
Malvern analyzer
MAM
 Mycoplasma arthritidis mitogen
mamanpian
mammal allergen
mammary
 m. cancer virus of mice
 m. Paget disease
 m. tumor virus of mice
mammilla, pl. **mammillae**
mammilliform
mammillitis
 bovine herpes m.
 bovine ulcerative m.
 bovine vaccinia m.
manager
 Integrated Wound M.
Manchurian
 M. hemorrhagic fever
 M. typhus
Mancini technique
mandibulae
 torus m.
mandibular
 m. movement
 m. torus
mandibuloacral dysplasia
mandibulofacial dysostosis
Mandol

mandrillaris
> *Balamuthia m.*

maneuver
> all-fours m.
> Apley m.
> arm duration m.
> arm raises m.
> arm straighten m.
> chair-rise m.
> floor-sit m.
> Gower m.
> leg-raise m.
> neck flexion m.
> pick-up m.
> Proetz m.
> stool-step m.
> straight-leg duration m.
> straight-leg lift m.
> supine-to-prone m.
> supine-to-sit m.
> touch object m.
> Valsalva m.

manganese superoxide dismutase gene

mange
> demodectic m.
> follicular m.
> sarcoptic m.

mango dermatitis

manifestation
> allergic m.
> clinical m.
> cutaneous m.
> mucocutaneous m.
> presenting clinical m.

manipulation
> gene m.

Mankin histologic/histochemical scale

mannan-binding
> m.-b. lectin (MBL)
> m.-b. lectin deficiency

mannequin

mannitol

mannose-binding
> m.-b. lectin (MBL)
> m.-b. molecule
> m.-b. protein

mannosidosis

Mann-Whitney U test

man-of-war
> Portuguese m.-o.-w.

MANOVA
> multivariate analysis of variance

Manson
> M. hemoptysis
> M. pyosis
> M. schistosomiasis

Mansonella
> *M. ozzardi*
> *M. streptocerca*

mansoni
> *Cladosporium m.*
> *Schistosoma m.*

Mantadil

Mantel-Haenszel
> M.-H. test
> M.-H. test for linearity
> M.-H. weighted odds ratio

M_1 antigen

mantle
> Acid M.
> m. cell lymphoma

Mantoux
> M. pit
> M. test

manubriosternal joint

manum

manus
> tinea pedis et m.

manuum
> keratolysis exfoliativa areata m.
> tinea m.

MAO
> monoamine oxidase
> MAO inhibitor

MAP
> mitogen-activated protein
> mitogen-activating protein
> multiantigenic peptide

map
> proteomic m.

Mapharsen organic arsenic

MAPK
> mitogen-activated protein kinase

maple
> m. bark disease
> box elder m.
> red m.
> sugar m.
> m. tree
> m. tree pollen

maple-bark stripper's disease

mapping
> epitope m.

M

NOTES

mapping *(continued)*
 fluorescence overlay antigen m.
  (FOAM)
Maprotiline
Maranox
marasmic kwashiorkor
marasmus
Marax
Marbaxin
marble
 m. cake hyperpigmentation
 m. skin
marblization
MarBlot test kit
Marburg
 M. virus
 M. virus disease
MARC
 Multicenter Airway Research
  Collaboration
Marcaine
Marcelle Sunblock
marcescens
 Serratia m.
march
 atopic m.
 m. fracture
Marcillin
Marek
 M. disease
 M. disease virus
Marena compression garment
Marezine
Marfan
 M. law
 M. syndrome
marfanoid habitus
margarine disease
margin
 free m.
 hidden m.
marginal
 m. alopecia
 m. band
 m. donor
 m. metallophilic macrophage
 m. nevus
 m. zone B-cell lymphoma (MZBL)
 m. zone macrophage
marginalis
 alopecia m.
 keratoelastoidosis m.
marginata
 alopecia m.
margination
 lesion m.
marginatum
 eczema m.

 erythema m.
 keratoacanthoma centrifugum m.
Marie-Bamberger syndrome
Marie-Strümpell disease
marigold
marine
 m. animal sting
 m. dermatitis
Marinesco-Sjögren syndrome
Marinesco succulent hand
Marinol
marinum
 Mycobacterium m.
marionette line
Marjolin ulcer
mark
 beauty m.
 dhobie m.
 ecchymotic m.
 erythematous m.
 port-wine m.
 strawberry m.
 stretch m.
 Unna m.
 washerman's m.
marked localized reaction
marker
 allotypic m.
 bone formation m.
 bone resorption m.
 bone turnover m.
 cell surface m.
 D'Assumpeau rhytidoplasty m.
 DR/MLC cell m.
 erythrocyte sheet rosette cell m.
 FAB-1 cell m.
 m. gene
 genetic m.
 highly polymorphic
  microsatellite m.
 Ia cell m.
 pan T-cell m.
 peroxidase cell m.
 serum m.
 solid-tumor m.
 Sudan cell m.
 surrogate m.
 T-cell m.
 tumor m.
market men disease
marking
 bronchovascular m.
Markov state-transition model
Marmine
 M. Injection
 M. oral
marmorata
 cutis m.
marmorated

marmorization
marmoset virus
marneffei
    Penicillium m.
Maroteaux-Lamy
    M.-L. mucopolysaccharidosis
    M.-L. syndrome
marrow
    m. failure syndrome
    m. space
Marseilles fever
Marshall syndrome
Marshall-White syndrome
marsh elder
marsupialization
Marthritic
Marzola flap
Mas antigen
mascara
    solvent-based m.
    water-based m.
maschalephidrosis
maschalyperidrosis
mask
    Acnomel Acne M.
    m. burn
    Hutchinson m.
    luetic m.
    Neutrogena Acne M.
    m. of pregnancy
    Swiss Therapy eye m.
    tropical m.
masked virus
Mason-Pfizer virus
masoprocol cream
masque biliaire
MASS
    mitral valve prolapse, aortic anomalies,
    skeletal changes, and skin changes
    MASS syndrome
mass
    body m.
    m. infection
    m. median aerodynamic diameter
    (MMD)
massive cerebral edema
massive-dose desensitization
Masson
    M. intravascular endothelial
    proliferation
    M. nevus
    M. pseudoangiosarcoma

M. trichrome
M. trichrome stain
mast
    m. cell
    m. cell degranulation test
    m. cell inhibitor
    m. cell proteinase
Mastadenovirus
mastectomy
    radical m.
master regulator gene
masticatory
    m. pain
    m. system
Mastisol
mastitis
    bovine m.
mastocyte
mastocytoma
    solitary m.
mastocytosis
    benign systemic m.
    cutaneous m.
    diffuse cutaneous m.
    malignant systemic m.
    papular m.
    pseudoxanthomatous m.
    m. syndrome
    systemic m.
    telangiectatic systemic m.
mastoiditis
Masugi nephritis
mat
    m. burn
    Harris pressure m.
    telangiectatic m.
Matarasso facelift scissors
matchbox sign
matched
    m. related donor (MRD)
    m. unrelated donor (MURD)
    m. unrelated donor stem cell
    transplant (mini-MUD)
material
    cross-reacting m.
    Cutinova Cavity wound filling m.
    DermAssist hydrocolloid
    dressing m.
    DermAssist wound filling m.
    Dermatell hydrocolloid dressing m.
    Epicel skin graft m.
    ExuDerm hydrocolloid dressing m.

M

NOTES

material *(continued)*
    keratinous m.
    keratotic m.
    periodic acid-Schiff-positive m.
    PolyWic wound filling m.
    RepliCare hydrocolloid dressing m.
    m. safety data sheet (MSDS)
    test m.
maternal immunity
maternus
    nevus m.
Matic UV-Optimize 555 skin reflectance meter
Matricaria recutita
matricectomy
matrices (*pl. of* matrix)
Matrigel
matrilin-1
matrilysin
    a disintegrin and m. (ADAM)
matrix, pl. matrices
    M. collagen
    m. component
    distal nail m.
    fibrin m.
    hair m.
    nail m.
    proximal nail m.
    m. synthesis
    m. unguis
    variance-covariance m.
matrix-assisted laser desorption ionization-time of flight (MALDI-TOF)
matrix-degrading enzyme
matter
    particulate m.
matting
    telangiectatic m. (TM)
mattress
    Akros extended care m.
    AkroTech m.
    convoluted foam m.
    kapok m.
    lateral rotation m.
    Roho m.
    vinyl-alternating air m.
Matuhasi-Ogata phenomenon
maturation
    affinity m.
    m. B cell
mature bacteriophage
maturity-onset diabetes of the young (MODY)
Maurer optimization test
Mauriac syndrome
Mauserung phenomenon

max
    AIR m.
    VO$_2$ m.
Maxacalcitol
Maxafil
Maxair Autohaler
Maxamine
Maxaquin oral
Max-Caro
Maxenal
Maxidex
Maxiflor topical
maxillary occlusal appliance
maximal
    m. oxygen consumption
    m. ventilation (MV)
    m. voluntary ventilation (MVV)
maximum
    m. breathing capacity (MBC)
    M. Strength Desenex Antifungal Cream
    M. Strength Nytol
    m. temperature
Maxi-Myst bronchodilator
Maxiphen DM
Maxipime
Maxitrol Ophthalmic
Maxivate topical
Maxivent
Maxon suture
Maxorb
    M. alginate wound cover
    M. alginate wound dressing
mayapple
    American m.
Mayaro virus
Mayer hemalum
Mayfly
maynei
    Euroglyphus m.
Mayo
    M. classification of rheumatoid elbow
    M. modified total elbow arthroplasty
May-Thurner syndrome
mazamorra
Mazon Medicated Soap
Mazzotti
    M. reaction
    M. test
MBC
    maximum breathing capacity
    minimal bactericidal concentration
MBL
    mannan-binding lectin
    mannose-binding lectin
MBP
    major basic protein

maltose-binding protein
myelin basic protein
MBT
Mycobacterium tuberculosis
McArdle disease
MCCN
McCune-Albright syndrome
McEwen Hyperventilation Questionnaire
MCF
monocyte chemotactic factor
McGill Pain questionnaire
MCGN
mesangiocapillary glomerulonephritis
McKeever and MacIntosh hemiarthroplasty
McKenzie test
McKrae strain of herpesvirus
McKusick
oculocerebral syndrome of Cross and M.
M. syndrome
McKusick-Kaufman syndrome
MCL
mucocutaneous leishmaniasis
McLean Limbic Somatic Symptom
3M Clean Seals bandage
McLeod phenotype
McMurray sign
MCN
minimal change nephropathy
McNeill-Goldman corneal transplant ring
McNemar
M. test
M-component hypergammaglobulinemia
MCP
monocyte chemotactic protein
MCP-1
monocyte chemoattractant protein-1
monocyte chemotactic peptide-1
m-cresyl acetate
mCsA
maintenance cyclosporine monotherapy
M-CSF
macrophage colony-stimulating factor
MCTD
mixed connective tissue disease
MCV
molluscum contagiosum virus
MDBK
Madin-Darby bovine kidney
MDBK cell

MDC
macrophage-derived chemokine
MDI
metered-dose inhaler
isocyanate MDI
MDR-TB
multidrug-resistant tuberculosis
MDS
myelodysplastic syndrome
MDT
multidrug therapy
meadow
m. dermatitis
m. fescue
m. fescue grass
m. foxtail
m. foxtail grass
M. syndrome
meadow-grass
m.-g. dermatitis
m.-g. dermatosis
meal
rye m.
soybean m.
mean (SD)
m. forced expiratory flow during the middle of FVC (FEF$_{25\text{-}75\%}$)
standardized response m. (SRM)
measles
atypical m.
bastard m.
black m.
confluent m.
m. convalescent serum
3-day m.
French m.
German m.
m. immune globulin human
m. immunoglobulin
modified m.
m., mumps and rubella vaccines, combined
m. and rubella virus vaccine (MR-VAX)
tropical m.
m. virus
m. virus vaccine
m. virus vaccine, live
measure
CD4+ M.
European Consensus Lupus Activity M. (ECLAM)

NOTES

M

measure *(continued)*
  m. mucociliary clearance (MMC)
  Systemic Lupus Activity M.
    (SLAM)
Measurin
meatus
mebendazole
Mecca balsam
mechanica
  acne m.
mechanical
  m. abrasion
  m. acne
  m. alopecia
  m. disorder of knee
  m. loading
  m. pleurodesis
  m. vector
  m. ventilation (MV)
  m. ventilator
  m. vessel blockage
mechanic hand
mechanism
  m. of action
  defense m.
  genomic glucocorticoid m.
  immunological m.
  interferon-independent m.
  jet-bubble m.
  nonadrenergic noncholinergic m.
    (NANC)
mechanoblister
mechanobullous disease
mechlorethamine
  cutaneous intolerance to m. (CIM)
  m. hydrochloride
Mecholyl skin test
Meclan topical
meclizine hydrochloride
meclocycline sulfosalicylate
meclofenamate
  m. sodium
meclofenamate sodium
Meclomen oral
MED
  minimal erythema dose
Mederma
MEDI-493
MEDI-507 anti-CD2 Mab
media
  acute otitis m. (AOM)
  chronic otitis m.
  otitis m.
  pneumococcal otitis m.
  radiographic contrast m. (RCM)
  secretory otitis m.
medial
  m. canaliform dystrophy
  m. hemijoint articular space

median
  m. canaliform dystrophy
  m. effective concentration (EC50)
  m. nail dystrophy
  m. nerve
  m. nerve disorder
  m. raphe cyst of the penis
  m. rhomboid glossitis (MRG)
  m. survival time (MST)
mediana
  glossitis rhombica m.
  glossitis rhomboidea m.
mediastinal
  m. amyloidosis
  m. fibrosis
  m. lipomatosis
mediastinoscopy
mediate contagion
mediation
  fibroblast m.
mediator
  m. cell
  downstream m.
  vasoactive m.
medical
  M. Dynamics 5990 needle
    arthroscope
  m. free electron laser (MFEL)
  M. Outcomes Study 36-Item Short
    Form Health Survey
  M. Research Council (MRC)
  M. Research Council Laboratories
    (MRCL)
  m. therapy
medicamentosa
  acne m.
  alopecia m.
  dermatitis m.
  dermatosis m.
  embolia cutis m.
  rhinitis m.
  stomatitis m.
  urticaria m.
medicamentosus
medication-induced hyperlipoproteinemia
medicinal eruption
medicine
  environmental M.
  European Confederation for
    Laboratory M. (ECLM)
  Reese's Pinworm M.
  sports M.
Medi-Facts system
Medifil collagen
Medihaler-Epi Ergotamine
Medihaler-Iso
Medihoney
Medi-Mist nebulizer
medina worm

medinensis
> *Dracunculus m.*

Medin poliomyelitis
Mediplast Plaster
Medipore Dress-it dressing
Medipren
Medi-Quick Topical Ointment
Medi-Strumpf support hose
Mediterranean
> M. erythematous fever
> M. exanthematous fever
> M. lymphoma
> M. spotted fever

medium
> BSK II m.
> Dulbecco modified eagle's m.
> excimer lasing m.
> HAT m.
> He-Ne lasing m.
> Iscove modified Dulbecco m.
> krypton lasing m.
> m. lesion
> Sabouraud m.
> serum-free m. (SFM)
> Thayer-Martin m.
> Tissue-Tek OCT m.

medium-grade drywall sanding screen
medi virus
Medix ultrasonic nebulizer
Medlar body
Medpor surgical implant
Medralone Injection
Medrol
> M. Dosepak
> M. oral
> M. Veriderm

medrysone
medulla
medullary
> m. carcinoma flush
> m. reticulosis

MedWatch
Mees
> M. line
> M. stripe

MEF
> middle ear fluid

mefenamic acid
mefloquine hydrochloride
Mefoxin
Megabombus **sting**
Megace

megacin
megacystic microcolon syndrome
megaloblastic anemia
megalonychia
megalonychosis
Megalopyge
> M. opercularis
> M. opercularis sting

megaterium
> *Bacillus m.*

megestrol acetate
meglumine diatrizoate enema study
MEGX
> monoethylglycinexylidide
> MEGX test/score

meibomian
> m. gland
> m. gland dysfunction

Meinicke test
Meirowsky phenomenon
Meischer syndrome
Meissner corpuscle
MEK
> methyl ethyl ketone

mekongi
> *Schistosoma m.*

Melacine vaccine
Melaleuca alternifolia
Melanex solution
melanidrosis
melanin
> hair m.
> m. synthesis
> m. transfer
> white m.

melaninogenica
> *Prevotella m.*

melanism
melanoacanthoma
> oral m.

melanoacanthosis
melanoblast
melanoblastoma
melanocarcinoma
melanocomous
melanocyte
> cultured autologous m.
> intradermal m.

melanocyte-stimulating hormone (MSH)
melanocytic
> m. activation

M

NOTES

melanocytic *(continued)*
    m. nevus
    m. proliferation
melanocytosis
    dermal m.
    oculodermal m.
melanoderma
    m. cachecticorum
    m. chloasma
    parasitic m.
    racial m.
    Riehl m.
    senile m.
melanodermatitis toxica lichenoides
melanodermia
melanodermic
melanodermicum
    erythema chronicum figuratum m.
melanogenesis
melanohidrosis
melanoid
melanoleukoderma colli
melanoma
    ACD features of m.
    amelanotic m.
    benign juvenile m.
    Breslow thickness in malignant m.
    m. cell adhesion molecule (Mel-
      CAM)
    m. cell lysate vaccine
    Cloudman m.
    cutaneous m.
    desmoplastic malignant m.
    halo m.
    juvenile m.
    lentigo m. (LM)
    lentigo maligna m. (LMM)
    malignant lentigo m.
    metastasizing thin m.
    minimal deviation m.
    multiple primary m. (MPM)
    nevoid malignant m. (NMM)
    nodular malignant m.
    ocular m.
    m. in situ
    spindle cell m.
    spitzoid malignant m.
    subungual m.
    superficial malignant m.
    superficial spreading m. (SSM)
    m. theraccine
    m. warning sign
melanoma-associated gene (MAGE)
melanoma-specific antigen
melanomatosis
melanomatous
melanonychia
    longitudinal m.
    m. striata

melanopathy
melanophage
    perifollicular m.
melanophore
melanoplakia
melanoprotein
melanorrhoea
    Anacardium m.
melanosis
    addisonian m.
    m. cachecticorum
    m. circumscripta precancerosa
    m. corii degenerativa
    m. diffusa congenita
    Dubreuilh precancerous m.
    generalized m.
    neonatal pustular m.
    neurocutaneous m.
    oculodermal m.
    primary acquired m. (PAM)
    pustular m.
    Riehl m.
    tar m.
    transient neonatal pustular m.
    universal acquired m.
melanosity
melanosome
melanotic
    m. ameloblastoma
    m. carcinoma
    m. freckle
    m. freckle of Hutchinson
    m. pigment
    m. progonoma
    m. protoporphyria
    m. prurigo of Borda
    m. prurigo of Hebra
    m. prurigo of Pierini
    m. sarcoma
    m. whitlow
melanotrichia
melanotrichous
melas
    icterus m.
melasma
    m. gravidarum
    m. universale
Melastatin
melatonin
Mel-CAM
    melanoma cell adhesion molecule
Meleda
    M. disease
    mal de M.
Meleney
    chronic undermining ulcer of M.
    M. chronic undermining ulcer
    M. gangrene
Melilotus officinalis

melioidosis
    Whitmore m.
Melissa officinalis
Melkersson-Rosenthal syndrome
Melkersson syndrome
Mellaril
mellifera
    Apis m.
mellitus
    diabetes m.
    insulin-dependent diabetes m.
      (IDDM)
    noninsulin-dependent diabetes m.
      (NIDDM)
    posttransplant diabetes m. (PTDM)
    type 1 diabetes m. (T1DM)
    type 2 diabetes m. (T2DM)
Melnick-Fraser syndrome
Meloidae
melorheostosis
meloxicam tablet
melphalan
Melzer reagent
membrane
    antiglomerular basement m. (anti-
      GBM)
    m. attack complex (MAC)
    basal cell m.
    basement m.
    bronchial mucous m.
    Bruch m.
    collodion m.
    croupous m.
    diphtheritic m.
    false m.
    m. filter
    focal rupture of basement m.
    hyaline basement m.
    immunoglobulin m.
    mucous m.
    Pall Biodyne m.
    PAN m.
    plasma m.
    m. ruffling
    semiimpermeable m.
    Seprafilm bioresorbable m.
    subbasement m. (SBM)
    subepithelial basement m. (SBM)
    synovial m.
    tuberculosis of serous m.
    tympanic m. (TM)
membrane-bound cytochrome b$_{558}$

membrane-coating granule
membrane-type matrix metalloproteinase
membranolytic attack complex (MAC)
membranoproliferative glomerulonephritis
membranous
    m. aplasia cutis
    m. desquamation
    m. glomerulonephritis
    m. lupus nephritis
    m. nephropathy (MN)
memory
    B-cell m.
    immune m.
    immunologic m.
MEN
    multiple endocrine neoplasm
    MEN syndrome
MEN 1
men
    Anti-Acne Formula for M.
Menadol
MEND
    minimum effective naproxen dose
Mendelson syndrome
Menest
Mengo
    M. encephalitis
    M. virus
Meni-D
méningéale
    tache m.
meningeal stage
meningioma
    cutaneous m.
meningitic streak
meningitidis
    Neisseria m.
meningitis, pl. meningitides
    African m.
    basal m.
    m. of the base
    basilar m.
    benign recurrent
      endothelioleukocytic m.
    brucellar m.
    m. carcinomatosa
    cerebrospinal m.
    chemical m.
    chronic posterior basic m.
    curable serous m.
    epidemic cerebrospinal m.
    external m.

M

NOTES

meningitis *(continued)*
gummatous m.
Haemophilus influenzae m.
influenzal m.
internal m.
localized tuberculous m.
meningococcal m.
Mollaret m.
m. necrotoxica reactiva
occlusive m.
otitic m.
otogenic m.
plasmodial m.
posttraumatic rheumatic m.
m. sympathica
Torula m.
torular m.
Wallgren aseptic m.
yeast m.
meningocele
atretic m.
rudimentary m.
meningococcal
m. arthritis
m. meningitis
m. polysaccharide vaccine, groups A, C, Y, W-135
m. vaccine
meningococcemia
acute m.
meningoencephalitis
acute primary hemorrhagic m.
biundulant m.
cryptococcal m.
herpetic m.
mumps m.
meningooculofacial angiomatosis
meningosepticum
Flavobacterium m.
meningovascular neurosyphilis
meningovasculitis
meniscal
m. disorder
m. fibrocartilage
meniscus, pl. **menisci**
Menkes kinky hair syndrome
menocelis
Menomune-A/C/Y/W-135
menopausal flushing
menopause
Menorest
menstrual
m. acne
m. dermatosis
menstrualis
herpes m.
mentagra
acne m.
Alibert m.

mentagrophytes
Trichophyton m.
mental
m. retardation, overgrowth, remarkable face, and acanthosis nigricans (MORFAN)
mentalis
herpes m.
Mentax
M. cream
Mentha spicata
menthol
camphorated m.
Mentholatum
MEP
mucoid exopolysaccharide
meperidine
mephenytoin
Mephyton oral
Mepiform self-adherent silicone dressing
Mepilex Transfer dressing
Mepitel
M. contact layer sheet
M. contact-layer wound dressing
mepivacaine hydrochloride
Mepore absorptive dressing
meprobamate
Mepron
mequinol and tretinoin
meralgia paresthetica
merbromin
2-mercaptoethane sulfonate sodium (mesna)
Mercapto mix
6-mercaptopurine (6-MP)
Mercedes
M. Benz incision
M. pattern
mercurial
m. compound
m. stomatitis
mercurials
organic m.
mercuric oxide
mercurochrome
Mercuroclear solution
mercury
ammoniated m.
m. arc
m. granuloma
m. hyperpigmentation
m. poisoning
meridian
Merkel
M. cell
M. cell carcinoma
M. cell tumor
Merkel-cell-neurite complex

Merkel-Ranvier
tactile cell of M.-R.
Merlenate topical
merocrine gland
meropenem for injection
merosin deficiency dystrophy
merozygote
Merrem IV
Mersol
Merthiolate
Meruvax II
mesalamine
Mesalt debridement dressing
mesangial complex formation
mesangiocapillary glomerulonephritis (MCGN)
mesangium
Mesantoin
mesenchymal
m. precursor
m. progenitor cell
m. tissue
mesenchyme
synovial m.
mesentericography
selective m.
mesenteric vasculitis
mesh
absorbable m.
mesher
Tanner m.
meshwork
coagulation m.
mesilate
nafamostat m.
mesna
2-mercaptoethane sulfonate sodium
Mesnex
mesoderm
mesodermal
m. dysplasia
m. nevus
mesodermogenic neurosyphilis
mesogenic
mesophilic
mesosyphilis
mesothelial cell
mesothelioma
mesquite tree
messenger RNA (mRNA)
mestranol

mesylate
bitolterol m.
dihydroergotamine m.
saquinavir m.
MET
minimum elicitation threshold
Metabisulfite
metabolic
m. acidosis
m. alteration
m. bone disease
m. disorder
m. enthesopathy
m. remission
m. study
metabolism
aberrant glycosaminoglycan m.
amino acid m.
arachidonic acid m.
chylomicron m.
copper m.
glycosphingolipid m.
P450 m.
phenylalanine m.
purine m.
transcellular m.
tyrosine m.
metabolite
arachidonic acid m.
16-hydroxylated m.
oxygen m.
metabolizer
poor m. (PM)
metacarpal index
metacarpophalangeal (MP)
m. joint subluxation
metachromasia
metachronous tissue lesion
Metadate ER
metaguazone
metal
m. dermatitis
m. fume fever
m. hyperpigmentation
m. intoxication
metal-catalyzed oxidative cleavage
metalloenzyme
metalloproteinase
membrane-type matrix m.
punctated m.
tissue m.
tissue inhibitor of m. (TIMP)

M

NOTES

metalloproteinase-2
metalloproteinase-3
metalloproteinase-7
metalloproteinase-8
metalloproteinase-9
metalloproteinase-10
metalloscopy
Metamucil
metaphysial, metaphyseal
    m. dysplasia
metaphysis, pl. metaphyses
metaplasia
    agnogenic myeloid m. (AMM)
    eccrine m.
    goblet cell m.
metaplastic mucus-secreting cell
Metaprel
metaproterenol
    Arm-a-Med M.
    Dey-Dose M.
    m. sulfate
metaraminol bitartrate
Metasep
metastasis, pl. metastases
    asymptomatic pulmonary
      melanoma m.
    biochemical m.
    contact m.
    hematogenous m.
    in-transit m.
    lymphogenous m.
    miliary m.
    tumor, nodes, m. (TNM)
metastasizing thin melanoma
metastatic
    m. calcification
    m. calcinosis cutis
    m. granuloma
    m. mumps
    m. tuberculous abscess
metatarsal (MT)
metatarsalgia
metatarsophalangeal (MTP)
    m. joint
metatypical carcinoma
Metazoa
metazoal parasite
metazoan infection
metazoonosis
Metchnikoff theory
Meted
meter
    AccuTrax peak flow m.
    Assess peak flow m.
    Astech peak flow m.
    AsthmaMentor peak flow m.
    Matic UV-Optimize 555 skin
      reflectance m.

    Mini-Wright peak flow m.
    peak flow m.
    Pocketpeak peak flow m.
    TruZone peak flow m.
metered-dose inhaler (MDI)
methacholine
    m. bronchoprovocation challenge
    m. challenge testing
    m. chloride
    m. chloride skin test
Methacin
methacrylate
    butyl m.
    ethyl m.
    polymethyl m.
methandrostenolone
methapyrilene hydrochloride
methdilazine
methenamine
methicillin-resistant *Staphylococcus*
    aureus (MRSA)
methicillin sodium
methionine
methocarbamol
method
    ABC m.
    avidin-biotin-peroxidase complex m.
    m. of Borrow
    Brehmer m.
    Buehler m.
    Cox-Spjotvoll m.
    Dick m.
    dipstick m.
    disc sensitivity m.
    double antibody m.
    Dual-Luciferase assay m.
    Fisher m.
    Genant m.
    heteroduplexing m.
    histoblot m.
    immunofluorescence m.
    Kaplan-Meier m.
    multinomial (polytomous) logistic
      regression m.
    N-geneous m.
    Ouchterlony m.
    pencil m.
    potato-peeler m.
    prick-test m.
    Ranawat triangle m.
    Sakaguchi-Kauppi m.
    Schick m.
    TUNEL m.
    van der Heijde modification of
      Sharp m.
    volumetric m.
methotrexate (MTX)
methoxsalen sterile solution

methoxycinnamate
    octyl m.
    m. and oxybenzone
methoxypromazine
methoxypsoralen
5-methoxypsoralen (5-MOP)
8-methoxypsoralen (8-MOP)
methyl
    m. ethyl ketone (MEK)
    m. nicotinate
    m. salicylate
methylation
    stochastic m.
methylbenzethonium chloride
methylcellulose
methylchloroisothiazoli-
    none/methylisothiazolinone
methyldopa
methylene blue
methylmalonic
methylmercury hydroxide
methylmethacrylate
methylphenidate
methylprednisolone
    m. acetate (MPA)
    pulse m.
methylrosaniline chloride
methylxanthine
methysergide maleate
Meticorten oral
Metimyd Ophthalmic
Metoprolol in Dilated Cardiomyopathy
    Trial
Metreton Ophthalmic
metric system
MetroCream topical cream
MetroGel
    M. topical
    M. topical gel
MetroGel-Vaginal
Metro IV Injection
MetroLotion topical lotion
metronidazole topical gel
Metzenbaum scissors
Mexican tea
mexiletine
Meyerson nevus
Meyhoeffer curette
Mezlin
mezlocillin sodium
MF
    mycosis fungoides

MFEL
    medical free electron laser
MFG-IRAP retrovirus
MFH
    malignant fibrous histiocytoma
MG
    myasthenia gravis
MGC
    multinucleated giant cell
MGT
    malignant glomus tumor
MGUS
    monoclonal gammopathy of
        undetermined significance
    monoclonal gammopathy of unknown
        significance
MHAQ
    Modified Health Assessment
        Questionnaire
MHA-TP
    microhemagglutination-*Treponema*
        pallidum
        MHA-TP test
MHC
    major histocompatibility complex
        restriction
        MHC antigen deficiency
        chromosome 6, class III MHC
        MHC class I, II
        MHC class (I, II) deficiency
        MHC contraction
        MHC molecule
        MHC restriction
Mi-2 antibody
Miacalcin
Miami STAR tissue expander
Mibelli
    angiokeratoma of M.
    M. angiokeratoma
    M. disease
    porokeratosis of M.
    M. porokeratosis
    M. syndrome
MIC
    minimal inhibitory concentration
    minimum inhibitory concentration
micaceous scale
Micanol cream
Micatin Topical
micdadei
    Legionella m.

M

NOTES

mice
- m. allergy
- back m.
- mammary cancer virus of m.
- mammary tumor virus of m.
- New Zealand m.
- pneumonia virus of m. (PVM)
- SCID m.
- severe combined immunodeficient m.
- transgenic m.

micelle

Michel solution

miconazole superabsorbent antifungal powder

micro
- Retin-A M.

microabscess
- intraepidermal m.
- Munro m.
- m. of mycosis fungoides
- Pautrier m.
- m. of psoriasis

Micro-Adson forceps with teeth

microaerophilic

microangiopathic hemolytic anemia

microaspiration

microbe

microbial
- m. associates
- m. genetics
- m. persistence
- m. vitamin

microbic

microbicidal

microbicide
- Pro 2000 topical m.

Microbid

microbiologic

microbiologist

microbiology

microbiotic

microbism
- latent m.

microceras
- *Dermatophagoides m.*

microcheilia

microchimeric
- m. antigen
- m. cell

microchimerism

microcircular

microcirculatory disturbance

Micrococcus

micrococcus, pl. **micrococci**
- coagulase-positive m.

microcontaminant

microcystic adnexal carcinoma (MAC)

microdermabrasion

MicroDigitrapper-HR, -S, -V

microdiskectomy

microdomain

microemulsion
- cyclosporine m.

microenvironment

microevolution

microfibril
- fibrillin-containing m.

microfilaria
- degenerated m.

microfine
- zinc oxide m.

microfocus, pl. **microfoci**

MicroGard

2-microglobulin-origin amyloid deposit

micrognathia

microhemagglutination

microhemagglutination-*Treponema*
- m. pallidum (MHA-TP)

microheterogeneity

microimmunofluorescence test (MIF)

MicroKlenz wound cleanser

microlymphocytotoxicity test

Micro-Mist nebulizer

microNefrin

micronodular tuberculid

micronychia

microorganism

micropapular tuberculid

microperfusion

microphage

microphagocyte

MicroPlaner soft tissue shaver

MicroPlus spirometer

Micropolyspora faeni

Micropore tape

microreactor
- immunoisolating m.

microsampling
- bronchoscopic m. (BMS)

microsatellite
- m. instability (MSI)
- m. polymorphism
- m. stable

microscope
- epiluminescent skin surface m.

microscopic
- m. agglutination test
- m. polyangiitis (MPA)

microscopically controlled surgery

microscopy
- confocal laser scanning m.
- darkfield m.
- dermatoscopy using epiluminescent m.
- dermoscopy using epiluminescent m.
- electron m.

epiluminescence light m. (ELM)
fluorescent m.
immune electron m. (IEM)
immunofluorescence m.
immunogold electron m.
light m.
proton magnetic resonance m.
surface m.
transmission electron m. (TEM)
microshaver
Stryker m.
microspherule
microspore
Microsporidia **diagnostic procedure**
microsporidiosis
microsporina
dermatomycosis m.
Microsporon (*var. of Microsporum*)
microsporon
Audouin m.
microsporosis
Microsporum, Microsporon
M. *audouinii*
M. *canis*
M. *canis, var distortum*
M. *felineum*
M. *ferrugineum*
M. *fulvum*
M. *furfur*
M. *gypseum*
M. *lanosum*
M. *minutissimum*
M. *nanum*
microsteatosis
microstomia
Microsulfon
microti
Babesia m.
MicroTrak test
microtrauma
postexertional m.
Microtrombidium
microtubule organizing center
microvascular abnormality
microvasculopathy
microvenular hemangioma
microvesicle
microvesicular steatosis
Microviridae
MID
minimal infecting dose

midazolam
benzodiazepine m.
middermal elastolysis
middle
m. ear
m. ear fluid (MEF)
midfoot problem
midge
m. bite
nimitti m.
midline
m. granulomatosis
m. lethal granuloma
Midol
M. IB
M. PM
midpoint skin test
midrange spectrum ultraviolet light
midrange-wavelength ultraviolet light
(UVB)
Midrin
Miescher
M. actinic granuloma
M. cheilitis granulomatosa
M. elastoma
M. granulomatous cheilitis
Miescher-Leder granulomatosis
MIF
microimmunofluorescence test
migration-inhibitory factor
Miglin method for arachnophlebectomy
migrans
anulus m.
cutaneous larva m.
erysipelas m.
erythema chronicum m. (ECM)
erythema nodosum m.
larva m.
ocular larva m.
spiruroid larva m.
ulcus m.
visceral larva m.
migrant erysipelas
migrating cheilitis
migration
m. inhibition test
m. inhibitory factor test
Jurkat cell m.
leukocyte m.
transendothelial neutrophil m.
migration-inhibitory factor (MIF)

M

NOTES

migratory
    m. glossitis
    m. panniculitis
Mikulicz
    M. aphtha
    M. disease
mild
    m. hypertension
    m. irritant
    silver protein, m.
    m. wheezy bronchitis (MWB)
Miles Nervine Caplets
milia
    m. cyst
    m. en plaque
Milian
    M. citrine skin
    M. disease
    M. erythema
    M. sign
    M. syndrome
miliaria
    m. alba
    apocrine m.
    m. crystallina
    occlusion m.
    m. papulosa
    m. profunda
    m. propria
    pustular m.
    m. pustulosa
    m. rubra
    sebaceous m.
    m. vesiculosa
miliaris
    acne necrotica m.
    tuberculosis cutis m.
    variola m.
miliary
    m. acne
    m. fever
    m. metastasis
    m. papular syphilid
    m. sarcoid
    m. tuberculosis
milium, pl. milia
    colloid m.
    juvenile colloid m.
    multiple eruptive milia
    m. neonatorum
    periocular milia
    pinhead-sized milia
    pinpoint-sized milia
milk
    acidophilus m.
    m. allergy
    cow's m.
    m. crust
    m. factor

    goat's m.
    lactobacillary m.
    m. scall
    soy m.
    m. tetter
milker's
    m. node
    m. nodule
    m. nodule virus
milk-induced colitis
milkpox
Millar asthma
Miller-Fisher variant
miller's asthma
millet
    M. phlebectomy hook
    m. seed
mill fever
milligram
millipede sting
millipore
Mills-Reincke phenomenon
milphosis
Milroy disease
Milton
    M. disease
    M. edema
    M. urticaria
Milwaukee
    M. knee syndrome
    M. shoulder
    M. shoulder syndrome
mimicry
    molecular m.
    poxviral m.
min
    AIR m.
mineralocorticoid
mineral oil
mineral-related nutritional disorder
Minerva cast
mini-allo
miniature scarlet fever
miniblade
    Beaver ES m.
    SP90 m.
minidose
minigene
Min-I-Jet
minimal
    m. bactericidal concentration (MBC)
    m. change nephropathy (MCN)
    m. deviation melanoma
    m. dose possible
    m. erythema dose (MED)
    m. infecting dose (MID)
    m. inhibitory concentration (MIC)
    m. lethal dose (MLD)
    m. phototoxic dose (MPD)

m. pigment (MP)
m. reacting dose (MRD)
minimal-pigment oculocutaneous albinism
mini-MUD
   matched unrelated donor stem cell
   transplant
minimum
   m. effective naproxen dose
      (MEND)
   m. elicitation threshold (MET)
   m. inhibitory concentration (MIC)
   m. temperature
MiniOX
   M. 1000
   M. 1A oxygen analyzer
Minipress
Miniscope MS-3
Mini Thin Asthma Relief
Mini-Wright peak flow meter
mink
   enteritis of m.
   m. enteritis virus
Minnesota antilymphoblast globulin
Minocin
   M. IV injection
   M. oral
minocycline
   m. hydrochloride
   m. hyperpigmentation
minor
   m. agglutinin
   aphthae m.
   M. Blue Dragon
   erythema multiforme m.
   M. iodine-starch test
   recurrent erythema multiforme m.
   variola m.
minoxidil
Minoxigaine
Mintezol
minus
   Spirillum m.
minute
   alveolar ventilation per m.
   oxygen consumption per m. (VO$_2$)
   physiological dead space ventilation
      per m.
   m. ventilation
   m. vesicle
minutissimum
   Corynebacterium m.
   Microsporum m.

miostagmin reaction
MIP
   macrophage inflammatory protein
MIPS
   myocardial isotopic perfusion scan
mirabilis
   Proteus m.
Mirchamp sign
Mirena
miscellaneous reaction
mismatch
   ABO m.
   CREG m.
   cross-reactive antigen group m.
   m. repair
missense mutation
missing self hypothesis
mist
   AsthmaHaler M.
   Bronitin M.
   Bronkaid M.
   ENTsol M.
   Primatene M.
Mitchell disease
mite
   m. bite
   m. control
   dust m.
   elevator grain dust m.
   hair follicle m.
   harvest m.
   house dust m. (HDM)
   house dust m. F, P
   m. infestation
   itch m.
   nevus flammeus human granulocytic
      ehrlichiosis m.
   pyroglyphid m.
   scabietic m.
   soybean grain dust m.
   m. typhus
   wheat grain dust m.
mite-borne typhus
mite-snail combined allergy
mithramycin
mitigata
   variola m.
mitior
   typhus m.
mitis
   junctional epidermolysis bullosa
      atrophicans generalisata m.

M

NOTES

mitis *(continued)*
    protoporphyria m.
    prurigo m.
Mitis-type Ehlers-Danlos syndrome
mitochondrial
    m. DNA syndrome
    m. membrane potential
    m. respiratory chain disorder
      (MRCD)
    m. targeting sequence (MTS)
mitochondrion, pl. **mitochondria**
mitogen
    Mycoplasma arthritidis m. (MAM)
    pokeweed m. (PWM)
mitogen-activated
    m.-a. protein (MAP)
    m.-a. protein kinase (MAPK)
mitogen-activating protein (MAP)
mitogenesis
mitogenetic
mitogenic
mitoguazone
Mitraflex
    M. Plus foam dressing
    M. SC foam dressing
    M. wound dressing
mitral
    m. leaflet
    m. valve prolapse, aortic
      anomalies, skeletal changes, and
      skin changes (MASS)
    m. valve prolapse, aortic
      anomalies, skeletal changes, and
      skin changes syndrome
Mitrazol
Mitsuda
    M. antigen
    M. radiation
    M. reaction
    M. test
Mitutoyo digital caliper
mix
    black rubber m.
    caine m.
    Carba m.
    juniper m.
    Mercapto m.
    paraben m.
    thiuram m.
mixed
    m. aerobic/anaerobic abscess
    m. agglutination
    m. agglutination reaction
    m. agglutination test
    m. asthma
    m. chancre
    m. connective tissue disease
      (MCTD)
    m. cryoglobulinemia

    m. feather
    m. hemangioma
    m. hematopoietic chimerism
    m. hepatic porphyria
    m. inflammatory granuloma
    m. interstitial and palisaded
      granuloma
    m. leprosy
    m. lymphocyte culture (MLC)
    m. lymphocyte culture reaction
    m. lymphocyte culture test
    m. nail infection
    m. seborrheic-staphylococcal
      blepharitis
    m. sore
    m. tumor
    m. tumor of skin
    m. vespid antigen
mixed-linker PCR (ML-PCR)
mixing
    phenotypic m.
Mixter forceps
Miyagawa body
mizolastine
mizoribine
Mkar disease
ML3000
MLC
    mixed lymphocyte culture
      MLC test
MLD
    minimal lethal dose
MLNS
    mucocutaneous lymph node syndrome
ML-PCR
    mixed-linker PCR
MM
    multiple myeloma
    mycophenolate mofetil
      MM virus
3MM
    Whatman 3MM
MMC
    measure mucociliary clearance
MMD
    mass median aerodynamic diameter
MMF
    mycophenolate mofetil
MMP
MMP-2
MMP-3
MMP-7
MMP-8
MMP-9
MMP-10
MMR
    MMR vaccine
MMS
    Mohs micrographic surgery

MN
    membranous nephropathy
Mnemonics
    Dermatology Education by Recall
    of M. (DERM)
MNS
    MNS antigen
    MNS blood group
MoAb
    monoclonal antibody
Mobic tablet
Mobidin
mobility
    syndrome of limited joint m.
    (SLJM)
Mobiluncus
moccasin
    m. foot
    m. snake bite
moccasin-type tinea pedis
model
    carrageenin-induced footpad
    inflammation m.
    Cholesky m.
    Markov state-transition m.
    Weibull regression m.
Modicon
modification
    posttranslational protein m.
modified
    cyclosporine capsules m.
    m. Draize test
    M. Health Assessment
    Questionnaire (MHAQ)
    m. Linton procedure for varicose
    veins
    m. measles
    m. Rodman skin thickness score
    m. smallpox
    m. vaccinia virus Ankara strain
    m. varicella-like syndrome (MVLS)
modulation
    antigenic m.
modulator
    immune m.
    immune system m.
    selective estrogen receptor m.
    (SERM)
module
    CO-Oximeter m.
    intercellular adhesion m. (ICAM)

MODY
    maturity-onset diabetes of the young
MODY2-glucokinase
MODY3 HNF-1-alpha mutation
Moeller
    M. glossitis
    M. itch
moensin
mofetil
    mycophenolate m. (MM, MMF)
MOG
    myelin-oligodendrocyte glycoprotein
mohair
Mohs
    M. chemosurgery
    M. fresh-tissue chemotherapy
    M. fresh-tissue technique
    M. micrographic surgery (MMS)
    M. procedure
MOI
    multiplicity of infection
moiety
moist
    m. gangrene
    Nasal M.
    m. papule
    m. tetter
    m. wart
Moi-Stir
moisture
    m. content
    M. Ophthalmic drops
    m. vapor transmission rate
    (MVTR)
Moisturel moisturizer
moisturizer
    Aquacare m.
    Betadine First Aid Antibiotics
    + M.
    body m.
    Eucerin Plus m.
    facial m.
    Keri m.
    Lubriderm m.
    Moisturel m.
    Nivea m.
    occlusive m.
    RoEzIt skin m.
    topical m.
    Vaseline Intensive Care m.
Mokola virus

M

NOTES

molar
>   mulberry m.

mold
>   m. aeroallergen
>   *Alternaria* m.
>   m. control
>   Smith-Pedersen m.
>   m. spore

mole
>   atypical m.
>   hairy m.
>   spider m.

molecular mimicry

molecule
>   accessory m.
>   adhesion m.
>   antiapoptotic m.
>   antiplatelet endothelial cell
>   adhesion m. (anti-PCAM)
>   apoptosis-associated m.
>   B7 costimulatory m.
>   costimulatory m.
>   effector m.
>   Fas-Fas ligand m.
>   FasL m.
>   fusin m.
>   heterotrimeric cell-membrane-
>   bound m.
>   ICOS m.
>   leukocyte cell adhesion m. (leu-
>   CAM)
>   mannose-binding m.
>   melanoma cell adhesion m. (Mel-
>   CAM)
>   MHC m.
>   multideterminant m.
>   multimeric m.
>   neural cell adhesion m. (NCAM)
>   precursor m.
>   soluble cell adhesion m.
>   vascular cell adhesion m. (VCAM)

molecule-1
>   endothelial leukocyte adhesion m.
>   (ELAM-1)
>   intercellular adhesion m. (ICAM-1)
>   vascular cell adhesion m. (VCAM-
>   1)

MoleMax

molgramostim

Mollaret
>   M. HSV
>   M. meningitis

molle
>   fibroma m.
>   heloma m.
>   papilloma m.

Moll gland

mollusciformis
>   nevus m.
>   verruca m.

molluscoid neurofibroma

molluscous

molluscum
>   m. body
>   cholesterinic m.
>   m. contagiosum virus (MCV)
>   m. corpuscle
>   m. epitheliale
>   m. fibrosum
>   m. giganteum
>   m. lipomatodes
>   m. pendulum
>   m. sebaceum
>   m. varioliformis
>   m. verrucosum

Moloney
>   M. murine leukemia virus
>   M. test

molt

MOLT-18, human T cell line

mometasone furoate

MOMP
>   major outer membrane protein

Monarch Mini Mask nasal interface

monarthritis

monarticular

Monazole-7

Mondor disease

mongolian
>   m. macula
>   m. macule
>   m. spot

mongolism

monilated

monilethrix

Monilia albicans

Moniliaceae

monilial
>   m. granuloma
>   m. intertrigo
>   m. onychia
>   m. paronychia

moniliasis

moniliforme
>   *Fusarium m.*

moniliform hair

moniliformis
>   lichen ruber m.
>   *Streptobacillus m.*

Moniliformis soni

moniliid

Monistat
>   M. IV Injection
>   M. Vaginal

Monistat-Derm topical

monitor
AirWatch Asthma m.
Digitrapper MkIII sleep m.
EcoCheck oxygen m.
Magellan M.
NoxBOX m.
Pick and Go m.
TINA m.
VenTrak respiratory mechanics m.
monitoring
cytoimmunologic m.
pulse oximetry m. (POM)
monkey
m. B virus
m. epithelium
m. facies
monkeypox virus
monk's cowl
monoamine oxidase (MAO)
monoarthritis (MA)
chronic m.
monoarticular
m. antigen-induced arthritis
m. arthritis
m. arthritis of unknown etiology
monoassociated
monobactam
monobenzone
monobenzyl ether of hydroquinone
monochloroacetic acid
monochromatic light source
Monocid
monoclonal
m. antibody (MoAb)
m. antibody to CD4, 5a8
m. antibody immobilization of
neutrophil antigens (MAINA)
m. antibody therapy
m. antiendothelial cell antibody
(mAECA)
m. autoantibody
m. B-cell neoplasm
m. gammopathy
m. gammopathy of undetermined
significance (MGUS)
m. gammopathy of unknown
significance (MGUS)
m. immunoglobulin
m. peak
m. protein
m. protein, skin

monocyte
m. chemoattractant protein
m. chemoattractant protein-1 (MCP-
1)
m. chemotactic factor (MCF)
m. chemotactic peptide-1 (MCP-1)
m. chemotactic protein (MCP)
monocyte-derived
m.-d. cytokine
m.-d. neutrophil chemotactic factor
monocyte-macrophage system
monocytic leukemia
monocytogenes
Listeria m.
monocytopoiesis
factor-inducing m.
monocytosis
avian m.
monodisperse aerosol
Monodox oral
monoecious
monoethylglycinexylidide (MEGX)
monogamous bivalency
Mono-Gesic
monohydrate
cefadroxil m.
cephalexin m.
monoinfection
monokine
monoleptic fever
monolisa test
monomer
Actin m.
monomeric
monomicrobic
monomorphous
mononeuritis multiplex
mononuclear
m. cell
m. phagocyte system (MPS)
mononucleosis
infectious m. (IM)
posttransfusion m. (PTM)
monooxygenase pathway
monophonic wheeze
monophosphate
cyclic guanosine m.
cyclic nucleotide adenosine m.
guanosine m. (GMP)
monoplast
monoplastic
monorecidive chancre

M

NOTES

355

monosodium
m. glutamate (MSG)
m. urate (MSU)
m. urate monohydrate crystal
monospecific antiserum
Monosporium apiospermum
monostearate
glyceryl m.
monosymptomatic hypochondriasis
monosyphilide
monotherapy
etanercept m.
maintenance cyclosporine m. (mCsA)
monotonous cell
monotypia
Mono-Vac test
monovalent antiserum
monoxide
carbon m.
monoxime
butanedione m.
Monro
foramen of M.
Monsel solution
monster
m. cell
Gila m.
montana
arnica m.
Hypericum m.
montelukast
Montenegro
M. reaction
M. test
Monterey
M. cypress
M. cypress tree
montevideo
Salmonella m.
Monurol
moon facies
5-MOP
5-methoxypsoralen
8-MOP
8-methoxypsoralen
morado
mal m.
Moraxella
M. catarrhalis
M. conjunctivitis
M. lacunata
morbilli
morbilliform
m. basal cell carcinoma
m. eruption
m. erythema
Morbillivirus
equine *M.*

morbus
cholera m.
m. Darier
mordax
calor m.
mordicans
calor m.
MORFAN
mental retardation, overgrowth, remarkable face, and acanthosis nigricans
MORFAN syndrome
Morgan
M. fold
M. line
Morganella morganii
morganii
Morganella m.
morning
m. glory anomaly
m. stiffness
morphea
acroteric m.
m. acroterica
Addison m.
m. alba
m. atrophica
generalized m.
m. guttata
m. herpetiformis
m. linearis
m. pigmentosa
m. pigmentosum
m. profunda
subcutaneous m.
m. variant
morpheaform
m. basal cell carcinoma
m. sarcoid
morphealike
morphine sulfate
morphogenesis
morphogenic protein 6
morphologic classification
morphology
dendritic m.
lesion m.
stellate m.
morphometric
morphonuclear
morpio, morpion, pl. **morpiones**
Morquio
M. mucopolysaccharidosis
M. syndrome
Morrey-Coonrad design
morrhuate
sodium m.
Morrow-Brown needle
morsicatio buccarum

mortality
mortification
mortified
Mortimer malady
Morton neuroma
morula cell
morus
    nevus m.
MoRu-Viraten
Morvan disease
mosaic
    m. fungus
    m. skin
    m. wart
mosaicism
Moschcowitz disease
Mosco callus and corn remover
Moscow typhus
MOSD
    multiple organ system dysfunction
MOSF
    multiple organ system failure
mosquito
    m. bite
    m. forceps
mosquito-borne disease
mossy foot
moth
    m. dermatitis
    m. patch
moth-eaten
    m.-e. alopecia
    m.-e. baldness
mother
    m. dermatitis
    infant of diabetic m. (IDM)
    m. lesion
    m. yaw
Mother2Be skin treatment
motif
    endosomal localization m.
    immunoreceptor tyrosine-based
        activation m. (ITAM)
    leucine zipper m.
    nonmethylated CpG m.
    YXXZ m.
motif-bearing cytokine
motion
    active range of m.
    continuous passive m. (CPM)
    joint alignment and m. (JAM)
    pain on m.

passive m.
range of m.
m. sickness
motor
    m. deconditioning
    m. neuron weakness
    m. neuropathy
motorized cutter
Motrin
    M. IB
    M. IB Sinus
    Junior Strength M.
MOTT
    mycobacteria other than tuberculosis
Mott cell
mottled
    m. opacity
    m. rarefaction
mottling
    netlike m.
moulage
mould
Moulin
    linear atrophoderma of M.
moult
mountain
    m. cedar
    m. cedar tree
mouse
    m. encephalomyelitis
    m. encephalomyelitis virus
    m. epithelium
    m. hepatitis
    m. hepatitis virus
    m. leukemia virus
    m. mammary tumor virus
    nude m.
    m. parotid tumor virus
    m. poliomyelitis
    m. poliomyelitis virus
    m. serum
    m. serum protein (MSP)
    m. thymic virus
    tight skin m.
    m. urine
    m. urine protein (MUP)
mousepox virus
mousse
    betamethasone m.
    RID M.
mousy odor

M

NOTES

mouth
>m. breathing
>burning m.
>dry m.
>m. erythema multiforme
>gaping m.
>painful m.
>purse-string m.
>scabby m.
>sore m.
>trench m.

mouthwash
>Zephiran m.

movement
>genistein-inhibited m.
>herbimycin-inhibited m.
>mandibular m.
>nonrapid eye m. (nonREM)
>periodic leg m.
>rapid eye m. (REM)

moxa
moxalactam
Moxam
moxibustion
moxifloxacin
>m. HCl
>m. HCl IV
>m. HCl tablet

Moynahan syndrome
MP
>machine preservation
>metacarpophalangeal
>minimal pigment

6-MP
>6-mercaptopurine

MPA
>methylprednisolone acetate
>microscopic polyangiitis

MPD
>minimal phototoxic dose

M-plasty
MPL vaccine adjuvant
MPM
>multiple primary melanoma
>>MPM antimicrobial wound cleanser
>>MPM composite dressing
>>MPM conductive gel pad
>>MPM GelPad impregnated gauze
>>MPM hydrogel dressing

MPO
>>MPO bone marrow stain
>>MPO deficiency

M-Prednisol Injection
MPS
>mononuclear phagocyte system
>myofascial pain syndrome

MPT
>multiple parameter telemetry
>multiple puncture test

MR
>multicentric reticulohistiocytosis
>muscle-relaxant
>>MR drug

MRC
>Medical Research Council

MRCD
>mitochondrial respiratory chain disorder

MRCL
>Medical Research Council Laboratories

MRD
>matched related donor
>minimal reacting dose

MRG
>median rhomboid glossitis

MRI
>magnetic resonance imaging

MRI-compatible hollow-fiber bioreactor
mRNA
>messenger RNA
>>cathepsin K mRNA

MRSA
>methicillin-resistant *Staphylococcus aureus*

MR-VAX
>measles and rubella virus vaccine

MS-3
>>Miniscope MS-3

MS-1, -2 agent
MSA
>myositis-specific autoantibody

MSD enteric-coated ASA
>musculoskeletal disorder enteric-coated aspirin

MSDS
>material safety data sheet

Mseleni disease
MSG
>monosodium glutamate

MSH
>melanocyte-stimulating hormone
>>beta-MSH

MSI
>microsatellite instability

MSP
>mouse serum protein

MST
>median survival time

MSTA
>mumps skin test antigen

MSU
>monosodium urate

MT
>metatarsal

MTC
>multilocular thymic cyst

MTD
>*Mycobacterium tuberculosis* Direct
>>MTD Test

MTI
magnetization transfer imaging
MTP
metatarsophalangeal
MTS
mitochondrial targeting sequence
MTX
methotrexate
Mu antigen
mucate
acetaminophen and
isometheptene m.
Mucha disease
Mucha-Habermann
M.-H. disease
M.-H. syndrome
Much granule
mucicarmine stain
mucilage-containing herb
mucin clot test
mucinoid
mucinosa
alopecia m.
mucinosis, pl. mucinoses
acral persistent papular m.
cutaneous focal m.
follicular m.
lymphoma-associated follicular m.
papular m.
plaque-like cutaneous m.
reticular erythematous m. (REM)
mucinous
m. cyst
m. degeneration
m. eccrine carcinoma
Muckle-Wells syndrome
mucoadhesive
bioerodible m.
mucocele
mucociliary clearance
mucocutaneous
m. candidiasis
m. disease
m. leishmaniasis (MCL)
m. lymph node syndrome (MLNS)
m. manifestation
m. sporotrichosis
Muco-Fen-LA
mucogenicum
Mycobacterium m.

mucoid
m. degeneration
m. exopolysaccharide (MEP)
mucolipidosis
mucolytic
Mucomyst
mucopolysaccharide
mucopolysaccharidosis
Hunter m.
Hurler-Scheie m.
Maroteaux-Lamy m.
Morquio m.
Sanfilippo m.
Scheie m.
Sly m.
type I–VII m.
X-linked m.
mucopurulent
mucormycosis
Mucor racemosus
mucosa, pl. mucosae
hyalinosis cutis et m.
nevus spongiosus albus m.
oral m.
reddening of oropharyngeal m.
ulceration of oral m.
upper respiratory tract m.
mucosa-associated
m.-a. lymphoid tissue (MALT)
m.-a. lymphoid tissue lymphoma
mucosal
m. disease
m. disease virus
m. inflammation
m. mast cell
m. neuroma
m. sloughing
mucositis
genital plasma cell m.
plasma cell m.
Mucosol
mucosum
stratum m.
mucous
m. cyst
m. desiccation
m. membrane
m. membrane pemphigoid
m. membrane ulceration
m. papule
m. patch
m. plaque

M

NOTES

mucous *(continued)*
> m. plug
> m. plugging
> m. stool

mucus
> ball of m.
> m. hypersecretion
> oyster mass of m.
> thick and sticky m.

Mudd acne

mud fever

Muehrcke
> M. band
> M. line
> M. sign

Mueller-Hinton agar

Muerto Canyon virus

mugwort weed pollen

mu-heavy chain disease

Muir-Torre syndrome

mulberry
> black m.
> m. molar
> paper m.
> m. pattern
> m. rash
> red m.
> m. spot
> white m.

Mulibrey nanism

mullein

Muller phlebectomy hook

multiantigenic peptide (MAP)

multibacillary

MultiBoot

multicellular helminth

Multicenter Airway Research Collaboration (MARC)

multicentric
> m. disease
> m. reticulohistiocytosis (MR)

multideterminant molecule

Multidex filler

multidigit dactylitis

multidrug-resistant tuberculosis (MDR-TB)

multidrug therapy (MDT)

multifactorial

multifidus

multifocal
> m. demyelinating motor neuropathy
> m. histiocytosis
> m. Langerhans cell
> m. lymphangioendotheliomatosis with thrombocytopenia

multiforme
> atypical erythema m.
> bullous erythema m.
> chronic erythema m.

> drug-associated erythema m.
> erythema m. (EM)
> granuloma m.
> Hebra erythema m.
> herpes-associated erythema m. (HAEM)
> herpes simplex-associated erythema m. (HAEM)
> mouth erythema m.
> oral erythema m.
> postherpetic erythema m.

multiformis
> dermatitis m.
> protoporphyria chronica m.

multifunctional extracellular glycoprotein

multigemini
> pili m.

multiinfection

MultiLight system

multilineage
> m. colony-stimulating factor
> m. macrochimerism
> m. reconstitution

multilocularis
> *Echinococcus m.*

multilocular thymic cyst (MTC)

multimembrane spanner

multimer

multimeric molecule

multinomial (polytomous) logistic regression method

multinucleate cell angiohistiocytoma

multinucleated giant cell (MGC)

MultiPad absorptive dressing

multipartial

multiple
> m. benign cystic epithelioma
> m. chemical sensitivity
> m. drug allergy syndrome
> m. endocrine neoplasia
> m. endocrine neoplasia type 1
> m. endocrine neoplasm (MEN)
> m. endocrine neoplasm syndrome
> m. epiphyseal dysplasia
> m. eruptive milia
> m. hamartoma syndrome
> m. hereditary hemorrhagic telangiectasis
> m. idiopathic hemorrhagic sarcoma
> m. keratoacanthoma
> m. lentigines syndrome
> m. minute digitate hyperkeratosis
> m. mucosal neuroma
> m. mucosal neuroma syndrome
> m. myeloma (MM)
> m. myositis
> m. organ system dysfunction (MOSD)
> m. organ system failure (MOSF)

m. parameter telemetry (MPT)
m. primary melanoma (MPM)
m. puncture test (MPT)
m. puncture tuberculin test
m. sclerosis
m. serositis
skin test antigens, m.
m. sulfatase deficiency
m. sulfatase deficiency syndrome
m. symmetrical lipomatosis
m. symmetric lipomatosis
m. trichoepithelioma
multiple-type hyperlipoproteinemia
multiplex
lymphangioma tuberosum m.
mononeuritis m.
m. nevus
steatocystoma m.
m. steatocystoma
trichoepithelioma papillosum m.
xanthoma tuberosum m.
multiplicity of infection (MOI)
multipotent hematopoietic cell
MultiPulse laser system
Multitest
M. CMI
M. test
multivalent
m. antigen
m. antiserum
m. vaccine
multivariant
multivariate
m. analysis of variance (MANOVA)
m. logistic regression
multocida
Pasteurella m.
mummification necrosis
mumps
m. meningoencephalitis
metastatic m.
m. sensitivity test
m. skin test antigen (MSTA)
m. virus
m. virus vaccine
Mumpsvax
Munchausen syndrome
Munro
M. abscess
M. microabscess
mu-opioid

MUP
mouse urine protein
mupirocin ointment
muramyl-tripeptide
MURD
matched unrelated donor
murex
m. hybrid capture assay
M. Suds
muriform
murine
m. hepatitis
m. homolog
m. leukemia
m. sarcoma virus
M. solution
m. thymoma
m. typhus
M. in vivo kit
Murine-CFSE Flow Kit
murmur
Carey Coombs m.
Murocel Ophthalmic solution
muromonab-CD3
Murray
M. test
M. Valley encephalitis (MVE)
M. Valley encephalitis virus
M. Valley rash
Murutucu virus
muscarinic receptor autoantibody
muscle
accessory m.
airway smooth m. (ASM)
arrectores pilorum m.
arrector pili m.
m. biopsy
bronchial smooth m.
cutaneous m.
dermal m.
m. relaxant
sacrospinalis m.
m. self-antigen
sternocleidomastoid m.
m. weakness
muscle-relaxant (MR)
m.-r. drug
Muscle-Wells syndrome
musculamine
muscular dystrophy
musculocutaneous nerve entrapment
musculoligamentous strain

M

NOTES

musculoskeletal
  m. disorder enteric-coated aspirin (MSD enteric-coated ASA)
  m. lupus
musculotendinous
  m. damage
  m. unit
musculus
  Mus m.
mushroom dust
mushroom-hook layer
mushroom-picker's lung
mushroom-worker's lung
musician's overuse syndrome
musk ambrette
Mus musculus
mussel
  blue m.
mustard
  l-phenylalanine m.
  nitrogen m.
  topical nitrogen m. (NH2)
  yellow m.
Mustargen Hydrochloride
Mustargen-MSD
mustelae
  Helicobacter m.
mutagen
  frame-shift m.
mutagenicity
mutant
  conditional-lethal m.
  conditionally lethal m.
  suppressor-sensitive m.
  temperature-sensitive m.
mutation
  addition-deletion m.
  CDKN2A m.
  CKR5 m.
  cyclin-dependent kinase inhibitor 2A m.
  factor V Leiden m.
  frame-shift m.
  IL-12 receptor beta-1 m.
  lysine m.
  missense m.
  MODY3 HNF-1-alpha m.
  novel missense m.
  point m.
  reading-frame-shift m.
  somatic m.
  transition m.
  transversion m.
mutilans
  m. arthritis
  arthritis m.
  keratoma hereditaria m.
  keratoma hereditarium m.
  lepra m.

  lupus m.
  psoriatic arthritis m.
mutilating
  m. keratoderma
  m. keratoderma of Vohwinkel
  m. leprosy
mutism
  tacrolimus-associated m.
MV
  maximal ventilation
  mechanical ventilation
M-Vax vaccine
MVE
  Murray Valley encephalitis
  MVE virus
MVLS
  modified varicella-like syndrome
MVP
  Centurion SiteGuard M.
MVTR
  moisture vapor transmission rate
MVV
  maximal voluntary ventilation
MWB
  mild wheezy bronchitis
MW 2000 microwave delivery system
myalgia
  eosinophilic m.
  epidemic m.
Myambutol
Myapap drops
myasthenia
  m. gravis (MG)
  m. gravis syndrome
Mycelex-7, -G
Mycelex troche
mycelium
mycetoma
  actinomycotic m.
  Bouffardi black m.
  Bouffardi white m.
  Brumpt white m.
  Carter black m.
  eumycotic m.
  Nicolle white m.
  Vincent white m.
mycetomi
  Madurella m.
mycid
Mycifradin
  M. Sulfate oral
  M. Sulfate Topical
Mycitracin Topical
Myclo-Derm
Myclo-Gyne
mycobacteria
  m. HSP
  nontuberculous m.

m. other than tuberculosis (MOTT)
rapidly growing m. (RGM)
mycobacterial
    m. abscess
    m. infection
mycobacteriosis
    environmental m.
Mycobacterium
    M. abscessus
    M. avium
    M. avium complex (MAC)
    M. avium-intracellulare (MAI)
    M. avium-intracellulare bacteremia
    M. balnei
    M. bovis
    M. chelonae
    M. fortuitum
    M. gordonae
    M. haemophilum
    M. kansasii
    M. leprae
    M. marinum
    M. mucogenicum
    M. peregrinum
    M. phlei
    M. smegmatis
    M. thermoresistable
    M. tuberculosis (MBT)
    M. tuberculosis detection
    M. tuberculosis Direct (MTD)
    M. tuberculosis Direct Test
    M. ulcerans
    M. vaccae
    M. xenopi
Mycobutin
mycodermatitis
Mycogen II Topical
Mycolog-II Topical
mycology
Myconel Topical
mycophage
mycophenolate mofetil (MM, MMF)
mycoplasma
    M. arthritidis
    M. arthritidis mitogen (MAM)
    m. disease
    M. faucium
    M. genitalium
    M. hominis
    m. IgM titer
    M. incognitus

M. pneumoniae
    m. pneumonia of pig
mycoplasmal pneumonia
mycosis, pl. **mycoses**
    m. cutis chronica
    deep m.
    m. favosa
    m. framboesioides
    m. fungoides (MF)
    m. fungoides d'emblée
    m. fungoides palmaris et plantaris
    Gilchrist m.
    m. interdigitalis
    opportunistic systemic m.
    Posada m.
    pulmonary m.
    rare m.
    subcutaneous m.
mycostatic
Mycostatin
    M. oral
    M. pastilles
    M. topical
mycotic dermatitis
mycovirus
Mydfrin Ophthalmic solution
mydriatic
myelin-associated glycoprotein antibody
    detection
myelin basic protein (MBP)
myelin-oligodendrocyte glycoprotein
    (MOG)
myelitic enterovirus
myelitis
    amyotrophic syphilitic m.
    transverse m.
myeloablative conditioning
myeloblastic protein
myeloblastosis
    avian m.
myelodysplastic syndrome (MDS)
myelofibrosis
    cutaneous m.
myelography
myeloid
    m. colony
    m. leukemia
    m. stem cell
myeloma
    m. growth factor
    multiple m. (MM)
    plasma cell m.

M

NOTES

myelomatosis
myelomonocytic leukemia
myelonecrosis
myelopathy
    vacuolar m.
myeloperoxidase
    m. bone marrow stain
    m. deficiency
myeloperoxidase bone marrow stain
myeloperoxidase-hydrogen peroxide
  halide system
myeloproliferative disease
myeloradiculopathy
myeloradiculopolyneuronitis
myelosis
myelosuppression
    azathioprine-induced m.
myelosuppressive
myelosyphilis
Myfortic
myiasis
    botfly facultative m.
    botfly obligate m.
    creeping m.
    facultative m.
    obligate m.
    m. oestruosa
    subcutaneous m.
    tumbu fly m.
    wound m.
Mylocel 1000 mg tablet
Myminic Expectorant
myoadenylate
    m. deaminase
    m. deaminase deficiency
myoblast
myoblastoma
    granular cell m.
myocardial
    m. dysfunction
    m. isotopic perfusion scan (MIPS)
myocarditis
    clinical m.
    giant cell m.
Myochrysine
myoclonus
    nocturnal m.
    progressive encephalomyelitis with
      rigidity and m. (PERM)
Myocrisin
myocyte
    Anitschkow m.
myoepithelial sialadenitis
myoepithelioma
myoepithelium
myofascial pain syndrome (MPS)
myofasciitis
    macrophagic m.
myofibril

myofibroblast
myofibroblastoma
    infantile digital m.
myofibromatosis
    infantile m.
myogenic paralysis
myoglobin
    quantitative immunoassay for
     urine m.
    m. release
myoglobinuria
myoma
myonecrosis
    clostridial m.
    m. syndrome
myopathy
    drug-related m.
    idiopathic inflammatory m. (IIM)
    noninflammatory m.
    sarcoid-like granulomatous m.
    steroid m.
    vacuolar m.
myophosphorylase deficiency
myorelaxant drug
myosin
    m. ATPase inhibitor
    m. heavy chain contraction
    m. light chain
myositis
    acute disseminated m.
    childhood m.
    dermatomyositis sine m.
    eosinophilic m.
    epidemic m.
    giant cell m.
    inclusion body m.
    juvenile m.
    multiple m.
    nodular m.
    orbital m.
    m. ossificans
    overlap m. (OVLP)
    m. with malignancy
myositis-associated autoantibody
myositis-specific
    m.-s. antibody
    m.-s. autoantibody (MSA)
myosynovitis
Myoviridae
Myphetapp
myringitis
    m. bulbosa
    bullous m.
myringodermatitis
myringotomy with aspiration
myristate
    isopropyl m.
myrmecia wart
myrmekiasm

myrtle
    wax m.
Mytrex F topical
myxadenitis labialis
myxedema
    circumscribed m.
    generalized m.
    pretibial m. (PTM)
myxedematosus
    lichen m.
myxedematous
    m. arthropathy
    m. facies
    m. lichen
myxoid
    m. cyst

    m. dermal dendrocytoma
    m. pseudocyst
myxolipoma
myxoma
    cardiocutaneous m.
    nerve sheath m.
myxomatosis virus
myxomatous degeneration
myxosarcoma
myxovirus
MZBL
    marginal zone B-cell leukemia
    marginal zone B-cell lymphoma
M-Zole 7 Dual Pack

NOTES

M

365

N

nitrogen
    Alferon N
    N segment

nabumetone

NAC

nasal allergen challenge

NACDG

North American Contact Dermatitis
Group

N-**acetylcysteine**

N-**acetylneuraminic acid**

N-**acetyl-4-S-cysteaminyl phenol**

nacreous ichthyosis

NAD

nevi with architectural disorder

Nadinola

nadolol

Nadopen-V

NADPH

nicotinamide adenine dinucleotide
phosphate
    NADPH oxidase
    NADPH oxidase system

Naegeli

chromatophore nevus of N.
N. syndrome

Naegeli-Franceschetti-Jadassohn
syndrome

Naegleria fowleri

NAEP

National Asthma Education Program

NAEPP

National Asthma Education and
Prevention Program Guidelines

naeslundii

Actinomyces n.

NAET

Nambudripad allergy elimination
technique

naevoid (*var. of* nevoid)

naevus (*var. of* nevus)

NAF

neutrophil-activating factor

nafamostat mesilate

nafarelin acetate

nafate

cefamandole n.

Nafcil injection

nafcillin sodium

Nafrine

naftifine hydrochloride

Naftin

    N. cream
    N. topical

Naga sore

nail

artificial n.
athletic n.
azure lunula of n.
n. biting
blue n.
brittle n.
n. change
Chevron n.
claw n.
clubbing of n.
n. clubbing
convex n.
double-edge n.
egg shell n.
n. fold
n. fold capillaroscopic instrument
n. fold capillaroscopy
n. fold capillaroscopy abnormality
n. fold capillary loop abnormality
geographic stippling of n.
green n.
green-striped n.
n. groove
half-and-half n.
herringbone n.
Hippocratic n.
n. horn
ingrown n.
INRO surgical prosthetic n.
n. keratin
n. matrix
omega n.
Ony-Clear N.
parrot-beak n.
pincer n.
n. pit
pitted n.
pitting of n.
n. pitting
n. plate
Plummer n.
n. polish
racket n.
racquet n.
ram's horn n.
reedy n.
ringworm of n.
n. root
sculptured n.
n. shedding
shell n.
n. skin
splitting n.

N

nail *(continued)*
    spoon n.
    stippled n.
    sulcus of matrix of n.
    n. technician
    Terry n.
    trumpet n.
    turtleback n.
    n. wall
    n. wart
    yellow n.
20-nail
    20-n. dystrophy
    20-n. involvement
nailbed cancer
10-nail dystrophy
nail-patella-elbow syndrome
nail-patella syndrome
Nairobi sheep disease virus
Nairovirus
naive B cell
Na⁺-K⁺ — Na^+-K^+
    sodium-potassium
    Na^+-K^+ ATPase pump
naked
    n. DNA encoding
    n. plasmid DNA
    n. tubercle
    n. virus
Nalcrom
Naldecon
Naldecon-EX Children's Syrup
Naldelate
Nalebuff classification
Nalfon
Nalgest
nalidixic acid
Nallpen injection
Nalmefene
naloxone hydrochloride
Nalspan
NALT
    nose-associated lymphoid tissue
naltrexone
Nambudripad allergy elimination technique (NAET)
NAME
    nevi, atrial myxoma, myxoid
    neurofibromas, and ephelides
    nevi, atrial myxomas, myxomas of skin
    and mammary glands, and ephelides
        NAME syndrome
nana
    Hymenolepis n.
NANB
    non-A non-B
        NANB hepatitis
NANC
    nonadrenergic noncholinergic mechanism

nanism
    Mulibrey n.
Nanophyetus salmincola
nanum
    Microsporum n.
NAP
    neutrophil-activating protein
nape nevus
Naphcon-A
naphthylalkalone
naphthylalkanone
napkin
    n. dermatitis
    n. psoriasis
    n. rash
Naprelan
Naprosyn
naproxen sodium
NAPRTCS
    North American Pediatric Rental
    Transplant Cooperative Study
NAR
    nonanaphylactic reaction
narcotic
NARES
    nonallergic rhinitis with eosinophilia
    syndrome
Narins cannula
naris, pl. **nares**
narium
narrowband
    n. ultraviolet B (NBUVB)
    n. UVB (NBUVB)
    n. UVB lamp
    n. UVB therapeutic light exposure
narrowing
    joint space n.
Nasabid
Nasacort AQ
Nasahist
    N. B
    N. B injection
nasal
    n. allergen challenge (NAC)
    n. allergy
    n. antigen challenge test
    n. cannula dermatitis
    n. canthus
    n. conditioning capacity (NCC)
    n. congestion
    n. congestion score (NCS)
    n. glioma
    n. herpes
    n. itching
    Kondon's N.
    N. Moist
    n. mucosal ulceration
    Otrivin N.
    n. polyp

n. provocation test
n. scraping
N. & Sinus Relief
n. smear
n. solar dermatitis
n. symptom score (NSS)
n. turbinate
Tyzine N.
n. verge
NasalCrom nasal solution
Nasalide nasal Aerosol
Nasarel Nasal Spray
NASBA
　nucleic acid sequence based amplification
nasi
　acne necroticans et exulcerans
　　serpiginosa n.
　alae n.
　granulosis rubra n.
　vestibulum n.
Nasik vibrio
nasoantral window
nasobronchial reflex
nasociliary
nasolabial fold (NLF)
Nasonex
nasopharyngeal
　n. aspirate (NPA)
　n. biopsy
　n. carcinoma
　n. leishmaniasis
　n. ulcer
nasopharyngoscopy
NASTRA
　North American Study of treatment for
　Refractory Ascites
　NASTRA study
Nasu-Hakola disease
Natacyn Ophthalmic
natalizumab
natamycin
natiform skull
national
　N. Asthma Education and
　Prevention Program Guidelines
　(NAEPP)
　N. Asthma Education Program
　(NAEP)
　N. Center for Health Statistics
　(NCHS)
　N. Committee for Clinical
　Laboratory Standards (NCCLS)

N. Immunization Program (NIP)
N. Institute of Arthritis and
　Metabolic Diseases (NIAMD)
N. Institute of Arthritis,
　Musculoskeletal and Skin
　Disorders (NIAMS)
N. Institutes of Health (NIH)
N. Marrow Donor Program
　(NMDP)
N. Psoriasis Foundation
N. Psoriasis Foundation/United
　States of America (NPF/USA)
N. Vaccine Advisory Committee
　(NVAC)
native
　n. anergy
　n. type anti-DNA antibody
natural
　n. anergy
　n. antibody
　n. cytotoxicity receptor
　n. focus of infection
　n. hemolysin
　n. immunity
　n. interferon alfa
　n. killer (NK)
　n. killer cell
　n. killer cell activation
　n. killer cell lymphoma
　n. killer cell-stimulating factor
　(NKSF)
　n. killer-mediated cytotoxicity
　n. rubber latex allergy
Naturale
　Tears N.
Nature's Tears solution
nausea
　epidemic n.
Nauseatol
Nausex
navy bean
Naxen
NBCCS
　nevoid basal cell carcinoma syndrome
NBT
　nitroblue tetrazolium
　NBT mosaic pattern
NBUVB
　narrowband ultraviolet B
　narrowband UVB
NCA
　nonspecific cross-reacting antigen

NOTES

369

NCAM
neural cell adhesion molecule
NCB
needle-core biopsy
NCC
nasal conditioning capacity
NCCLS
National Committee for Clinical
Laboratory Standards
NCHS
National Center for Health Statistics
NCS
nasal congestion score
nerve conduction study
ND
Newcastle disease
Congestac ND
ND virus
N.D.
Chlor-Tripolon N.D.
Nd
neodymium
NDDH
neutrophilic dermatosis of the dorsal
hand
NDO
nondigestible oligosaccharide
ND-Stat injection
Nd:YAG
neodymium:yttrium-aluminum-garnet
Nd:YAG laser
near-fatal asthma
Nebcin injection
Nebraska calf scours virus
Nebuhaler inhaler
nebules
Ventolin n.
nebulin
nebulization
nebulize
nebulized
n. bronchodilator
n. inhaler
n. isoproterenol
nebulizer
Aerochamber n.
AeroSonic personal ultrasonic n.
AeroTech II n.
Ailos n.
DeVilbiss Pulmon-Aid n.
Fisoneb ultrasonic n.
jet n.
John Bunn Mini-Mist n.
Medi-Mist n.
Medix ultrasonic n.
Micro-Mist n.
Pulmo-Aide n.
Respirgard II n.
Schuco 2000 n.

Shuco-Myst n.
turbo n.
Twin Jet n.
ultrasonic n.
Wright n.
NebuPent Inhalation
NEC
necrotizing enterocolitis
Necator americanus
necatoriasis
neck
n. dermatitis
farmer's n.
fiddler n.
n. flexion maneuver
n. pain
sailor's n.
necklace
Casal n.
n. of Venus
necrobiosis
n. granulomatosis
n. lipoidica
n. lipoidica diabeticorum
necrobiotic
n. granuloma
n. xanthogranuloma
necrogenic
n. tubercle
n. wart
necrogenica
verruca n.
necrolysis
epidermal n.
toxic epidermal n. (TEN)
necrolytic migratory erythema
necrosis
acute tubular n.
aseptic n.
aspirin-induced papillary n.
caseation n.
central fibrinoid n.
cold-induced n.
coumarin n.
fat n.
fibrinoid n.
ischemic bone n.
late centrilobar n.
liquefaction n.
mummification n.
neutrophilic n.
papillary n.
piecemeal n.
n. progrediens
progressive outer retinal n. (PORN)
radium n.
subcutaneous fat n.
traumatic fat n.

necrosum
  vaccinia n.
necrotic
  n. arachnidism
  n. center
  n. cutaneous loxoscelism
  n. excoriation
  n. pocket
  n. tissue
  n. ulcer
necrotica
  acne n.
  dermatitis nodularis n.
necroticans
  erythema n.
necrotisans
  sycosis nuchae n.
necrotized chilblain
necrotizing
  n. angiitis
  n. enterocolitis (NEC)
  n. fasciitis
  n. granuloma
  n. infection
  n. lymphadenitis
  n. scleritis with adjacent
    inflammation
  n. scleritis without adjacent
    inflammation
  n. sialometaplasia
  n. vasculitis
nectary of floral unit
nedocromil sodium
needle
  Accuhair n.
  ADG n.
  adjustable-depth gauge n.
  Allerprick n.
  arachnophlebectomy n.
  n. arthroscopy
  n. biopsy
  Colorado microdissection n.
  Davis and Geck systemic plastic
    reconstruction P3 or PS3 n.
  Davis and Geck systemic PR and
    PRE P3 or PS3 n.
  Ethicon P and PS n.
  FS reverse cutting n.
  Hagedorn n.
  Morrow-Brown n.
  No-Kor n.
  Osterballe precision n.

  Parker-Pearson n.
  precision-point n.
  Pricker n.
  reverse cutting n.
  for skin reverse cutting n.
  Stallerpointe n.
  Thomas n.
  Wyeth bifurcated n.
needle-core biopsy (NCB)
Needleman-Wunsch algorithm
needlestick
Needs Evaluation Questionnaire (NEQ)
Neer II implant
Neethling virus
Nef protein
NEG
  nonenzymatic glycation
negative
  n. anergy
  n. control test
  n. cross-match
  n. nevus
  n. patch test
  n. phase
  n. predictive value (NPV)
  n. pressure wound therapy
  n. reaction
  n. Schick test
  n. selection
  n. strand virus
NegGram
Negishi virus
Negri
  N. body
  N. corpuscle
NEH
  neutrophilic eccrine hidradenitis
Neill-Mooser reaction (NMR)
Neisseria
  N. gonorrhoeae
  N. meningitidis
  N. meningitidis B
nelfinavir
Nellcor Symphony N-3000 pulse oximeter
Nelson syndrome
nematocyst
  venom-bathed n.
nematode
  n. dermatitis
  filarial n.
  intestinal n.

NOTES

N

neoangiogenesis
neoangiomatous
neoantigen
neoarsphenamine organic arsenic
NEOB
    New England Organ Bank
Neocate formula
Neo-Cortef
    N.-C. Ophthalmic
    N.-C. Topical
NeoDecadron Ophthalmic
NeoDerm
Neo-Dexameth Ophthalmic
neodymium (Nd)
neodymium:yttrium-aluminum-garnet
  (Nd:YAG)
    n.-a.-g. laser
neoepidermis
neoepithelium
neoepitope
    aggrecanase-induced aggrecan n.
NeoFed
neoformans
    Cryptococcus n.
    Saccharomyces n.
Neo-fradin oral
neomembrane
Neo-Metric
Neomixin topical
neomycin
    n. dermatitis
    n. and hydrocortisone
    n. and polymyxin b
    n., polymyxin b, and
      dexamethasone
    n., polymyxin b, and gramicidin
    n., polymyxin b, and
      hydrocortisone
    n., polymyxin b, and prednisolone
    n. sulfate
neonatal
    n. acne
    n. anemia
    n. biotin deficiency
    n. calf diarrhea virus
    n. citrullinemia
    n. giant congenital nevus
    n. herpes
    n. herpes simplex virus
    n. hypoxia
    n. lupus
    n. lupus erythematosus (NLE)
    lupus erythematosus, n.
    n. pustular melanosis
    n. skin allograft
    n. systemic candidiasis
    n. tyrosinemia
neonatalis
    herpes n.

neonatal-onset multisystem inflammatory
  disease (NOMID)
neonate
neonatorum
    acne n.
    adiponecrosis subcutanea n.
    anemia n.
    blennorrhea n.
    dermatitis exfoliativa n.
    edema n.
    erythema toxicum n.
    ichthyosis congenita n.
    icterus n.
    impetigo n.
    keratolysis n.
    milium n.
    ophthalmia n.
    pemphigus n.
    scleredema n.
    sclerema n.
    seborrhea squamosa n.
Neopap
neoplasia
    cutaneous n.
    malignant n.
    multiple endocrine n.
    vulvar intraepithelial n.
neoplasm
    monoclonal B-cell n.
    multiple endocrine n. (MEN)
    plasma cell n.
    Revised European-American
      Classification of Lymphoid N.
neoplastic
    n. angioendotheliomatosis
    n. cell
    n. disease
neoplastica
    acrokeratosis n.
    alopecia n.
NEOPO
    Northeast Organ Procurement
    Organization
Neo-Polycin ointment
neopterin
Neoral
    N. oral
    N. soft gelatin capsule
Neosar injection
Neospora canium
Neosporin
    N. Cream
    N. Ophthalmic Ointment
    N. Ophthalmic Solution
    N. scar solution
    N. Topical Ointment
Neosten

NeoStrata
    N. HQ
    N. Skin Lightening gel
NeoSynalar
Neo-Synephrine
    N.-S. 12-Hour Nasal solution
    N.-S. Ophthalmic solution
Neo-Tabs oral
Neothylline
Neotopic
Neotricin HC Ophthalmic Ointment
Neova Eye Therapy
neovascularization
Neo-Zol
nephelometry
nephrectomy
    laparoscopic donor n. (LDN)
    laparoscopic live donor n. (LLDN)
nephritic factor
nephritis, pl. nephritides
    acute interstitial n.
    antibasement membrane n.
    antikidney serum n.
    immune complex n.
    immune-mediated membranous n.
    interstitial n.
    lupus n. (LN)
    Masugi n.
    membranous lupus n.
    nephrotoxic serum n. (NSN)
    Polyomavirus-associated
      interstitial n.
    scarlatinal n.
    serum n.
    silent lupus n.
    streptococcal n.
    transfusion n.
    tuberculous n.
    tubulointerstitial n. (TIN)
    World Health Organization
      classification of lupus n. (I, IIA,
      IIB, III, IV, V)
nephritogenic
    n. effector
    n. process
nephritogenicity
Nephrocaps
nephrogenic
    n. diabetes insipidus
    n. fibrosing dermopathy
nephrogenicity
nephrolithiasis

nephrolysin
nephrolysis
nephrolytic
nephropathia epidemica
nephropathic
    n. immune response
    n. immunoglobulin
nephropathy
    amyloidotic n.
    Berger IgA n.
    chronic cyclosporine n.
    familial juvenile hyperuricemic n.
    IgA n.
    IgM n.
    membranous n. (MN)
    minimal change n. (MCN)
    urate n.
nephrosis
    hemoglobinuric n.
    toxic n.
nephrotic-range proteinuria
nephrotic syndrome
nephrotoxicity
    chronic n.
nephrotoxic serum nephritis (NSN)
nephrotoxin
NEQ
    Needs Evaluation Questionnaire
NERDS
    nodules, eosinophilia, rheumatism,
      dermatitis, and swelling
      NERDS syndrome
nerve
    common peroneal n.
    n. compression-degeneration
      syndrome
    n. conduction study (NCS)
    n. conduction velocity
    n. deafness
    digital n.
    n. entrapment
    n. entrapment syndrome
    femoral n.
    n. growth factor (NGF)
    n. growth factor antiserum
    median n.
    peripheral n.
    phrenic n.
    radial n.
    sciatic n.
    n. sheath
    n. sheath myxoma

N

NOTES

nerve *(continued)*
    sinuvertebral n.
    tibial n.
    ulnar n.
    vagus n.
Nervocaine
nervorum
    lepra n.
    vasa n.
nervosa
    lepra n.
    lues n.
    onychalgia n.
    purpura n.
    rhinitis n.
nervosus
    nevus n.
nervous
    n. exhaustion
    n. system
    n. system involvement
Nesacaine-MPF
nests of nevus cells
Netherton syndrome (NS)
N-ethyl-o-crotonotoluide
netilmicin sulfate
netlike mottling
Netromycin injection
netted pattern
nettle rash
Nettleship disease
Nettleship-Falls ocular albinism
Nettleship-Falls-type ocular albinism
nettling hair
network
    People of Color Against AIDS N.
    (POCAAN)
Neucalm
Neucalm-50 Injection
Neufeld
    N. capsular swelling
    N. reaction
Neumann disease
Neupogen injection
neural
    n. cell adhesion molecule (NCAM)
    n. foramina
    n. leprosy
    n. nevus
    n. theory
    n. tissue
neuralgia
    postherpetic n. (PHN)
    red n.
neural-mediated flushing
neuraminidase
neurapraxia
neurasthenia
neuridine

neurilemmoma, neurolemmoma
neuritic atrophoderma
neuriticum
    atrophoderma n.
    eczema n.
neuritis
    optic n.
    peripheral n.
neuroallergy
neuroarthropathy
Neurobehavioral Cognitive Status examination
neuroblastoma
    infantile n.
NeuroCell-HD, -PD
neurocirculatory asthenia
neurocristic hamartoma
neurocutaneous
    n. melanosis
    n. syndrome
neurocysticercosis
neurodegenerative disease
neurodermatitic
neurodermatitis
    circumscribed n.
    n. disseminata
    disseminated n.
    exudative n.
    genital n.
    localized n.
    nodular n.
    nummular n.
neurodermatosis
neurodermite dissemine
neuroectodermal
    n. defect
    n. melanolysomonal disease
neuroendocrine tumor
neuroepidermal
neurofibroma
    molluscoid n.
    pacinian n.
    plexiform n.
neurofibromatosis
    abortive n.
    central type n.
    classic n.
    elephantiasis n.
    incomplete n.
    late onset n.
    segmental n.
    n. type 1–8
    n., type 1 syndrome
    variant n.
neurofibrosarcoma
neurofilament promoter
neurogenic claudication
neuroid nevus
neuroimmune dysfunction

neuroimmunomodulation
neurokinin A, B
neurolabyrinthitis
    viral n.
neurolemmoma (*var. of* neurilemmoma)
neuroleprosy
neurolipomatosis dolorosa
neurologic
    n. disorder
    n. genodermatosis
    n. lupus
neurolues
neurolymphomatosis gallinarum
neurolysin
neuroma
    amputation n.
    n. cutis
    encapsulated n.
    Morton n.
    mucosal n.
    multiple mucosal n.
    palisaded encapsulated n.
    plexiform n.
    traumatic n.
    Verneuil n.
neuromatosa
    elephantiasis n.
neuromatosis elephantiasis
neuromatous
neuromelanin
neuromuscular junction disorder
neuromyelitis optica
neuromyoarterial glomus
neuromyopathy
    peripheral n.
neuromyotonia
neuron
    GABAergic n.
neuronal sensitization
neuronevus
neuronophage
neuronophagia
neuron-specific
    n.-s. enolase (NSE)
    n.-s. enolase stain
Neurontin
neuropathic
    n. amyloidosis
    n. arthritis
    n. arthropathy
    n. foot
    n. joint disease

neuropathica
    plica n.
neuropathy
    asymmetric peripheral sensory n.
    cranial n.
    entrapment n.
    hereditary sensory radicular n.
    motor n.
    multifocal demyelinating motor n.
    peripheral n.
    posterior interosseous n.
neuropeptide
neuropsychiatric
    n. disease
    n. symptom
    n. syndrome of systemic lupus
      erythematosus (NPSLE)
    n. systemic lupus erythematosus
      (NPSLE)
neurorelapse
neuroretinitis
Neuro-smooth needle holder
Neurospora sitophila
neurosurgery needle holder
neurosyphilis
    ectodermogenic n.
    meningovascular n.
    mesodermogenic n.
    parenchymatous n.
    paretic n.
    tabetic n.
neurotabes diabetica
neurothekeoma
neurotica
    alopecia n.
neurotic excoriation
neurotoxicity
    cyclosporine-induced n.
neurotoxin
    eosinophil-derived n.
neurotransmitter
    GABA inhibitory n.
    nociceptive n.
neurotrophic
    n. ulcer
    n. virus
neurotropic virus
neurovaccine
neurovirus
Neut injection
neutral
    n. lipid

N

NOTES

neutral *(continued)*
    n. lipid storage
    n. lipid storage disease
    n. protease
    n. proteinase
neutralization
    serum n.
    n. test
    viral n.
neutralizing (Nt)
    n. murine monoclonal antitumor
        necrosis factor antibody
Neutrexin
Neutrogena
    N. Acne Mask
    N. fresh foaming cleanser
    N. hand cream
    N. Healthy Scalp Anti-Dandruff
    N. Healthy Skin anti-wrinkle cream
    N. Healthy Skin face lotion
    N. Oil-Free acne Wash
    N. On-The-Spot Acne Lotion
    N. Sensitive Skin sunblock lotion
    N. T/Derm
    T/Gel N.
    N. T/Gel
    T/Sal N.
neutropenia
    autoimmune n.
    cyclic n.
    immune n.
    isoimmune neonatal n.
neutrophil
    n. antibody and transfusion reaction
    n. chemotactant factor
    n. chemotaxis
    n. dysplasia
    n. elastase
    n. ingress
    polymorphonuclear n. (PMN)
    n. polynucleosis
    rolling n.
neutrophil-activating
    n.-a. factor (NAF)
    n.-a. peptide-1
    n.-a. protein (NAP)
neutrophilic
    n. dermatosis of the dorsal hand
        (NDDH)
    n. eccrine hidradenitis (NEH)
    n. inflammation
    n. intraepidermal IgA dermatosis
    n. necrosis
neutrophil-mediated joint inflammation
**neutrophil-specific (secondary) granule
    deficiency**
NeuVisc
nevi *(pl. of* nevus)
nevirapine

nevocellular nevus
nevocyte
nevocytic nevus
nevoid, naevoid
    n. anomaly
    n. basal cell carcinoma
    n. basal cell carcinoma syndrome
        (NBCCS)
    n. elephantiasis
    n. hyperkeratosis of nipple and
        areola
    n. hypermelanosis
    n. hypertrichosis
    n. keratosis
    n. lentigo
    n. malignant melanoma (NMM)
    n. telangiectasia
nevolipoma
nevomelanocyte
    banal-appearing n.
nevomelanocytic (NM)
nevose
nevoxanthoendothelioma
nevus, naevus, pl. **nevi**
    n. acneiformis unilateralis
    acquired melanocytic n.
    active n.
    agminated atypical n.
    amelanotic n.
    n. anemicus
    n. angiectodes
    n. angiomatodes
    angiomatoid Spitz n.
    angiomatous n.
    n. arachnoideus
    n. araneosus
    n. araneus
    nevi, atrial myxoma, myxoid
        neurofibromas, and ephelides
        (NAME)
    nevi, atrial myxomas, myxomas of
        skin and mammary glands, and
        ephelides (NAME)
    n. avasculosus
    balloon cell n.
    basal cell n.
    bathing-trunk n.
    Becker n.
    benign junctional n.
    blue rubber-bleb n.
    Blue + SpITZ n.
    capillary n.
    n. cavernosus
    n. cell
    n. cell, A-, B-, C-type
    cellular blue n.
    n. cerebelliformis
    combined nevi
    comedo n.

comedones epidermal n.
comedonicus n.
common blue n.
compound n.
congenital giant pigmented n.
connective tissue n.
deep penetrating n.
n. depigmentosus
dermoepidermal n.
desmoplastic Spitz n.
dysplastic n.
n. elasticus of Lewandowski
epidermal n.
epidermic-dermic n.
epithelial n.
epithelioid blue n.
epithelioid cell n.
n. epitheliomatocylindromatosus
erectile n.
fatty n.
faun tail n.
n. fibrosus
flame n.
n. flammeus
flammeus n.
n. flammeus human granulocytic
  ehrlichiosis mite
n. flammeus nuchae
n. follicularis keratosis
n. fragarius
n. fuscoceruleus
n. fuscoceruleus acromiodeltoideus
  fuscoceruleus ophthalmomaxillaris
garment n.
giant congenital pigmented n.
hair follicle n.
hairy n.
halo n.
hard n.
hepatic n.
honeycomb n.
inflamed linear verrucous
  epidermal n. (ILVEN)
inflammatory linear verrucous
  epidermal n. (ILVEN)
intracutaneous n.
intradermal n.
intraepidermal n.
Ito n.
n. of Ito
Jadassohn sebaceous n.
Jadassohn-Tièche n.

junction n.
junctional n.
lentigines, atrial myxoma,
  mucocutaneous myxomas, and
  blue nevi (LAMB)
lichen striatus epidermal n.
linear epidermal n.
n. lipomatodes
n. lipomatodes superficialis
n. lipomatosus
n. lipomatosus cutaneus superficialis
lymphatic n.
n. lymphaticus
n. maculosus
malignant blue n.
marginal n.
Masson n.
n. maternus
melanocytic n.
mesodermal n.
Meyerson n.
n. mollusciformis
n. morus
multiplex n.
nape n.
negative n.
neonatal giant congenital n.
n. nervosus
neural n.
neuroid n.
nevocellular n.
nevocytic n.
nodular connective tissue disease n.
nonpigmented n.
nuchal n.
n. oligemicus
oral epithelial n.
organoid n.
Ota n.
n. of Ota
n. papillaris
n. papillomatosus
pigmented hair epidermal n.
n. pigmentosus
n. pigmentosus et pilosus
n. pilosus
plane n.
plexiform spindle cell n. (PSCN)
polypoid n.
port-wine n.
n. profundus
raspberry n.

NOTES

N

nevus (continued)
    resting n.
    n. sanguineus
    scarf n.
    n. sebaceous
    sebaceous n.
    n. sebaceus
    n. sebaceus of Jadassohn (NSJ)
    segmental n.
    soft n.
    speckled lentiginous n.
    spider n.
    n. spilus
    n. spilus lentigo
    n. spilus tardus
    spindle and epithelioid cell n.
    Spitz n.
    n. spongiosus albus mucosa
    stellar n.
    stocking n.
    straight hair n.
    strawberry n.
    subcutaneous n.
    n. sudoriferous
    Sutton n.
    n. syringocystadenosus papilliferus
    systematized n.
    Tièche n.
    n. unilateralis comedonicus
    n. unius lateralis
    n. unius lateris
    Unna n.
    vascular n.
    n. vascularis
    n. vascularis fungosus
    n. vasculosus
    n. venosus
    venous n.
    n. verrucosus
    verrucous n.
    n. vinosus
    vulvar n.
    Werther n.
    white sponge n.
    nevi with architectural disorder
      (NAD)
    woolly-hair n.
    zoniform n.
    zosteriform lentiginous n. (ZLN)
new
    N. Beginnings topical gel sheeting
    N. Decongestant
    N. England Organ Bank (NEOB)
    N. Star model 130 laser
    N. World leishmaniasis
    N. Zealand mice
newborn
    bullous impetigo of n.
    hemolytic anemia of n.

    hemolytic disease of n.
    lamellar exfoliation of the n.
    spontaneous gangrene of n.
    subcutaneous fat necrosis of n.
    transient bullous dermolysis of
      the n.
Newcastle
    N. disease (ND)
    N. disease virus
Newman-Keuls test
newsprint
nexin-1
    protease n.
nexine
Nexium
Nezelof
    N. syndrome
    N. type of thymic alymphoplasia
NF1
    neurofibromatosis type I
NF-κB
    nuclear factor-kappa B
NFAT
    nuclear factor of activated T cell
NF-ATc protein
N-geneous method
NGF
    nerve growth factor
    NGF antiserum
N.G.T. Topical
NH2
    topical nitrogen mustard
NHBD
    nonheart-beating donor
    NHBD transplantation
NHL
    non-Hodgkin leukemia
    non-Hodgkin lymphoma
NHP
    Nottingham Health Profile
Niacels
niacinamide
niacin deficiency
NIAMD
    National Institute of Arthritis and
      Metabolic Diseases
NIAMS
    National Institute of Arthritis,
      Musculoskeletal and Skin Disorders
NiCad
    nickel-cadmium
nickel
    n. allergy
    n. and dime lesion
    n. hand dermatitis
    n. sensitivity
    n. sulfate
nickel-cadmium (NiCad)
Niclocide

niclosamide
Nicobid
Nicolar
Nicolau syndrome
Nicolle-Novy-MacNeal culture
Nicolle white mycetoma
nicotinamide adenine dinucleotide phosphate (NADPH)
nicotinate
    methyl n.
nicotine stomatitis
Nicotinex
nicotinic acetylcholine receptor
Nico-Vert
NICU
    nonconimmunological contact urticaria
NidaGel
NIDDM
    noninsulin-dependent diabetes mellitus
nidogen
Nidryl oral
nidulans
    Aspergillus n.
Nieden syndrome
Niemann-Pick disease
nifedipine
nifurtimox
niger
    Aspergillus n.
    Peptococcus n.
NightBird nasal CPAP
night blindness
nightshade
    bittersweet n.
nighttime
    Arthritis Foundation N.
nigra
    acanthosis papulosa n.
    dermatosis papulosa n.
    linea n.
    lingua n.
    pityriasis n.
    seborrhea n.
    tinea n.
    trichomycosis n.
nigricans
    drug-induced acanthosis n.
    familial acanthosis n.
    hyperandrogenism, insulin resistance, and acanthosis n. (HAIR-AN)
    keratosis n.
    malignant acanthosis n.

    mental retardation, overgrowth, remarkable face, and acanthosis n. (MORFAN)
    pseudoacanthosis n.
    Rhizopus n.
    type A, B, C acanthosis n.
nigrities lingua
Nigrospora
NIH
    National Institutes of Health
Nijmegen breakage syndrome
Nikolsky sign
Nilstat topical
NIMA
    noninherited maternal antigen
Nimble Fingers glove
nimitti midge
nimodipine
Nimotop
nines
    rule of n.
    n. rule
ninth-day erythema
NIP
    National Immunization Program
Nipah virus
nipper
    Amico nail n.
nipple
    jogger's n.'s
NIR
    noninfectious rhinitis
nit
nitazoxanide (NTZ)
2-nite
    Sleepwell 2-n.
nitidus
    lichen n.
nitrate
    econazole n.
    intravesical silver n.
    oxiconazole n.
    sertaconazole n.
    silver n.
    sulconazole n.
nitric oxide
nitritoid reaction
nitroblue
    n. tetrazolium (NBT)
    n. tetrazolium test
nitrofurantoin

NOTES

N

nitrofurazone
nitrogen (N)
    n. mustard
2-(2-nitro-4-trifluromethylbenzoyl)-3-cyclohexanedione
nitrotyrosine
nitrous oxide
Nivea moisturizer
Nix Creme Rinse
Nizoral
    N. A-D Shampoo
    N. oral
    N. Topical
NK
    natural killer
      NK cell
      NK cell activation
      NK cell lysis
      NK cell-mediated cytotoxicity
NKSF
    natural killer cell-stimulating factor
NK/T-cell lymphoma
NLE
    neonatal lupus erythematosus
NLF
    nasolabial fold
N-linked pattern
NLite laser
NLS
    nuclear localization signal
NM
    nevomelanocytic
NMDP
    National Marrow Donor Program
308-nm Excimer laser
NMM
    nevoid malignant melanoma
NMR
    Neill-Mooser reaction
NMRL
    normal-mode ruby laser
NMSC
    nonmelanoma skin cancer
NNM
    Nicolle-Novy-MacNeal culture
NNRTI
    nonnucleoside reverse transcriptase
    inhibitor
no
    no observed adverse effect level
    (NOAEL)
    No Pain-HOT PACKS
    No Pain-HP
    No Sting barrier film
NO-AD Sunscreen
NOAEL
    no observed adverse effect level
NOAR
    Norfolk Arthritis Register

Nocardia
    N. asteroides
    N. brasiliensis
    N. caviae
    N. farcinica
    N. tenuis
    N. transvalensis
nocardia
nocardiosis
nociception
nociceptive neurotransmitter
nocodazole
nocturnal
    n. asthma
    n. hemoglobinuria
    n. myoclonus
    n. wheezing
NOD
    nonobese diabetic
nodal fever
node
    Bizzozero n.
    Bouchard n.
    funicular n.
    Heberden n.
    juxtaarticular n.
    lymph n.
    milker's n.
    Osler n.
    Parrot n.
    Schmorl n.
    sentinel lymph n. (SLN)
nodi (*pl. of* nodus)
nodosa
    cutaneous polyarteritis n.
    dermatitis n.
    periarteritis n.
    polyarteritis n. (PAN)
    systemic polyarteritis n.
    tinea n.
    trichomycosis axillaris n.
    trichorrhexis n.
nodose
nodositas crinium
nodosity
nodosum
    erythema n. (EN)
nodous
nodular
    n. basal cell carcinoma
    n. chondrodermatitis
    n. connective tissue disease nevus
    n. elastosis
    n. episcleritis
    n. granulomatous vasculitis
    n. hidradenoma
    n. leprosy
    n. malignant melanoma
    n. migratory panniculitis

n. myositis
n. neurodermatitis
n. nonsuppurative panniculitis
n. non-X histiocytosis
n. panencephalitis
n. pattern
n. pseudosarcomatous fasciitis
n. pulmonary amyloidosis
n. scabies
n. scleritis
n. sclerosing Hodgkin disease (NSHD)
n. shadow
n. subepidermal fibrosis
n. synovitis
n. syphilid
n. tuberculid
n. xanthoma
nodularis
chondrodermatitis helicis n.
dermatitis psoriasiformis n.
prurigo n.
trichomycosis axillaris n.
nodulated
nodulation
nodule
apple jelly n.
athlete's n.
Bohn n.
Busacca n.
Caplan n.
cutaneous n.
cutaneous-subcutaneous n.
dark-staining n.
embolic n.
n.'s, eosinophilia, rheumatism, dermatitis, and swelling (NERDS)
n. eosinophilia, rheumatism, dermatitis, and swelling
n.'s, eosinophilia, rheumatism, dermatitis, and swelling syndrome
glial n.
Jeanselme n.
juxtaarticular n.
Koeppe n.
lepromatous n.
Lisch n.
lymph n.
milker's n.
paraumbilical n.
picker's n.
pulmonary necrobiotic n.

red papule and n.
rheumatoid n.
sharply circumscribed n.
Sister Mary Joseph n.
Stockman n.
subcutaneous granulomatous n.
subcutaneous rheumatoid n.
subepidermal calcified n.
noduli (*pl. of* nodulus)
nodulocystic acne
nodulosis
pulmonary n.
rheumatoid n.
noduloulcerative
n. basal cell carcinoma
n. syphilis
n. tertiary syphilis
nodulous
nodulus, pl. noduli
n. cutaneus
nodus, pl. nodi
noir
talon n.
noire
atrophie n.
tache n.
No-Kor needle
Nolahist
Nolamine
Nolex LA
noma
nomenclature
binary n.
linnaean system of n.
NOMID
neonatal-onset multisystem inflammatory disease
nominal allotype
non-A
n.-A. non-B (NANB)
n.-A. non-B hepatitis
n.-A. non-B hepatitis virus
nonacetylated salicylate
nonacnegenic
nonadherent cell
nonadrenergic noncholinergic mechanism (NANC)
non-A-E hepatitis
nonalcoholic white shake lotion
nonallergic
n. asthma

N

NOTES

nonallergic *(continued)*
>   n. rhinitis with eosinophilia
>   syndrome (NARES)

No-Name Dandruff Treatment
nonamer
nonamide
nonanaphylactic reaction (NAR)
nonantiinflammatory analgesic agent
nonarticular
>   n. rheumatism
>   n. syndrome

non-B
>   n.-B cell
>   non-A n.-B (NANB)

nonblanchable, abnormally colored lesion
nonblanching purpura
nonbullous
>   n. congenital erythrodermic
>   ichthyosis
>   n. congenital ichthyosiform
>   erythroderma
>   n. impetigo

noncaseating granuloma
noncatecholamine
noncavitary
noncicatrizing alopecia
noncomedogenic
nonconimmunological contact urticaria (NICU)
nonconjugative plasmid
noncorticosteroid antiinflammatory agent
noncross-reactive drug
noncytolytic
nondenaturing condition
nondermatophyte fungal infection
nondigestible oligosaccharide (NDO)
Non-Drowsy
>   Contac Cold N.-D.
>   Drixoral N.-D.

nondrug-related reaction
noneczematous persistent papular gold eruption
nonenzymatic glycation (NEG)
nonesterified PABA
non-fish-sensitive Prausnitz skin
nonfunction
>   primary n. (PRNF)

nongenomic glucocorticoid effect
nongonococcal
>   n. bacterial arthritis
>   n. urethritis

nonheart-beating
>   n.-b. donor (NHBD)
>   n.-b. donor liver transplantation

nonhemophiliac patient
nonhistone protein
non-Hodgkin lymphoma (NHL)

nonidentity
>   reaction of n.

nonimmediate-type immunologic drug reaction
nonimmune
>   n. agglutination
>   n. serum

nonimmunity
nonimmunologic
>   n. basis
>   n. complication
>   n. drug reaction

noninfectious rhinitis (NIR)
noninflammatory
>   n. arthritis
>   n. edema
>   n. myopathy

noninherited maternal antigen (NIMA)
Nonin Onyx pulse oximeter
noninsulin-dependent diabetes mellitus (NIDDM)
nonirritating test substance
nonlinear IgA deposition
nonlymphocytic cell
nonmelanoma
>   n. cutaneous malignancy
>   n. skin cancer (NMSC)

nonmeningeal
nonmethylated CpG motif
nonmyeloablative
>   n. conditioning regimen
>   n. HSCT

nonnecrotizing angiitis
Nonne-Milroy-Meige syndrome
nonneoplastic disease
nonneuropathic systemic amyloidosis
nonnucleoside reverse transcriptase inhibitor (NNRTI)
nonobese diabetic (NOD)
nonoccluded virus
nonocclusive dressing
nonoxynol-9 cream
nonpalpable purpura
nonparasitic sycosis
nonpathogenic fungus
nonpharmacologic measure of treatment
nonpigmented nevus
nonpoisonous
nonpolio enterovirus
nonprecipitable antibody
nonprecipitating antibody
nonprecipitation antibody
nonproductive cough
nonradicular
nonrandom X chromosome inactivation
nonrapid eye movement (nonREM)
nonREM
>   nonrapid eye movement
>   nonREM sleep

nonresponder tolerance
nonrestorative sleep
nonrheumatoid
    n. episcleritis
    n. scleritis
nonscarring alopecia
nonsecretor
nonsedating antihistamine
nonselective adenosine receptor
  antagonist
nonsense triplet
nonshedding dog
nonspecific
    n. absorption
    n. anergy
    n. bronchial hyperreactivity
    n. climatic change
    n. cross-reacting antigen (NCA)
    n. dermatitis
    n. esterase (NSE)
    n. esterase stain
    n. protein
    n. therapy
nonsteroidal
    n. antiinflammatory
    n. antiinflammatory drug (NSAID)
nonstick gauze
nonsuction grasper
nonsyncytium-inducing variant of the
  AIDS virus
nonsyphilitic treponematosis
nonthrombocytopenic purpura
nontreponemal flocculation test
nontropical sprue
nontuberculous
    n. mycobacteria
    n. mycobacterial infection
nonunion
    ankylosis n.
    supracondylar n.
nonunited olecranon
nonvellus hair
nonvenereal
    n. bubo
    n. syphilis
    n. treponematosis
noon
    noon unit
    N. pollen unit
Noonan syndrome
norastemizole
Nordimmun IGIV

Norditropine
Nordryl
    N. injection
    N. oral
Norel
norepinephrine bitartrate
norethindrone
norfloxacin
Norfolk Arthritis Register (NOAR)
norgestimate
Norisodrine
Noritate cream
norlupinane
normal
    n. animal
    n. antibody
    n. antitoxin
    n. cornification
    n. horse serum
    n. opsonin
    n. toxin
normal-mode ruby laser (NMRL)
Normlgel hydrogel dressing
normocapnia
normocholesteremic xanthoma
normochromic
normocomplementemic
normocytic
normolipemic xanthomatosis
normolipoproteinemic xanthomatosis
normouricemia
Noroxin oral
Norpramin
Nor-tet oral
north
    N. American antisnakebite serum
    N. American blastomycosis
    N. American Contact Dermatitis
    Group (NACDG)
    N. American Pediatric Rental
    Transplant Cooperative Study
    (NAPRTCS)
    N. American Study of treatment
    for Refractory Ascites (NASTRA)
    N. American Study of Treatment
    for Refractory Ascites study
    N. Asian tick typhus
    N. Queensland tick typhus
Northbent scissors
Northeast Organ Procurement
  Organization (NEOPO)

NOTES

N

northern
>N. blot analysis
>n. rat flea
>n. rat flea bite
>N. Research Laboratories

Northland bone density machine
nortriptyline
Norvir
Norwalk
>N. agent
>N. virus

Norwalk-like agent
Norway itch
Norwegian scabies
Norwood classification system
nose
>bunny n.
>saddle n.
>total water gradient across the n.
>(TWG)

nose-associated lymphoid tissue (NALT)
Nosema
>*N. connori*
>*N. corneum*
>*N. ocularum*

nosematosis
nose-pad dermatitis
nosocomial
>n. candidemia
>n. gangrene
>n. infection
>n. pneumonia (NP)

nosocomialis
>phagedena n.

Nosopsyllus
>*N. fasciatus*
>*N. fasciatus* bite

nosotoxic
nosotoxin
nostras
>cholera n.
>n. elephantiasis
>elephantiasis n.
>piedra n.

Nostrilla
notalgia paresthetica
notatum
>*Penicillium n.*

Notch signaling pathway
Nothnagel-type acroparesthesia
Notoedres
Nottingham Health Profile (NHP)
Notuss PD
Novacet topical
Novafed
Novafil suture
Novahistine
Novamoxin
Nova Perfecting Lotion

Novasen
Novasome creme
novel missense mutation
novo
>de n.

Novo-AZT
Novobetamet
Novocaine
Novocain injection
Novo-Cimetine
Novo-Cromolyn
Novo-Difenac-K
Novo-Difenac-SR
Novo-Diflunisal
Novo-Dimenate
Novo-Doxylin
Novo E
Novo-Famotidine
Novo-Flurprofen
Novo-Keto
Novo-Ketoconazole
Novo-Keto-EC
Novo-Methacin
Novo-Naprox
Novo-Nidazol
Novo-Pen-VK
Novo-Pheniram
Novo-Pirocam
Novo-Piroxicam
Novo-Prednisolone
Novo-Profen
Novo-Purol
Novo-Pyrazone
Novo-Ranidine
Novo-Rythro Encap
Novo-Sundac
Novo-Tetra
Novo-Tolmetin
noxa, pl. noxae
NoxBOX monitor
noxythiolin
NP
>nosocomial pneumonia

NPA
>nasopharyngeal aspirate

NPF/USA
>National Psoriasis Foundation/United
>States of America

NPSLE
>neuropsychiatric syndrome of systemic
>lupus erythematosus
>neuropsychiatric systemic lupus
>erythematosus

NPV
>negative predictive value

NR
>Tussi-Organidin NR

NRTI
>nucleoside analog RT inhibitor

NS
   Netherton syndrome
NSAID
   nonsteroidal antiinflammatory drug
      NSAID gastropathy
NSE
   neuron-specific enolase
   nonspecific esterase
      NSE stain
NSHD
   nodular sclerosing Hodgkin disease
NSJ
   nevus sebaceus of Jadassohn
NSN
   nephrotoxic serum nephritis
NSS
   nasal symptom score
Nt
   neutralizing
NTBC therapy
N-telopeptide
      cross-linked N-t.
      N-t. urine test
N-Terface
      N-T. contact layer sheet
      N-T. contact layer wound dressing
      N-T. gauze
N-terface
NTPPH, NTPPPH
   nucleoside triphosphate
      pyrophosphohydrolase
NTZ
   nitazoxanide
      NTZ Long Acting Nasal Solution
Nu-Amoxi
Nu-Ampi
Nu-Beclomethasone
nuchae
      acne keloidalis n.
      cutis rhomboidalis n.
      erythema n.
      lichen n.
      ligamentum n.
      nevus flammeus n.
      sycosis n.
nuchal
      n. hemangioma
      n. nevus
Nu-Cimet
nuclear
      n. dot pattern
      n. factor

      n. factor of activated T cell
      (NFAT)
      n. factor-kappa B (NF-κB)
      n. factor-kappa B ligand
      n. inclusion body
      n. lamin B1
      n. localization signal (NLS)
nucleated endothelial cell
nucleatum
      Fusobacterium n.
nuclei (*pl. of* nucleus)
nucleic
      n. acid probe
      n. acid sequence based
      amplification (NASBA)
nucleocapsid
nucleohistone
nucleoid
nucleolar staining
Nucleopore filter
nucleoside
      n. analog RT inhibitor (NRTI)
      n. phosphorylase
      n. reverse transcriptase inhibitor
      n. triphosphate
      pyrophosphohydrolase (NTPPH,
      NTPPPH)
nucleosome
      n. antibody
      n. ladder
nucleotidase
nucleotide
      antisense n.
      n. polymorphism
      sense n.
nucleotoxin
nucleus, pl. **nuclei**
      droplet n.
      n. pulposus
Nucofed
nude
      n. bone graft transplantation
      n. mouse
Nu-Derm
      N.-D. hydrocolloid
      N.-D. hydrocolloid dressing
      Obagi N.-D.
      N.-D. System
Nu-Diclo
Nu-Diflunisal
Nu-Doxycycline
Nu-Famotidine

N

NOTES

Nu-Flurprofen
Nu Gauze dressing
Nu-Gel
    N.-G. hydrogel sheet
    N.-G. hydrogel wound dressing
    N.-G. synthetic dressing
Nu-Hope skin barrier strip
Nu-Ibuprofen
Nu-Indo
Nu-Ketocon
Nu-Ketoprofen
Nu-Ketoprofen-E
NuLev oral
null
    n. allele
    n. cell
    n. cell leukemia
null-type non-Hodgkin lymphoma
number
    chromosome n.
numbness
numerical taxonomy
nummular
    n. eczema
    n. eczematous dermatitis
    n. erythema
    n. lesion
    n. neurodermatitis
    n. syphilid
nummulare
    eczema n.
nummularis
    psoriasis n.
Nu-Naprox
Nu-Pen-VK
Nupercainal
Nu-Pirox
Nuprin
Nu-Ranit

nurse cell
Nursoy formula
NuSieve agarose gel
nut
    Brazil n.
Nu-Tears II solution
Nu-Tetra
nutraceuticals
Nutracort topical
Nu-Trake Weiss emergency airway
  system
Nutramigen formula
Nutraplus Topical
nutrient artery
nutritional
    n. deficiency dermatitis
    n. deficiency eczema
    n. disorder
Nutrol AD
Nutrotropin
Nuvion
NUVO barrier film
Nuvolase 660 laser system
NVAC
    National Vaccine Advisory Committee
Nydrazid injection
Nylexogrip cohesive long stretch
  bandage
nylon
    n. stocking dermatitis
    n. suture
nystagmus
nystatin and triamcinolone
Nystat-Rx
Nystex topical
Nyst-Olone II topical
Nytol
    Maximum Strength N.
    N. oral

O

O agglutinin
O antigen
padimate O
O to T flap
O to Z flap

OA

occupationally induced asthma
ocular albinism
osteoarthritis

OAF

osteoclast-activating factor

oak

Gambel o.
live o.
o. moss absolute
poison o.
o. tree
o. tree pollen
western poison o.
white o.

oakridgensis

Legionella o.

OAS

oral allergy syndrome
OAS 1000

Oasis wound dressing

oatmeal

colloidal o.
o. treatment

oat straw

Obagi Nu-Derm

obconica

Primula o.

obesity

protein-energy-related o.
vitamin-related o.

objective

O. Severity Assessment of Atopic
dermatitis (OSAAD)
o. synonym

obligate

o. aerobe
o. myiasis

oblique advancement flap

obliterans

arteriosclerosis o.
balanitis xerotica o.
bronchiolitis o.
keratosis o.
thromboangiitis o. (TAO)

obliterative

o. airway disease
o. granulomatous fibrosis

O'Brien

O. actinic granuloma
O. scissors

obstruction

episodic bronchial o.
fixed airflow o.
severe o.
upper airway o.

obstructive

o. liver disease
o. purpura
o. sleep apnea (OSA)

obturator

o. internus bursitis
o. nerve entrapment

obtusa

Malassezia o.

obtusus

lichen o.

obvious physical exhaustion

OCA

oculocutaneous albinism

occidentale

Anacardium o.

occidentalis

Dermacentor o.

occipital

o. forelock
o. horn syndrome

occipitoaxial joint

occlude

occluded virus

occludens

zonula o.

occlusal appliance therapy

Occlusal-HP Liquid

occlusion

o. miliaria
portal o.

occlusive

o. dressing
o. meningitis
o. moisturizer
o. patch test
o. phase
o. sheeting
o. therapy

occuloglandular syndrome

occult

o. blood
o. bowel inflammation

occupational

o. acne
o. allergen
o. allergic alveolitis

O

occupational *(continued)*
- o. allergic contactant
- o. contact dermatitis
- o. dermatosis
- o. exposure
- o. immunologic lung disease (OLD)
- o. koilonychia
- o. leukoderma
- o. non-IgE-dependent asthma
- o. rubber dermatitis
- o. therapy (OT)
- o. vitiligo

occupationally induced asthma (OA)
occupation-related syndrome
Ochrobacterium anthropi
ochrodermia
ochronosis
- endogenous o.
- exogenous o.
- ocular o.

ochronotic
- o. arthritis
- o. arthropathy
- o. spondylosis

Ockelbo disease
octamer
octapeptide
Octicair Otic
Octocaine injection
octreotide acetate
octulosonic acid
2-octylcyanoacrylate topical bandage
octyl methoxycinnamate
OcuClear Ophthalmic
OcuCoat PF Ophthalmic solution
Ocufen Ophthalmic
ocular
- o. adnexa
- o. albinism (OA)
- o. allergy
- o. atopic dermatitis
- o. basal cell carcinoma
- o. cicatricial pemphigoid
- o. herpes simplex
- o. herpes simplex virus infection
- o. herpes zoster virus infection
- o. hypertelorism
- o. immune disease
- o. inflammatory disease
- o. inflammatory disorder
- o. larva migrans
- o. lesion
- o. lymphomatosis
- o. melanoma
- o. ochronosis
- o. pemphigus
- o. rosacea
- o. sarcoidosis
- o. toxicity

ocular-mucous membrane syndrome
ocular-scoliotic type Ehlers-Danlos syndrome
ocularum
- *Nosema o.*

oculi
- orbicularis o.

oculocerebral syndrome of Cross and McKusick
oculocutaneous
- o. albinism (OCA)
- o. telangiectasia

oculodermal
- o. melanocytosis
- o. melanosis

oculoglandular
oculoleptomeningeal amyloidosis
oculo-oral-genital syndrome
oculopharyngeal dystrophy
Ocu-Merox
Ocutricin
- O. HC Otic
- O. Topical Ointment

Ocu-Tropine Ophthalmic
odaxetic
ODD
- once daily dosing

odeus
- herpes o.

Odland body
ODN
- oligodeoxynucleotide

odontoid process displacement
odonto-tricho-ungual-digital-palmar syndrome
odor
- o. control
- mousy o.
- volatile o.

odorans
- *Alcaligenes o.*

odoriferous
ODTS
- organic dust toxic syndrome

O'Duffy criteria
Odulimomab
oedema
- purpura en cocarde avec o.

Oesch
- O. perforation invagination stripper
- O. phlebectomy hook

Oesophagostomum
oestrosa
- dermamyiasis linearis migrans o.

oestruosa
- myiasis o.

OET
   open epicutaneous test
OFC
   open food challenge
   oral food challenge
Off-Ezy
officinalis
      Calendula o.
      Melilotus o.
      Melissa o.
      poxvirus o.
ofloxacin
Ofuji
   O. disease
   papuloerythroderma of O.
Ohara disease
OHL
   oral hairy leukoplakia
Ohmeda handheld oximeter
ohne Hauch
OI
   opportunistic illness
oidiomycin
oidiomycosis
"oid-oid" disease
oil
   o. acne
   Alpha-Keri o.
   bath o.
   o. bath
   o. of bergamot
   Cade o.
   Cajuput o.
   citronella o.
   clove o.
   coal tar, lanolin, and mineral o.
   Derma-Smoothe O.
   o. drop change
   o. drop lesion
   o. drop sign
   essential o.
   eucalyptus o.
   evening primrose o.
   fish o.
   o. folliculitis
   o. gland
   o. immersion
   jojoba o.
   Lubath o.
   mineral o.
   O. of Olay soap
   patchouli o.
   petitgrain o.
   pine o.
   RoBathol o.
   silicone o.
   o. staining
   tea tree o.
   trypsin, balsam Peru, and castor o.
   Turpentine o.
   o. vaccine
   ylang-ylang o.
Oilated Aveeno
oil-based facial foundation
Oil-Free
   O.-F. Acne Wash
   Coppertone O.-F.
oiliness
oil-in-water cream
oil-spot discoloration
oily
   o. granuloma
   o. skin
ointment
   absorbent o.
   A and D O.
   AK-Spore H.C. Ophthalmic O.
   Aloe Vesta antifungal o.
   Amerigel topical o.
   ApexiCon o.
   Baby's Own O.
   Cavilon barrier o.
   Cormax O.
   Cortisporin Ophthalmic O.
   Cortisporin Topical O.
   Denavir o.
   Dermagran o.
   Efalith o.
   emulsifiable o.
   Ethezyme Papain-Urea Debriding o.
   fluocinolone o.
   Hebra o.
   HydroSkin o.
   James C. White tar o.
   Jarisch o.
   Kligman's o.
   Medi-Quick Topical O.
   mupirocin o.
   Neo-Polycin o.
   Neosporin Ophthalmic O.
   Neosporin Topical O.
   Neotricin HC Ophthalmic O.
   Ocutricin Topical O.
   Panscol o.

O

NOTES

ointment *(continued)*
> Protopic o.
> rose water o.
> Salacid O.
> Septa Topical O.
> tacrolimus o.
> tacrolimus o.
> tacrolimus o.
> o. of tar
> Terak Ophthalmic O.
> Terramycin w/Polymyxin B
>   Ophthalmic O.
> triamcinolone o. (TAO)
> Tronothane o.
> water-in-oil o.
> water-repellent o.
> water-soluble o.
> Whitfield o.
> Xenaderm o.

ointment/dressing
> Dermagran o.

Oka vaccine
OKT
> Ortho-Kung T
> OKT3 antibody
> OKT cell

OKT3
> 5 OKT3 antilymphocyte therapy
> Orthoclone OKT3

olamine
> ciclopirox o.

Olay Sensitive Skin bar
OLD
> occupational immunologic lung disease

old
> o. ecchymosis
> o. tuberculin (OT)
> O. World leishmaniasis

old-man's pemphigus
Olea europa
olecranon
> o. bursitis
> o. fossa
> nonunited o.
> o. procedure
> o. process

Oleeva
oleic acid
oleoresin
> capsaicin o.
> plant o.

oleosa
> hyperhidrosis o.
> seborrhea o.

oleosus
Oligella
oligemicus
> nevus o.

olighidria

oligoadenylate synthase
oligoarthritis
> asymmetric o.
> seronegative o.

oligoarthropathy
> asymmetric o.

oligoarticular seronegative rheumatoid arthritis
oligoclonal
oligocystic
oligodendrocyte
> o. destruction
> o. injury

oligodeoxynucleotide (ODN)
> antisense o.
> immunostimulatory o. (ISS-ODN)
> unmethylated o.

oligodynamic
oligoglysine
oligohidria
oligohidrosis
oligonucleotide
> antisense phosphorothioate o.
> o. probe

oligophrenia
> phenylpyruvic o.

oligoprobe
oligosaccharide
> asparagine-linked o.
> hyaluronan o.
> Lewis X o.
> nondigestible o. (NDO)

oligosymptomatic
oligotrichia
oligotrichosis
oligotyping
O-linked
> O-l. pattern
> O-l. saccharide

olivae
> vellus o.

olive
> Russian o.
> o. tree
> o. tree pollen

Ollendorf syndrome
Olmsted syndrome
olopatadine hydrochloride
olsalazine sodium
Olsen-Hegar needle holder
OLT
> orthotopic liver transplantation

Olux foam
omalizumab
Ombrelle
> O. sunscreen
> O. sunscreen lotion

omega-3, -6 fatty acid
omega nail

Omenn syndrome
omeprazole
Omiderm
Ommaya reservoir
Omniderm
    O. synthetic dressing
    O. transparent film
Omnipen
Omnipen-N
omphalocele
Omsk
    O. hemorrhagic fever
    O. hemorrhagic fever virus
OMU
   ostiomeatal unit
once daily dosing (ODD)
Onchocerca
    O. caecutiens
    O. volvulus
onchocerciasis
onchocercosis
oncofetal antigen
oncogene
    BNLF-1 o.
    Kirsten-MSV Ras o.
oncogenic
    o. hypophosphatemic osteomalacia
    o. virus
oncology
Oncolym radiolabeled monoclonal
  antibody
Onconase
oncornaviruses
oncostatin M (OSM)
Oncovin
Oncovirinae
oncovirus
oncus
Ondine curse, periodic breathing
ongles en raquette
onion mite dermatitis
only
    Faces O.
onset
    insidious o.
    pauciarticular o.
Ontak protein
ontogeny
onychalgia nervosa
onychatrophia
onychatrophy
onychauxis

onychectomy
onychia
    Candida o.
    o. craquelé
    o. lateralis
    o. maligna
    monilial o.
    o. parasitica
    o. periungualis
    o. piannic
    o. punctata
    o. sicca
    syphilitic o.
onychitis
onychoclasis
onychocryptosis
onychodystrophy
onychogenic
onychogryphosis, onychogryposis
onychoheterotopia
onychoid
onychology
onycholysis
    distal o.
onychoma
onychomadesis
onychomalacia
onychomycosis
onychonosus
onychoosteodysplasia
onychopachydermoperiostitis
    psoriatic o. (POPP)
onychopathic
onychopathology
onychopathy
onychophagia
onychophagy
onychophosis
onychophyma
onychoptosis
onychorrhexis
onychoschizia
onychosis
onychotillomania
onychotomy
onychotrophy
Ony-Clear
    O.-C. Nail
    O.-C. Spray
o'nyong-nyong
    o.-n. fever
    o.-n. virus

O

NOTES

Onyvul · ophthalmic

Onyvul
onyx
onyxis
onyxitis
oocyst
    Cryptosporidium o.
oomycetes
oozing dermatitis
O&P
    ova and parasites
    test for O&P
opacification
    amorphous parenchymal o.
    corneal o.
    ground-glass o.
opacity
    mottled o.
opaline patch
Opcon-A
OPD
    optical penetration depth
open
    o. application test
    o. comedo
    o. epicutaneous test (OET)
    o. food challenge (OFC)
    o. lung biopsy
    o. patch test
    o. reduction and internal fixation
      (ORIF)
    o. tuberculosis
    o. wet dressing
opera-glass deformity
operator
    Boolean o.
opercula
opercularis
    Megalopyge o.
operculate
ophiasic alopecia areata
ophiasis
ophritis
ophryitis
ophryogenes
    ulerythema o.
Ophthacet Ophthalmic
Ophthalgan Ophthalmic
ophthalmia
    gonococcal o.
    o. neonatorum
    spring o.
    sympathetic o.
ophthalmic
    Achromycin O.
    Acular O.
    AK-Chlor O.
    AK-Cide O.
    AK-Dex O.
    AK-Homatropine O.

AK-Neo-Dex O.
AK-Poly-Bac O.
AK-Pred O.
AK-Sulf O.
AKTob O.
AK-Tracin O.
AK-Trol O.
Alomide O.
Atropair O.
Atropine-Care O.
Atropisol O.
Betimol O.
Bleph-10 O.
Blephamide O.
Cetamide O.
Cetapred O.
Chloroptic O.
Chloroptic-P O.
Ciloxan O.
Collyrium Fresh O.
Dexacidin O.
Dexasporin O.
Econopred Plus O.
Flarex O.
Fluor-Op O.
FML O.
Garamycin O.
Genoptic S.O.P. O.
Gentacidin O.
Gentak O.
Herplex O.
HMS Liquifilm o.
Ilotycin O.
Inflamase Forte O.
Inflamase Mild O.
Isopto Atropine O.
Isopto Cetapred O.
Isopto Homatropine O.
Isopto Hyoscine O.
I-Sulfacet O.
I-Tropine O.
Livostin o.
Maxitrol o.
Metimyd o.
Metreton o.
Natacyn O.
Neo-Cortef O.
NeoDecadron o.
Neo-Dexameth O.
OcuClear O.
Ocufen O.
Ocu-Tropine O.
Ophthacet O.
Ophthalgan O.
Ophthocort O.
Osmoglyn O.
Polysporin O.
Polytrim O.
Pred Forte O.

Pred-G o.
Pred Mild O.
Sodium Sulamyd O.
Sulf-10 O.
Sulfair O.
Tetrasine Extra O.
Timoptic O.
Timoptic-XE O.
TobraDex O.
Tobrex O.
Vasocidin O.
Vasosulf O.
Vira-A O.
Viroptic O.
Visine L.R. O.

ophthalmica
  zona o.
ophthalmicus
  herpes zoster o.
ophthalmic zoster
ophthalmomaxillaris
  nevus fuscoceruleus
    acromiodeltoideus fuscoceruleus o.
ophthalmomyiasis
ophthalmopathy
  thyroid-associated o. (TAO)
Ophthocort Ophthalmic
opiate
opioid
O-plasty to Z-plasty
OPO
  optical parametric oscillator
  organ procurement organization
oppilation
opportunistic
  o. fungus
  o. illness (OI)
  o. organism
  o. pathogen
  o. systemic fungal infection
  o. systemic mycosis
opposition-versus-pressure relation
oprelvekin
OPSI
  overwhelming postsplenectomy infection
opsinogen
OpSite
  O. Flexigrid adhesive dressing
  O. Flexigrid transparent film
  O. Plus
  O. Plus composite dressing
  O. Post-Op

O. postop composite dressing
O. semipermeable dressing
opsogen
opsonic
  o. deficiency
  o. receptor
opsonin
  common o.
  immune o.
  normal o.
  specific o.
  thermolabile o.
  thermostable o.
opsonization
opsonizing antibody
opsonocytophagic
opsonometry
opsonophagocytic defect
opsonophilia
opsonophilic
optic
  o. atrophy
  o. glioma
  o. neuritis
optica
  neuromyelitis o.
optical
  o. coherent tomography
  o. parametric oscillator (OPO)
  o. penetration depth (OPD)
OptiChamber
Opticrom
Opti-Flex
OptiHaler
Optimine
optimum temperature
Optimyd
Optipore Sponge wound cleanser
Opti 1 portable pH/blood gas analyzer
Optivar
Optotechnik
  Heine O.
OPV
  oral polio vaccine
Orabase
  O. HCA
  O. HCA topical
  Kenalog in O.
  O. with benzocaine
Oracit
Orafen
Ora-Jel

O

NOTES

oral

Achromycin V O.
o. administration of psoralen and subsequent exposure to long wavelength ultraviolet light (PUVA)
Aller-Chlor O.
o. allergy syndrome (OAS)
AllerMax O.
AL-Rr O.
Amino-Opti-E O.
Ansaid O.
o. antihistamine
Anxanil O.
o. aphthous ulcer
Aquasol E O.
Aristocort O.
Asacol O.
Atarax O.
Atolone O.
Atozine O.
Bactocill O.
Banophen O.
Beepen-VK O.
Belix O.
Benadryl O.
Betapen-VK O.
Bio-Tab O.
Blocadren O.
Brethine O.
Bricanyl O.
Calciferol O.
o. calcitonin
Calm-X O.
o. candidiasis
Cataflam O.
o. cavity abnormality
CeeNU O.
Ceftin O.
Celestone O.
o. challenge
Chlo-Amine O.
Chlorate O.
Cipro O.
Cleocin HCl O.
Cleocin Pediatric O.
Coly-Mycin S O.
o. condyloma planus
Cortone Acetate O.
Cytoxan O.
Decadron O.
Delta-Cortef O.
Deltasone O.
Diamine T.D. O.
Diflucan O.
Dimetabs O.
Dimetane O.
Dormarex 2 O.
Dormin O.

Doryx O.
Doxychel O.
Dramamine O.
Drisdol O.
Dynacin O.
E.E.S. O.
E-Mycin O.
o. epithelial nevus
o. erosive lichen planus
Eryc O.
EryPed O.
Ery-Tab O.
o. erythema multiforme
Erythrocin O.
o. erythromycin ethylsuccinate
Eryzole O.
Flagyl O.
o. florid papillomatosis
Floxin O.
Flumadine O.
o. food challenge (OFC)
Gantrisin O.
Gastrocrom O.
Genahist o.
o. hairy leukoplakia (OHL)
hyoscyamine sulfate o.
Hy-Pam o.
o. hyposensitization
Ilosone O.
Imitrex O.
Indocin SR o.
o. iron therapy
Kantrex O.
Kenacort o.
o. keratosis
Lamisil o.
Laniazid O.
Ledercillin VK O.
Liquid Pred O.
Loniten o.
Marmine o.
Maxaquin O.
Meclomen O.
Medrol o.
o. melanoacanthoma
Mephyton O.
Meticorten O.
Minocin O.
Monodox O.
o. mucosa
Mycifradin Sulfate O.
Mycostatin O.
Neo-fradin O.
Neoral O.
Neo-Tabs O.
Nidryl O.
Nizoral O.
Nordryl o.
Noroxin O.

Nor-tet o.
NuLev o.
Nytol o.
Orasone O.
Panmycin O.
PCE O.
PediaCare o.
Pediapred o.
Pediazole O.
Penetrex O.
Pentasa O.
Pen-Vee K O.
Pepcid O.
Phenameth O.
Phendry O.
Phenergan O.
Phenetron O.
o. polio vaccine (OPV)
poliovirus vaccine, live,
  trivalent, o.
o. postinflammatory
  hyperpigmentation
Prednicen-M O.
Prelone o.
Prostaphlin O.
Prothazine O.
Protostat o.
Retrovir O.
Rifadin o.
Rimactane O.
Robicillin VK O.
Robitet o.
Salagen O.
Sandimmune O.
Siladryl o.
Sleep-eze 3 O.
Sominex O.
Sporanox O.
Sterapred O.
Sumycin O.
o. tattoo
Tega-Vert O.
Telachlor O.
Teldrin O.
Teline O.
Terramycin O.
Tetracap o.
Tetralan O.
Tetram O.
o. thrush
o. tolerance
Trisoralen O.

o. tuberculosis
Twilite o.
o. ulceration
Unipen O.
Uri-Tet O.
Valium O.
Valrelease o.
Vancocin o.
V-Cillin K o.
Veetids o.
VePesid o.
Vibramycin o.
Videx o.
Vistaril o.
Vivotif Berna o.
Voltaren o.
Voltaren-XR o.
Wellcovorin o.
Zantac o.
Zovirax o.
oral-ocular-genital syndrome
Oraminic II injection
orange
  o. blossom
  o. peel appearance
Orap
Orasone oral
Orbasone system
orBec
orbiculare
  Pityrosporum o.
orbicular eczema
orbicularis
  alopecia o.
  o. oculi
  psoriasis o.
orbital
  o. granuloma
  o. inflammatory disease
  o. myositis
  o. pseudotumor
Orbivirus
orchard
  o. grass
  o. grass pollen
orchitis
  allergic o.
ordinal designation of the exanthemata
Oregon ash
Orentreich punch
Orex
3'orf gene

NOTES

organ
    o. culture
    o. parking
    o. procurement organization (OPO)
    o. system failure index (OSFI)
    o. transplantation system
    o. xenograft
organ-cultured corneal tissue
organelle
Organex
organic
    o. dust toxic syndrome (ODTS)
    o. extracts of diesel exhaust
      particles
    o. mercurials
Organidin
organism
    Cox o.
    culprit o.
    encapsulated o.
    gram-negative o.
    gram-positive o.
    group JK o.
    hypothetical mean o.
    opportunistic o.
    pleuro-pneumoniae-like o. (PPLO)
    prokaryotic extracellular o.
    transgenic o.
organization
    Food Agricultural O. (FAO)
    health maintenance o. (HMO)
    International Labor O. (ILO)
    Northeast Organ Procurement O.
      (NEOPO)
    organ procurement o. (OPO)
    World Health O. (WHO)
organoclay
organoid nevus
organotaxis
organotropic
organotropism
organotropy
organ-specific
    o.-s. antigen
    o.-s. tolerance
Orgotein
Oriboca virus
Oriental
    O. boil
    O. button
    O. rat flea
    O. rat flea bite
    O. ringworm
    O. sore
    O. ulcer
orientalis
    Amycolatopsis o.
    furunculosis o.
    Leishmania o.

ORIF
    open reduction and internal fixation
orifice
    follicular o.
orificialis
    tuberculosis cutis o.
orificial tuberculosis
origin
    antirabies serum, equine o.
    fever of unknown o. (FUO)
original
    Doan's, O.
Orimune
Orinidyl
Orion
    O. device
    O. inhaler
oris
    adenomatosis o.
    cancrum o.
    fetor o.
    leukokeratosis o.
Ormazine
Ornade
Ornex Cold
ornidazole
Ornidyl injection
ornithine
    o. carbamyl transferase compound
    o. transcarbamylase deficiency
**ornithine-ketoacid transaminase 3
antibody**
Ornithodoros
ornithosis virus
orofacial
    o. herpes simplex
    o. tuberculosis
orolabial herpes
oronasal
oropharyngeal
    o. candidiasis
    o. gonorrhea
oropharynx
orosomucoid
orotic aciduria
orotidinuria
Oroya fever
orphan
    chicken embryo lethal o. (CELO)
    o. disease
    o. drug
    enteric cytopathogenic bovine o.
      (ECBO)
    enteric cytopathogenic human o.
      (ECHO)
    enteric cytopathogenic monkey o.
      (ECMO)
    enteric cytopathogenic swine o.
      (ECSO)

respiratory enteric o. (REO)
   o. virus
orris root
Ortho-Cept
Orthoclone
   O. OKT3
   O. OKT3 anti-CD3 monoclonal
   antibody
Ortho-Ice Multipaks system
orthokeratinization
orthokeratosis
Ortho-Kung
   O.-K. T (OKT)
   O.-K. T cell
orthologue
orthomolecular therapy
Orthomune monoclonal antibody
Orthomyxoviridae virus
orthophosphate (P1)
orthopnea
Orthopoxvirus vaccinia
orthosis, pl. **orthoses**
   patellar tendon-bearing o.
   spring-assisted knee extension o.
   thoraco-lumbar-sacral o.
orthostatic
   o. acrocyanosis
   o. hypotension
   o. purpura
orthotic
orthotopic
   o. heart transplantation
   o. liver transplantation (OLT)
Orthovisc
Orudis KT
Oruvail
oryzae
   Aspergillus o.
   Rhizopus o.
orzihabitans
   Flavimonas o.
OS
   oxidative stress
OSA
   obstructive sleep apnea
OSAAD
   Objective Severity Assessment of Atopic
   dermatitis
Oscar virus
oscillation
   high frequency o.

oscillator
   Hayek o.
   optical parametric o. (OPO)
OSFI
   organ system failure index
Osler
   O. disease
   O. hemangiomatosis
   O. node
   O. sign
   O. syndrome II
   O. triad
Osler-Weber-Rendu
   O.-W.-R. disease
   O.-W.-R. syndrome
OSM
   oncostatin M
OSMED
   otospondylometaphyseal dysplasia
   OSMED syndrome
osmidrosis
osmiophilic crystal structure
Osmitrol injection
OsmoCyte
   O. pillow
   O. pillow wound dressing
Osmoglyn Ophthalmic
osmolality
osmophil
osmotic shock
OspA primer-probe
ospB
   outer surface protein B
OspB primer-probe
ospC
   outer surface protein C
osseous
   o. choristoma of the tongue
   o. heteroplasia
   o. lesion
   o. syphilis
   o. tumor
   o. yaw
ossicle
   intraarticular o.
ossificans
   myositis o.
ossification
   entheseal o.
   paraarticular o.
   periarticular o.

O

NOTES

ossium
  fibrogenesis imperfecta o.
osteitis
  o. condensans ilii
  o. fibrosa
  o. fibrosa cystica disseminata
  o. pubis
  synovitis, acne, pustulosis,
    hyperostosis, o. (SAPHO)
osteoarthritis (OA)
  erosive o. (EOA)
  facet joint o.
  glenohumeral o.
  idiopathic hypertrophic o.
  patellofemoral o.
  radiologic o. (ROA)
osteoarthropathy
  hypertrophic o.
  tabetic o.
osteoarticular
  o. candidiasis
  o. tuberculosis
Osteo Bi-Flex
osteoblast-lineage cell
osteocalcin
osteochondral
  o. graft
  o. implant
osteochondritis
  o. dissecans
  parrot syphilitic o.
osteochondrodysplasia
osteochondromatosis
osteoclast-activating factor (OAF)
osteoclast differentiation factor
osteoclastogenesis
osteocyte lacunae
osteodermatopoikilosis
osteodermatous
osteodermia
osteodystrophy
  Albright hereditary o.
osteogenesis
  o. imperfecta
  o. imperfecta syndrome
  o. imperfecta tarda
OsteoGram bone density test
osteohypertrophic nevus flammeus
osteoid osteoma
osteolytic bone lesion
osteoma
  o. cutis
  intraarticular osteoid o.
  osteoid o.
osteomalacia
  oncogenic hypophosphatemic o.
Osteomark
  O. NTx point-of-care device
  O. urine-based test

osteomatoid
osteomatosis
osteomyelitis
  Aspergillus o.
  blastomycotic o.
  Candida o.
  candidal o.
  chronic multifocal o.
  coccidioidal o.
  pyogenic o.
  Salmonella o.
  typhoid o.
  o. variolosa
osteon
osteonecrosis
osteonectin
osteoonychodysplasia
  hereditary o. (HOOD)
osteopenia
  juxtaarticular o.
  periarticular o.
osteopetrosis gallinarum
osteophyte
osteopoikilosis
osteopontin
osteoporosis
  age-related o.
  o. circumscripta
  glucocorticoid-induced o.
  juxtaarticular o.
  periarticular o.
  type (I, II) o.
osteoprotegerin ligand
osteosis cutis
osteotabes
osteotomy
  Bernese periacetabular o.
  periacetabular o.
  proximal femoral o.
Osterballe precision needle
ostia (*pl. of* ostium)
ostial
  porokeratotic eccrine o.
ostiomeatal unit (OMU)
ostium, pl. **ostia**
  pilosebaceous o.
ostracea
  parakeratosis o.
ostraceous
  o. psoriasis
  o. scale
ostreacea
  psoriasis o.
OT
  occupational therapy
  old tuberculin
Ota
  nevus of O.
  O. nevus

Ot antigen
Otic
>Acetasol HC O.
>AK-Spore H.C. O.
>AntibiOtic O.
>Bacticort O.
>Cortatrigen O.
>Cortisporin O.
>O. Domeboro
>Dri-Ear O.
>Drotic O.
>LazerSporin-C O.
>Octicair O.
>Ocutricin HC O.
>Otobiotic O.
>Otocort O.
>Otomycin-HPN O.
>Otosporin O.
>Pediotic O.
>Swim-Ear O.
>VoSol HC O.

oticus
>herpes zoster o.

otitic meningitis
otitis
>o. externa
>external o.
>o. media

Otobiotic Otic
Otocalm Ear
Otocort Otic
otogenic meningitis
Otomycin-HPN Otic
otomycosis
otoscopy
>pneumatic o.

otospondylometaphyseal dysplasia (OSMED)
Otosporin Otic
ototoxicity
Otrivin Nasal
Ouchterlony
>O. double diffusion technique
>O. method
>O. test

Oudin current
Out of Africa
Outcome Measures in Rheumatology Clinical Trial
outer
>o. canthus
>o. root sheath

>o. surface protein A (pspA)
>o. surface protein B (ospB)
>o. surface protein C (ospC)

Outerbridge scale
output
>adequate urine o.

OVA
>ovalbumin
>OVA antigen

ova and parasites (O&P)
ovalbumin (OVA)
>o. antigen

ovalbumin-derived epitope
ovalbumin-induced arthritis
ovale
>*Pityrosporum o.*
>*Plasmodium o.*

ovalis
>*Malassezia o.*

Ovarex MAb monoclonal antibody
ovarian failure
Ovcon
overdosage
overdose
>drug o.

overexpression
>gene o.

Overhauser effect
overlap
>o. disease
>eosinophilic syndrome o.
>o. myositis (OVLP)
>o. syndrome

overlay
>PAL pump for air mattress o.

overmoisturization
overriding maxillary incisor
over-the-door device
overt hyperthyroidism
overuse syndrome
overwhelming postsplenectomy infection (OPSI)
overwintering
Ovide topical
ovine progressive pneumonia
ovinia
oviposit
OVLP
>overlap myositis

ovomucoid
ovulation induction
Owens Surgical dressing

O

NOTES

OX-2, -19 test
oxacillin
    o. disk diffusion test
    o. sodium
oxalate crystal
oxalosis
oxamniquine
Oxandrin
oxandrolone
oxaprozin
oxazepam
oxeye, ox-eye
    e. daisy
Oxford unit
oxiconazole nitrate
oxidase
    lysyl o.
    monoamine o. (MAO)
    NADPH o.
    urate o.
oxidative
    o. burst
    o. stress (OS)
oxide
    aluminum o.
    endothelial-derived nitric o.
    ethylene o.
    mercuric o.
    nitric o.
    nitrous o.
    yellow mecuric o.
    zinc o.
oxidized cellulose
OxiFlow
oximeter
    Cricket recording pulse o.
    INVOS Cerebral O.
    Nellcor Symphony N-3000 pulse o.
    Nonin Onyx pulse o.
    Ohmeda handheld o.
    Oxypleth pulse o.
    OxyTemp handheld pulse o.
    SpotCheck+ handheld pulse o.
oxipurinol
Oxistat topical
OX-K proteus antigen
Oxsoralen topical
Oxsoralen-Ultra oral
oxtriphylline
Oxy
    O. Control
    O. Deep Pore
    O. Medicated Pads
    O. Night Watch
    O. Power Pads
    O. 10 Wash

Oxy-5
    Oxy-5 Advanced Formula for
      Sensitive Skin
    Oxy-5 Tinted
Oxy-10 Advanced Formula for Sensitive Skin
OxyBalance Facial Cleansing Wash
oxybenzone
    methoxycinnamate and o.
Oxybutazone
Oxycel
oxychlorosene sodium
OxyContin
Oxyderm
Oxyfil oxygen refilling system
oxygen
    o. consumption per minute (VO_2)
    continuous low-flow o.
    fraction of inspired o. (FIO_2)
    o. free radical
    humidified o.
    hyperbaric o. (HBO)
    o. metabolite
    partial pressure of o. (PO_2)
    partial pressure alveolar o. (PAO_2)
    partial pressure arterial o. (PaO_2)
    supplemental o.
oxygenase
    enzyme heme o.
oxygenation
oxygenator
oxyhemoglobin (HbO_2)
Oxyl
oxymetazoline hydrochloride
oxymetholone
oxyphenbutazone
Oxypleth pulse oximeter
oxypurinol
oxysporum
    Fusarium o.
OxyTemp handheld pulse oximeter
oxytetracycline
    o. hydrochloride
    o. and hydrocortisone
    o. and polymyxin b
OxyTip
oxytoca
    Klebsiella o.
Oxytrex
oxyuriasis
Oxyuris vermicularis
oyster mass of mucus
oyster-shell crust
Oz
    O. antigen
    O. isotypic determinant
ozochrotia
ozone

ozzardi
  Mansonella o.

NOTES

O

P

P antigen
P blood group antigen
P and PD
P & S plus

P1

orthophosphate

p24

p24 antigen
p24 antigen testing

P450

cytochrome P450
P450 metabolism

P53 tumor suppressor gene
p56 Lck deficiency
PA

persistent asthma
polyarthritis

P-450-3A4

cytochrome P.

PABA

paraaminobenzoic acid
PABA ester
esterified PABA
nonesterified PABA

PAC

papular acrodermatitis of childhood

PACD

photoallergic contact dermatitis

Pacheco parrot disease virus
pachydactyly
pachyderma

p. lymphangiectatica
p. verrucosa
p. vesica

pachydermatis

Malassezia p.

pachydermatocele
pachydermatosis
pachydermatous
pachydermia
pachydermic
pachydermoperiostosis plicata
pachyglossia
pachyhymenia
pachyhymenic
pachylosis
pachymenia
pachymenic
pachymeningitis

hypertrophic cervical p.
rheumatoid p.

pachyonychia congenita
pachyotia
Pacific tick

pacificus

Ixodes p.

pacinian neurofibroma
Pacis BCG
pack

ice p.
interferon alfa-2b and ribavirin
combination p.
M-Zole 7 Dual P.

packed red cell transfusion
packet

ENTsol P.'s

PACKS

No Pain-HOT P.

paclitaxel
pad

Clearasil P.'s
Elbowlift suspension p.
grounding p.
herniated presacral fat p.
impregnated p.
knuckle p.
MPM conductive gel p.
Oxy Medicated P.'s
Oxy Power P.'s
STD-E P.'s
Tegaderm transparent dressing with
absorbent p.

PADI

posterior atlantodental interval

padimate O
PAEC

pig aortic endothelial cell

Paecilomyces

P. lilacinus
P. variotii

Paederus

P. dermatitis
P. gemellus
P. gemellus sting
P. limnophilus
P. limnophilus sting

Paenibacillus popilliae
Paeonia lactiflora
PAF

platelet activating/aggregating factor
platelet-activating factor
platelet-aggregating factor

PAF-AH

platelet-activating factor acetylhydrolase

PAFD

percutaneous abscess and fluid drainage

PAG

pregnancy alpha-2 glycoprotein

P

PAGE
   polyacrylamide gel electrophoresis
Paget
   P. abscess
   P. abscess syndrome
   P. cell
   P. disease
pagetic petrous bony invasion
pagetoid
   p. cell
   p. reticulosis
PAH
   p-aminohippurate
Pahvant
   P. Valley fever
   P. Valley plague
pain
   chronic widespread p.
   facial p.
   global rating of p.
   heel p.
   ischemic bone p.
   limb p.
   low back p.
   masticatory p.
   neck p.
   p. on motion
   paranasal sinus p.
   pleuritic chest p.
   p. spot
   subchondral bone p.
Painaid
   P. BRF
   P. ESF
   P. PMF
painful
   p. adiposity
   p. mouth
   p. piezogenic pedal papule
   p. tongue
painful-bruising syndrome
Pain-HP
   No P.-HP
painless thyroiditis
paint
   Castellani p.
   keratolytic p.
   SAL p.
   salicylic acid-lactic acid p.
pair
   base p. (bp)
   recipient-donor p.'s
paired venom gland
PAIS
   punctate area of increased signal
PAK
   pancreas-after-kidney
   pancreas after kidney transplant
   PAK transplant

Pak
   Benzamycin P.
   Shingles Relief P.
palatal
   p. clicking
   p. papillomatosis
palate
   ankyloblepharon, ectodermal defect,
      and cleft lip and/or p. (AEC)
   hard p.
   high-arched p.
   itchy soft p.
palatinus
   torus p.
pale
   p. cell acanthoma
   p. color
palestinensis
   Acanthamoeba p.
palindromic rheumatism
palisade
   p. cell
   p. layer
palisaded
   p. encapsulated neuroma
   p. granuloma
palisading
   p. granuloma
   p. histiocyte
palivizumab antibody
Pall Biodyne membrane
pallescense
pallesthesia
pallida
   Spirochaeta p.
pallidum
   direct fluorescent antibody test for
      Treponema p. (DFA-TP)
   microhemagglutination-*Treponema p.*
      (MHA-TP)
   Treponema p.
Pallister-Hall syndrome
Pallister mosaic aneuploid syndrome
pallor
palm
   black p.
   hyperlinear p.
   liver p.
   queen p.
   reddening of p.
   p. tree
   tripe p.
   triple p.
palmar
   p. aponeurosis
   p. crease
   p. erythema
   p. fascia

p. fasciitis and polyarthritis
syndrome
p. hyperlinearity
p. psoriasis
p. subluxation
p. syphilid
p. wart
p. xanthoma
palmare
erythema p.
xanthoma multiplex striatum p.
palmaris
acanthosis p.
pyosis p.
xanthochromia striata p.
xanthoma striata p.
palmellina
trichomycosis p.
palmitate
cetyl p.
clofazimine p.
palmoplantar
p. eccrine hidradenitis (PEH)
p. erythrodysesthesia syndrome
p. fibromatosis
p. keratoderma (PPK)
p. pustulosis
palmoplantaris
pustulosis p.
palm-sole involvement
Palomar
P. E2000 ruby laser hair reduction
P. EsteLux
P. SLP1000 diode laser system
palpable purpura
palpebral
p. blotch
p. edema
palpebrarum
dermatolysis p.
pediculosis p.
xanthelasma p.
xanthoma p.
p. xanthoma
PAL pump for air mattress overlay
palsy
axillary nerve p.
Bell p.
facial nerve p.
handlebar p.
long thoracic nerve p.
spinal accessory nerve p.

suprascapular nerve p.
transitory p.
PAM
primary acquired melanosis
Pamelor
pamidronate
p-aminohippurate (PAH)
pamoate
pyrantel p.
PAMP
pathogen-associated molecular pattern
Pamprin IB
PAN
polyacrylonitrile
polyarteritis nodosa
PAN membrane
Panadol
Panafil
P. enzymatic debrider
P. enzymatic debriding agent
Panafil-White
P.-W. enzymatic debrider
P.-W. enzymatic debriding agent
panagglutinable
panagglutinin
panallergen
panama
Salmonella p.
panaritium
Panasol
P. II home phototherapy system
panatrophy of Gower
panbronchiolitis
P-ANCA
perinuclear antineutrophil cytoplasmic
antibody
P-ANCA titer
pancreas
p. after kidney transplant (PAK)
p. transplant alone (PTA)
p. transplantation
pancreas-after-kidney (PAK)
pancreatic
p. disorder
p. lobular panniculitis
p. oncofetal antigen (POA)
pancreaticoduodenal transplantation
pancreaticoduodenectomy
pancreatitis
pancuronium bromide
pancytopenia
familial p.

NOTES

P

405

Pandel
pandemic
pandemicity
panel
    ABPA p.
    acute bronchopulmonary
      aspergillosis p.
    anergy p.
    cellular immune p.
    humoral immunity status p.
    hypersensitivity pneumonitis p.
    latex RIA p.
panel-reactive
    p.-r. antibody (PRA)
    p.-r. antibody testing
panencephalitis
    nodular p.
    subacute sclerosing p. (SSPE)
Paneth cell granule
panhidrosis
panhypogammaglobulinemia
panhypopituitarism
    autoimmune p.
    idiopathic p.
    secondary p.
panidrosis
panimmunity
panleukopenia virus of cats
panmictic
Panmycin Oral
panmyelophthisis
    familial p.
panniculalgia
panniculitides
panniculitis
    alpha$_1$-antitrypsin deficiency p.
    chemical p.
    cold p.
    connective tissue p.
    cytophagic histiocytic p.
    cytophagic lobular p.
    enzyme-related p.
    eosinophilic p.
    equestrian p.
    factitial p.
    gouty p.
    histiocytic cytophagic p. (HCP)
    idiopathic lobular p.
    lobular p.
    lupus erythematosus p.
    migratory p.
    nodular migratory p.
    nodular nonsuppurative p.
    pancreatic lobular p.
    physical lobular p.
    popsicle p.
    poststeroid p.
    relapsing febrile nodular
      nonsuppurative p.

    scleroderma septal p.
    sclerosing p.
    septal p.
    subacute nodular migratory p.
    traumatic p.
    vessel-based lobular p.
pannus
    p. cell
    cellular p.
    fibrous p.
    rheumatoid p.
pannus-cartilage junction
PanoGauze
    P. hydrogel-impregnated gauze
    P. impregnated gauze
panophthalmitis
Panoplex
Panoplex hydrogel dressing
Panosol II home phototherapy device
PanOxyl-AQ
PanOxyl Bar
panreactive monoclonal antibody
Panretin topical gel
Panscol
    P. Lotion
    P. ointment
pansinusitis
panspermia
pansy flower
pan T-cell marker
Pantoloc+
pantoprazole sodium
pantothenic acid deficiency
pantropic virus
pants paresthesia syndrome
panuveitis
    idiopathic p.
PAO$_2$
    partial pressure alveolar oxygen
PaO$_2$
    partial pressure arterial oxygen
pao ferro wood
PAP
    Guaifenex PPA 75
Pap
    pyrophosphate arthritis-pseudogout
    Pap test
PAPA
    pyogenic sterile arthritis, pyoderma
    gangrenosum and acne
    PAPA syndrome
papain
Papain enzymatic débridement
Papanicolaou test
papaverine
paper
    p. dermatitis
    Diazo p.
    litmus p.

p. mulberry
p. mulberry tree
p. radioimmunosorbent test (PRIST)
p. wasp
paper-thin scar
papilla, pl. **papillae**
anogenital vestibular p.
dermal p.
hypertrophy of tongue p.
vestibular p.
papillaris
nevus p.
pars p.
papillary
p. atrophy
p. dermal fibroplasias
p. dermis
p. eccrine adenoma
p. ectasia
p. hidradenoma
p. hypertrophy
p. necrosis
p. tumor
papillation
papilliferous
papilliferum
hidradenoma p.
syringoadenoma p.
syringocystadenoma p.
papilliferus
nevus syringocystadenosus p.
papilliform
papillitis
papilloadenocystoma
papillocarcinoma
papilloma
p. acuminatum
basal cell p.
canine oral p.
p. diffusum
p. durum
hard p.
p. inguinale tropicum
p. molle
Shope p.
soft p.
p. venereum
p. virus
zymotic p.
papillomatosis
confluent and reticulate p.

familial confluent and reticulated p.
florid oral p.
p. of Gougerot-Carteaud
juvenile p.
laryngeal p.
malignant p.
oral florid p.
palatal p.
recurrent respiratory laryngeal p.
reticulated p.
papillomatosus
lupus p.
nevus p.
papillomatous
papillomavirus
human p. (HPV)
Hybrid Capture II DNA-based test
for human p.
Papillon-Lèfevre syndrome
Papineau graft
Papovaviridae
papovavirus
pappataci
p. fever
p. fever virus
pappose
pappus
paprika-splitter's lung
papula
papular
p. acne
p. acrodermatitis
p. acrodermatitis of childhood
(PAC)
p. dermatitis
p. dermatitis of pregnancy
p. fever
p. fibroplasia
p. mastocytosis
p. mucinosis
p. sarcoid
p. scrofuloderma
p. stomatitis virus of cattle
p. syphilid
p. syphiloderma
p. tuberculid
p. urticaria
p. xanthoma
papular-purpuric
p.-p. gloves and socks syndrome
p.-p. stocking and glove syndrome

NOTES

P

407

papulation
    granular p.
    perifollicular p.
papulatum
    erythema p.
papule
    Celsus p.
    discrete umbilicated p.
    fibrous p.
    follicular p.
    Gottron p.
    indolent p.
    indurated p.
    keratotic p.
    moist p.
    mucous p.
    painful piezogenic pedal p.
    penile pearly p.
    persistent pearly penile p.
    piezogenic pedal p.
    polygonal p.
    prurigo p.
    pruritic p.
    purple-red p.
    red p.
    satellite erythematous p.
    split p.
    yellow p.
Papulex
papuliferous
papuloerosive erythema
papuloerythematous
papuloerythroderma of Ofuji
papulonecrotic
    p. eruption
    p. tuberculid
papulonecrotica
    tuberculosis cutis p.
papulopustular lesion
papulopustule
papulosa
    acne p.
    miliaria p.
    p. nigra dermatosis
    parakeratosis p.
    stomatitis p.
    urticaria p.
papulose atrophicante maligne
papulosis
    atrophic p.
    p. atrophicans maligna
    bowenoid p.
    clear cell p.
    malignant atrophic p.
papulosquamous
    p. dermatitis
    p. disorder
    p. eruption

    p. lesion
    p. syphilid
papulosum
    eczema p.
    erythema p.
papulovesicle
papulovesicular
    p. acrolocated syndrome
    p. lesion
    p. rash
Papworth heart donor survey
papyraceous scar
PAR
    protease-activated receptor
    pseudoallergic reaction
paraaminobenzoic acid (PABA)
paraaminosalicylate sodium
paraaminosalicylic acid
paraarticular ossification
paraben mix
parachlorometaxylenol (PCMX)
parachlorophenylalanine
parachroma
parachromatosis
paracoccidioidal granuloma
Paracoccidioides brasiliensis
paracoccidioidin skin test
paracoccidioidomycosis
paracrine
paradox
    thoracoabdominal p.
paradoxical
    p. pulse
    p. sleep
paradoxus
    pulsus p.
paraffin
    p. breast augmentation
    Liquid p.
paraffinoma
parafollicularis
    hyperkeratosis follicularis et p.
paragonimiasis
Paragonimus
    P. kellicotti
    P. westermani
parahaemolyticus
    Haemophilus p.
parahidrosis
parainfluenzae
    Haemophilus p.
parainfluenza virus
parakeet feather
parakeratosis
    p. ostracea
    p. papulosa
    p. psoriasiformis
    p. pustulosa

p. scutularis
p. variegata
parallel furrow
parallergic
paraluis-cuniculi
    Treponema p.-c.
paralysis, pl. **paralyses**
    acute atrophic p.
    fowl p.
    immune p.
    immunological p.
    infectious bulbar p.
    myogenic p.
    parotitic p.
    phrenic nerve p.
    postdiphtheric p.
    Pott p.
    syphilitic spastic spinal p.
    tick p.
paramesonephric rest
parameter
    spatiotemporal gait p.
paramethasone acetate
paramyloidosis
Paramyxoviridae virus
Paramyxovirus
paranasal
    p. sinus drainage
    p. sinus pain
paraneoplastic
    p. acrokeratosis
    p. pemphigus (PNP)
    p. subacute cerebellar degeneration
    p. syndrome
paraneoplastica
    acrokeratosis p.
parangi
Para-Pak Ultra Ecofix system
paraparesis
    areflexic p.
    HTLV-1-associated myelopathy or
      tropical spastic p. (HAM/TSP)
    tropical spastic p. (TSP)
parapertussis
    Bordetella p.
paraphenylenediamine (PPDA)
    p. dermatitis
paraphimosis
paraplegia
    Pott p.
parapneumonic effusion
Parapoxvirus

paraproteinemia
parapsilosis
    Candida p.
parapsoriasis
    p. acuta et varioliformis
    p. en gouttes
    p. en plaque
    p. guttata
    guttate p.
    large-plaque p.
    p. large-plaque
    p. lichenoid
    p. lichenoides
    p. lichenoides et varioliformis acuta
    p. maculata
    poikilodermatous p.
    retiform p.
    p. retiform
    p. small-plaque
    small-plaque p. (SPP)
    p. variegata
    p. varioliformis acuta
pararama
pararenal abscess
pararosaniline hydrochloride
parascarlatina
parasitaria
parasite
    metazoal p.
    ova and p.'s (O&P)
parasitic
    p. cyst
    p. disease
    p. granuloma
    p. melanoderma
    p. sycosis
parasitica
    achromia p.
    glossitis p.
    onychia p.
parasiticum
    eczema p.
parasitophobia
parasitosis
    delusion of p.
paraspinal abscess
paraspinous abscess
parasympathetic nerve fiber
parasyphilis
parathyroidectomy
paratope
paratracheal region

NOTES

P

paratrichosis
paratrimma
    erythema p.
paratripsis
paratriptic
paratyphi
    Salmonella p.
paratyphoid fever
paraumbilical nodule
paraungual
paravaccinia
    p. virus
    p. virus infection
Paravespula **sting**
parchment skin
Par Decon
parenchyma
parenchymal
    p. amyloidosis
    p. fibrosis
parenchymatous
    p. glossitis
    p. neurosyphilis
    p. syphilis
parenteral
    p. absorption
    Coly-Mycin M P.
    p. corticosteroid
    p. diphenhydramine
    p. gold
paresis
paresthesia
paresthetica
    meralgia p.
    notalgia p.
paretic neurosyphilis
paridrosis
parietalis
    decidua p.
Parietaria-**induced rhinoconjunctivitis**
Parietaria judacia
Parinaud oculoglandular syndrome
Paris green
Parker-Pearson needle
Parker retractor
Parkes-Weber hemangiomatosis
parking
    organ p.
Parkinson disease
Parkland
    P. burn resuscitation formula
    P. formula for fluid resuscitation
      for burn trauma
Park-Williams bacillus
paromomycin sulfate
paronychia
    acute p.
    bacterial p.
    Candida p.

    candidal p.
    chronic p.
    herpetic p.
    monilial p.
paronychial wart
paronychomycosis
paronychosis
parotid
    p. gland
    p. sialography
parotiditis
    epidemic p.
parotitic paralysis
parotitis
paroxetine
    p. HCl
    p. hydrochloride
paroxysmal
    p. cold hemoglobinuria
    p. flushing
    p. hand hematoma
    p. nocturnal hemoglobinuria (PNH)
    p. pruritus
    p. sneezing
paroxysm of coughing
PARP
    poly(ADP-ribose)polymerase
    PARP autoantibody
parrot
    p. feather
    P. node
    P. pseudoparalysis
    P. sign
    p. syndrome
    p. syphilitic osteochondritis
    P. ulcer
    p. virus
parrot-beak nail
Parry-Romberg syndrome
pars
    p. papillaris
    p. reticularis
Parsol 1789 sunscreen
parthenium dermatitis
partial
    p. agglutinin
    p. albinism
    p. albinism with immunodeficiency
    p. antigen
    p. combined immunodeficiency
      disorder
    p. face-sparing lipodystrophy
    p. leukonychia
    p. lipoatrophy
    p. pressure alveolar oxygen (PAO_2)
    p. pressure arterial oxygen (PaO_2)
    p. pressure of carbon dioxide
      (PCO_2)

p. pressure of oxygen (PO$_2$)
p. thromboplastin time (PTT)
partialis
hypertrichosis p.
partial-thickness burn
particle
anti-signal recognition p. (anti-SRP)
Dane p.
defective interfering p.
DI p.
organic extracts of diesel
exhaust p.'s
signal recognition p. (SRP)
particulate matter
Partuss LA
parvilocular cyst
Parvoviridae
parvovirus
p. B19
human p. (HPV)
human p. B19
parvum bovine Ig concentrate
PAS
periodic acid-Schiff
PAS stain
PAS technique
P.A.S.
P.A.S. Port catheter
Sodium P.A.S.
Paschen body
Paser
PASI
Psoriasis Area and Severity Index
Psoriasis Area Severity Index
Pasini epidermolysis bullosa
Pasini-Pierini
P.-P. idiopathic atrophoderma
P.-P. syndrome
passage
blind p.
percutaneous p.
serial p.
passant
en p.
passenger leukocyte
passion purpura
passive
p. agglutination
p. cutaneous anaphylactic reaction
p. cutaneous anaphylaxis (PCA)
p. cutaneous anaphylaxis test
p. hemagglutination (PHA)

p. immunity
p. immunization
p. immunoprophylaxis
p. immunotherapy
p. motion
p. prophylaxis
p. range of motion exercise
p. transfer
p. transference
p. transfer test
Passy-Muir tracheostomy speaking valve
paste
baking soda p.
Camcreme ECG p.
Emplasterium urea p.
Lassar betanaphthol p.
Lassar plain zinc p.
Triple P.
Unna p.
Veiel p.
zinc chloride p.
Pasteurella
P. aerogenes
P. multocida
P. pestis
P. tularensis
pasteurellosis
Pasteur vaccine
Pastia
P. line
P. sign
pastilles
Mycostatin p.
patagium
cervical p.
Patanol eye drops
patch
Alora transdermal p.
Ben-Gay p.
butterfly p.
Carrel p.
cotton-wool p.
eczematous p.
herald p.
moth p.
mucous p.
opaline p.
peau d'orange p.
PediaPatch Transdermal P.
Peyer p.
pruritic erythematous p.
salmon p.

NOTES

411

patch *(continued)*
  shagreen p.
  smoker p.
  soldier p.
  p. stage
  p. test
  p. testing
  p. test interpretation
  Testoderm p.
  p. test scarring
  Tinamed plantar p.
  Transderm Scōp P.
  Trans-Plantar Transdermal P.
  Trans-Ver-Sal Transdermal P.
    Verukan solution
Patched gene (PTC)
patchouli oil
patchy
  p. airspace consolidation
  p. infiltrate
Pate d'Unna
patellae
  chondromalacia p.
patellar
  p. tendinitis
  p. tendon-bearing orthosis
patellofemoral
  p. alignment
  p. arthritis
  p. disease
  p. joint
  p. osteoarthritis
  p. pain syndrome
pathergy
pathoanatomy
Pathocil
pathoclisis
pathogen
  Cunninghamella p.
  opportunistic p.
pathogen-associated molecular pattern
  (PAMP)
pathogenesis
  peripheral prion p.
pathogenetic
pathogenic blastomycetes
pathogenicity
pathognomic
pathognomonic
pathologically confirmed complete
  remission (PCR)
pathologic feature
pathology
  allograft p.
  bite p.
pathometric
pathometry
pathophysiology

pathway
  arachidonic acid p.
  classic p.
  classical p. (CP)
  cross-priming p.
  cyclooxygenase p.
  effector p.
  endotoxin signaling p.
  Fas-based killing p.
  inositol triphosphate p.
  lectin p.
  lipoxygenase p.
  monooxygenase p.
  Notch signaling p.
  perforin killing p.
  perforin-mediated p.
  proinflammatory p.
  Raf/mitogen-activated protein kinase
    signaling p.
  Raper-Mason p.
  Ras p.
  Ras-Raf-Mek-Erk p.
  Vav/Rac p.
patient
  p. advocate
  p. education
  p. global assessment of disease
    activity
  hemophiliac p.
  nonhemophiliac p.
  p. patch test record sheet
Patois virus
patronymic
pattern
  apron p.
  ball-in-claw p.
  bimodal immunofluorescent p.
  cannonball p.
  Christmas tree p.
  church spire p.
  clock-face p.
  differential expression p.
  p. of distribution
  fir-tree-like p.
  geographic p.
  ground-glass p.
  herringbone p.
  honeycomb staining p.
  p. of inheritance
  livedo p.
  lymphocutaneous p.
  Mercedes p.
  mulberry p.
  NBT mosaic p.
  netted p.
  N-linked p.
  nodular p.
  nuclear dot p.
  O-linked p.

pathogen-associated molecular p. (PAMP)
polycyclic p.
polygenic inheritance p.
p. recognition receptor (PRR)
restrictive ventilatory p.
reticular p.
rheumatoid p.
serpiginous p.
sporotricoid p.
p. of staining
starry-sky p.
stellate p.
webbed p.
zosteriform p.
patterned
  p. alopecia
  p. leukoderma
pauciarthritis
pauciarticular
  p. juvenile chronic arthritis
  p. juvenile rheumatoid arthritis
  p. onset
  p. presentation
paucibacillary leprosy
pauciimmune glomerulonephritis
pauciinflammatory
paucimobilis
  Sphingomonas p.
Paul
  P. reaction
  P. test
paul
  Salmonella st. p.
Paul-Bunnell test
Paulo
  exanthematic typhus of São P.
Paulus
  P. composite score
  P. composite score criteria
  P. criteria
paurometabolum
  Tsukamurella p.
Pautrier
  P. abscess
  P. microabscess
Paxene
Paxil
paxillin
Paxton disease
PBC
  primary biliary cirrhosis

PBL
  peripheral blood lymphocyte
pBlueScript vector
PBMC
  peripheral blood mononuclear cell
PBMTx
  porcine bone marrow transplantation
PBPC
  peripheral blood progenitor cell
PBS
  phosphate-buffered saline
PBSC
  peripheral blood stem cell
PBSCT
  peripheral blood stem cell transplantation
PBV
  pulmonary blood volume
PBZ
  pyribenzamine
    PBZ-SR
PC
  pilomatrix carcinoma
PCA
  passive cutaneous anaphylaxis
    PCA test
PCB
  polychlorobiphenyl
PCE
  pseudocholinesterase
    PCE oral
p-chloro-meta-xylenol (PCMX)
PCMX
  parachlorometaxylenol
  p-chloro-meta-xylenol
PCNA
  proliferating cell nuclear antigen
PCO$_2$
  partial pressure of carbon dioxide
PCPs
  pollen-coat proteins
PCR
  pathologically confirmed complete remission
  polymerase chain reaction
    PCR assay
    PCR for HIV DNA
    mixed-linker PCR (ML-PCR)
    repetitive PCR (Rep-PCR)
    TB test by PCR
    PCR testing
PCT
  porphyria cutanea tarda

NOTES

P

PD
  Bromfenex PD
  Iofed PD
  Notuss PD
  P and PD
PDA
  Indocid PDA
PDAF
  platelet-derived angiogenesis factor
PDEGF
  platelet-derived epidermal growth factor
PDGF-A
  platelet-derived growth factor A
    isoform P.-A.
PDGF-B
  platelet-derived growth factor B
    isoform PDGF-B
Pdi
  transdiaphragmatic pressure
PDL
  pulsed-dye laser
PDS
  polydioxanone
    PDS suture
PDT
  photodynamic therapy
  provocative dose test
PE
  phycoerythrin
    Guiatuss PE
    Halotussin PE
P-E
  portal (venous and) enteric
    P-E technique
peach fuzz
peak
  biclonal p.
  p. expiratory flow (PEFR)
  p. expiratory flow rate
  p. flow meter
  p. flow sensitivity
  p. inspiratory ventilator pressure
  monoclonal p.
  p. nasal inspiratory flow (PNIF)
  p. serum level
  p. and trough
  widow's p.
peak-plateau response
peanut allergy (PN)
pearl
  collar of p.'s
  Epstein p.'s
  p. oyster shell pneumonitis
Pearson chi square test
peau
  p. de chagrin
  p. d'orange
  p. d'orange patch
pebbly surface

pecan tree
Peck-Joseph scissors
Pecquet
  P. cistern
  P. duct
  P. reservoir
pectoris
  pseudoangina p.
pectus excavatum
Pedameth
PediaCare oral
Pediacof
PediaPatch Transdermal Patch
Pediapred oral
Pedia-Profen
pediatric
  Cleocin P.
  p. dermogram
  Fedahist Expectorant p.
  p. infectious disease developmental
    screening test (PIDDST)
  p. scleroderma
Pediazole oral
pedicellaria
  triple-jawed p.
pedicled flap
Pedi-Cort V topical
pediculation
pediculicide
Pediculoides ventricosus
pediculosis
  p. capillitii
  p. capitis
  p. corporis
  p. corporis vel vestimentorum
  eyelash p.
  p. palpebrarum
  p. pubis
  p. vestimenti
pediculous
Pediculus
  P. corporis
  P. humanus
  P. humanus capitis
  P. humanus capitis infestation
Pedi-Dri
Pedinol
Pediotic Otic
Pedi-Pro topical
pedis (*gen. of* pes)
Pedituss
pedrosoi
  compacta Jeanselmei p.
  Fonsecaea p.
  Hormodendron p.
peduncle
pedunculated
  p. fibroma
  p. seborrheic keratosis

peel
  chemical p.
  face p.
  familial continuous skin p.
  freshening p.
  Jessner P.
  lunch-time p.
  phenol p.
  Pulse P.
  skin p.
peeling
  chemical p.
peeling-skin syndrome
PEEP
  positive end-expiratory pressure
Pefabloc SC
pefloxacin
PEFR
  peak expiratory flow
peg
  rete p.
pegademase bovine
pegvisomant
pegylated
  p. interferon
  p. p55 TNF-R
PEH
  palmoplantar eccrine hidradenitis
PEL
  permissible exposure limit
pelade
pelage
pelidnoma
pelioma
peliosis hepatitis
pellagra
  glossitis of p.
  wet p.
pellagra-associated dermatitis
pellagrin
pellagroid
  p. dermatitis
  p. erythema
pellagrous
pellet
  chondrin p.
  house dust mite fecal p. (HDMFP)
pelletieri
  Actinomadura p.
pellicle
  acquired p.

pellitory
  wall p.
Pelodera **dermatitis**
pelt
peltation
peltatum
  Podophyllum p.
pelvic inflammatory disease (PID)
PEM
  protein-energy malnutrition
pemphigoid
  benign mucosal p.
  Brunsting-Perry p.
  bullous p. (BP)
  cicatricial p. (CP)
  p. gestationis
  lichen planus p.
  mucous membrane p.
  ocular cicatricial p.
  p. syphilid
pemphigoides
pemphigosa
  variola p.
pemphigus
  p. acutus
  benign familial chronic p.
  Brazilian p.
  p. contagiosus
  p. erythematosus
  familial benign chronic p.
  foliaceous p.
  p. foliaceus (PF)
  p. gangrenosus
  p. hemorrhagicus
  herpetiform p. (HP)
  p. leprosus
  p. malignus
  p. neonatorum
  ocular p.
  old-man's p.
  paraneoplastic p. (PNP)
  p. syphiliticus
  p. vegetans
  p. vulgaris (PV)
  p. vulgaris acantholysis
pemphigus-like eruption
pen
  Pilot Spotlighter p.
penciclovir
pencil
  p. and cup deformity
  p. method

NOTES

P

pencil *(continued)*
　　solid carbon dioxide p.
　　styptic p.
pendula
　　cutis p.
pendulum
　　fibroma p.
　　molluscum p.
Penecort topical
penetrans
　　hyperkeratosis follicularis et
　　　parafollicularis in cutem p.
　　Tunga p.
penetrant
Penetrex oral
penicillamine
penicillin
　　p. aqueous
　　p. desensitization
　　p. g benzathine
　　p. g, benzathine and procaine,
　　　combined
　　p. g procaine
　　phenoxymethyl p.
　　p. therapy
　　unit of p.
　　p. V potassium
　　p. V suspension
penicillin-induced anaphylaxis
**penicillin-penicilloyl human serum
　albumin (PPO-HSA)**
penicillin-resistant *Streptococcus
　pneumoniae* **(PRSP)**
penicilliosis
Penicillium
　　P. casseii
　　P. marneffei
　　P. notatum
penicilloyl G, G/V, V
penicilloyl-polylysine (PPL)
penile
　　p. pearly papule
　　p. sclerosing lymphangitis
penis
　　Bowen disease of the glans p.
　　glans p.
　　induratio p. plastica
　　kraurosis p.
　　median raphe cyst of the p.
Pen-Kera lotion
Penlac nail lacquer
Pennsaid topical lotion
pensilis
　　cutis p.
Pentacarinat injection
Pentacef
Pentam-300 Injection
pentamer

pentamidine
　　p. in aerosol form
　　p. isethionate
Pentasa oral
Pentastomida
Pentatrichomonas hominis
pentavalent gas gangrene antitoxin
pentazocine
penton antigen
pentosan
　　p. polysulfate sodium
　　sodium p.
pentoxifylline (PTX)
Pentrax
pentraxin protein family
Pen-Vee K oral
**People of Color Against AIDS Network
　(POCAAN)**
PEP
　　positive expiratory pressure
　　postexposure prevention
　　postexposure prophylaxis
Pepcid
　　P. AC Acid Controller
　　P. oral
　　P. RPD
peplomer
peplos
pepper
　　betel p.
　　black p.
　　green p.
peppertree
Pepscan study
pepsinogen-secreting zymogenic cell
peptide
　　anaphylatoxin p.
　　p. antigen
　　arthritogenic p.
　　chemotactic p.
　　class II invariant chain-derived p.
　　　(CLIP)
　　COOH-terminal p.
　　cyclic citrullinated p.
　　deamidated gliadin p.
　　immunogenic p.
　　p. ligand
　　multiantigenic p. (MAP)
　　procollagen type III
　　　aminoterminal p.
　　signal p.
　　substance P p.
　　synovial antigenic p.
　　P. T
　　thymic p.
　　p. transporter protein
　　trefoil family p.'s
　　vasoactive intestinal p. (VIP)

peptide-1
>monocyte chemotactic p. (MCP-1)
>neutrophil-activating p.

peptidoglycan
>bacterial p.

peptidoglycan-polysaccharide complex
Pepto-Bismol
Peptococcus niger
Peptol
Peptostreptococcus
>*P. anaerobius*
>*P. asaccharolyticus*
>*P. magnus*
>*P. prevotii*
>*P. productus*
>*P. saccharolyticus*

peracute
perambulating ulcer
percent reactive antibody/panel reactive antibody (PRA)
perch
perchlornaphthalin
perchloroethylene
Percogesic
percussion and postural drainage
percutaneous
>p. abscess and fluid drainage (PAFD)
>p. absorption
>p. conchotome biopsy technique
>p. passage
>p. test
>p. transfemoral renal angioplasty (PTRA)

peregrinum
>*Mycobacterium p.*

perennial
>p. allergic rhinitis
>p. rye
>p. rye grass

Perfectoderm Gel
perfloxacin
perfluoroalkylpolyether (PFAPE)
perfluorocarbon
perforans
>folliculitis nares p.
>mal p.
>malum p.
>scleromalacia p.

perforant
>mal p.

perforating
>p. calcific elastosis
>p. disease
>p. disease of hemodialysis
>p. disorder of uremia
>p. folliculitis
>p. granuloma annulare
>p. ulcer of foot

perforin
>p. killing pathway
>p. pore

perforin-mediated pathway
performance
>Western Ontario and McMaster Universities Osteoarthritis Index Physical Functioning subscale and chair-stand p. (WOMAC-PF)

perfosfamide
perfrigeration
perfume dermatitis
perfusion
>exsanguinous metabolic support p.
>ex-vivo liver p.
>hypothermic p.
>isolated limb p.

periacetabular osteotomy
Periactin
periadenitis mucosa necrotica recurrens
periadnexal dermis
perianal
>p. condylomata lata
>p. pruritus
>p. streptococcal cellulitis

perianth
periaortitis
periapical
periarteritis nodosa
periarthritis
>calcific p.
>shoulder p.

periarticular
>p. disorder
>p. ossification
>p. osteopenia
>p. osteoporosis
>p. syndrome

periauricular
peribronchial desquamation
peribronchiolar lymphocyte infiltration
péribuccale
>erythrose pigmentaire p.

pericarditis

NOTES

P

417

pericardium
perichondrial implant
perichondritis
    auricular p.
    infectious p.
pericyte
periderm
perifollicular
    p. accentuation
    p. fibroma (PFF)
    p. fibrosis
    p. granuloma
    p. melanophage
    p. papulation
perifolliculitis
    p. capitis abscedens et suffodiens
    dissecting p.
    pustular p.
    superficial pustular p.
periglandular fibrosis
perigranulomatous fibrotic change
perihilar
perikarya
Perimed PeriFlux Doppler probe system
perimyocarditis
    rheumatic p.
perimyositis
perinatal
    p. gangrene of buttocks
    p. septicemia
Perineal Skin Cleanser
perineural fibrosis
perinevic vitiligo
perinevoid vitiligo
perinuclear
    p. antineutrophil cytoplasmic
      antibody (P-ANCA)
    p. zone
periocular
    p. area
    p. dermatitis
    p. milia
period
    eclipse p.
    honeymoon p.
    incubation p. (IP)
    induction p.
    latent p.
    prepatent p.
    refractory p.
periodic
    p. acid-Schiff (PAS)
    p. acid-Schiff-positive material
    p. acid-Schiff stain
    p. acid-Schiff technique
    p. edema
    p. fever syndrome
    p. leg movement

    p. peritonitis
    p. polyserositis
periodontitis-type Ehlers-Danlos
  syndrome
perionychia
perionyxis
perioral
    p. area
    p. dermatitis
periorbital
    p. area
    p. dermatitis
    p. hyperpigmentation
    p. purpura
    p. violaceous erythema
periorificial
    p. dermatitis
    p. lentiginosis
Periostat tablet
periosteal implant
periostosis
    idiopathic p.
peripheral
    p. airspace
    p. ameloblastoma
    p. anergy
    p. arthritis
    p. blood count
    p. blood eosinophilia
    p. blood lymphocyte (PBL)
    p. blood mononuclear cell (PBMC)
    p. blood progenitor cell (PBPC)
    p. blood stem cell (PBSC)
    p. blood stem cell rescue
    p. blood stem cell transplantation
      (PBSCT)
    p. fibrosis
    p. gangrene
    p. giant cell granuloma
    p. joint
    p. nerve
    p. nerve entrapment disorder
    p. nerve involvement
    p. nerve sheath tumor
    p. nervous system (PNS)
    p. neuritis
    p. neuromyopathy
    p. neuropathy
    p. ossifying fibroma
    p. prion pathogenesis
    p. staining
    p. T-cell lymphoma
    p. type
    p. vascular system
periphlebitis
periplakin
periplasmic
periporate
periporitis

periporoma
Peri-Strips Dry
peritendinitis crepitans
peritonitis
    acute p.
    benign paroxysmal p.
    feline infectious p.
    periodic p.
periumbilical perforating
  pseudoxanthoma elasticum
periungual
    p. erythema
    p. fibroma
    p. telangiectasia
    p. wart
periungualis
    onychia p.
perivascular infiltrate
perivasculitis
    retinal p.
Perlane wrinkle treatment
perlecan
perlèche
Perles
    Tessalon P.
PERM
    progressive encephalomyelitis with
    rigidity and myoclonus
permanent-press finish clothing
  dermatitis
permanganate
    potassium p.
Permapen injection
permeability
    vascular p.
permethrin
permissible exposure limit (PEL)
permissive
    p. hypercapnia
    p. MHC allele
Permitil
perna disease
pernicious anemia
pernio
    Besnier lupus p.
    p. cyanosis
    erythema p.
    lupus p.
perniosis
Pernox
peroneal
    p. nerve entrapment

    p. tendinitis
    p. tendon
    p. tendon dislocation
peroral intestinal biopsy
peroxidase
    p. cell marker
    eosinophil p.
    thyroid p. (TPO)
peroxidation
    lipid p.
peroxide
    benzoyl p.
    clindamycin/benzoyl p.
    erythromycin and benzoyl p.
    hydrogen p.
Peroxin
    P. A5
    P. A10
peroxisome proliferator-activated
  receptor-gamma (PPAR-gamma)
peroxynitrite
perphenazine
Persa-Gel
Persantine
Persian Gulf syndrome
persistence
    microbial p.
persistent
    p. acantholytic dermatosis
    p. asthma (PA)
    p. edema
    p. generalized lymphadenopathy
    (PGL)
    p. light reaction
    p. light reactor
    p. pearly penile papule
    p. pyoderma
    p. reactivity to light (PLR)
persister
Personal Best Peak Flowmeter
Persona ovulation predicting kit
perspiration
    insensible p.
    sensible p.
perspire
perstans
    acrodermatitis p.
    Dipetalonema p.
    erysipelas p.
    erythema dyschromicum p.
    erythema figuratum p.
    erythema gyratum p.

NOTES

P

perstans *(continued)*
    hyperkeratosis lenticularis p.
    telangiectasia macularis eruptiva p.
      (TMEP)
    urticaria p.
    xanthoerythrodermia p.
persufflation
persulcatus
    Ixodes p.
persulfate salt
pertechnetate
    technetium p.
pertenue
    Treponema p.
Pert Plus
pertrichosis
pertussis
    p. agglutination test
    Bordetella p.
    p. immune globulin
    p. immunoglobulin
    p. vaccine
Peru
    balsam of P.
peruana
    verruca p.
    verruga p.
peruviana
    verruca p.
Peruvian wart
PERV
    porcine endogenous retrovirus
pes, gen. **pedis**
    p. anserinus bursa
    bicho dos p.
    dermatomycosis pedis
    p. febricitans
    malum perforans pedis
    moccasin-type tinea pedis
    p. planus
    spina pedis
    tinea pedis
pest
    fowl p.
    swine p.
pesticemia
pestifer
    Salsola p.
pestiferous
pestilence
pestilential bubo
pestis
    Pasteurella p.
    Yersinia p.
Pestivirus
PET
    positron emission tomography
    problem elicitation technique
petechia, pl. **petechiae**

    calcaneal p.
    linear p.
    Tardieu p.
petechial
    p. eruption
    p. hemorrhage
    p. typhus
petechiasis
petitgrain oil
Petriellidium boydii
petrolatum
    hydrated p.
    hydrophilic p.
    lanolin, cetyl alcohol, glycerin,
      and p.
    Liquid p.
    red veterinary p. (RVP)
    white p.
petroleum
    p. acne
    p. jelly
Pette-Döring disease
Peutz-Jeghers syndrome
pexiganan acetate
Peyer patch
Peyronie disease
PF
    pemphigus foliaceus
    pulmonary function
PF4
    platelet factor 4
PFAPE
    perfluoroalkylpolyether
PFB
    pseudofolliculitis barbae
Pfeiffer
    P. phenomenon
    P. syndrome
PFF
    perifollicular fibroma
PFGE
    pulsed field gel electrophoresis
    pulse-field gel electrophoresis
Pfizerpen-AS injection
Pfizerpen injection
PFS
    Folex P.
    Tarabine P.
    Vincasar P.
PFT
    pulmonary function test
PFU
    plaque-forming unit
PG
    prostaglandin
    pyoderma gangrenosum
P/G
    Fulvicin P/G

PGD
  prostaglandin D
PGD$_2$
  prostaglandin D$_2$
PGE
  prostaglandin E
PGE$_1$
  prostaglandin E$_1$
PGE$_2$
  prostaglandin E$_2$
  purine-stimulated prostaglandin E$_2$
    PGE$_2$ synthase
PGF$_2$
  prostaglandin F2
    PGF$_2$ alpha
    PGF$_2$ synthase
PGH$_2$
  prostaglandin H2
PGHS-1, -2
  prostaglandin H synthase-1, -2
    PGHS-1, -2 cDNA
PGI
  prostaglandin I
PGI$_2$
  prostacyclin
    PGI$_2$ synthase
PGL
  persistent generalized lymphadenopathy
Ph
  Philadelphia chromosome
    Ph positive
pH
  blood p.
  low urine p.
  Propa p.
PHA
  passive hemagglutination
  phytohemagglutinin
phacoanaphylactic uveitis
phacoanaphylaxis
phacomatosis
Phadezym
  P. PRIST
  P. RAST
phaeohyphomycosis
phage
  beta p.
  defective p.
phagedena
  p. gangrenosa
  p. nosocomialis
  sloughing p.

p. tropica
  tropical p.
  tropical sloughing p.
phagedenic ulcer
phagedenis
  direct fluorescent antibody for
    Treponema p. (DFA-TP)
    Treponema p.
phagocyte
  p. dysfunction
  frustrated p.
  p. oxidative burst
  sinusoidal p.
phagocytic
  p. deficiency
  p. dysfunction disorders
    immunodeficiency
  p. function
  p. index
  p. thrombus
phagocytin
phagocytize
phagocytoblast
phagocytolysis
phagocytolytic
phagocytosable debris
phagocytose
phagocytosis
  frustrated p.
  induced p.
  spontaneous p.
phagocytotic
phagolysis
phagolysosome
phagolytic
phagosome
phagotype
phakoma
phakomatosis pigmentovascularis
phakomatous choristoma
phalanges
  proximal p.
phalloidin staining
phaneroscope
phanerozoite
phantom tumor
Pharmacia lancet
pharmacokinetic
  Dapsone P.'s
pharmacologic
  p. mediators of anaphylaxis
  p. therapy

NOTES

P

pharyngeal
  p. gonorrhea
  p. pouch syndrome
pharyngitis
  arcanobacterial p.
  herpangina p.
  herpes p.
  streptococcal p.
pharyngoconjunctival
  p. fever
  p. fever virus
phase
  accelerated p. (AP)
  anagen growth p.
  chronic
    myelocytic/myelogenous/myeloid
    leukemia accelerated p. (CML AP)
  eclipse p.
  growth p.
  horizontal growth p.
  p. (I, II) rheumatoid arthritis
  lag p.
  lichenoid p.
  logarithmic p.
  negative p.
  occlusive p.
  positive p.
  prepulseless p.
  presensitization p.
  pulseless p.
  resting p.
  stationary p.
  telogen p.
  vertical growth p.
  walk cycle p.
Phazet lancet
Phemister triad
phenacetin
Phenameth oral
PhenaVent
  P. D
  P. LA
Phenazine Injection
phenazopyridine
  sulfisoxazole and p.
Phendry Oral
Phenelzine
Phenerbel-S
Phenergan
  P. Injection
  P. Oral
  P. Rectal
Phenetron oral
phenindamine tartrate
pheniramine
  p., phenylpropanolamine, and
    pyrilamine

phenyltoloxamine,
    phenylpropanolamine, pyrilamine,
    and p.
phenobarbital
  theophylline, ephedrine, and p.
phenol
  camphor, menthol and p.
  N-acetyl-4-S-cysteaminyl p.
  p. peel
phenolated disinfectant
phenolformaldehyde
phenology
phenolphthalein
phenol-preserved extract
phenomenon, pl. **phenomena**
  adhesion p.
  anaphylactoid p.
  angry back p.
  Arthus p.
  autoimmune p.
  Azzopardi p.
  booster p.
  Bordet-Gengou p.
  Chase-Sulzberger p.
  cheek p.
  Danysz p.
  Debré p.
  Denys-Leclef p.
  d'Herelle p.
  Ehrlich p.
  epitope-spreading p.
  erythrocyte adherence p.
  experimentally induced Köbner p.
    (KP-e)
  fall-and-rise p.
  gel p.
  gelling p.
  generalized Shwartzman p.
  Gengou p.
  Gerhardt p.
  Gordon p.
  Hata p.
  Hecht p.
  Hektoen p.
  hunting p.
  immune adherence p.
  isomorphic p.
  jodbasedow p.
  Kasabach-Merritt p.
  Köbner p. (KP)
  Koch p.
  Koebner p.
  LE cell p.
  Leede-Rumpel p.
  Leichtenstern p.
  Liacopoulos p.
  Lucio leprosy p.
  lupus erythematosus p.
  Matuhasi-Ogata p.

Mauserung p.
Meirowsky p.
Mills-Reincke p.
Pfeiffer p.
pseudo-Koebner p.
quellung p.
Raynaud p.
red cell adherence p.
Rumpel-Leede p.
Sanarelli p.
Sanarelli-Shwartzman p.
satellite p.
Schultz-Charlton p.
Shwartzman p.
Splendore-Hoeppli p.
spreading p.
Sulzberger-Chase p.
Theobald Smith p.
Twort p.
Twort-d'Herelle p.
vacuum p.
phenothiazine
phenotype
Bombay p.
dominant p.
Fairbanks arthritis p.
McLeod p.
PiZZ p.
Ribbing arthritis p.
Turner p.
unexpected p.
VanA p.
phenotypic mixing
Phenoxine
phenoxybenzamine hydrochloride
phenoxymethyl penicillin
phenylalanine metabolism
phenylbutazone
Phenyldrine
phenylephrine
brompheniramine and p.
chlorpheniramine, phenyltoloxamine,
  phenylpropanolamine, and p.
guaifenesin, phenylpropanolamine,
  and p.
p. hydrochloride
isoproterenol and p.
sodium sulfacetamide and p.
Phenylfenesin L.A.
phenylketonuria
phenylpropanolamine
brompheniramine and p.

chlorpheniramine, phenylephrine,
  and p.
chlorpheniramine, pyrilamine,
  phenylephrine, and p.
clemastine and p.
guaifenesin and p.
p. hydrochloride
phenylpyruvic oligophrenia
phenyltoloxamine
acetaminophen and p.
chlorpheniramine, phenylephrine,
  and p.
p., phenylpropanolamine, and
  acetaminophen
p., phenylpropanolamine, pyrilamine,
  and pheniramine
phenytoin
pheochromocytoma
pheohyphomycosis
pheomelanin
pheomycotic cyst
pheresis catheter
Phialophora
  P. richardsiae
  P. verruca
  P. verrucosa
Philadelphia
  P. chromosome (Ph)
  P. chromosome positive
Philip gland
Philips
  24, 50 P. 100W TL-01 lamp
philtrum
phimosis
pHisoDerm
pHisoHex
phi-X174
  bacteriophage phi-X174
phlebectasia
  congenital generalized p.
  corona p.
phlebectomy
phlebodissector
phlebography
phlebology
Phlebotomus
  Phlebotomus fever
  Phlebotomus fever virus
  Phlebotomus sandfly bite
phlebotomy
Phlebovirus

NOTES

P

423

phlegmasia
    p. alba
    p. alba dolens
    p. malabarica
phlegmon
    diffuse p.
phlegmonous
    p. abscess
    p. cellulitis
    p. erysipelas
    p. ulcer
phlei
    Mycobacterium p.
Phleum pratense
phlogistic
phlogosin
phlogotherapy
phloxine-tartrazine stain
phlyctaenodes
    herpes p.
phlyctena, pl. **phlyctenae**
phlyctenar
phlyctenoid
phlyctenosis
phlyctenous
phlyctenular
phlyctenule
phlyctenulosis
    allergic p.
    tuberculous p.
PHN
    postherpetic neuralgia
Phoma
    P. betae
    P. species
Phoma **fungus**
phorbol
    p. ester
    p. myristate acetate (PMA)
Phormia
phosophoinositol-3 (PI3)
phosphatase
    tartrate-resistant acid p. (TRAP)
phosphate
    antazoline p.
    Aralen phosphate with
     primaquine p.
    chloroquine p.
    Decadron P.
    dexamethasone sodium p.
    Hexadrol p.
    histamine p.
    Hydrocortone P.
    nicotinamide adenine dinucleotide p.
     (NADPH)
    potassium titanyl p. (KTP)
    primaquine p.
phosphate-buffered saline (PBS)

phosphatidylcholine-specific phospholipase C
phosphatidylinositol
phosphatidylserine
phosphatidylserine-prothrombin complex
phosphatidyl serine receptor
5-phospho-alpha-d-ribosyl 1-
   pyrophosphate (PP-ribose-P)
phospho-c-Jun
phosphodiester
phosphodiesterase isoenzyme inhibitor
phosphofructokinase
phosphoglycerolmutase
phosphoinositide 3 kinase
phospholipase
    p. A, A2, C
    p. enzyme
phospholipase A$_2$ (PLA$_2$)
phospholipid
phosphonoformate
    trisodium p.
phosphorhidrosis
phosphoribosylaminoimidazole-
   carboxamide
phosphoribosyltransferase
    hypoxanthine-guanine p. (HGPRT)
phosphoridrosis
Phosphorimaging
phosphorus
phosphorylase
    nucleoside p.
    purine nucleoside p. (PNP)
phosphorylated serine/arginine splicing
phosphorylation
    chondrocyte mitochondrial
     oxidative p.
    protein kinase A-dependent p.
    tyrosine p.
phosphotransferase deficiency
phossy jaw
photo
    p. aging
    p. epilation
    p. protection
photoacoustic injury
photoaged
photoaging, photo aging
photoallergen
photoallergic
    p. contact dermatitis (PACD)
    p. drug reaction
    p. sensitivity
photoallergy
    soap p.
photobiologic reaction
photobiology
photochemical
    p. reaction
    p. smog

photochemistry
photochemotherapy
    extracorporeal p.
    p. with oral methoxypsoralen
      therapy followed by UVA
      (PUVA)
photocontact dermatitis
photodamage
PhotoDerm
    P. filtered, flashlamp-pumped light
      source
    P. laser
    P. machine
    P. MultiLight system
    P. VL light source
photodermatitis
    contact p.
    drug-induced p.
photodermatosis
photodistribution
photodrug reaction
photodynamic
    p. sensitization
    p. therapy (PDT)
photoepilation
    flashlamp p.
photoerythema
Photofrin porfimer sodium
photogenica
    P. laser
    P. laser system
    urticaria p.
photoinactivation
photoingestant dermatitis
photoirritant contact dermatitis (PICD)
photology
photomechanical
photometry
    reflectance p.
photomicrography
photomicroscope
    Leitz periplan p.
photon absorptiometry
photoncia
2-Photon Excitation
photonic stimulator
photonosus
photoonycholysis
photo-patch test
photopathy
photopheresis
photophobia

photophoresis
    extracorporeal p. (ECP)
photophytodermatitis
photoplethysmography (ppg)
photoradiation
photosensitive
    p. nonscarring dermatitis
    p. rash
photosensitivity
    p. dermatitis
    drug-induced bullous p.
       , p. ichthyosis, brittle hair,
      impaired intelligence, decreased
      fertility, and short stature
    p., ichthyosis, brittle hair, impaired
      intelligence, decreased fertility,
      and short stature
       , p. ichthyosis, brittle hair,
      intellectual impairment, decreased
      fertility, and short stature
    p., ichthyosis, brittle hair,
      intellectual impairment, decreased
      fertility, and short stature
    p. reaction
photosensitization
    contact p.
phototherapy
    UVB p.
photothermolysis
    selective p.
phototoxic
    p. contact dermatitis
    p. drug reaction
    p. sensitivity
    p. textile dermatitis
phototoxicity
phototoxis
PHP
    pseudohypoparathyroidism
phragmospore
phrenic
    p. nerve
    p. nerve paralysis
phrynoderma
phthalate
phthalic anhydride
phthiriasis
Phthirus
phthisicorum
    chloasma p.
phycoerythrin (PE)

NOTES

P

phycomycosis
subcutaneous p.
phycomycotic infection
phylacagogic
phylaxis
Phyllocontin Tablet
phylogenetic atavism
phyma, pl. **phymata**
phymatosis
physical
p. allergy
p. barrier
p. deconditioning
p. lobular panniculitis
p. stimulus
p. sunscreen
p. therapy
p. urticaria
physician global assessment of disease activity
physiologic
p. alopecia
p. test
physiological
p. dead space
p. dead space ventilation per minute
physiology
sleep p.
physostigmine
phytanic
p. acid
p. acid storage
p. acid storage disease
phytoagglutinin
phytodermatitis
Phytodolor
phytohemagglutinin (PHA)
phytomitogen
phytonadione
Phytophathoria infestans
phytophlyctodermatitis
phytophotodermatitis
phytophototoxic dermatitis
phytosterolemia
phytotoxic
phytotoxin
PI3
phosophoinositol-3
pian
p. bois
hemorrhagic p.
piannic
onychia p.
piano-key deformity
PIBF
progesterone-induced blocking factor
PIBIDS
PIBIDS syndrome

PICD
photoirritant contact dermatitis
picker's
p. acne
p. nodule
Pick and Go monitor
pickle weed pollen
pick-up maneuver
picomolar
Picornaviridae virus
picornavirus
picrate
butamben p.
PID
pelvic inflammatory disease
primary immune deficiency
PIDDST
pediatric infectious disease developmental screening test
PIE
pulmonary infiltrate with eosinophilia
PIE syndrome
piebald
p. albinism
p. skin
piebaldism
piebaldness
piece
Fab p.
Fc p.
piecemeal
p. degranulation (PMD)
p. necrosis
piechaudii
Alcaligenes p.
pied
mal perforant du p.
p. rond rheumatism
piedra
black p.
p. nostras
white p.
Piedraia hortae
Pierini
atrophoderma of Pasini and P.
idiopathic atrophoderma of Pasini and P.
melanotic prurigo of P.
piesesthesia
piezogenic pedal papule
Piffard curette
pig
p. aortic endothelial cell (PAEC)
guinea p.
mycoplasma pneumonia of p.
p. skin
virus pneumonia of p.
pigeon
p. breeder's disease

p. droppings
p. feather
p. serum protein (PSP)

pigment
abnutzung p.
age p.
p. cell transplantation
p. change
incontinence of p.
iron oxide p.
melanotic p.
minimal p. (MP)

pigmentaire
Brocq erythrose peribuccale p.

pigmentary
p. abnormality
p. atopic dermatitis
p. demarcation line
p. syphilid

pigmentation
Addison p.
addisonian dermal p.
amiodarone p.
arsenic p.
blue-gray p.
epidermolysis bullosa simplex with mottled p.
exogenous p.

pigmented
p. ameloblastoma
p. basal cell carcinoma
p. hair epidermal nevus
P. Lesion Study Group (PLSG)
p. purpura
p. purpuric lichenoid dermatitis
p. purpuric lichenoid dermatitis of Gougerot
p. purpuric lichenoid dermatosis
p. skin lesion (PSL)
p. spindle cell (PSC)
p. villonodular synovitis (PVNS)

pigmenti
incontinentia p.

pigmenting agent
pigmentolysin
pigmentosa
familial urticaria p.
morphea p.
urticaria p.

pigmentosum
morphea p.

urticaria p.
xeroderma p.

pigmentosus
lichen planus p.
nevus p.

pigmentovascularis
phakomatosis p.

pig-to-primate model of xenotransplantation
pigweed
redroot p.
spiny p.
p. weed pollen

pilar
p. cyst
p. neurocristic hamartoma
p. sheath acanthoma
p. tumor of scalp

pilaris
favus p.
juvenile pityriasis rubra p.
keratosis p.
lichen p.
pityriasis rubra p.

pilar neurocristic hamartoma
pilary
pileous
pili (*pl. of* pilus)
piliferous cyst
piliform
pill
Asiatic p.
Doan's Backache P.
Ge Jie Anti-asthma P.
prom p.

pillow
OsmoCyte p.

pilocarpine iontophoresis sweat test
piloerection
piloid
piloleiomyoma
pilomatricoma
pilomatrix carcinoma (PC)
pilomatrixoma carcinoma
pilomotor reflex
pilonidal
p. cyst
p. fistula
p. sinus

pilorum
p. agenesis
arrectores p.

NOTES

P

pilorum (*continued*)
scissura p.
vortices p.
pilose
pilosebaceous
p. apparatus
p. follicle
p. ostium
p. structure
p. unit
pilosis
pilosus
nevus p.
nevus pigmentosus et p.
Pilot Spotlighter pen
pilus, pl. **pili**
p. annulatus
arrector p.
pili bifurcati
p. bifurcatus
F p.
I p.
p. incarnatus
pili multigemini
pili pseudoannulati
R p.
scapus pili
pili torti
pili tortus
pili triangulati et canaliculi
pili trianguli et canaliculi
Pima
pimecrolimus cream
pimozide
Pimpinella anisum
pimple
PIMS
psychological irritable bowel/migraine syndrome
pincer
p. jaw
p. nail
pinch
devil's p.
p. graft
pulp-to-pulp tip p.
p. purpura
pincushioning
pine
Australian p.
loblolly p.
lodgepole p.
p. oil
ponderosa p.
p. resin
p. resin-colophony
slash p.
p. tree pollen
white p.

pineapple
Pinellia
ping-pong
p.-p. infestation
p.-p. syphilis
pinhead-sized milia
pink
p. disease
p. salmon
p. spot
pinkeye
Pinkus
fibroepithelioma of P.
P. tumor
pinna
pinocyte
pinocytosis
active p.
pinosome
pinpoint electrocoagulation
pinpoint-sized milia
Pin-Rid
pinta treponematosis
pintid
pinto
P. cannula
mal del p.
pintoid
pintos
mal de los p.
pinworm
Pin-X
pioglitazone HCl
PIP
positive inspiratory pressure
proximal interphalangeal
piperacillin sodium and tazobactam sodium
piperazine
p. citrate
p. hydrochloride
piper beetle
piperidine derivative
piperonyl butoxide
Pipracil
pique
pirbuterol acetate
piriformis syndrome
Pirital virus
piritrexim isethionate
piroxicam
Pirquet
P. reaction
P. test
pistachio
pistillate
pit
discrete p.
ear p.

Mantoux p.
nail p.
tooth p.
p. viper bite
p. viper snake
pitch wart
Pitrex
pitted
p. keratolysis
p. nail
pitting
p. edema
nail p.
p. of nail
pituitary
p. disorder
p. snuff taker's lung
pityriasic alopecia
pityriasis
p. alba
p. alba atrophicans
p. amiantacea
p. capitis
p. circinata
p. folliculorum
p. furfuracea
Gibert p.
Hebra p.
p. lichenoid
lichenoid acute p.
p. lichenoides
p. lichenoides chronica (PLC)
p. lichenoides et varioliformis acuta
(PLEVA)
p. lingua
p. maculata
p. nigra
p. rosea (PR)
p. rosea-like eruption
p. rotunda
p. rubra
p. rubra pilaris
p. sicca
p. simplex
p. simplex faciei
p. steatoides
p. versicolor
pityriasis-type scale
pityrodes
alopecia p.
pityroid

Pityrosporum
P. orbiculare
P. ovale
Pityrosporum **folliculitis**
pivalate
pivampicillin
pivoxil
cefditoren p.
Pixy321
Piz Buin
pizotifen
PiZZ phenotype
P-K
Prausnitz-Kustner
P-K antibody
P-K reaction
P-K test
PKA
protein kinase A
PLA$_2$
phospholipase A$_2$
PLA$_2$ isoenzyme (type IIA, IV, V)
PLA$_2$ isozyme
placebo
placebo-controlled oral challenge testing
(DPOC)
placenta-eluted gamma globulin
placental
p. sulfatase deficiency
p. sulfatase deficiency syndrome
p. syncytiotrophoblast
placentation
pladaroma
plague
bubonic p.
cattle p.
duck p.
fowl p.
Pahvant Valley p.
rabbit p.
p. vaccine
vector of p.
plain
Citanest P.
p. gut suture
Ultraquin P.
plakin
plakoglobin
plana
verruca p.
planar xanthoma

NOTES

P

planci
> *Acanthaster p.*

Planck law

plane
> p. angioma
> diffuse p.
> Frankfort horizontal p.
> p. nevus
> p. wart
> p. xanthoma

planing

planopilaris

plant
> p. agglutinin
> p. antitoxin
> arum p.
> datura p.
> p. dermatitis
> p. oleoresin
> p. toxin
> p. virus
> wind-pollinated p.

planta, pl. **plantae**
> verruca p.

Plantago lanceolata

plantain
> English p.

plantaire
> chromidrose p.

plantar
> p. dermatitis
> p. desquamation
> p. fascia
> p. fasciitis
> p. fibromatosis
> p. hyperlinearity
> p. inoculum
> p. maceration
> p. nerve syndrome
> p. syphilid
> p. talalgia
> p. wart

plantare
> keratoma palmare et p.

plantaris
> epidermolytic keratosis palmaris
>   et p.
> ichthyosis palmaris et p.
> keratoderma palmaris et p.
> keratosis palmaris et p.
> mycosis fungoides palmaris et p.
> pustulosis palmaris et p.
> tylosis palmaris et p.
> verruca palmaris et p.

plantibody

planum
> xanthoma p.

planus
> actinic lichen p. (ALP)

anular lichen p.
atrophic lichen p.
bullous lichen p.
condyloma p.
erosive lichen p.
follicular lichen p.
genital erosive lichen p.
hepatitis-associated lichen p.
hypertrophic lichen p.
lichen ruber p.
linear lichen p.
oral condyloma p.
oral erosive lichen p.
pes p.
ulcerative lichen p.
zosteriform lichen p.

plaque
> anular erythematous p.
> atrophic p.
> attachment p.
> bacterial p.
> centrofacial p.
> cytoplasmic p.
> degenerative collagenous p.
> dental p.
> disseminées parapsoriasis en p.'s
> eczematoid pruritic p.
> erythematosquamous p.
> erythematous vulvitis en p.
> honeycomb p.
> p. index
> inflammatory p.
> lichenified p.
> milia en p.
> mucous p.
> parapsoriasis en p.
> p. psoriasis
> psoriatic p.
> red-purple p.
> shadow p.
> p. stage
> submucosal p.
> ulcerovegetating p.
> urticarial p.
> violaceous p.
> warty keratotic p.

plaque-forming unit (PFU)

plaque-like cutaneous mucinosis

Plaquenil

plaque-type psoriasis

plasma
> p. cell
> p. cell balanitis
> p. cell dyscrasia with
>   polyneuropathy, organomegaly,
>   endocrinopathy, monoclonal protein
> p. cell mucositis
> p. cell myeloma
> p. cell neoplasm

p. cell pneumonia
p. cellularis
p. cell vulvitis
p. fibronectin
fresh frozen p.
frozen p.
p. kallikrein
p. membrane
poor platelet p. (PPP)
p. protein autoantibody
p. therapy
zoster immune p. (ZIP)

plasmablast
rapidly dividing p.'s
plasmacellularis
balanitis p.
plasmacyte
plasmacytoapheresis
plasmacytoma
plasmapheresis
exchange p.
plasmid
bacteriocinogenic p.
conjugative p.
F p.
infectious p.
nonconjugative p.
R p.
resistance p.
transmissible p.
plasmin
plasminogen
p. activator
kringle 4 domain of p.
plasmoacanthoma
plasmodia
plasmodial meningitis
Plasmodium
P. falciparum
P. malariae
P. ovale
P. vivax
plasmodium embolism
plaster
Mediplast P.
Sal-Acid P.
Plastibase
plastic
p. adhesive dressing
p. iritis
p. occlusive wrap
p. worker's lung

plastica
plastid
Plastizote shoe
**Plast-O-Fit thermoplastic bandage
system**
plate
BioPress p.
Jaeger p.
lamellar p.
nail p.
V-type microtiter p.
white spots of the nail p.
plateau bronchodilation
platelet
p. activating/aggregating factor
(PAF)
p. basic protein
p. concentrate
p. factor 4 (PF4)
hemolysis, elevated liver enzymes,
low p. (HELLP)
p. neutralization procedure
p. neutralization test
washed maternal p.
platelet-activating
p.-a. factor (PAF)
p.-a. factor acetylhydrolase (PAF-
AH)
platelet-aggregating factor (PAF)
platelet-derived
p.-d. angiogenesis factor (PDAF)
p.-d. epidermal growth factor
(PDEGF)
p.-d. growth factor A (PDGF-A)
p.-d. growth factor B (PDGF-B)
plate-like crystal
Platelin, phospholipid platelet substitute
platform
Profile p.
Platinol
Platinol-AQ
platinum
salt of p.
platonychia
platybasia
Platycodon
Platyhelminthes
platyonychia
platypnea
platysma
platyspondylia
Plaut-Vincent disease

NOTES

P

PLC
pityriasis lichenoides chronica
pleckstrin homology domain
pledget
alcohol p.
pleiotropic cytokine
pleocytosis
pleomorphic
p. lipoma
p. lymphoma
Plesiomonas shigelloides
plethysmograph
plethysmography
pleura, pl. **pleurae**
pleural
p. abrasion
p. amyloidosis
p. friction rub
p. tag
pleurectomy
pleurisy
benign dry p.
diaphragmatic p.
epidemic benign dry p.
epidemic diaphragmatic p.
rheumatoid p.
tuberculous p.
pleuritic chest pain
pleuritis
pleurodesis
doxycycline p.
mechanical p.
pleurodynia
epidemic p.
pleuropericarditis
pleuroperitonitis
pleuro-pneumoniae-like organism (PPLO)
PLEVA
pityriasis lichenoides et varioliformis
acuta
plexiform
p. angioma
p. neurofibroma
p. neuroma
p. spindle cell nevus (PSCN)
Plexion
P. cleanser
P. SCT
plexopathy
plexus
branchial p.
Kiesselbach p.
supragaleal p.
plica
p. neuropathica
p. polonica
p. syndrome

plicata
lingua p.
pachydermoperiostosis p.
plicatic acid
PLK
Polo-like kinase
PLL
prolymphocytic leukemia
plombage
plot
Wu-Kabat p.
PLR
persistent reactivity to light
PLSG
Pigmented Lesion Study Group
PLSI
Psoriasis Life Stress Inventory
plucked
p. chicken papules appearance
p. chicken skin
plug
follicular p.
keratotic p.
laminated epithelial p.
mucous p.
plugging
mucous p.
plume
laser p.
Plummer nail
Plummer-Vinson syndrome
pluriorificialis
ectodermosis erosiva p.
pluripotent
pluripotential cell
pluriresistant
plus
AeroHist P.
Amvisc p.
Clearasil B.P. p.
Cold-Eezer P.
Compound W p.
Cutifilm P.
Duramist p.
Ionil-T p.
OpSite P.
Pert P.
P & S p.
P. Sinus
Soluver p.
p. strand
Sustacal P.
Vivonex P.
PM
polymyositis
poor metabolizer
Midol PM
PM 81 monoclonal antibody

P.M.
Excedrin P.M.
PMA
phorbol myristate acetate
premenstrual exacerbation of asthma
PMD
piecemeal degranulation
pMDI
pressurized metered-dose inhaler
PMF
Painaid PMF
PML
polymorphonuclear leukocyte
progressive multifocal
leukoencephalopathy
PMLE
polymorphous light eruption
eczematous PMLE
familial PMLE
PMN
polymorphonuclear neutrophil
PMR
polymyalgia rheumatica
proportionate morbidity ratio
PM-Scl antigen
PMS-Cyproheptadine
PMS-Dexamethasone
PMS-Erythromycin
PMS-Ketoprofen
PMS-Lindane
PMS-Pseudoephedrine
PMS-Sodium Cromoglycate
PN
peanut allergy
PncCRM vaccine
PNCS
primary neuroendocrine carcinoma of
skin
PND
postnasal drip
pneumatic otoscopy
pneumatosis intestinalis
pneumococcal
p. antigenuria
p. C-polysaccharide (CPS)
p. infection
p. otitis media
p. pneumolysin
p. pneumonia
p. polysaccharide
p. polysaccharide/protein conjugate
vaccine

p. polysaccharide vaccine
p. pyomyositis
p. stain
pneumococcic abscess
pneumococcidal
pneumococcolysis
Pneumococcus
pneumoconiosis
Pneumocystis carinii
pneumocystosis
extrapulmonary p.
pneumocyte
hydropic change in p.
type II p.
pneumolysin
pneumococcal p.
pneumomediastinum
pneumonia
atypical p.
bacterial pneumococcal p.
drug-induced p.
Eaton agent p.
eosinophilic p.
Friedländer p.
Hecht p.
idiopathic acute eosinophilic p.
lipoid p.
mycoplasmal p.
nosocomial p. (NP)
ovine progressive p.
plasma cell p.
pneumococcal p.
polymicrobial p.
primary atypical p.
progressive p.
recurrent bacterial p.
recurrent viral p.
usual interstitial p. (UIP)
ventilator-associated p.
viral p.
p. virus of mice (PVM)
pneumoniae
Chlamydia p.
Klebsiella p.
Mycoplasma p.
penicillin-resistant *Streptococcus p.*
(PRSP)
pneumonitis
acute hypersensitivity p.
acute lupus p.
acute radiation p.
chronic hypersensitivity p.

NOTES

P

pneumonitis *(continued)*
    desquamative interstitial p.
    hypersensitivity p. (HP)
    lymphocytic interstitial p. (LIP)
    pearl oyster shell p.
    radiation p.
    summer p.
    summer-type hypersensitivity p.
      (SHP)
    uremic p.
Pneumopent
pneumoperitoneum
pneumophila
    Legionella p.
Pneumo-Sleeve
pneumotachograph
pneumothorax, pl. **pneumothoraces**
    iatrogenic p.
Pneumovax 23
Pneumovirus
PNH
    paroxysmal nocturnal hemoglobinuria
PNIF
    peak nasal inspiratory flow
PNP
    paraneoplastic pemphigus
    purine nucleoside phosphorylase
PNS
    peripheral nervous system
PNU
    protein nitrogen unit
Pnu-Imune 23
PO$_2$
    partial pressure of oxygen
POA
    pancreatic oncofetal antigen
Poa pratensis
POCAAN
    People of Color Against AIDS Network
pock
pocket
    necrotic p.
    P. Scrubz
    p. SPO$_2$T
Pockethaler
    Vancenase P.
Pocketpeak peak flow meter
POCkit herpes test
pockmark
podagra
Pod-Ben-25
Podiatrix-TFM
Podiatrx-AF
podobromidrosis
Podocon-25
podofilox
Podofin
podophyllin and salicylic acid
podophyllotoxin cream

podophyllum
    P. peltatum
    p. resin
PodoSpray nail drill system
Podoviridae
POEMS
    polyneuropathy, organomegaly,
    endocrinopathy, monoclonal
    gammopathy, and skin changes
    POEMS syndrome
POF
    premature ovarian failure
poikiloderma
    acrokeratotic p.
    p. atrophicans and cataract
    p. atrophicans vasculare
    p. of Civatte
    Civatte p.
    p. congenitale
    crepey p.
    hereditary sclerosing p. (HSP)
    Jacobi p.
    reticulated pigmented p.
poikilodermatomyositis
poikilodermatous parapsoriasis
point
    Castellani p.
    fibromyalgia trigger p.
    Kienböck-Adamson p.
    p. mutation
    tender p.
pointed
    p. condyloma
    p. wart
pointing
4-,5-,7-point Likert scale
6-point vitiligo disease activity scale
poison
    p. bun sponge dermatitis
    contact p.
    corrosive p.
    p. ivy
    p. ivy dermatitis
    p. oak
    p. oak dermatitis
    p. sumac
    p. sumac dermatitis
poisoning
    ciguatera p.
    lead p.
    mercury p.
    scombroid fish p.
    silver p.
    strychnine p.
    systemic p.
poisonous
Poisson-Pearson formula
pokeweed mitogen (PWM)
Poladex

polar
  p. lepromatous
  p. lepromatous leprosy
Polaramine
pol gene
polidocanol
poliglecaprone suture
polio
polioencephalitis infectiva
poliomyelitis
  acute anterior p.
  acute bulbar p.
  chronic anterior p.
  p. immune globulin (human)
  p. immunoglobulin
  Medin p.
  mouse p.
  p. vaccine
  p. virus
poliosis
  p. circumscripta
  p. eccentrica
poliovirus
  p. hominis
  p. vaccine
  p. vaccine, inactivated
  p. vaccine, live, trivalent, oral
polish
  nail p.
Polistes **sting**
polka-dot technique
polka fever
pollen
  acacia tree p.
  alder tree p.
  alfalfa weed p.
  p. antigen
  ash tree p.
  aspen p.
  Bermuda grass p.
  birch tree p.
  black walnut tree p.
  blue grass p.
  box elder tree p.
  brome grass p.
  canary grass p.
  cattail p.
  cheat grass p.
  cocklebur weed p.
  cottonwood tree p.
  curly dock weed p.
  elm tree p.
  English plantain weed p.
  English walnut tree p.
  eucalyptus tree p.
  p. extract
  false ragweed weed p.
  goldenrod p.
  goosefoot weed p.
  grass p.
  hazelnut tree p.
  June grass p.
  lamb's quarters weed p.
  locust tree p.
  maple tree p.
  mugwort weed p.
  oak tree p.
  olive tree p.
  orchard grass p.
  pickle weed p.
  pigweed weed p.
  pine tree p.
  poplar tree p.
  red top grass p.
  Russian thistle weed p.
  rye grass p.
  sage weed p.
  saltbush weed p.
  salt grass p.
  sheep sorrel weed p.
  spruce p.
  sweet vernal grass p.
  tree p.
  tumbleweed weed p.
  Western ragweed weed p.
  wild oat grass p.
  willow tree p.
  windborne p.
pollen-coat proteins (PCPs)
pollen-induced allergic rhinitis
pollination
pollinosis, pollenosis
  Cupressaceae p.
pollution
  air p.
Polocaine injection
Polo-like kinase (PLK)
polonica
  plica p.
poloxamer 188, 331
POL sclerosing solution
polyacrylamide gel electrophoresis (PAGE)
polyacrylonitrile (PAN)

NOTES

P

polyad
polyadenylylation
  alternative p.
  canonical p.
poly(ADP-ribose)polymerase autoantibody
polyangiitis
  microscopic p. (MPA)
  p. overlap syndrome
polyarteritis
  p. in childhood
  p. nodosa (PAN)
  p. nodosa syndrome
polyarthralgia
  systemic p.
polyarthritis (PA)
  asymmetric p.
  cutaneous p.
  epidemic p.
  erosive p.
  juvenile chronic p.
polyarticular
  p. gonococcal arthritis
  p. juvenile rheumatoid arthritis
  p. septic arthritis
  p. synovitis
polychemotherapy
polychlorobiphenyl (PCB)
polychlorodioxins
polychondritis
  relapsing p.
polychotomous
polychromatic
Polycillin
Polycillin-N
Polycillin-PRB
polyclonal
  p. activator
  p. antibody
  p. B cell
  p. gammopathy
  p. hypergammaglobulinemia
polycyclic
  p. distribution of lesion
  p. pattern
polycystic
  p. ovary disease
  p. ovary syndrome
polycythemia vera
polydactylia
Polyderm foam dressing
polydioxanone (PDS)
polydioxanone suture
polydysplastic epidermolysis
polydystrophy
  pseudo-Hurler p.
polyene
polyethylene glycol precipitation assay
Polygam S/D
polygenic inheritance pattern

polyglactin 910 suture
polyglandular autoimmune endocrine
  disease
polyglutamate
polyglycolic acid suture
polyglyconate suture
polygonal papule
polygonum
polyhedral body
PolyHeme blood replacement product
polyhidrosis
Poly-Histine-D Capsule
polykaryon
polyleptic fever
polymastia
PolyMem
  P. alginate dressing
  P. alginate wound cover
  P. foam dressing
polymer
  collagen p.
  p. film dressing
  p. foam dressing
polymerase
  p. chain reaction (PCR)
  p. chain reaction assay
  p. chain reaction-based detection of
    hepatitis G virus
  p. chain reaction testing
  DNA p.
  RNA p.
  Taq p.
polymerization
  chondrocyte cytoskeletal actin p.
polymerized antigen
polymethyl methacrylate
polymicrobial
  p. arthritis
  p. bacteremia
  p. pneumonia
polymicrobic
polymorphe
  erythema p.
polymorphic
  p. eruption of pregnancy
  p. light eruption
  p. protein
  p. protoporphyria
  p. reticulosis
polymorphism
  allelic p.
  biallelic p.
  functional p.
  Hind III p.
  iatrogenic p.
  lipoprotein p.
  microsatellite p.
  nucleotide p.

restriction fragment length p.
(RFLP)
single-strand conformation p.
(SSCP)
polymorphonuclear
p. cell
p. leukocyte (PML)
p. leukocyte collagenase
p. leukocyte-dependent tissue
destruction
p. leukocyte elastase
p. neutrophil (PMN)
polymorphous
p. exanthema
p. light eruption (PMLE)
p. rash
Polymox
polymyalgia
p. rheumatica (PMR)
p. rheumatica syndrome
polymyositis (PM)
juvenile dermatomyositis/p.
(JDMS/PM)
polymyositis-scleroderma antigen
polymyxa
Bacillus p.
polymyxin
bacitracin and p. b
bacitracin, neomycin, and p. b
p. b and hydrocortisone
p. b-hydrocortisone suspension
p. b sulfate
neomycin and p. b
oxytetracycline and p. b
polynesic
polyneuritiformis
heredopathia atactica p.
polyneuritis
acute idiopathic p.
infectious p.
polyneuropathic amyloidosis
polyneuropathy
amyloidotic p.
familial amyloidotic p. (FAP)
p., organomegaly, endocrinopathy,
monoclonal gammopathy, and skin
changes (POEMS)
polynucleosis
neutrophil p.
polynucleotide antibody
polyolprepolymer
Polyomavirus

Polyomavirus-associated interstitial nephritis
polyonychia
polyostotic fibrous dysplasia
polyp
fibroepithelial p.
intestinal p.
nasal p.
polypapilloma
polypectomy
polypeptide
CD4, human truncated-365 AA p.
p. chain
cyclic p.
glutamine-rich p.
p. hormone
p. inhibitor
islet amyloid p. (IAPP)
proline-rich p.
polyphaga
Acanthamoeba p.
polyphenol
green tea p. (GTP)
Polyphenon E
polypi (*pl. of* polypus)
polypoid
p. lesion
p. nevus
polypophyrin
polyposis
Poly-Pred Ophthalmic suspension
polypropylene suture
polypus, pl. polypi
polyquaternium-1
polyradiculoneuropathy
polyradiculopathy
polysaccharide
p. antigen
pneumococcal p.
specific soluble p.
polyserositis
familial paroxysmal p.
familial recurrent p.
idiopathic p.
periodic p.
recurrent p.
tuberculous p.
Polyskin
P. II dressing
P. II transparent film
P. M.R. transparent film

NOTES

P

polysomnograph
polysomnography (PSG)
Polysporin
    P. Ophthalmic
    P. Topical
polystichia
polystyrene latex
polysulfate
    calcium pentosan p.
Polytar
Polytec PI LaseAway
polytetrafluoroethylene
    expanded p. (ePTFE)
polythelia
polytomous
polytrichia
polytrichosis
Polytrim Ophthalmic
polyunguia
polyurethane film (PUF)
polyvalent
    p. allergy
    p. antiserum
    antivenin p.
    p. serum
    p. vaccine
polyvinyl chloride (PVC)
polyvinyldifluoride
PolyWic
    P. filler
    P. wound filling material
POM
    pulse oximetry monitoring
pomade acne
Pompe disease
pomphoid
pompholyx
pomphus
Poncet
    P. disease
    P. rheumatism
ponderosa
    p. pine
    p. pine tree
Pondocillin
Ponds Prevent
Ponstel
Pontocaine
    P. injection
    P. topical
pool
    thapsigargin p.
pooled serum
poona
    Salmonella p.
poor
    p. marrow function
    p. metabolizer (PM)
    p. platelet plasma (PPP)

poorly reversible asthma
Popeye sign
popilliae
    Paenibacillus p.
poplar
    p. tree
    p. tree pollen
    white p. tree
popliteal
    p. cyst
    p. fossa
    p. pterygium syndrome
popliteal-arcuate complex
POPP
    psoriatic onychopachydermoperiostitis
poppers' dermatitis
popsicle
    p. dermatitis
    p. panniculitis
population-based testing
porate
Porcelana Sunscreen
porcine
    p. bone marrow transplantation
    (PBMTx)
    p. endogenous retrovirus (PERV)
    p. fetal lateral ganglionic eminence
    cell
    p. hemagglutinating
    encephalomyelitis virus
    p. transmissible gastroenteritis
    p. xenograft
porcupine
    p. disease
    p. skin
pore
    dilated p.
    Kohn p.
    Oxy Deep P.
    perforin p.
    p. of Winer
Porges-Meier test
PORN
    progressive outer retinal necrosis
porocarcinoma
poroid hidradenoma
porokeratosis
    actinic p.
    disseminated superficial actinic p.
    (DSAP)
    linear p.
    malignant p.
    Mibelli p.
    p. of Mibelli
    p. palmaris plantaris et disseminata
    p. plantaris discreta
    p. punctata
porokeratotic eccrine ostial

poroma
> apocrine p.
> eccrine p.
> follicular p.
> malignant eccrine p.

porphobilinogen

porphyria
> ALA dehydratase deficiency p.
> p. cutanea tarda (PCT)
> erythropoietic p. (EPP)
> hepatic p.
> hepatoerythrocytic p. (HEP)
> hepatoerythropoietic p.
> mixed hepatic p.
> South African genetic p.
> symptomatic p.
> p. variegata
> variegate p. (VP)

porphyric

porphyrin

porrigo
> p. decalvans
> p. favosa
> p. furfurans
> p. larvalis
> p. lupinosa
> p. scutulata

portal
> p. occlusion
> p. tract fibrosis
> p. (venous and) enteric (P-E)
> p. venous and enteric drainage technique

portoenterostomy
> hepatic p.

portopulmonary hypertension (PPHTN)

Portuguese
> P. jellyfish
> P. man-of-war
> P. man-of-war sting

port-wine
> p.-w. hemangioma
> p.-w. mark
> p.-w. nevus
> p.-w. stain (PWS)

Posada mycosis

Posada-Wernicke disease

position
> left side down-head up p.

positive
> p. anergy
> biologic false p. (BFP)

> CALLA p.
> common acute lymphocytic leukemia antigen p.
> p. end-expiratory pressure (PEEP)
> p. expiratory pressure (PEP)
> p. inspiratory pressure (PIP)
> p. patch test
> Ph p.
> p. phase
> Philadelphia chromosome p.
> p. predictive value (PPV)
> p. reaction
> p. rheumatoid factor
> p. selection

positron emission tomography (PET)

posology

possible
> minimal dose p.

postanesthetic effect

postbiopsy fistula

postcardiotomy syndrome

postdiphtheric paralysis

postencephalitic trophic ulcer

posterior
> p. atlantodental interval (PADI)
> p. interosseous nerve syndrome
> p. interosseous neuropathy
> p. rhinomanometry
> p. scleritis
> superior labrum anterior and p. (SLAP)
> p. synechia formation
> p. tarsal tunnel syndrome

posteriores
> limbi palpebrales p.

posteroanterior radiograph

postexertional microtrauma

postexposure
> p. prevention (PEP)
> p. prophylaxis (PEP)

postgrafting immunosuppression

postherpetic
> p. erythema multiforme
> p. neuralgia (PHN)

posthitis

post hoc analysis

postinfection lipoatrophy

postinfectious
> p. encephalomyelitis syndrome
> p. glomerulonephritis
> p. steatorrhea

NOTES

P

postinflammatory
    p. hyperpigmentation
    p. hypopigmentation
    p. pigment alteration
post-kala-azar dermal leishmanoid
postmastectomy lymphangiosarcoma
postmenopausal frontal fibrosing alopecia
postmiliarial hypohidrosis
postmortem
    p. core protein degradation
    p. pustule
    p. tubercle
    p. wart
postnasal drip (PND)
postnatal therapy
Post-Op
    OpSite P.-O.
postoperative pressure alopecia
postosteotomy deformity
postpartum
    p. alopecia
    p. effect
    p. thyroiditis (PPT)
postphlebitic syndrome
postprimary tuberculosis
postpyodermal acute glomerulonephritis
poststeroid panniculitis
poststreptococcal
    p. glomerulonephritis (PSGN)
    p. reactive arthritis (PSRA)
postsynaptic terminal
postthrombotic disease
posttransfusion
    p. hepatitis (PTH)
    p. mononucleosis (PTM)
    p. purpura
posttranslation
posttranslationally modified arginine residue
posttranslational protein modification
posttransplant
    p. diabetes
    p. diabetes mellitus (PTDM)
    p. erythrocytosis
    p. lymphoproliferative disease (PTLD)
    p. lymphoproliferative disorder (PTLD)
posttransplantation
    p. lymphoproliferative disease (PTLD)
    p. lymphoproliferative disorder (PTLD, PT-LPD)
posttraumatic
    p. arthritis
    p. pustular eruption
    p. rheumatic meningitis

postulate
    Ehrlich p.
    Henle-Koch p.
    Koch p.
postural drainage
postvaccinal encephalitis
postvenereal reactive arthritis
potassium
    p. chloride stain (KOH)
    p. hydroxide (KOH)
    p. hydroxide preparation
    p. iodide
    p. iodide enseals
    penicillin V p.
    p. permanganate
    p. permanganate bath
    p. permanganate crystal
    p. permanganate solution
    p. titanyl phosphate (KTP)
    p. titanyl phosphate laser (KTP laser)
potato
    sweet p.
potato-peeler method
potential
    extravasation p.
    mitochondrial membrane p.
    sensory nerve action p. (SNAP)
    stress-generated electric p.
    zeta p.
    zoonotic p.
potentially fatal asthma
Potentilla chinensis
potion
    Donizetti p.
    Wagner p.
Pott
    P. gangrene
    P. paralysis
    P. paraplegia
    P. puffy tumor
poultice
poultry handler's disease
poultryman's itch
poverty weed
povidone-iodine
Powassan
    P. encephalitis
    P. virus
powder
    Absorbine Antifungal Foot p.
    Arglaes p.
    p. bed
    Bluboro p.
    Columbia Antiseptic p.
    facial p.
    Flovent Rotadisk p.
    full-coverage facial p.
    Lotrimin AF Spray P.

miconazole superabsorbent
antifungal p.
Surgifoam absorbable p.
transparent facial p.
Zeasorb-AF superabsorbent
antifungal p.
power
P. Doppler ultrasonography
p. spectral analysis
powered air loss
pox
chicken p.
farmyard p.
Kaffir p.
zinc p.
poxviral mimicry
Poxviridae
poxvirus officinalis
pp65(UL83) antigen
PPAR-gamma
peroxisome proliferator-activated
receptor-gamma
PPD
purified protein derivative
PPD test
PPDA
paraphenylenediamine
pp′-DDE
pp′-dichlorodiphenyldichloroetene
**pp′-dichlorodiphenyldichloroetene (pp′-
DDE)**
PPD-S
purified protein derivative-standard
ppg
photoplethysmography
PPH
primary pulmonary hypertension
p-phenylenediamine
PPHP
pseudopseudohypoparathyroidism
PPHTN
portopulmonary hypertension
PPi
pyrophosphate
PPIX
protoporphyrin IX
PPK
palmoplantar keratoderma
PPL
penicilloyl-polylysine
PPL skin test

PPLO
pleuro-pneumoniae-like organism
PPMS
primary-progressive multiple sclerosis
PPO-HSA
penicillin-penicilloyl human serum
albumin
PPP
poor platelet plasma
PP-ribose-P
5-phospho-alpha-d-ribosyl 1-
pyrophosphate
PPT
postpartum thyroiditis
PPV
positive predictive value
PR
pityriasis rosea
PR3
proteinase 3
PRA
panel-reactive antibody
percent reactive antibody/panel reactive
antibody
PRA test
PRA test
PRA testing
practice
Advisory Committee on
Immunization p. (ACIP)
Prader-Willi syndrome
praecox
icterus p.
lymphedema p.
praepuffalis
herpes p.
Pragmatar
prairie itch
pralnacasan
PrameGel
Pramosone cream
pramoxine
p., camphor, zinc acetate
p. HCl
p. hydrochloride
prasterone
pratense
Phleum p.
pratensis
dermatitis bullosa striata p.
Poa p.

NOTES

P

Pratt procedure
Prausnitz-Kustner (P-K)
    P.-K. antibody
    P.-K. reaction
    P.-K. syndrome
    P.-K. test
pravastatin
Prax
prayer sign
praziquantel
prazosin hydrochloride
PRCA
    pure red cell aplasia
preauricular
    p. cyst
    p. sinus
pre-B
    p.-B cell
    p.-B cell expansion
precancer
precancerosa
    melanosis circumscripta p.
precancerous
    p. dermatitis
    p. lesion
    p. melanosis of Dubreuilh
    p. tumor
precipitate
    p. in gel
    p. in solution
precipitating antibody
precipitation
    double antibody p.
    hapten inhibition of p.
    immune p.
    p. test
precipitin
    p. assay
    p. reaction
    rheumatoid arthritis p. (RAP)
    serum p.
    p. test
precipitinogen
precipitinogenoid
precipitoid
precipitophore
Precise stapler
precision-point needle
precocious puberty
precursor
    abnormal localization of
      immature p.'s (ALIP)
    mesenchymal p.
    p. molecule
Pred
    P. Forte Ophthalmic
    Liquid P.
    P. Mild Ophthalmic
Predaject injection

Predalone injection
Predcor injection
Pred-G Ophthalmic
Predicort-50 injection
predictive
    p. patch test
    p. testing
predispose
predisposition
    genetic p.
prednicarbate
Prednicen-M oral
prednisolone
    chloramphenicol and p.
    p. and gentamicin
    neomycin, polymyxin b, and p.
    sodium sulfacetamide and p.
    p. tebutate
Prednisol TBA injection
prednisone
    p. burst
    p. pulse
    p. taper
predominant
    p. DIP joint involvement
    p. distal interphalangeal joint
      involvement
    p. spondylitis
preelastic fiber
preemptive therapy
preeruptive
preexisting antibody
preformed
    p. antibody
    p. granule-associated mast cell
Prefrin Ophthalmic solution
Pregestimil
pregnancy
    p. alpha-2 glycoprotein (PAG)
    intrahepatic cholestasis of p.
    linea IgM dermatosis of p.
    mask of p.
    papular dermatitis of p.
    polymorphic eruption of p.
    pruritic folliculitis of p.
    pruritic inflammatory dermatosis
      of p.
    pruritic urticarial papules and
      plaques of p. (PUPPP)
pregnancy-associated glycoprotein
prehydration
preicteric fever
Preiser disease
preleukemia
Prelone oral
premalignant tumor
prematura
    alopecia p.

premature
p. aging
p. alopecia
p. ovarian failure (POF)
prematurity
anetoderma of p.
premenstrual
p. acne
p. exacerbation of asthma (PMA)
p. flare
Premier H. pylori assay
Premium stapler
premorbid
Premphase
premunition
premunitive
premycotic
prenatal therapy
preoperative anesthetic
preosteoblast
preosteoclast
prep
touch p.
Xylol p.
preparation
alum-precipitated p.
hyperimmune gamma globulin p.
KOH p.
leukocyte-poor p.
potassium hydroxide p.
scabies p.
Scholl Athlete's Foot P.
Scholl Corn, Callus Plaster P.
tar p.
Tzanck p.
prepatellar bursitis
prepatent period
Pre-Pen
prepolypoid
prepriming effect
prepro-von Willebrand factor
prepuce
prepulseless phase
preputiale
sebum p.
Prescription Strength Desenex
presenile spontaneous gangrene
presenilis
alopecia p.
presensitization phase
presentation
pauciarticular p.

presenting clinical manifestation
preservation
machine p. (MP)
p. perfusion injury
pulsatile p.
p. reperfusion injury
preservative
benzoate p.
pressure
p. alopecia
bilevel positive airway p. (BiPAP)
p. blister
blood p.
p. bulla
continuous positive airway p.
(CPAP)
p. gangrene
inspiratory positive airway p.
(IPAP)
interstitial p.
intracranial p. (ICP)
intragraft p.
peak inspiratory ventilator p.
positive end-expiratory p. (PEEP)
positive expiratory p. (PEP)
positive inspiratory p. (PIP)
pulmonary artery p.
p. sore
p. support ventilation (PSV)
transdiaphragmatic p. (Pdi)
p. ulcer
P. Ulcer Scale for Healing
(PUSH)
p. Ulcer Scale for Healing tool
p. urticaria
zero end-expiratory p. (ZEEP)
**pressure-controlled inverse ratio
ventilation**
pressure-induced urticaria
**pressure-regulated volume control
ventilation**
**pressurized metered-dose inhaler
(pMDI)**
Prestara
PreSun lotion and gel
presynaptic terminal
prethrombotic
pretibial
p. fever
p. myxedema (PTM)
pretransplant donor blood transfusion
Pretz-D

NOTES

P

443

Prevent
    Gaviscon P.
    Ponds P.
prevention
    bone loss p.
    Centers for Disease Control and P.
    postexposure p. (PEP)
preventive treatment
Preveon
Prevex
    P. B
    P. Diaper Rash cream
    P. HC
Preview treatment planning software
Prevotella melaninogenica
prevotii
    Peptostreptococcus p.
Prexige
prezone
prick
    p. puncture test
    p. test concentration
    p. testing
Pricker needle
prickle
    p. cell
    p. cell layer
prickle-cell
    p.-c. carcinoma
    p.-c. epithelioma
prickly heat
prick-prick test
prick-test method
prick-to-prick test
Prieur-Griscelli syndrome
prilocaine
    lidocaine and p.
Primaderm dressing
Primapore absorptive wound dressing
primaquine
    chloroquine and p.
    p. phosphate
primary
    p. acquired melanosis (PAM)
    p. adrenocortical failure
    p. amyloid
    p. amyloidotic arthropathy
    p. angiitis of the central nervous
      system
    p. areola
    p. atypical pneumonia
    p. biliary cirrhosis (PBC)
    p. bubo
    p. cell-mediated deficiency
    p. complex
    p. cutaneous adenoid cystic
      carcinoma
    p. cutaneous amyloidosis
    p. cutaneous aspergillosis

    p. cutaneous B-cell lymphocytic
      leukemia
    p. cutaneous B-cell lymphoma
    p. cutaneous blastomycosis
    p. cutaneous T-cell lymphoma
    p. effusion lymphoma
    p. epithelial germ
    p. genital herpes simplex virus
    p. herpes simplex infection
    p. herpetic stomatitis
    p. hyperaldosteronism
    p. hyperhidrosis
    p. hyperlipoproteinemia
    p. hypogammaglobulinemia
    p. idiopathic macular atrophy
    p. immune deficiency (PID)
    p. immune response
    p. immunodeficiency disorder
    p. inoculation tuberculosis
    p. irritant
    p. irritant dermatitis
    p. irritant reaction
    p. lesion
    p. localized amyloidosis
    p. lymphedema
    p. macular atrophy of skin
    p. neuroendocrine carcinoma
    p. neuroendocrine carcinoma of
      skin (PNCS)
    p. neuroendocrine tumor
    p. nonfunction (PRNF)
    p. pauciimmune necrotizing
      glomerulonephritis
    p. pulmonary histoplasmosis
    p. pulmonary hypertension (PPH)
    p. pulmonary parenchymal disease
    p. pyoderma
    p. rejection
    p. sclerosing cholangitis (PSC)
    p. Sjögren syndrome
    p. sore
    p. syphilis
    p. systemic amyloidosis
    p. systemic vasculitides (PSV)
    p. systemic vasculitis (PSV)
    p. telangiectasia
**primary-progressive multiple sclerosis
(PPMS)**
Primatene Mist
Primatized
Primaxin
prime-boost strategy
Primed cell
primer
    P. leg compression dressing
    sequence-specific p. (SSP)
primer-probe
    3 p.-p.

OspA p.-p.
OspB p.-p.
priming renal dialysis unit
primrose
    evening p.
Primula obconica
Principen
principle
    Castaneda p.
    diagnostic p.
Pringle disease
print
    scent p.
    tentacle p.
Prioderm
prion
    p. protein
    p. protein-origin amyloid deposit
prior drug exposure
priority
    law of p.
PRIST
    paper radioimmunosorbent test
    Phadezym PRIST
Pristine-100 allergy control product
private antigen
privet tree
PRNF
    primary nonfunction
pro
    P. residue
    P. 2000 topical microbicide
proactivator
    C3 p.
Pro-Air
proalpha-chain
Pro-Amox
Proampacin
proapoptotic gene
probacteriophage
    defective p.
Probalan
proband
probe
    Acradinium-ester-labeled nucleic
      acid p.
    Arthro-BST arthroscopic p.
    cDNA p.
    IntraDop p.
    nucleic acid p.
    oligonucleotide p.

    radioactive p.
    viral p.
Proben-C
probenecid
    ampicillin and p.
    colchicine and p.
probiosis
probiotic
problem
    p. elicitation technique (PET)
    hindfoot p.
    midfoot p.
problem-oriented
    p.-o. algorithm
    p.-o. diagnosis
procainamide
procaine
    p. hydrochloride
    penicillin g p.
procapsid
Procaryotae (*var. of* Prokaryotae)
procaryote (*var. of* prokaryote)
procaryotic (*var. of* prokaryotic)
procaterol
procedure
    arachnophlebectomy p.
    Caldwell-Luc p.
    cheilectomy p.
    Darrach p.
    domino p.
    elimination p.
    fluorometric p.
    hemicallotasis p.
    Hoffman-Clayton p.
    "Laser bra" p.
    Microsporidia diagnostic p.
    Mohs p.
    olecranon p.
    platelet neutralization p.
    Pratt p.
    Rotazyme diagnostic p.
    streptavidin-biotinperoxidase p.
    Z-plasty p.
procera
    Calotropis p.
process
    airspace p.
    AuTolo Cure P.
    complement-mediated host
      defense p.
    exocrinopathic p.
    host-immune p.

NOTES

P

process *(continued)*
    nephritogenic p.
    olecranon p.
    recapitulation of ontogenesis p.
    SoftLight laser/skin resurfacing p.
Pro-Clude
    P.-C. transparent film
    P.-C. transparent film wound
      dressing
procoagulant
procollagen
    p. suicide
    p. type II
    p. type III aminoterminal peptide
Procort
Procrit
proctitis
    dietary protein p.
    pseudoinfectious p.
proctocolitis
    ulcerative p.
Proctocort
procurement
    regional organ p. (ROP)
Procuven solution
ProCyte
    P. transparent adhesive film
      dressing
    P. transparent film
Procytox
Pro-Depo injection
prodromal
    p. stage
    p. symptom
prodromon, pl. **prodroma**
Prodrox injection
product
    AllerCare allergy control p.
    Blue Peel skin health p.
    cyclooxygenase p.
    Exact skin p.
    ginger-based p.
    Gly Derm skin care p.
    HLA-B27 gene p.
    home cleaning p.
    hypoallergenic p.
    Lantiseptic skin care p.
    latex p.
    lipoxygenase interaction p.
    PolyHeme blood replacement p.
    Pristine-100 allergy control p.
    Refinity skin p.
    Xcellerate T-cell p.
production
    cytokine p.
    p. of lymphokine
    prostanoid p.
    purulent sputum p.

productus
    Peptostreptococcus p.
Proetz maneuver
Profen
    P. II
    P. LA
Profeta law
profile
    angioedema p.
    P. of Mood States Scale
    Nottingham Health P. (NHP)
    P. platform
    relapsing-remitting p.
    Sickness Impact P. (SIP)
    Western blot vaccine p.
Profore
    P. 4-layer bandage
    P. leg compression dressing
    P. wound contact layer
profunda
    miliaria p.
    morphea p.
    tinea p.
profundus
    larva migrans p.
    lupus erythematosus p.
    nevus p.
profundus/panniculitis
    lupus p.
profusa
    lentiginosis p.
progenitalis
    herpes p.
progenitor lymphoid cell
progeria
    Hutchinson-Gilford p.
    true p.
progeroid Ehlers-Danlos syndrome
progesterone
progesterone-induced blocking factor (PIBF)
prognosis, pl. **prognoses**
prognostic
progonoma
    melanotic p.
Prograf
    P. capsule
    P. injection
program
    Lipman-Pearson protein
      alignment p.
    National Asthma Education P.
      (NAEP)
    National Immunization P. (NIP)
    National Marrow Donor P.
      (NMDP)
    Rush-Presbyterian St. Luke's Heart
      Failure and Transplant P.

progrediens
    necrosis p.
progression
    damaged joint p.
    malignant p.
progressiva
    acromelanosis p.
    fibrodysplasia ossification p.
    granulomatosis disciformis et p.
    junctional epidermolysis bullosa p.
    leukopathia symmetrica p.
progressive
    p. acinar consolidation
    p. azotemia
    p. bacterial synergistic gangrene
    p. disseminated histoplasmosis
    p. encephalomyelitis with rigidity and myoclonus (PERM)
    p. facial hemiatrophy
    p. idiopathic atrophoderma
    p. interstitial fibrosis
    p. lipodystrophy
    p. multifocal leukoencephalopathy (PML)
    p. outer retinal necrosis (PORN)
    p. pigmentary dermatosis
    p. pneumonia
    p. pneumonia virus
    p. symmetrical verrucous erythrokeratodermia
    p. symmetric erythrokeratodermia (PSEK)
    p. symptom sclerosis (PSS)
    p. synovial hypertrophy
    p. systemic sclerosis (PSS)
    p. vaccinia
proguanil
ProGuide
prohormone
Pro-Indo
proinflammatory
    p. cytokine
    p. cytokine response
    p. effect
    p. immunoreactant
    p. pathway
project
    Rochester Epidemiology P. (REP)
Prokaryotae, Procaryotae
prokaryote, procaryote
prokaryotic, procaryotic
    p. extracellular organism

prolactin
Prolastin
Prolene suture
Proleukin
prolidase deficiency
proliferans
    angioendotheliomatosis p.
proliferating
    p. cell nuclear antigen (PCNA)
    p. pilar cyst
    p. systematized angioendotheliomatosis
    p. trichilemmal cyst
proliferation
    acanthotic epidermal p.
    p. assay
    p. disorder
    endothelial cell p.
    gliomatous p.
    homeostasis-driven p.
    intravascular endothelial p.
    Masson intravascular endothelial p.
    melanocytic p.
proliferation-associated antigen
proliferative
    p. cell
    p. dermatitis
    p. fasciitis
    p. glomerulonephritis
    p. inflammatory disease
    p. intimitis
    p. lesion
    p. synovitis
    p. synovium
    p. tenosynovitis
    p. verrucous leukoplakia
prolificans
    Scopulariopsis p.
ProLine endoscopic instrument
proline-rich polypeptide
prolixus
    Rhodnius p.
prolongation
    p. of expiration
    expiratory p.
prolonged
    p. diarrhea
    p. pulmonary eosinophilia
Proloprim
prolyl
prolymphocytic leukemia (PLL)
Prometa

NOTES

promethazine
    p. HCl
    p. hydrochloride
Prometh injection
Promit
Promogran matrix wound dressing
promoter
    IL-10 gene p.
    neurofilament p.
promotor
    p. allele
    p. element
prom pill
pronator teres syndrome
Pronto Shampoo
Propaderm
Propadrine
Propagest
Propa pH
Propecia
properdin
    p. deficiency
    p. factor A, B, D, E
    p. system
property
    degreasing p.'s
prophage
    defective p.
prophylactic
    p. antibody
    p. treatment
prophylaxis
    active p.
    p. agent
    chemical p.
    malaria p.
    passive p.
    postexposure p. (PEP)
Prophyllin
propidium iodide
propionate
    clobetasol p.
    halobetasol p.
propionate/salmeterol
    flucatisone p. (FP/Salm Combo)
Propionibacterium
    P. acnes
    P. propionicus
propionicus
    Propionibacterium p.
Pro-Piroxicam
propolis
proportional assist ventilation
proportionate morbidity ratio (PMR)
propranolol hydrochloride
propria
    atrophia pilorum p.
    lamina p.
    miliaria p.

propylene
    p. glycol
    p. glycol allergy
    p. glycol dermatitis
propylthiouracil
proquazone
Prorex Injection
prosector's
    p. tubercle
    p. wart
prosodemic
Prosorba column device
prostacyclin (PGI$_2$)
    p. I3
    p. synthase
prostaglandin (PG)
    p. D (PGD)
    p. D$_2$ (PGD2)
    p. E (PGE)
    p. E$_1$ (PGE$_1$)
    p. E$_2$ (PGE$_2$)
    p. H2 (PGH$_2$)
    p. H synthase-1, -2 (PGHS-1, -2)
    p. I (PGI)
    p. synthesis inhibition
prostanoid
    p. biosynthetic enzyme
    p. production
Prostaphlin
    P. injection
    P. oral
ProstaScint monoclonal antibody
prostatitis
prosthesis, pl. **prostheses**
    silicone rubber p.
prosthetic joint
protease
    Hirudin-sensitive p.
    neutral p.
    p. nexin-1
    serine p.
    thiol p.
protease-activated receptor (PAR)
protease-antiprotease imbalance
proteasome
protectant
    LiquiShield-A Skin P.
protection
    photo p.
    Sundown Extra P.
    Sun Management Lip P.
    Sun Management Sensible P.
    p. test
    topical skin p. (TSP)
protective
    p. protein
    p. therapy
protector
    Heelbo decubitus p.

protegrin rinse
protein
    acetylation of cellular p.
    acetylation of serum p.
    actin-binding p.
    activator p. 1 (AP1)
    acute phase p.
    adhesion p.
    AL p.
    amyloid A p.
    amyloid fibril p.
    antibiotic p.
    p. antigen
    arthritogenic p.
    Australian parrot p.
    azurophil granule p.
    B7 p.
    Bence Jones p.
    BPI p.
    BvgS p.
    p. C
    C p.
    cartilage matrix p.
    cartilage oligomeric p.
    CD28 p.
    p. C deficiency
    CD40 soluble p.
    cell adhesion p.
    p. C1 esterase inhibitor
    c-fos p.
    p. chip
    c-jun p.
    p. contact dermatitis
    control p.
    CREB p.
    CTLA-4 soluble p.
    cytoskeletal p.
    eosinophil granule cationic p.
    eosinophil p. X
    ErbB-2 p.
    p. fever
    p. filaggrin
    F12-MABP fusion p.
    p. folding
    foreign p.
    freeze-dried p.
    fusion p.
    G p.
    glucocorticoid-inducible p.
    glycosylphosphatidylinositol-
      anchored p.
    GP47 p.

    GP67 p.
    GPI-anchored p.
    haptenated p.
    heat-shock p. (HSP)
    heat-shock p. 70 (HSP-70)
    HEL p.
    hen egg lysozyme p.
    heterologous p.
    homeobox p.
    immune p.
    immunogenic p.
    220-kD p.
    38-kd P_o p.
    45-kilodalton p.
    p. kinase A (PKA)
    p. kinase A-dependent
      phosphorylation
    latex ELISA for antigen p.
      (LEAP)
    5-LO-activating p.
    M p.
    MacMARCKS p.
    macrophage inflammatory p. (MIP)
    major basic p. (MBP)
    major outer membrane p. (MOMP)
    maltose-binding p. (MABP, MBP)
    mannose-binding p.
    mitogen-activated p. (MAP)
    mitogen-activating p. (MAP)
    monoclonal p.
    monocyte chemoattractant p.
    monocyte chemotactic p. (MCP)
    mouse serum p. (MSP)
    mouse urine p. (MUP)
    myelin basic p. (MBP)
    myeloblastic p.
    Nef p.
    neutrophil-activating p. (NAP)
    NF-ATc p.
    p. nitrogen unit (PNU)
    nonhistone p.
    nonspecific p.
    Ontak p.
    p. origin amyloid deposit
    peptide transporter p.
    pigeon serum p. (PSP)
    plasma cell dyscrasia with
      polyneuropathy, organomegaly,
      endocrinopathy, monoclonal p.
    platelet basic p.
    pollen-coat p.'s (PCPs)
    polymorphic p.

NOTES

P

protein *(continued)*
    prion p.
    protective p.
    Ras p.
    ras-mitogen-activated p.
    rat serum p. (RSP)
    rat urine p. (RUP)
    Rb p.
    receptor interacting p. (RIP)
    recombinant human p.
    recombinant human tumor necrosis
      factor receptor fusion p.
    recombinant LFA-3/IgG1 human
      fusion p.
    retinoblastoma tumor suppressor p.
    RFX-associated p. (RFXAP)
    rhoGDI p.
    p. S
    SCA p.
    secretory leukoprotease inhibitor p.
    p. shock
    p. shock therapy
    single-chain antigen-binding p.
    Sma- and Mad-related p. (SMAD)
    Structural Classification of P.'s
      (SCOP)
    Tamm-Horsfall p.
    TAP1, TAP2 p.
    TATA-binding p.
    testis-specific binding p. (TSBP)
    ToxR p.
    p. transglutamination
    variant amyloidogenic p.
    Wiskott-Aldrich syndrome p.
      (WASP)
    zinc finger p.
protein-1
    human monocyte chemoattractant p.
    monocyte chemoattractant p. (MCP-
      1)
proteinase
    p. 3 (PR3)
    aspartic p.
    connective tissue p.
    cysteine p.
    disintegrin p.
    ECM-degrading p.
    extracellular matrix-degrading p.
    p. inhibitor
    lysosomal p.
    mast cell p.
    neutral p.
    serine p.
protein-energy malnutrition (PEM)
protein-energy-related obesity
protein-losing
    p.-l. enteropathy
    p.-l. gastroenteropathy

proteinosis
    lipoid p.
proteinuria
    nephrotic-range p.
proteoglycan
    cartilage p.
    human stromelysin aggregated p.
      (H-SLAP)
    surface p.
proteolysis
proteolytic enzyme
proteomic map
Proteque SPS
Proteus
    P. mirabilis
    P. syndrome
    P. vulgaris
Prothazine
    P. injection
    P. oral
protist
protistologist
protistology
protobe
protobiology
protocol
    2-day ultrarush p.
    triple-drug therapy
      immunosuppression p.
Protoctista
ProtoDerm
proton
    p. leak
    p. magnetic resonance microscopy
protooncogene
    c-myc p.
    Fos p.
    Jun p.
protopianoma
Protopic ointment
protoplast fusion
protoporphyria
    Besnier p.
    p. chronica multiformis
    erythropoietic p.
    p. estivalis
    p. ferox
    p. gestationis
    p. of Hebra
    Hutchinson summer p.
    melanotic p.
    p. mitis
    polymorphic p.
    p. prurigo agria
    p. simplex
    p. universalis
    winter p.

protoporphyrin
  p. IX (PPIX)
  zinc p. (ZPP)
protoporphyrinogen
Protostat oral
Prototheca wickerhamii
protothecosis
Protovir
Protox
protozoa
  extraintestinal p.
  intestinal p.
  unicellular p.
protozoal
  p. abscess
  p. parasitic disease
protozoan infection
protracta
  Triatoma p.
Protropin II
protrusio acetabuli
protrusion
  infantile perianal pyramidal p.
protuberans
  dermatofibroma p.
  dermatofibrosarcoma p. (DFSP)
proud flesh
Provascar
Provatene
Pro-Vent arterial blood sampling kit
Proventil
  P. HFA
  P. Repetabs
Providence clamp
provirus
provocation
  bronchial p.
  colonoscopic allergen p. (COLAP)
  p. typhoid
provocation-neutralization test
provocative
  p. dose test (PDT)
  p. dose testing
  p. use test (PUT)
Provocholine
Prowazek body
Prowazek-Greeff body
prowazekii
  Rickettsia p.
proxetil
  cefpodoxime p.

proximal
  p. bronchiectasis
  p. femoral osteotomy
  p. interphalangeal (PIP)
  p. nail matrix
  p. phalange
  p. pseudoarthrosis
  p. tubular epithelial cells (PTEC)
Proximate
  P. II, III stapler
  P. RH stapler
Prozac Weekly
prozone reaction
PRR
  pattern recognition receptor
PRSP
  penicillin-resistant *Streptococcus*
    pneumoniae
Prudoxin cream
pruinosum
  Chrysosporium p.
prune
pruriginosus
  strophulus p.
pruriginous
prurigo
  actinic p.
  p. agria
  Besnier p.
  p. diathsique
  p. estivalis
  p. ferox
  p. gestationis
  p. gestationis of Besnier
  p. gravidarum
  Hebra p.
  p. hiemalis
  Hutchinson summer p.
  p. infantilis
  p. mitis
  p. nodularis
  p. papule
  p. simplex
  p. simplex subacuta
  summer p.
pruritic
  p. dermatosis
  p. erythematous patch
  p. folliculitis of pregnancy
  p. inflammatory dermatosis of
    pregnancy
  p. lesion

NOTES

P

pruritic *(continued)*
    p. papule
    p. urticarial papules and plaques
      of pregnancy (PUPPP)
pruritica
    puncta p.
pruritogenic
pruritus
    p. ani
    aquagenic p.
    p. balnea
    bath p.
    biliary p.
    brachioradial p.
    central p.
    Duhring p.
    essential p.
    p. estivalis
    generalized p.
    genital p.
    p. hiemalis
    paroxysmal p.
    perianal p.
    psychogenic p.
    p. scroti
    seasonal p.
    senile p.
    p. senilis
    symptomatic p.
    uremic p.
    p. vulva
    winter p.
psammoma
PSC
    pigmented spindle cell
    primary sclerosing cholangitis
PSCN
    plexiform spindle cell nevus
PSE
    PSE CPM chewable tablet
    Entex PSE
    Guaifenex PSE
PSEK
    progressive symmetric
      erythrokeratodermia
P-selectin ligand
Pseudallescheria boydii
pseudallescheriasis
pseudarthrosis
    Girdlestone p.
pseudoacanthosis nigricans
pseudoachondroplasia
pseudoagglutination
pseudoainhum
pseudoallergic reaction (PAR)
pseudoalopecia areata
pseudoanaphylactic shock
pseudoanaphylaxis

pseudoaneurysm
    ventricular p. (VPA)
pseudoangina pectoris
pseudoangiomatosis
    eruptive p.
pseudoangiosarcoma
    Masson p.
pseudoannulati
    pili p.
pseudoarthrosis
    proximal p.
pseudobacteremia
pseudobacteriuria
pseudocavitation
pseudochancre redux
pseudocholinesterase (PCE)
pseudochromidrosis
pseudocolloid of lip
pseudocowpox virus
pseudocyst
    digital mucinous p.
    myxoid p.
pseudocystic rheumatoid arthritis
pseudodermachalasis
pseudodiphtheria
pseudodiphtheriticum
    Bacillus p.
pseudodysentery
pseudoedema
pseudoemperipolesis
pseudoephedrine
    acetaminophen, chlorpheniramine,
      and p.
    acrivastine and p.
    brompheniramine and p.
    carbinoxamine and p.
    chlorpheniramine and p.
    p. and dextromethorphan
    diphenhydramine and p.
    fexofenadine and p.
    guaifenesin and p.
    p. HCl
    p. and ibuprofen
    loratadine and p.
    terfenadine and p.
    triprolidine and p.
pseudoepitheliomatous
    p. hyperplasia
    p. keratotic and micaceous balanitis
pseudoerysipelas
pseudoexfoliation
pseudofolliculitis barbae (PFB)
pseudofracture
Pseudofrin
pseudogene
Pseudo-Gest Plus Tablet
pseudoglandular squamous cell
    carcinoma
pseudogout

pseudogynecomastia
pseudohorned cyst
pseudo-Hurler polydystrophy
pseudo-Hutchinson sign
pseudohyphae
pseudohypoparathyroidism (PHP)
pseudoicterus
pseudoinfection
pseudoinfectious proctitis
pseudojaundice
pseudo-Kaposi sarcoma
pseudo-Koebner phenomenon
pseudolaxity
pseudolepromatous leishmaniasis
pseudoleukonychia
pseudolymphocytic choriomeningitis virus
pseudolymphoma
    B-cell p.
    cutaneous p.
    Spiegler-Fendt p.
    T-cell p.
pseudolysogenic strain
pseudolysogeny
pseudomalignant lymphoma
pseudomallei
    Burkholderia p.
    Malleomyces p.
    Pseudomonas p.
pseudomembrane
pseudomembranous colitis
pseudomeningitis
pseudomilium
    colloid p.
Pseudomonas
    P. aeruginosa
    P. aeruginosa bacteremia
    P. cepacia dermatitis
    P. elastase
    P. maltophilia
    P. pseudomallei
    P. putida
    P. stutzeri
pseudomonic acid
pseudomonilethrix
pseudoneuropathic joint
pseudonit
pseudoobstruction
pseudoparalysis
    Parrot p.
pseudopelade
    Brocq p.
    p. of Brocq

pseudopelade-type alopecia
pseudophlegmon
    Hamilton p.
pseudophytophotodermatitis
pseudopilus, pl. pseudopili
    p. annulatus
pseudopneumonia
pseudopod
pseudopodagra
pseudoporphyria
pseudoproteinuria
pseudopseudohypoparathyroidism (PPHP)
pseudopseudothrombophlebitis
pseudorabies virus
pseudoradicular syndrome
pseudoreaction
pseudorecidive
pseudoreplica
pseudorheumatism
pseudorheumatoid
pseudorubella
pseudosarcomatous fasciitis
pseudoscar
    spontaneous p.
    stellate p.
pseudoscarlatina
pseudoseptic arthritis
pseudosmallpox
pseudosyndactyly
pseudotattooing
pseudothrombophlebitis
pseudotrichinosis
pseudotuberculosis
    Yersinia p.
pseudotumor
    p. cerebri
    orbital p.
pseudotumoral mediastinal amyloidosis
pseudo-Turner syndrome
pseudovariola
Pseudovent PED capsule
pseudoxanthoma elasticum (PXE)
pseudoxanthomatous mastocytosis
PSG
    polysomnography
PSGN
    poststreptococcal glomerulonephritis
psilate
psilosis
psilostachya
    Ambrosia p.
psilothin

NOTES

P

psilotic
psittaci
    Chlamydia p.
psittacosis
    p. inclusion body
    p. virus
PSL
    pigmented skin lesion
psoas
PsoE
    erythrodermic psoriasis
psora
psoralen
    p. compound
    p.'s plus ultraviolet A
      radiation/ultraviolet B radiation
      (PUVA/UVB)
    p. ultraviolet A (PUVA)
    p. ultraviolet A-range (PUVA)
    p. ultraviolet A regimen/therapy
Psoraxine
PsorBan
Psorcon
    P. e
    P. topical
    P. topical steroid
psorelcosis
psoriasic
psoriasiform
    p. dermatitis
    p. epidermal hyperplasia
    p. eruption
    p. lesion
psoriasiformis
    parakeratosis p.
psoriasis
    p. annularis
    p. annulata
    anti-CD11a humanized monoclonal
      antibody for p.
    P. Area and Severity Index (PASI)
    P. Area Severity Index (PASI)
    p. arthropathica
    p. arthropica
    Barber p.
    p. buccalis
    p. circinata
    circinate p.
    p. diffusa
    p. discoidea
    p. discoides
    drop-like p.
    erythrodermic p. (PsoE)
    exfoliative p.
    p. figurata
    figurate p.
    flexural p.
    generalized pustular p.
    genital p.

p. geographica
geriatric p.
p. guttata
guttate p.
p. gyrata
gyrate p.
Ingram regimen for p.
intertriginous p.
intraepidermal microabscess of p.
inverse p.
p. inveterata
P. Life Stress Inventory (PLSI)
p. lingua
localized pustular p.
microabscess of p.
napkin p.
p. nummularis
p. orbicularis
ostraceous p.
p. ostreacea
palmar p.
plaque p.
plaque-type p.
p. punctata
pustular p.
rupioid p.
p. rupioides
p. spondylitica
treatment of p.
p. universalis
volar p.
von Zumbusch pustular p.
psoriatic
    p. arthritis
    p. arthritis mutilans
    p. arthritis with spinal involvement
    p. arthropathy
    p. nail change
    p. onychopachydermoperiostitis
      (POPP)
    p. plaque
    p. sacroiliitis
    p. spondylitis
psoriatica
    arthropathia p.
psoriatic-type scale
psoriaticum
    erythroderma p.
psoric
psoriGel
Psorion
    P. Cream
    P. topical
psoroid
psorophthalmia
psoroptic acariasis
psorous
PSP
    pigeon serum protein

pspA
  outer surface protein A
PSRA
  poststreptococcal reactive arthritis
PSS
  progressive symptom sclerosis
  progressive systemic sclerosis
P&S Shampoo
PSV
  pressure support ventilation
  primary systemic vasculitides
  primary systemic vasculitis
    Quantum PSV
psychocutaneous disease
Psychodidae
psychogalvanic
psychogalvanometer
psychogenic
  p. factor
  p. pain syndrome
  p. pruritus
  p. purpura
  p. reaction
psychoitchical
psychological
  p. irritable bowel/migraine
    syndrome (PIMS)
  p. stimulus
psycho-neuro-immuno-endocrine axis
psychoneuroimmunology
psychophysiologic disorder
psychosis
psychosocial intervention
psychotropic
  p. agent
  p. agent therapy
psyllium seed
PTA
  pancreas transplant alone
PTC
  Patched gene
PTDM
  posttransplant diabetes mellitus
PTEC
  proximal tubular epithelial cells
pteronyssinus
  Dermatophagoides p.
pterygium
  p. colli
  p. inversum unguis
PTH
  posttransfusion hepatitis

pthiriasis
  p. capitis
  p. corporis
  p. pubis
Pthirus
  P. pubis
  P. pubis infestation
PTLD
  posttransplantation lymphoproliferative
    disease
  posttransplantation lymphoproliferative
    disorder
  posttransplant lymphoproliferative
    disease
  posttransplant lymphoproliferative
    disorder
PT-LPD
  posttransplantation lymphoproliferative
    disorder
PTM
  posttransfusion mononucleosis
  pretibial myxedema
ptosis
PTRA
  percutaneous transfemoral renal
    angioplasty
PTT
  partial thromboplastin time
PTX
  pentoxifylline
puberty
  precocious p.
pubes
pubescence
pubic
  p. baldness
  p. louse
pubis
  osteitis p.
  pediculosis p.
  pthiriasis p.
  Pthirus p.
public antigen
pubomadesis
pudenda (*pl. of* pudendum)
pudendal ulcer
pudendi
  granuloma p.
pudendum, pl. pudenda
  ulcerating granuloma of p.
pudicitiae
  erythema p.

NOTES

P

pudore
    erythema a p.
pudoris
    erythema p.
puellaris
    erythrocyanosis crurum p.
puellarum
    erythrocyanosis frigida crurum p.
Puente disease
puerorum
    hydroa p.
puerperal
    p. bacteremia
    p. fever
puerperium
PUF
    polyurethane film
puff
    buff p.
Pulex irritans
pulicans
    purpura p.
pulicicide
pulicide
pulicosa
    purpura p.
pulicosistungiasis
pulicosis tungiasis
pull cell
pulling boat hand
pullulans
    Aureobasidium p.
Pullularia
Pulmanex
Pulmicort Turbuhaler
Pulmo-Aide
    P.-A. nebulizer
    P.-A. Traveler
pulmonale
    cor p.
pulmonary
    p. adenomatosis of sheep
    p. agenesis
    p. amyloidosis
    p. artery pressure
    p. aspergillosis
    p. blood volume (PBV)
    p. capillary hemangiomatosis
    p. disease anemia syndrome
    p. embolism
    p. fibrosis
    p. flushing
    p. function (PF)
    p. function test (PFT)
    p. hemorrhage
    p. hemosiderosis
    p. hypertension
    p. infiltrate with eosinophilia (PIE)
    p. lesion

    p. lymphoma
    p. mycosis
    p. necrobiotic nodule
    p. nodulosis
    p. occlusive vasculopathy
    p. sarcoidosis
    p. sling syndrome
    p. surfactant
    p. toilet
    p. vascular resistance (PVR)
    p. venoocclusive disease (PVOD)
Pulmonet spirometer
pulmonic valve closure sound
PulmoSonic
Pulmowrap
Pulmozyme
pulp abscess
pulpal abscess
pulposus
    herniated nucleus p. (HNP)
    nucleus p.
pulp-to-pulp tip pinch
pulsatile preservation
pulse
    p. dosing
    p. methylprednisolone
    p. oximetry device
    p. oximetry monitoring (POM)
    paradoxical p.
    P. Peel
    prednisone p.
    p. rate
    spin-echo p.
    steroid p.
    p. test
pulsed-dye
    p.-d. laser (PDL)
    p.-d. laser therapy
pulsed field gel electrophoresis (PFGE)
PulseDose oxygen delivery technology
pulse-field gel electrophoresis (PFGE)
pulseless
    p. disease
    p. phase
pulsus paradoxus
pultaceous
Pulvules
    Cinobac P.
    Co-Pyronil 2 P.
    Ilosone P.
    Seromycin P.
pumice stone
pumilus
    Bacillus p.
pump
    Alpha 1 p.
    Alzet osmotic p.
    elastomeric p.
    Klein p.

Na⁺-K⁺ ATPase p.
Wells Johnson p.
pump-bumps bursitis
pumpkin
punch
Accuderm p.
Australian p.
Baker-Cummings p.
p. biopsy
Dyonics suction p.
Keyes p.
Loo p.
Orentreich p.
skin p.
upcurved p.
punched-out erosion
puncta pruritica
punctata
acne p.
chondrodysplasia p.
keratosis palmoplantaris p.
onychia p.
porokeratosis p.
psoriasis p.
punctate
p. area of increased signal (PAIS)
p. bleeding
erythema p.
p. hemorrhage
p. keratoderma
p. porokeratotic keratoderma
punctated metalloproteinase
punctatum
erythema p.
keratoderma p.
punctum
puncture wound
pupate
pupil
Adie tonic p.
Argyll Robertson p.
PUPPP
pruritic urticarial papules and plaques of
pregnancy
pura (*pl. of* pus)
Puralube Tears solution
PuraPly wound dressing
pure
p. neural leprosy
p. red cell aplasia (PRCA)

purging
tumor cell p.
in vitro p.
Puricase
Puri-Clens wound cleanser
purified
p. protein derivative (PPD)
p. protein derivative-standard (PPD-S)
p. protein derivative test
p. protein derivative of tuberculin
p. talc
purine
p. analog
p. metabolism
p. nucleoside phosphorylase (PNP)
p. nucleoside phosphorylase deficiency
p. nucleotide adenosine triphosphate
p. nucleotide cycle
p. ribonucleotide
p. ring
purine-stimulated prostaglandin E₂ (PGE₂)
purinoceptor
Purinol
purple-red papule
purple sail dermatitis
Purpose cleanser
purpura
actinic p.
acute idiopathic thrombocytopenic p.
acute vascular p.
allergic nonthrombocytopenic p.
anaphylactoid p.
p. angioneurotica
p. annularis telangiectodes
p. annularis telangiectodes of Majocchi
autoimmune thrombocytopenic p.
Bateman p.
p. bullosa
p. cachectica
chronic idiopathic thrombocytopenic p.
p. cryoglobulinemia
cutaneous p.
drug-induced p.
Ducas and Kapetanakis pigmented p.
dysproteinemic p.

NOTES

purpura *(continued)*
    p. en cocarde avec oedema
    essential thrombocytopenic p.
    factitious p.
    fibrinolytic p.
    p. fulminans
    Gardner-Diamond p.
    p. hemorrhagica
    Henoch p.
    Henoch-Schönlein p. (HSP)
    hypergammaglobulinemic p.
    hyperglobulinemic p.
    idiopathic thrombocytopenic p.
      (ITP)
    p. iodica
    itching p.
    Landouzy p.
    macular p.
    p. maculosa
    Majocchi p.
    p. nervosa
    nonblanching p.
    nonpalpable p.
    nonthrombocytopenic p.
    obstructive p.
    orthostatic p.
    palpable p.
    passion p.
    periorbital p.
    pigmented p.
    p. pigmentosa chronica
    pinch p.
    posttransfusion p.
    psychogenic p.
    p. pulicans
    p. pulicosa
    p. rheumatica
    Schamberg p.
    Schönlein p.
    scorbutic p.
    senile p.
    p. senilis
    p. simplex
    skin p.
    solar p.
    stasis p.
    steroid p.
    p. symptomatica
    thrombocytopenic p.
    thrombotic thrombocytopenic p.
      (TTP)
    traumatic p.
    p. urticans
    p. variolosa
    Waldenström p.
    Werlhof p.
purpurascens
    Epicoccum p.

purpureum
    Trichophyton p.
purpuric
    p. halo
    p. lesion
    p. phototherapy-induced eruption
    p. pigmented lichenoid dermatitis
pursed lips breathing
purse-string mouth
purulent
    p. arthritis
    p. sputum
    p. sputum production
puruloid
pus, pl. **pura**
    p. tube
Pusey emulsion
PUSH
    Pressure Ulcer Scale for Healing
      PUSH tool
puss
    p. caterpillar
    p. caterpillar sting
pustula, pl. **pustulae**
    p. maligna
pustulant
pustular
    p. acne
    p. acrodermatitis
    p. bacterid
    p. dermatosis
    p. eruption
    p. folliculitis
    p. lesion
    p. melanosis
    p. miliaria
    p. patch-test reaction
    p. perifolliculitis
    p. psoriasis
    p. psoriasis of the palms and
      soles of Barber
    superficial p.
    p. syphilid
    p. vasculitis
    p. vesicle
pustulation
pustule
    deep-seated p.
    denudation of p.
    desquamation of p.
    follicular p.
    Kogoj p.
    malignant p.
    postmortem p.
    spongiform p.
    sterile p.
pustuliform
pustulocrustaceous

pustulosa
    acne p.
    acrodermatitis p.
    miliaria p.
    parakeratosis p.
    trichomycosis p.
    varicella inoculata p.
pustulosis
    acute generalized exanthematous p.
      (AGEP)
    cephalic p.
    Malassezia furfur p.
    p. palmaris et plantaris
    palmoplantar p.
    p. palmoplantaris
    sterile eosinophilic p.
    p. vacciniformis acuta
pustulosum
    eczema p.
    erysipelas p.
pustulotic arthrosteitis
PUT
    provocative use test
putative oxidative cleavage site
putida
    Pseudomonas p.
putrescentiae
    Tyrophagus p.
Puumala virus
PUVA
    oral administration of psoralen and
      subsequent exposure to long
      wavelength ultraviolet light
    photochemotherapy with oral
      methoxypsoralen therapy followed by
      UVA
    psoralen ultraviolet A
    psoralen ultraviolet A-range
      foil bath PUVA
      PUVA regimen/therapy
      topical PUVA
PUVA-induced lentigo
PUVA/UVB
    psoralens plus ultraviolet A
      radiation/ultraviolet B radiation
PV
    pemphigus vulgaris
PVAC treatment
PVC
    polyvinyl chloride
PVM
    pneumonia virus of mice

PVNS
    pigmented villonodular synovitis
PVOD
    pulmonary venoocclusive disease
PVR
    pulmonary vascular resistance
PV virus
PWM
    pokeweed mitogen
PWS
    port-wine stain
PXE
    pseudoxanthoma elasticum
pycnidia
pycnidium
pyemia
pyemic abscess
Pyemotes ventricosus
pyknodysostosis
pyknosis
pyknotic cell
pylori
    Campylobacter p.
    Helicobacter p.
    ImmunoCard used for diagnosis of
      Helicobacter p.
Pym fever
Pyocidin-Otic
pyocin
pyocyanine
pyocyanolysin
pyoderma
    blastomycosis-like p.
    chancriform p.
    p. chancriforme faciei
    p. faciale
    p. gangrenosum (PG)
    granulomatous p.
    intractable p.
    malignant p.
    persistent p.
    primary p.
    secondary p.
    superficial follicular p.
    superficial granulomatous p.
    p. ulcerosum tropicalum
    p. vegetans
    p. verrucosum
pyodermatitis
pyodermatosis

NOTES

P

pyodermatous
    p. infection
    p. skin lesion
pyodermia
    p. facialis
    p. gangrenosa
pyogenes
    Streptococcus p.
pyogenic
    p. abscess
    p. arthritis
    p. bacterium
    p. fever
    p. granuloma
    p. infection
    p. osteomyelitis
    p. sacroiliitis
    p. sterile arthritis, pyoderma
       gangrenosum and acne (PAPA)
pyogenicum
    granuloma p.
pyohemia
pyomyositis
    pneumococcal p.
    tropical p.
pyosis
    Corlett p.
    Manson p.
    p. palmaris
    p. tropica
pyostomatitis vegetans
Pyradone
Pyral
    Jaa P.
pyrantel pamoate
pyrazinamide (PZA)
    rifampin, isoniazid, and p.
pyrethrin and piperonyl butoxide
pyrethroid
    synthetic p.
pyrethrum
pyrexia
    tick p.
pyribenzamine (PBZ)

pyridinoline cross-link
pyridoxine deficiency
pyridoxol deficiency
pyriformis syndrome
pyrilamine
    pheniramine, phenylpropanolamine,
      and p.
pyrimethamine
    sulfadoxine and p.
pyrimidine
    fluorinated p.
Pyrinate
    A-200 P.
pyrindinyl imidazole
Pyrinex Pediculicide Shampoo
Pyrinyl
    P. II
    P. II Liquid
    P. Plus Shampoo
pyrithione
    zinc p.
    p. zinc
Pyrobombus **sting**
pyrogen
    endogenous p.
pyroglobulin
pyroglyphid mite
pyrophosphate (PPi)
    alkaline phosphatase and p.
    p. arthritis-pseudogout (Pap)
    p. arthropathy
pyrophosphohydrolase
    nucleoside triphosphate p. (NTPPH,
      NTPPPH)
pyrotoxin
pyruvate kinase deficiency
pyruvic acid
PZA
    pyrazinamide

Q
Q albumin
amyloid Q
Q fever
6q
chromosome 6q
QA antigen
QALY
quality-adjusted life-year
Q-angle
QCT
quantitative computed tomography
1q duplication
QIE
quantitative immunoelectrophoresis
QOL
quality of life
QPCR assay
(q23q31)
trisomy of chromosome II, dup(1) (q23q31)
QSRL
Q-switched ruby laser
Q-switched
Q-s. alexandrite laser
Q-s. Nd:YAG laser
Q-s. neodymium:YAG laser (QSYAG)
Q-s. ruby laser (QSRL)
QSYAG
Q-switched neodymium:YAG laser
Quad-A-Hist
quadrilateral space syndrome
Quadrinal
quadroma
quail bronchitis virus
quality
q. of life (QOL)
Q. of Life score
Q. of Upper Extremities Test (QUEST)
Q., Utilization, Effectiveness, Statistically Tabulated (QUEST)
quality-adjusted life-year (QALY)
Quant broth
Quantikine ELISA kit
quantitation of B cell
quantitative
q. complement assay
q. computed tomography (QCT)
q. HCV RNA
q. immunoassay for urine myoglobin
q. immunoelectrophoresis (QIE)
q. immunoglobulin analysis

q. polymerase chain reaction
q. polymerase chain reaction assay
q. precipitin reaction
Quanti-Test System
Quantum PSV
Quaranfil virus
quarantine
quarter
lamb's q.'s
quarter-evil
quarter-ill
quartz-iodine lamp
quartz lamp
quasicontinuous-wave laser
quaternary
q. ammonium
q. syphilis
quaternium-15
quaternium-18 bentonite
queen
q. palm
q. palm tree
Queensland tick typhus
quellung
q. phenomenon
q. reaction
q. test
quenching
fluorescence q.
Quercus rubor
QUEST
Quality of Upper Extremities Test
Quality, Utilization, Effectiveness, Statistically Tabulated
Quest
Tranquility Q.
questionnaire
Childhood Health Assessment Q. (CHAQ)
EQ-5D EuroQol q.
Health Assessment Q. (HAQ)
McEwen Hyperventilation q.
McGill Pain q.
Modified Health Assessment Q. (MHAQ)
Needs Evaluation Q. (NEQ)
revised Skindex Q.
Rhinitis Outcomes Q. (ROQ)
rhinoconjunctivitis-specific quality of life q. (RQLQ)
Skindex q.
Stanford Health Assessment Q. (HAQ)
QUEST study

Queyrat
    erythroplasia of Q.
Quibron-T, -T/SR
Quickscreen assay
QuickVue One-Step Allergen Screen
Quiess
quinacrine
Quincke
    Q. disease
    Q. edema
    Q. I syndrome
quinidine
quinine
    q. fever
    q. sulfate

quinolizidine
quinolones
Quinquaud disease
Quinsana Plus topical
quintana
    Rochalimaea q.
quinti
    adductor digiti q.
quinupristin/dalfopristin
Quotidian fever
QUS-2 calcaneal ultrasonometer
Qvar

R

R antigen
R factor
R gene
Night Cast R
R pilus
R plasmid

r24 antibody

RA

rheumatoid arthritis
rhinocerebral aspergillosis
RA synoviocyte line

rabbit

r. antithymocyte globulin (RATG)
r. bush
r. epithelium
r. fibroma
fibromatosis virus of r.
r. fibroma virus
r. myxoma virus
r. plague
virus III of r.

rabbitpox virus
rabid
rabies

r. immune globulin, human
r. immunoglobulin
r. vaccine, Flury strain egg-passage
r. virus
r. virus, Flury strain
r. virus, Kelev strain
r. virus vaccine

Rabson-Mendenhall syndrome
raccoon eyes
racemosa

livedo r.

racemosus

Mucor r.

Racet Topical
racial melanoderma
racket nail
racquet nail
RAD 001
radial

r. immunodiffusion (RID)
r. nerve
r. nerve entrapment
r. scar

radiation

r. burn
cold quartz r.
r. dermatitis
r. dermatosis
dopa r.
electromagnetic r.

r. erythema
foreign body r.
ionizing r.
Jones-Mote r.
Mitsuda r.
r. pneumonitis
psoralens plus ultraviolet A
radiation/ultraviolet B r.
(PUVA/UVB)
r. spectrum
r. therapy
ultraviolet r.
wheal and erythema r.

radical

free r.
r. mastectomy
oxygen free r.

radicans

Rhus r.
Toxicodendron r.

radiciform
radicular nerve root
radiculitis
radiculoganglionitis
radiculoneuritis
radiculopathy
radioactive probe
radioallergosorbent test (RAST)
radioassay

C1qR r.

radiobacter

Agrobacterium r.

radiocarpal joint
radiocontrast
radiodermatitis

acute r.
chronic r.
r. emulsion (RE)

radiodurans

Deinococcus r.

radioepidermitis
radioepithelitis
radiograph

posteroanterior r.

radiographic

r. contrast media (RCM)
r. erosion

radioimmunoassay (RIA)

Raji cell r.

radioimmunodiffusion
radioimmunoelectrophoresis
radioimmunoprecipitation assay (RIPA)
radioimmunosorbent test (RIST)
radiolabeled iodine

radioligand assay
radiologic osteoarthritis (ROA)
radiolunate
radiometric resin system
radiometry
    BACTEC r.
radionuclide ventriculography
radioreceptor assay
radiosensitivity
radiotherapy (RT)
    eosinophilic, polymorphic, and
    pruritic eruption associated
    with r. (EPPER)
radium necrosis
RADS
    reactive airways dysfunction syndrome
RAEB
    refractory anemia with excess blasts
RAEB-t
    refractory anemia with excess blasts in
    transformation
Raf/mitogen-activated protein kinase
  signaling pathway
RAG
    recombination activation gene
RAG1, RAG2 gene
Ragnell scissors
ragweed (RW)
    canyon r.
    desert r.
    false r.
    giant r.
    r. oil dermatitis
    slender r.
    Western r.
ragwort
rail
    Railguard bed r.
Railguard bed rail
railroad tracking
Rainbow vacuum
rain splash
raised border
raisin
Raji
    R. cell
    R. cell radioimmune assay
    R. cell radioimmunoassay
Rajka and Langeland scoring system
rales
    coarse r.
raloxifene
Raman shifting
Ramelet phlebectomy hook
Ramirez
    ashy dermatosis of R.
Ramos B-cell line
Ramsay Hunt syndrome
ram's horn nail

ranarum
    Basidiobolus r.
Ranawat triangle method
random breeding
randomized controlled trial (RCT)
range
    interquartile r. (IQR)
    r. of motion
Ranikhet disease
ranitidine hydrochloride
RANKL
    receptor activator of nuclear factor kappa
    B ligand
RANTES
    regulated on activation, normal T-cell
    expressed and secreted
    regulated upon activation, normal T-cell
    expressed and secreted
ranula
RAP
    rheumatoid arthritis precipitin
Rapamune
rapamycin
Raper-Mason pathway
rapid
    r. canities
    r. cooling
    r. eye movement (REM)
    r. eye movement sleep
    r. eye movement sleep-related
    hypoxemia
    r. plasma reagin (RPR)
    r. whole blood test (RWBT)
Rapide
    Voltaren R.
rapidly
    r. dividing plasmablasts
    r. growing mycobacteria (RGM)
    r. progressive necrotizing
    glomerulonephritis (RPNG)
Rappaport classification
Rapp-Hodgkin ectodermal dysplasia
Raptiva
raquette
    ongles en r.
rare
    r. mycosis
    r. system reaction
rarefaction
    mottled r.
Ras
    Ras pathway
    Ras protein
rash
    ammonia r.
    antitoxin r.
    astacoid r.
    atopic dermatitis r.
    black currant r.

brown-tail r.
butterfly r.
cable r.
caterpillar r.
crystal r.
diaper r.
discoid r.
drug r.
ecchymotic r.
generalized maculopapular r.
gum r.
heat r.
heliotrope r.
hemorrhagic r.
hydatid r.
juvenile rheumatoid arthritis r.
lupus erythematous-like r.
macular r.
maculopapular r.
malar butterfly r.
mulberry r.
Murray Valley r.
napkin r.
nettle r.
papulovesicular r.
photosensitive r.
polymorphous r.
red r.
rose r.
serum r.
skin r.
slapped-cheek r.
summer r.
sunburn-like r.
tooth r.
violaceous shawl pattern r.
violaceous V-neck pattern r.
wandering r.
wildfire r.
ras-mitogen-activated protein
raspberry
   r. lesion
   r. nevus
   r. tongue
Ras-Raf-Mek-Erk pathway
RAST
   radioallergosorbent test
     Phadezym RAST
rat
   r. flea bite
   r. mite dermatitis
   r. serum protein (RSP)

   r. urine protein (RUP)
   Wistar r.
rat-bite fever
rate
   Clean Air Delivery R. (CADR)
   erythrocyte sedimentation r. (ESR)
   graft survival r.
   low absolute glomerular filtration r.
   low flow r.
   moisture vapor transmission r. (MVTR)
   peak expiratory flow r.
   pulse r.
   respiratory r.
   Westergren sedimentation r.
   zeta sedimentation r.
RATG
   rabbit antithymocyte globulin
     RATG polyclonal antibody
ratio
   carpal to metacarpal r.
   CD4/CD8 r.
   dead space:tidal volume r.
   helper-suppressor cell r.
   I:E r.
   inspiratory to expiratory r. (I:E ratio)
   International Normalization R. (INR)
   Mantel-Haenszel weighted odds r.
   proportionate morbidity r. (PMR)
   residual volume to total lung capacity r. (RV/TLC)
   risk r. (RR)
   standardized incidence r. (SIR)
   standardized mortality r. (SMR)
   Standard Morbidity R. (SMR)
   therapeutic r.
   ventilation/perfusion r.
   zinc protoporphyrin:heme r.
rattlesnake bite
Rauscher leukemia virus
rauwolfia drug
RAV
   Rous-associated virus
raw vegetables
ray
   grenz r.
Rayer disease
Rayleigh scattering
Raynaud
   R. disease

R

NOTES

Raynaud *(continued)*
   R. phenomenon
   R. syndrome
razor bump
RBC surface
Rb protein
RCA
  reactive cutaneous
    angioendotheliomatosis
rCD4
   CD4, human recombinant soluble
    rCD4
RCE
  renal cholesterol embolization
RCM
  radiographic contrast media
RCR
  replication-competent retrovirus
   RCR assay
   RCR testing
R&C Shampoo
RCT
  randomized controlled trial
RD
  rhabdomyosarcoma
   human RD
RDEB
  recessive dystrophic epidermolysis
   bullosa
RDS
  respiratory distress syndrome
rDsg
  recombinant desmoglein
RE
  radiodermatitis emulsion
   Biafine RE
ReA
  reactive arthritis
reacher
   long-handled dressing r.
reactant
Reactine
reaction
   absent r.
   accelerated r.
   acute anaphylactic r.
   acute phase r.
   acute pulmonary r.
   acute transfusion r.
   adverse drug r.
   adverse drug-induced r. (ADR)
   adverse food r.
   allergic drug r.
   anamnestic r.
   anaphylactic hypersensitivity r.
   anaphylactoid r.
   angry back r.
   antigen-antibody r.
   Arthus r.

Arthus-type r.
Ascoli r.
associative r.
autoimmune type of r.
autologous mixed leukocyte r.
Bloch r.
bullous drug r.
capsular precipitation r.
Casoni r.
cell-mediated immunologic drug r.
Chantemesse r.
cholera-red r.
cocarde r.
complement-fixation r.
constitutional r.
cross r.
cutaneous graft-versus-host r.
cytotoxic immunologic drug r.
Dale r.
delayed hypersensitivity
  immunologic drug r.
delayed systemic r.
delayed transfusion r.
demarcated r.
depot r.
dermatophytid r.
dermotuberculin r.
Dick r.
diffuse histiocytic r.
dopa r.
drug r.
early r.
early-phase r. (EPR)
eczematous r.
endotoxic r.
epicutaneous r.
false-negative r.
false-positive r.
Fernandez r.
fixation r.
fixed drug r.
flocculation r.
focal r.
foreign-body r.
Forssman antigen-antibody r.
Frei-Hoffmann r.
fungal id r.
gel diffusion r.
Gell and Coombs r.
Gerhardt r.
graft-versus-host r.
granulomatous inflammatory r.
Griess r.
group r.
Gruber r.
Gruber-Widal r.
Haber-Weiss r.
Hapten-type r.
hematologic r.

Herxheimer r.
homocytotropic r.
homograft r.
hunting r.
hypersensitivity r.
hysterical r.
id r.
idiosyncratic drug r.
IgE-dependent immunologic drug r.
immediate hypersensitivity r.
immediate phase r. (IPR)
immediate transfusion r.
immediate wheal r.
immune complex immunologic
  drug r.
immune complex-mediated drug r.
immunologic drug r.
incompatible blood transfusion r.
inflammation r.
insulin r.
interstitial granulomatous drug r.
  (IGDR)
intracutaneous r.
intradermal r.
irritant patch-test r.
Janus r.
Jarisch-Herxheimer r.
Jones-Mote r.
Koebner r.
late-phase allergic r. (LPAR)
late-phase cutaneous r. (LPCR)
latex fixation r.
lepromatous r.
lepromin r.
ligase chain r.
Loewenthal r.
marked localized r.
Mazzotti r.
miostagmin r.
miscellaneous r.
Mitsuda r.
mixed agglutination r.
mixed lymphocyte culture r.
Montenegro r.
negative r.
Neufeld r.
neutrophil antibody and
  transfusion r.
nitritoid r.
nonanaphylactic r. (NAR)
nondrug-related r.
r. of nonidentity

nonimmediate-type immunologic
  drug r.
nonimmunologic drug r.
r. of partial identity
passive cutaneous anaphylactic r.
Paul r.
persistent light r.
photoallergic drug r.
photobiologic r.
photochemical r.
photodrug r.
photosensitivity r.
phototoxic drug r.
Pirquet r.
P-K r.
polymerase chain r. (PCR)
positive r.
Prausnitz-Kustner r.
precipitin r.
primary irritant r.
prozone r.
pseudoallergic r. (PAR)
psychogenic r.
pustular patch-test r.
quantitative polymerase chain r.
quantitative precipitin r.
quellung r.
rare system r.
reversed Prausnitz-Küstner r.
reverse transcriptase-polymerase
  chain r. (RT-PCR)
ribonucleic acid-polymerase chain r.
  (RNA-PCR)
Roger r.
Schultz-Charlton r.
Schultz-Dale r.
self-limited allergic r.
serum r.
severe acute allergic r.
severe immediate r.
severe systemic r.
Shwartzman r.
skin r.
specific r.
2-stage r.
suprasternal r.
symptomatic r.
systemic r.
thiuram-alcohol r.
toxic systemic r.
TPI r.
transfusion r.

NOTES

reaction *(continued)*
>type I–III hypersensitivity r.
type III immune complex drug r.
type I–IV immunologic drug r.
type IV delayed hypersensitivity r.
vaccinoid r.
vascular r.
vasomotor r.
vasovagal r.
in vivo r.
Wassermann r. (W.r.)
Weil-Felix r.
Weinberg r.
well-demarcated skin r.
wheal and erythema r.
wheal and flare r.
whitegraft r.
Widal r.
zonal type r.

reactional leprosy
reactiva
>meningitis necrotoxica r.

reactivate
reactivation
>sunburn r.

reactive
>r. airways disease
r. airways dysfunction syndrome (RADS)
r. arthritis (ReA)
r. cutaneous angioendotheliomatosis (RCA)
r. lysis
r. oxygen intermediate (ROI)
r. oxygen species (ROS)
r. perforating collagenosis (RPC)
r. postinfectious synovitis
r. salpingitis
R. Skin Decontamination Lotion

reactivity
>airway r.
antihost r.
immediate skin r.
specific alteration in immunologic r.

reactor
>persistent light r.

reading
>delayed patch test r.

reading-frame-shift mutation
reagent
>Melzer r.
TriZol r.

reagin
>atopic r.
rapid plasma r. (RPR)
r. screen test (RST)
unheated serum r. (USR)

reaginic
>r. antibody
r. hypersensitivity

REAL
>Revised European-American Lymphoma
Revised European-American leukemia
REAL classification

Rea-Lo
rearfoot valgus
rearrangement
>immunoglobulin gene r.

Reatine
Rebetron
rebound dermatitis
Rebuck
>R. skin window
R. skin window technique

recalcitrant wart
recall
>ultraviolet r.
r. urticaria (RU)

recapitulation of ontogenesis process
Receptin
receptor
>r. activator of nuclear factor kappa B ligand (RANKL)
antigenic binding r.
antimuscarinic acetylcholine r.
B-cell antigen r.
bone morphogenetic protein r.
brush border r.
C3b r.
C4b r.
C3bBb r.
C3/C4 r.
CD44 Hyaluronic acid r.
CD26/vitronectin r.
costimulatory r.
C1q r.
r.'s for endogenous danger signals (REDS)
Fc r.
Fc gamma r. III
fibronectin r.
G-protein-coupled r.
homing r.
IL-1 r.
r. interacting protein (RIP)
killer cell inhibitory r. (KIR)
lymphocyte homing r.
natural cytotoxicity r.
nicotinic acetylcholine r.
opsonic r.
pattern recognition r. (PRR)
phosphatidyl serine r.
protease-activated r. (PAR)
r. site
soluble r.

soluble tumor necrosis factor-a r.
(sTNFR)
soluble type 1 interleukin-1 r.
(sIL-1R)
surface r.
T-cell antigen r.
thyroid-stimulating hormone r.
(TSH-R)
Toll r.
transmembrane r.
TSH r. (TSH-R)
tumor necrosis factor r.
receptor-gamma
peroxisome proliferator-activated r.-
g. (PPAR-gamma)
receptor-ligand interaction
recessive
autosomal r.
r. dystrophic epidermolysis bullosa
(RDEB)
r. trait
r. X-linked ichthyosis
recidivans
leishmaniasis r.
r. leishmaniasis (RL)
recidive
chancre r.
recipient
cross-match-positive r.
elective low-risk r.
high-risk r. (HRR)
renal transplant r. (RTR)
single-lung transplant r.
SLT r.
recipient-donor pairs
reciprocal transfusion
recirculation
lymphocyte r.
Recklinghausen disease type I
reclusa
Loxosceles r.
Reclus disease
recognition
cognate r.
r. factor
recoil
elastic r.
recombinant
r. allergen
r. desmoglein (rDsg)
r. gamma interferon
r. human IL-10

r. human interleukin-1 receptor
antagonist
r. human protein
r. human relaxin
r. human tissue factor pathway
inhibitor (r-hT-FPI)
r. human tumor necrosis factor
receptor fusion protein
r. immunoblot assay (RIBA)
r. LFA-3/IgG1 human fusion
protein
r. platelet-derived growth factor
r. strain
r. vector
recombinase-activating gene
recombination
r. activation gene (RAG)
genetic r.
high frequency of r.
recombinational activity
recombinatorial
Recombivax HB
recommended exposure level (REL)
reconstitution
hematopoietic r.
multilineage r.
reconstruction
recorder
sensory nerve action potential
sleep r.
SNAP sleep r.
recovery
short tau inversion r. (STIR)
recrudescent
r. typhus
r. typhus fever
recruitment
host-generated neutrophils r.
rectal
r. gonorrhea
Phenergan R.
Rowasa R.
r. ulceration
rectus abdominis syndrome
recurrens
herpes simplex r.
periadenitis mucosa necrotica r.
recurrent
r. aspiration
r. bacterial pneumonia
r. cutaneous abscess
r. erythema multiforme minor

NOTES

recurrent *(continued)*
  r. genital herpes simplex virus
  r. infection
  r. infundibulofolliculitis
  r. intraoral herpes simplex virus
  r. labial herpes simplex virus
  r. palmoplantar hidradenitis
  r. polyserositis
  r. respiratory laryngeal
    papillomatosis
  r. ulcer
  r. urticaria
  r. viral pneumonia
recurrentis
  Borrelia r.
recutita
  Matricaria r.
red
  r. albinism
  r. alder
  r. alder tree
  r. balls
  basic r. 46
  r. birch
  r. blood cell
  r. blood cell surface
  r. bug bite
  r. cedar
  r. cedar tree
  r. cell adherence phenomenon
  r. cell adherence test
  r. cell antigen
  r. cell membrane alteration
  r. eye
  r. feed dermatitis
  r. ginseng
  r. granulation
  r. half-moon
  r. halo
  r. imported fire ant
  r. imported fire ant sting
  r. lunula
  r. man syndrome
  r. maple
  r. maple tree
  r. moss dermatitis
  r. mulberry
  r. mulberry tree
  r. neuralgia
  r. papule
  r. papule and nodule
  r. rash
  r. sponge dermatitis
  r. sweat
  r. tide dermatitis
  r. top
  r. top grass pollen
  r. veterinary petrolatum (RVP)

reddening
  r. of oropharyngeal mucosa
  r. of palm
  r. of sole of foot
RediTabs
  Claritin R.'s
redox stress
red-purple plaque
redroot pigweed
REDS
  receptors for endogenous danger signals
redtop A grass
reduced
  r. cold ischemic time
  r. joint survey (RJS)
  r. liver transplant (RLT)
reduced-size
  r.-s. liver transplant (RSLT)
  r.-s. liver transplantation (RSLT)
reducing substance
reductase
  5 alpha r.
  thioredoxin r. (TR)
5α-reductase type 1, 2
reduction
  leukotriene r.
  Palomar E2000 ruby laser hair r.
Redutemp
Reduviidae
redux
  chancre r.
  pseudochancre r.
redwood tree
reed
  r. canary
  common r.
Reed-Sternberg cell
reedy nail
reenameling
Reenstierna antiserum
reepithelialization
Reese dermatome
Reese's Pinworm Medicine
reference nutrient intake (RNI)
Refinity
  R. Coblation system
  R. skin care solution
  R. skin product
reflectance-guidance laser selection
reflectance photometry
reflex
  r. cough
  nasobronchial r.
  pilomotor r.
  stretch r.
  submersion r.
  r. sympathetic dystrophy (RSD)
  r. sympathetic dystrophy syndrome
reflux

refractoriness
    exercise-induced r.
refractory
    r. anemia with excess blasts
    (RAEB)
    r. anemia with excess blasts in
    transformation (RAEB-t)
    r. pemphigus vulgaris
    r. period
Refresh Plus Ophthalmic solution
Refsum
    R. disease
    R. syndrome
regia
    Juglans r.
regimen
    Goeckerman r.
    immunomodulating drug r.
    nonmyeloablative conditioning r.
    steroid-sparing r.
    The Epidemiology and Natural
    History of Asthma: Outcome
    and Treatment R.'s (TENOR)
    TL-01 UV-B r.
regimen/therapy
    psoralen ultraviolet A r./t.
    PUVA r./t.
region
    constant r.
    hinge r.
    hypervariable r.
    I r.
    intertriginous r.
    L2 linker r.
    paratracheal r.
    ringworm of genitocrural r.
    switch r.
    upstream regulatory r. (URR)
    variable r.
regional
    r. granulomatous lymphadenitis
    r. organ procurement (ROP)
    R. Organ Procurement Agency
    (ROPA)
Register
    Norfolk Arthritis R. (NOAR)
Registry
    Cord Blood R.
    International Pancreas Transplant R.
    (IPTR)
    R. of the International Society for
    Heart and Lung Transplantation

Regranex
regressing atypical histiocytosis
regression
    Cox r.
    multivariate logistic r.
    spontaneous r.
regular
    r. Aveeno
    Esotcrica R.
    Iodex R.
regulated
    r. on activation, normal T-cell
    expressed and secreted (RANTES)
    r. upon activation, normal T-cell
    expressed and secreted (RANTES)
regulation
    leukotriene r.
    tolerance through r.
regulator
regulatory CD4+ T cell
regulon
    BvgAS r.
Rehmannia glutinosa
reinfection
    graft r.
    r. tuberculosis
reinoculation
Reiter
    R. disease
    R. syndrome
    R. test
rejection
    accelerated r.
    acute cellular xenograft r.
    allograft r.
    cardiac r.
    r. cascade
    cellular xenograft r.
    chronic allograft r.
    delayed xenograft r. (DXR)
    ductopenic r.
    first-set r.
    graft r.
    hyperacute organ r.
    islet allograft r.
    primary r.
    second set r.
    steroid-resistant acute r.
    xenograft r.
REL
    recommended exposure level
Relafen

R

NOTES

relapsing
  r. febrile nodular nonsuppurative
    panniculitis
  r. fever
  r. polychondritis
relapsing-remitting
  r.-r. multiple sclerosis (RRMS)
  r.-r. profile
related transplant
relation
  opposition-versus-pressure r.
relationship
  temporal r.
relative
  r. immunity
  immunochemical r.
  r. risk
relaxant
  muscle r.
relaxation
  smooth muscle r.
Relaxed Skin Tension Line (RSTL)
relaxin
  recombinant human r.
relaxometry
release
  allergen-induced mediator r.
  delayed anagen r.
  delayed telogen r.
  GFN 1000/DM50 sustained r.
  GFN 550/PSE 60/DM30
    sustained r.
  immediate antigen r.
  immediate telogen r.
  leukocyte histamine r.
  myoglobin r.
  sustained r. (SR)
releaser
  direct histamine r.
releasing factor (RF)
relevant sting history
Reliable Change Index
relief
  Allergy R.
  Claritin Hives R.
  DayQuil Sinus with Pain R.
  Mini Thin Asthma R.
  Nasal & Sinus R.
  R. Ophthalmic solution
  Vicks DayQuil Sinus Pressure &
    Congestion R.
reliever
  Arthritis Foundation Pain R.
ReLume system
REM
  rapid eye movement
  reticular erythematous mucinosis
  REM sleep

REM sleep-related hypoxemia
REM syndrome
Remak sign
remedy
  home r.
  Scholl 2-Drop Corn R.
Remicade
Reminyl
remission
  brief metabolic r.
  metabolic r.
  pathologically confirmed
    complete r. (PCR)
remitting
  r. necrotizing acrocyanosis
  r. seronegative symmetrical
    synovitis
  r. seronegative symmetrical
    synovitis with pitting edema
    (RS3PE)
remodeling
  extracellular matrix r.
  tissue r.
removal
  excisional r.
  laser hair r.
  Lasertrolysis hair r.
  LightSheer diode laser system for
    permanent hair r.
remover
  Histofreezer cryosurgical wart r.
  Mosco callus and corn r.
  Scholl Wart R.
  Tinamed wart r.
  Wart R.
renal
  r. biopsy
  r. cholesterol embolization (RCE)
  r. cyst
  r. failure
  r. involvement
  r. lupus
  r. stone
  r. transplant
  r. transplantation (RTx)
  r. transplant recipient (RTR)
  r. tubular acidosis
Rendu-Osler-Weber
  R.-O.-W. disease
  R.-O.-W. syndrome
Renova cream
REO
  respiratory enteric orphan
    REO virus
ReoPro monoclonal antibody
Reoviridae
Reovirus-like agent
REP
  Rochester Epidemiology Project

repair
    abnormal DNA r.
    DNA r.
    Lich-Gregoire r.
    mismatch r.
    staged abdominal r. (STAR)
    tissue r.

repeat
    r. open-application testing (ROAT)
    r. open reaction application test
    short consensus r.'s
    tetratricopeptide r.
    variable numbers of tandem r.'s
    (VNTR)

repeated
    r. exposure
    r. respiratory infection

repellent
    Cutter insect r.
    dimethyl carbate butopyropoxyl
    insect r.
    dimethyl phthalate insect r.
    UltraThon insect r.

repens
    dermatitis r.
    erythema gyratum r.

reperfusion
    hepatic ischemia and r. (HIR)
    r. injury
    ischemia and r. (I/R)

Repetabs
    Proventil R.

repetitive PCR (Rep-PCR)
Repifermin
repigmentation
replacement
    enzyme r.
    r. therapy

replica
RepliCare
    R. hydrocolloid
    R. hydrocolloid dressing
    R. hydrocolloid dressing material

replicase
replicate
replication
replication-competent
    r.-c. retrovirus (RCR)
    r.-c. retrovirus assay

replicative
    r. form (RF)
    r. senescence

replicator
Repliderm
repository therapy
Rep-PCR
    repetitive PCR

Re-PUVA
requirement
    immunization r.

RES
    reticuloendothelial system

Rescriptor
rescue
    peripheral blood stem cell r.

Resectisol Irrigation solution
reserve
    bone marrow r.
    breathing r. (BR)
    heart rate r. (HRR)

reservoir
    r. host
    r. of infection
    Ommaya r.
    Pecquet r.

ResiDerm
residual
    r. thermal damage (RTD)
    r. volume
    r. volume to total lung capacity
    ratio (RV/TLC)

residue
    aliphatic r.
    posttranslationally modified
    arginine r.
    Pro r.

resin
    Chelex r.
    epoxy r.
    ethyleneurea melamine
    formaldehyde r.
    formaldehyde r.
    InstaGene Matrix r.
    pine r.
    podophyllum r.
    thermosetting r.

resin-colophony
    pine r.-c.

resistance
    adenovirus-induced steroid r.
    airway r.
    bacteriophage r.
    r. factor
    insulin r.

NOTES

resistance *(continued)*
  r. plasmid
  pulmonary vascular r. (PVR)
resistance-inducing factor
resistance-transfer factor
resistance-transferring episome
resistant bacterium
resistentiae
  locus minoris r.
Resnick criteria
Resorcin
resorcinol
resorption
  Weichselbaum lacunar r.
resorptive arthropathy
Respaire-60 SR
Respaire-120 SR
Respa-1st
Respbid
RespiGam
Respihaler
  Decadron Phosphate R.
Respinol-G
respiration
  Cheyne-Stokes r.
respirator
  BABYbird r.
respiratory
  r. acidosis
  r. burst
  r. change
  r. distress
  r. distress syndrome (RDS)
  r. enteric orphan (REO)
  r. enteric orphan virus
  r. failure
  r. rate
  r. syncytial virus (RSV)
  r. syncytial virus immune globulin
    intravenous (RSV-IGIV)
  r. syncytial virus IV immune
    globulin
Respirgard II nebulizer
Respitrace machine
responder T cell
response
  anamnestic r.
  antigen-specific immune r.
  autoimmune r.
  biphasic r.
  booster r.
  bronchoconstrictor r.
  cholinergic r.
  delayed nasal r. (DYNR)
  delayed-type hypersensitivity r.
  early allergic r. (EAR)
  early asthmatic r. (EAR)
  early-phase r.
  endogenous immune r.

  exaggerated bronchoconstrictor r.
  high inflammatory r.
  histiocytic r.
  host r.
  humoral immune r.
  IgE-mediated r.
  immediate nasal r. (INR)
  immediate skin r. (ISR)
  immune r. (Ir)
  immunologic r.
  irritant patch-test r.
  isomeric r.
  isomorphic r.
  late asthmatic r. (LAR)
  late-phase r.
  late pulmonary r. (LPR)
  Lewis triple r.
  low inflammatory r.
  nephropathic immune r.
  peak-plateau r.
  primary immune r.
  proinflammatory cytokine r.
  secondary immune r.
  seroconversion r.
  somatosensory evoked r.
  sympathoneural r.
  T-dependent r.
  Th-1 mediated immune r.
  T-independent r.
  transferred immune r.
  triple r.
  in vitro proliferative lymphocyte r.
  white line r.
  xenogeneic cellular immune r.
responsiveness
  airway r.
rest
  bed r.
  r. hypoxemia
  r., ice, compresses, elevation
    (RICE)
  paramesonephric r.
restaurant syndrome
resting
  r. nevus
  r. phase
  r. splint
restitope
Reston
  R. foam
  R. foam wound dressing
  R. hydrocolloid dressing
  R. subtype
restorative sleep
restore
  R. alginate dressing
  R. alginate wound cover
  R. hydrocolloid
  R. hydrocolloid dressing

R. hydrogel dressing
R. impregnated gauze
R. wound cleanser

restricta
    Malassezia r.

restriction
    r. fragment length
    r. fragment length polymorphism
    (RFLP)
    major histocompatibility complex r.
    (MHC)
    MHC r.

restrictive
    r. cardiomyopathy
    r. dermopathy
    r. functional impairment
    r. lung disease
    r. ventilatory pattern

restrictus
    Aspergillus r.

Restylane Fine Lines wrinkle treatment
result
    Surveillance, Epidemiology and
    End R.'s (SEER)

resurfacing
    facial r.
    laser skin r. (LSR)
    Skinlight erbium:YAG laser system
    for skin r.

resuscitation
    cardiopulmonary r.

retardation
    r. and ear defect
    growth r.

rete
    r. peg
    r. ridge
    r. ridge hyperplasia

retention
    bromsulfophthalein r.
    r. cyst
    r. triad

reticular
    r. degeneration
    r. dermis
    r. dysgenesis
    r. erythematous mucinosis (REM)
    r. erythematous mucinosis syndrome
    r. lesion
    r. pattern

reticularis
    acropigmentatio r.

angiitis livedo r.
dermatopathia pigmentosa r.
idiopathic livedo r.
livedo r.
pars r.
zona r.

reticulata
    folliculitis ulerythema r.
    folliculitis ulerythematosa r.

reticulate
    r. array
    r. body
    r. hyperpigmentation
    r. hypopigmentation
    r. pigmented anomaly

reticulated
    r. black solar lentigo
    r. papillomatosis
    r. pigmented poikiloderma

reticulatum
    atrophoderma r.

reticule
reticulin fiber
reticulocyte count
reticuloendothelial
    r. blockade
    r. cell
    r. hyperplasia
    r. system (RES)

reticuloendothelioma
reticuloendotheliosis
    avian r.
    familial r.
    leukemic r.

reticuloendothelium
reticulogranuloma
reticulohistiocytic granuloma
reticulohistiocytoma
reticulohistiocytosis
    congenital self-healing r.
    r. disease
    multicentric r. (MR)
    self-healing r.

reticuloid
    actinic r.

reticulosis
    benign inoculation r.
    disseminated pagetoid r.
    epidermotropic r.
    histiocytic medullary r.
    lipomelanic r.
    localized pagetoid r.

R

NOTES

reticulosis *(continued)*
    medullary r.
    pagetoid r.
    polymorphic r.
    Sézary r.
reticulum
    r. cell carcinoma
    r. cell sarcoma
    endoplasmic r.
    r. fiber
retiform
    r. erythema
    r. hemangioendothelioma
    parapsoriasis r.
    r. parapsoriasis
Retin-A
    R.-A Micro
    R.-A Micro gel
    R.-A Micro topical
retina
retinaculum of ankle
retinal
    r. examination
    r. exudate
    r. hemorrhage
    r. perivasculitis
    r. pigment epithelial cell (RPE)
    r. thrombophlebitis
retinitis
    cytomegalovirus r.
    varicella-zoster virus r.
    VZV r.
retinoblastoma tumor suppressor protein
retinochoroidopathy
    birdshot r.
retinoic acid
retinoid
    gold r.
    r. therapy
    r. X receptor-selective ligand
Retinol-A
retinopathy
retinovirus
    HTLV-1 r.
retinyl acetate-induced arthritis
retractor
    Desmarres r.
    Langenbeck r.
    Parker r.
    Roux r.
    Upper Hands self-retaining r.
retransplantation (Re-Tx)
retrocalcaneal bursitis
retroelement
retroperitoneal fibrosis
retropharyngeal
Retrovir
    R. injection
    R. oral

retroviral vector
Retroviridae
retrovirus
    r. group
    human r.
    lymphotropic r.
    MFG-IRAP r.
    porcine endogenous r. (PERV)
    replication-competent r. (RCR)
    zoonotic r.
retrovirus-associated lymphoma
Re-Tx
    retransplantation
Reu curette
revaccination
reverse
    r. cutting needle
    r. endocytosis
    r. passive hemagglutination
    r. tetracycline transactivator
    r. transcriptase
    r. transcriptase-polymerase chain
      reaction (RT-PCR)
reversed
    r. passive anaphylaxis
    r. passive latex agglutination
    r. Prausnitz-Küstner reaction
reversible posterior leukoencephalopathy (RPLE)
reversion
Reversionex
revertant
Reviderm wrinkle treatment
revised
    R. European-American Classification
      of Lymphoid Neoplasms
    R. European-American Lymphoma
      (REAL)
    R. European-American Lymphoma
      classification
    r. Skindex Questionnaire
Rev-responsive element (RRE)
revulsion
Reye syndrome
Rezine
RF
    releasing factor
    replicative form
    rheumatoid factor
      IgG RF
      IgM RF
      RF test
RFLA
    rheumatoid factor-like activity
RFLP
    restriction fragment length polymorphism
RFXAP
    RFX-associated protein
RFX-associated protein (RFXAP)

R-Gel
RGM
  rapidly growing mycobacteria
RH
  rheumatoid
Rh
  rhesus
    Rh antigen
    Rh blocking test
    Rh factor
    Rh immune globulin intravenous
      (RhIGIV)
    Rh isoantigen
rhabditic dermatitis
rhabdomyolysis syndrome
rhabdomyoma
rhabdomyosarcoma (RD)
  human r.
Rhabdoviridae
rhabdovirus
rhacoma
rhagades
rhagadiform
rhagas
$RH_o(D)$
    $RH_o(D)$ globulin
    $RH_o(D)$ immunoglobulin
rheometer
    Haake r.
rheophoresis
rheostat
    ceramide-S1P r.
rhesus (Rh)
    r. factor
    r. rotavirus (RRV)
    r. theta defensin 1 (RTD-1)
rheum
    salt r.
Rheumatex
    R. test
    R. test for rheumatoid factor
rheumatic
    r. disorder
    r. erythema
    r. fever
    r. heart disease
    r. perimyocarditis
rheumatica
    polymyalgia r. (PMR)
    purpura r.
    scarlatina r.

rheumaticum
    erythema annulare r.
rheumatism
    European League Against R.
      (EULAR)
    nonarticular r.
    palindromic r.
    pied rond r.
    Poncet r.
    tuberculous r.
rheumatocelis
rheumatoid (RH)
    r. arthritis (RA)
    r. arthritis precipitin (RAP)
    r. arthritis vaccine
    r. atlantoaxial subluxation
    r. cachexia
    r. clawing
    r. disease
    r. episcleritis
    r. factor (RF)
    r. factor-like activity (RFLA)
    r. factor test
    r. factor titer
    r. nodule
    r. nodulosis
    r. pachymeningitis
    r. pannus
    r. pattern
    r. pleurisy
    r. rheumatic vasculitis
    r. scleritis
    r. syndrome
    r. synovial fibroblast
    r. synovial macrophage-like/dendritic
      cell
rheumatologist
rheumatology
    American College of R. (ACR)
    World Health
      Organization/International League
      of Associations for R.
      (WHO/ILAR)
Rheumaton
    R. test
    R. test for rheumatoid factor
Rheumatrex
RhIGIV
    Rh immune globulin intravenous
Rhinalar
Rhinaris-F

NOTES

477

rhinitis
    acute r.
    allergic r.
    endocrine r.
    foreign body r.
    granulomatosis r.
    gustatory r.
    idiopathic r. (IR)
    infectious r.
    r. medicamentosa
    r. nervosa
    noninfectious r. (NIR)
    R. Outcomes Questionnaire (ROQ)
    perennial allergic r.
    pollen-induced allergic r.
    seasonal allergic r. (SAR)
    vasomotor r. (VMR)
    r. VS symptom score
rhinobronchitis
    allergic r.
rhinocerebral
    r. aspergillosis (RA)
    r. infection
Rhinocladiella aquaspera
rhinoconjunctivitis
    allergic r.
    Parietaria-induced r.
rhinoconjunctivitis-specific quality of life questionnaire (RQLQ)
Rhinocort
rhinomanometry
    posterior r.
rhinometry
rhinophyma
rhinopneumonitis
    equine r.
rhinoprobe
rhinorrhea
    cerebrospinal r.
rhinoscleroma
rhinoscleromatis
    Klebsiella r.
rhinoscopy
rhinosinusitis
rhinosporidiosis
Rhinosporidium seeberi
Rhinosyn Liquid
Rhinosyn-PD Liquid
rhinotracheitis
    feline viral r.
    infectious bovine r. (IBR)
rhinovirus
    bovine r.'s
    r. challenge test
    equine r.'s
Rhizopus
    R. arrhizus
    R. nigricans
    R. oryzae

Rhodacine
rhodamine isothiocyanate
Rhodis
Rhodis-EC
Rhodnius prolixus
Rhodococcus
    R. equi
    R. erythropolis
rhodopsin-type coupling
Rhodotorula rubra
Rhodurea
rhoGDI protein
Rholosone
rhombic flap
rhomboencephalitis
rhomboid
    r. glossitis
    r. swelling
rhonchus, pl. **rhonchi**
rhopheocytosis
Rhoprolene
Rhoprosone
Rhovail
r-hT-FPI
    recombinant human tissue factor pathway inhibitor
rhupus
Rhus
    R. diversiloba
    R. radicans
    R. toxicodendron
    R. toxicodendron antigen
    R. venenata
    R. venenata antigen
    R. vernix
rhus dermatitis
rhusiopathiae
    Erysipelothrix r.
rhyparia
rhysodes
    Acanthamoeba r.
rhythmical dermatosis
rhytide
rhytidectomy
    cervicofacial r.
rhytidoplasty
RIA
    radioimmunoassay
RIBA
    recombinant immunoblot assay
    HCV by RIBA
    RIBA HCV
    RIBA II antibody testing
Ribas-Torres disease
ribavirin
Ribbing arthritis phenotype
riboflavin deficiency
ribonuclease protection assay (RPA)

R

ribonucleic
> r. acid (RNA)
> r. acid-polymerase chain reaction (RNA-PCR)

ribonucleoprotein (RNP)
> r. antigen
> small nuclear r. (snRNP)
> U3 small nuclear r.

ribonucleotide
> purine r.

riboprobe
ribosomal
ribosome
ribosylated
ribotide
ribovirus
ribozyme
RICE
> rest, ice, compresses, elevation

rice
> r. body
> r. itch

richardsiae
> *Phialophora* r.

Richner-Hanhart
> R.-H. keratoderma
> R.-H. syndrome

richteria
> *Solenopsis saevissima* r.

Richter syndrome
ricin
> R. A
> anti-B4 blocked r.
> B4 blocked r.

ricinus
> *Ixodes* r.

rickets
Rickettsia
> R. akari
> R. australis
> R. conorii
> R. prowazekii
> R. rickettsii
> R. tsutsugamushi
> R. typhi
> R. vaccine, attenuated

rickettsial infection
rickettsialpox
rickettsii
> *Rickettsia* r.

rickettsiosis
> Eastern tick-borne r.

rickettsiostatic
Ricobid
Ricord chancre
RID
> radial immunodiffusion
> RID Mousse
> RID Shampoo

Ridaura
Rida virus
Ridenol
ridge
> broad-based rete r.
> interpapillary r.
> rete r.

ridged wart
Ridley classification
RIE
> rocket immunoelectrophoresis

Riedel struma
Rieger anomaly
Riehl
> R. melanoderma
> R. melanosis

rifabutin
Rifadin
> R. Injection
> R. oral

Rifamate
rifampin
> r. and isoniazid
> r., isoniazid, and pyrazinamide

rifampin-isoniazid-streptomycin-ethambutol (RISE)
rifampin-isoniazid-streptomycin-ethambutol-resistant tuberculosis
rifamycin
rifapentine
Rifater
rifaximin
Rift
> R. Valley fever
> R. Valley fever virus

right
> Breathe R.
> r. renal vein (RRV)

rigid thoracoscope
rigidus
> hallux r.

rigor
Riley-Day syndrome
Riley-Smith syndrome
Rilutek

NOTES

riluzole
Rimactane Oral
rimantadine hydrochloride
rimexolone
rinderpest virus
ring
>Kayser-Fleischer r.
>McNeill-Goldman corneal
> transplant r.
>r. precipitin test
>purine r.
>r. shadow
>tracheal vascular r.
>r. ulcer
>Walsh pressure r.
>Wessely r.
>Woronoff r.

ringed hair
ringhook method of Feuerstein
ringworm
>r. of axilla
>r. of beard
>black-dot r.
>r. of body
>crusted r.
>r. of the face
>r. of foot
>r. of genitocrural region
>gray-patch r.
>r. of the groin
>r. of the hand
>honeycomb r.
>hypertrophic r.
>r. of nail
>Oriental r.
>r. of the scalp
>scaly r.
>Tokelau r.
>r. yaw

Rinkel
>R. serial endpoint titration
>R. testing

Rinne test
RinoFlow nasal wash and sinus system
rinse
>Nix Creme R.

Rio rosewood
RIP
>receptor interacting protein

RIPA
>radioimmunoprecipitation assay

ripe lesion
rippled pattern sebaceoma
rippling muscle disease
Risdon incision
RISE
>rifampin-isoniazid-streptomycin-
> ethambutol

RISE-resistant tuberculosis

risk
>r. ratio (RR)
>relative r.

RIST
>radioimmunosorbent test

RIT
>rush immunotherapy

Ritchie articular index
ritonavir
>lopinavir and r.

Ritter disease
Rituxan monoclonal antibody
rituximab
Rivasone
river
>r. birch
>r. blindness

RJS
>reduced joint survey

RL
>recidivans leishmaniasis

RLT
>reduced liver transplant

RNA
>ribonucleic acid
>>antisense RNA
>>RNA glycosidase toxin
>>HAV RNA
>>HCV RNA
>>messenger RNA (mRNA)
>>RNA polymerase
>>quantitative HCV RNA
>>RNA tumor virus

RNA-PCR
>ribonucleic acid-polymerase chain
> reaction

Rnase P
RNeasy
>R. Maxi kit
>R. Mini kit
>R. spin column

RNI
>reference nutrient intake

RNP
>ribonucleoprotein
>>RNP antigen

ROA
>radiologic osteoarthritis

road burn
Ro antigen
ROAT
>repeat open-application testing

RoBathol oil
Robaxin
robe
>Hunter r.

Robicillin VK oral
Robidrine
Robinson disease

R

Robinul Forte
Robitet oral
Robitussin-PE
Robitussin Severe Congestion Liqui-Gels
Robles disease
Robomol
robustus
 arthritis r.
Rocaltrol
Rocephin
Rochalimaea
 R. henselae
 R. quintana
Rocha-Lima inclusion
Roche Amplicor CMV DNA assay
Rochester Epidemiology Project (REP)
rocket immunoelectrophoresis (RIE)
Rockwool dermatitis
Rocky
 R. Mountain spotted fever
 R. Mountain spotted fever vaccine
 R. Mountain tick
rod
 gram-negative r.
 gram-positive r.
rodent
 r. allergy
 sigmodontine r.
 r. ulcer
rodhaini
 Babesia r.
Rodnan skin thickness score
rodonalgia
Rodriguez-Castellanos study
Roederer ecchymosis
roentgen alopecia
roentgenogram
roentgen-ray dermatitis
roetheln
RO-Eye drops
RO-Eyewash
RoEzIt skin moisturizer
Rofact
rofecoxib
Roferon-A
Rogaine topical
Roger
 R. reaction
 R. symptom
Roho mattress
ROI
 reactive oxygen intermediate

Roitter disease
Rokitansky-Aschoff sinus
rolipram
roll
 banana r.
rolled shoulder lesion
Rollet chancre
rolling neutrophil
Romaña sign
Romanus lesion
Romberg
 R. hemiatrophy
 R. sign
 R. syndrome
Rombo syndrome
Römer test
Rondec
 R. drops
 R. Filmtab
 R. Syrup
Rondec-TR
Rondo inhaler
ronds
 corps r.
room temperature
root
 life r.
 nail r.
 orris r.
 radicular nerve r.
ROP
 regional organ procurement
ROPA
 Regional Organ Procurement Agency
rope
 r. burn
 r. sign
RO-Predphate
ROQ
 Rhinitis Outcomes Questionnaire
roquinimex
ROS
 reactive oxygen species
Rosac cream
rosacea
 acne r.
 corticosteroid r.
 granulomatous r.
 hypertrophic r.
 keratitis r.
 ocular r.
 tuberculoid r.

NOTES

rosaceaform dermatitis
rosacea-like
    r.-l. tuberculid
    r.-l. tuberculid of Lewandowski
Rosai-Dorfman
    R.-D. disease
    R.-D. syndrome
rose
    r. bengal stain
    r. cold
    r. fever
    r. rash
    r. spot
    r. water ointment
rosea
    atypical pityriasis r.
    inverse pityriasis r.
    pityriasis r. (PR)
Rosenbach
    R. disease
    erysipeloid of R.
    R. erysipeloid
Rosen papular eruption
Rosenthal-French dosimeter
roseola
    epidemic r.
    idiopathic r.
    r. infantilis
    r. infantum
    syphilitic r.
    r. vaccinia
roseola-like illness
roseolous
rosette
    r.'s of cell
    E r.
    EAC r.
    T-cell r.
    r. test
rosette-forming cell
Rose-Waaler test
rosewood
    Rio r.
rosin
Ross
    R. River fever
    R. River virus
RoSSA/RoSSB antibody test
rostratum
    Exserohilum r.
Rosula
    R. aqueous cleanser
    R. aqueous gel
rosuvastatin
rot
    Barcoo r.
    jungle r.
Rotacaps
    Ventolin R.

Rotahaler inhaler
Rotamune vaccine
RotaShield vaccine
rotating
    r. air impactor
    r. arm impactor
    r. wire brush
rotation
    r. flap
    timed intermittent r.
rotator
    r. cuff
    r. cuff tendinitis
rotavirus
    r. gastroenteritis
    group C r.
    rhesus r. (RRV)
Rotazyme diagnostic procedure
röteln
Roth-Bernhardt disease
Rothia dentocariosa
Rothmann-Makai syndrome
Rothmund syndrome
Rothmund-Thomson syndrome
Roth spot
Rotorod sampler
rotoslide
rotunda
    pityriasis r.
rouge
    homme r.
    L'Homme r.
rough marsh elder
Roujeau
    DRESS syndrome of Bocquet
      and R.
rouleaux
round
    r. body
    r. facies
    r. fingerpad sign
roundworm
Rous
    R. sarcoma
    R. sarcoma virus (RSV)
    R. sarcoma virus immune globulin
      intravenous (RSV-IGIV)
    R. tumor
Rous-associated virus (RAV)
Roux
    R. retractor
    R. spatula
Roux-en-Y hepaticojejunostomy
Roux-Y loop
Rovighi sign
Rowasa Rectal
Rowe elimination diet for food allergies
Rowell syndrome
roxithromycin

Royl-Derm wound hydrogel dressing
RPA
  ribonuclease protection assay
RPC
  reactive perforating collagenosis
RPD
    Pepcid RPD
RPE
  retinal pigment epithelial cell
RPLE
  reversible posterior leukoencephalopathy
RPNG
  rapidly progressive necrotizing
    glomerulonephritis
RPR
  rapid plasma reagin
    RPR circle card test
RQLQ
  rhinoconjunctivitis-specific quality of life
    questionnaire
RR
  risk ratio
RRE
  Rev-responsive element
RRMS
  relapsing-remitting multiple sclerosis
RRV
  rhesus rotavirus
  right renal vein
RSD
  reflex sympathetic dystrophy
    RSD syndrome
RSLT
  reduced-size liver transplant
  reduced-size liver transplantation
RSP
  rat serum protein
RS3PE
  remitting seronegative symmetrical
    synovitis with pitting edema
RST
  reagin screen test
RSTL
  Relaxed Skin Tension Line
RSV
  respiratory syncytial virus
  Rous sarcoma virus
RSV-IGIV
  respiratory syncytial virus immune
    globulin intravenous
  Rous sarcoma virus immune globulin
    intravenous

Rs virus
RT
  radiotherapy
RTD
  residual thermal damage
RTD-1
  rhesus theta defensin 1
RT-PCR
  reverse transcriptase-polymerase chain
    reaction
RTR
  renal transplant recipient
RTx
  renal transplantation
RU
  recall urticaria
rub
    pleural friction r.
    tendon friction r.
    r. test
Rubarth
    R. disease
    R. disease virus
rubber
    r. additive dermatitis
    r. allergy
    Brazilian r.
    r. elongation factor (Hev b1)
    r. man syndrome
rubedo
rubefacient
rubefaction
rubella
    r. arthritis
    congenital r.
    r. HI test
    r. IgG ELISA test
    r. and mumps vaccines, combined
    r. vaccine virus
    r. virus vaccine, live
rubelliform
rubeola virus
rubeosis
ruber
    lichen r.
ruberous
rubescent
Rubinstein-Taybi syndrome
Rubivirus
rubor
    Quercus r.
    skin r.

R

NOTES

rubra
keratosis pilaris r.
miliaria r.
pityriasis r.
Rhodotorula r.
stria r.
trichomycosis r.
rubricytes
rubrifacient
rubrum
eczema r.
tinea r.
Trichophyton r.
ruby
r. laser
r. spot
rudiment
calcaneal r.
hair r.
rudimentary
r. cephalocele
r. meningocele
r. supernumerary digit
Rud syndrome
ruffling
membrane r.
rufous oculocutaneous albinism
ruga, pl. **rugae**
Rugger-jersey spine
rugosa
Candida r.
rugose
rugous
rule
nines r.
r. of nines
Rumalon
ruminantium
Cowdria r.
Rumpel-Leede
R.-L. phenomenon
R.-L. sign
R.-L. test
running
r. intradermal stitch
long-distance r.
r. simple stitch
runt disease
runting syndrome
Runyon classification
RUP
rat urine protein
rupia escharotica
rupial syphilid
rupioides
psoriasis r.
rupioid psoriasis

rupture
apertural pore r.
disc r.
rural cutaneous leishmaniasis
Ruscus aculeatus
rush immunotherapy (RIT)
Rush-Presbyterian St. Luke's Heart Failure and Transplant Program
Russell
R. body
R. sign
R. viper venom time
Russian
R. autumn encephalitis
R. autumn encephalitis virus
R. olive
R. olive tree
R. spring-summer encephalitis
R. spring-summer encephalitis Eastern subtype
R. spring-summer encephalitis virus
R. spring-summer encephalitis Western subtype
R. thistle
R. thistle weed pollen
R. tick-borne encephalitis
Rust
R. disease
R. syndrome
rusting
Ru-Tuss
R.-T. DE
Ruvalcaba-Myhre-Smith syndrome
Ru-Vert-M
RVP
red veterinary petrolatum
RVPaba
RVPaque
RV/TLC
residual volume to total lung capacity ratio
RW
ragweed
RWBT
rapid whole blood test
RWJ 57504
rye
R. classification
r. grass pollen
r. meal
perennial r.
wild r.
Rymed
Rymed-TR
Rynacrom
Ryna Liquid
Rynatan
Rynatuss

S

S antigen
Bel-Phen-Ergot S
S unit of streptomycin

SA

severe asthma
Sinutab SA
Targel SA

SAA

severe aplastic anemia

Saalfield expressor

SAARD

slow-acting antirheumatic drug

sabdariffa

Hibiscus s.

saber shin

Sabin-Feldman dye test

Sabin vaccine

Sabouraud

S. agar
S. medium

sabre

coup de s.
en coup de s.

SAC

seasonal allergic conjunctivitis

sac

s. fungus
venom s.

sacbrood

sacchari

Fusarium s.

saccharide

O-linked s.

saccharolyticus

Peptostreptococcus s.

Saccharomyces

S. cerevisiae
S. neoformans

sacer ignis

Sachs-Georgi test

Sackett criteria

sacral

s. agenesis syndrome
s. agenesis type 1 syndrome
Hydrocol s.
s. root sheath ectasia
s. spot

sacroiliitis

psoriatic s.
pyogenic s.

sacrospinalis muscle

Sactimed-I-Sinald disinfectant

SAD

specific antibody deficiency

SADBE

squaric acid dibutylester

saddle

s. nose
s. nose deformity

saddleback

s. caterpillar
s. caterpillar sting
s. fever

Saenger macula

SAF-Clens wound cleanser

Safe Tussin

safety-pin appearance

SAF-Gel

Saf-Gel hydrogel dressing

Safranin

S. O/Fast-Green staining
S. O stain

sage

coast s.
s. weed pollen

sagebrush

saginata

Taenia s.

sailor's

s. neck
s. skin

saimiri

Herpesvirus s.
herpesvirus s. (HVS)

Saint, St.

S. Anthony fire
S. Anthony's fire
S. Ignatius itch
S. John's wort
S. Joseph Adult Chewable Aspirin
S. Louis encephalitis
S. Louis encephalitis virus
S. Thomas solution

Saizen

Sakaguchi-Kauppi method

sakazakii

Enterobacter s.

SAL

salicylic acid-lactic acid
SAL paint

Salac

Salacid Ointment

Sal-Acid Plaster

Salagen oral

Salazopyrin

salbutamol

Saleto-200, -400

Salflex

Salgesic

S

salicylanilide
halogenated s.'s
salicylate
choline s.
glucuronidation s.
magnesium s.
methyl s.
nonacetylated s.
trolamine s.
salicylic
s. acid collodion
s. acid-lactic acid (SAL)
s. acid and lactic acid
s. acid-lactic acid paint
s. acid and propylene glycol
salicylism
saligenin compound
saligna
eucalyptus s.
salina
Artemisia s.
saline
s. agglutinin
Broncho S.
s. isohemagglutinin
phosphate-buffered s. (PBS)
s. sodium citrate (SSC)
tris-buffered s. (TBS)
Salisbury common cold virus
saliva
enzymatic s.
s. substitute
Salivart
salivary
s. gland
s. gland virus
s. gland virus disease
s. scintigraphy
Salk vaccine
salmeterol xinafoate
salmincola
Nanophyetus s.
salmon
s. calcitonin
s. patch
pink s.
Salmonella
S. arizonae
S. arthritis
S. bredeney
S. choleraesuis
S. enteritidis
S. montevideo
S. osteomyelitis
S. panama
S. paratyphi
S. poona
S. st. paul

S. typhi
S. typhimurium
salmonellosis
salmonicolor
Sporobolomyces s.
salpingitis
reactive s.
salsalate
Salseb
Salsitab
Salsola pestifer
SALT
skin-associated lymphoid tissue
salt
aluminum s.
s. cedar
s. cedar tree
Epsom s.'s
gold s.'s
s. grass
s. grass pollen
s. and pepper lesion
persulfate s.
s. of platinum
s. rheum
s. sensitivity
silver s.
sodium s.
s. solution
theophylline s.
s. water boil
saltbush weed pollen
salts
saltwater catfish
saltwort
salute
allergic s.
saluting
salvage therapy
Salve
Callus S.
Scholl Corn S.
SAM-e nutritional supplement
sampler
Anderson s.
gravitational s.
impaction s.
inertial suction s.
Rotorod s.
Sartorious air s.
suction s.
Samter syndrome
San
S. Joaquin Valley fever
S. Miguel sea lion virus
Sanarelli phenomenon
Sanarelli-Shwartzman phenomenon

sand
  s. flea
  s. flea bite
sandal
  keratodermic s.
  s. strap dermatitis
sandfly
  s. bite
  s. fever
  s. fever virus
Sandimmune (SIM)
  S. injection
  S. oral
Sandoglobulin
sandpaper dermabrader
sandwich assay
sandworm disease
Sanfilippo
  S. mucopolysaccharidosis
  S. syndrome
SangCya oral solution
sanguineus
  Allodermanyssus s.
  nevus s.
  sudor s.
sanguisuga
  Triatoma s.
Sanochrysin
Sansert
Santyl
  S. enzymatic debrider
  S. enzymatic debriding agent
SAP-1
  stress-activated protein 1
SAPASI
  self-administered Psoriasis Area and
    Severity Index
saphenous nerve entrapment
SAPHO
  synovitis, acne, pustulosis, hyperostosis,
    osteitis
  SAPHO syndrome
saponin
Sapporo criteria
saprophytic
  s. disease
  s. flora
  s. fungi
saquinavir mesylate
SAR
  seasonal allergic rhinitis

SARA
  sexually acquired reactive arthritis
Saran Wrap therapy
sarcoid
  s. arthritis
  Boeck s.
  Darier-Roussy s.
  s. granuloma
  miliary s.
  morpheaform s.
  papular s.
  Spiegler-Fendt s.
sarcoidal
sarcoid-like granulomatous myopathy
sarcoidosis
  Boeck s.
  cardiac s.
  cutaneous s.
  Danielssen-Boeck s.
  erythrodermic s.
  extraocular s.
  extrapulmonary s.
  ichthyosiform s.
  ocular s.
  pulmonary s.
  thyroiditis, Addison disease, Sjögren
    syndrome, s. (TASS)
sarcolemma
sarcoma
  Abernethy s.
  African cutaneous Kaposi s.
  African lymphadenopathic Kaposi s.
  African-variety Kaposi s.
  avian s.
  disseminated Kaposi s.
  epithelioid s.
  Kaposi s. (KS)
  melanotic s.
  multiple idiopathic hemorrhagic s.
  pseudo-Kaposi s.
  reticulum cell s.
  Rous s.
sarcomatosis cutis
sarcomatous
sarcomere
Sarcophaga
sarcophagi fly
Sarcopsylla
Sarcoptes
  S. hominis
  S. scabiei

NOTES

sarcoptic
    s. acariasis
    s. mange
sarcosepsis
sarcosis
sarcosporidiosis
sardine
sargassum
    Japanese s.
sargramostim
Sarna HC
SARS
    severe adult respiratory syndrome
Sartorious air sampler
SAS
    statistical analysis system
saseloides
    Ledebouriella s.
SASSAD
    Six-Area, Six-Sign Atopic Dermatitis
    SASSAD severity index
SAStid Plain Therapeutic Shampoo and Acne Wash
satellite
    s. buboes
    s. cell
    s. erythematous papule
    s. lesion
    s. phenomenon
satellitosis
satia
    vena s.
Satinique Anti-Dandruff
sativum
    Allium s.
saturated solution of potassium iodide (SSKI)
saturation analysis
saturnine gout
saucerization technique
sauna suit
Saunders-Zwilling hypothesis
sauriasis
sauriderma
saurine
sauriosis
sauroderma
    ichthyosis s.
sausage
    s. digit
    s. finger
    s. toe
sausage-shaped bulla
SAV
    specific allergy vaccination
savitum
    Helminthosporium s.
sawdust
sawtooth strategy

saxitoxin
SBE
    subacute bacterial endocarditis
SBM
    subbasement membrane
    subepithelial basement membrane
SBTx
    small bowel transplantation
SC
    spindle cell carcinoma
    stratum corneum
        LightSheer SC
        Pefabloc SC
sc
    subcutaneous
SCA
    single-chain antigen-binding
    SCA protein
scab
scabby mouth
Scabene
    S. Lotion
    S. Shampoo
scabetic
scabicidal
scabicide
scabiei
    Sarcoptes s.
scabies
    animal s.
    Boeck s.
    crusted s.
    environmental s.
    hair follicle mite s.
    hyperkeratotic s.
    s. incognito
    keratotic s.
    nodular s.
    Norwegian s.
    s. preparation
scabieticide
scabietic mite
scabious
scabrities unguium
scaffold
    cytoskeletal s.
    knottin s.
scald
scalded skin syndrome
scale
    aluminum density step s.
    Borg s.
    branny s.
    carpet-tack s.
    Chisholm s.
    Chisolm s.
    expanded disability status s. (EDSS)
    Greenspan s.

illness attitude s. (IAS)
lamellar s.
lichen-type s.
Likert s.
Lund-Browder burn s.
Mankin histologic/histochemical s.
micaceous s.
ostraceous s.
Outerbridge s.
pityriasis-type s.
4-point Likert s.
5-point Likert s.
7-point Likert s.
6-point vitiligo disease activity s.
Profile of Mood States S.
psoriatic-type s.
Sessing pressure ulcer
  assessment s.
Shea pressure ulcer assessment s.
Shea s. (stages I-IV)
silver-white s.
silver-white-colored s.
silvery s.
Tarpley s.
visual analog s. (VAS)
Ways of Coping S.
WOMAC stiffness s.

scaling
s., erythema, and induration (SEI)
s., erythema, and induration scoring
  system

scaling skin-colored lesion
scall
milk s.

scalp
dissecting cellulitis of s.
dissection cellulitis of s.
s. folliculitis
hair and s.
s. infection
s. louse
pilar tumor of s.
ringworm of the s.
scurfy s.
seborrheic dermatitis of the s.

scalpel
Shaw hemostatic s.
s. skimming

Scalpicin topical
scaly
s. ringworm
s. tetter

scan
high-resolution computed
  tomography s.
HRCT s.
indium chloride s.
myocardial isotopic perfusion s.
  (MIPS)
single-photon emission computed
  tomography s.
SPECT s.
Tc polyphosphate s.
technetium s.
V/Q lung s.

scanner
DermaTemp DT-1000 infrared
  temperature s.
ECAT 951/33 PET s.
SilkTouch CO_2 Flash S.
Softscan laser s.

scanning
indium-labeled s.

Scanpor
S. acrylate adhesive
S. tape

scapi (*pl. of* scapus)
scapularis
Ixodes s.

scapulocostal syndrome
scapulothoracic
s. articulation
s. syndrome

scapus, pl. scapi
s. pili

scar
atrophic white s.
cigarette-paper s.
s. formation
hypertrophic s.
ice-pick type s.
keloidal type s.
paper-thin s.
papyraceous s.
radial s.
shilling s.
white s.

scarf nevus
scarification test
scarificator
scarifier
Berkeley s.

scarify

NOTES

S

scarlatina
anginose s.
s. hemorrhagica
s. latens
s. maligna
s. rheumatica
s. simplex
scarlatinal nephritis
scarlatinella
scarlatiniform
s. eruption
s. erythema
scarlatiniforme
erythema s.
scarlatinoid
scarlet
s. fever
s. fever antitoxin
s. fever erythrogenic toxin
scarring
cigarette-paper s.
keloidal s.
patch test s.
s. vertex alopecia
SCAS
Self-Care Assessment Schedule
SCAT
short-contact treatment
scattering
Rayleigh s.
Thomson s.
scavenger
s. cell
s. macrophage
SCB
DuoDerm S.
SCC
squamous cell carcinoma
SCD
sickle cell disease
Scedosporium apiospermum
scent print
SCF
stem cell factor
Schafer-Branauer syndrome
Schäfer syndrome
Schamberg
S. comedo extractor
S. dermatitis
S. disease
S. expressor
S. fever
S. progressive pigmented purpuric
   dermatosis
S. purpura
Schaumann
S. benign lymphogranulomatosis
S. body

Schedule
Diagnostic Interview S.
Self-Care Assessment S. (SCAS)
Scheie
S. mucopolysaccharidosis
S. syndrome
Scheinpharm Triamcine-A
scheme
Kauffmann-White s.
Schenck disease
schenckii
Sporothrix s.
Sporotrichum s.
Scheuermann disease
Schick
S. method
S. sign
S. test
S. test toxin
Schilder disease
Schimmelpenning syndrome
Schirmer test
schistocyte
Schistosoma
S. haematobium
S. japonicum
S. mansoni
S. mekongi
schistosomal
s. dermatitis
s. granuloma of scrotum
schistosome
s. cercarial dermatitis
s. granuloma
schistosomiasis
ectopic cutaneous s.
hepatosplenic s.
Manson s.
visceral s.
Schizonepeta tenuifolia
schizonychia
schizotrichia
Schmidt syndrome
Schmorl node
Schnitzler syndrome
Schober
S. test
S. test for spondylitis
schoenleinii
Achorion s.
Trichophyton s.
Scholl
S. Athlete's Foot Preparation
S. Corn, Callus Plaster Preparation
S. Corn Salve
S. 2-Drop Corn Remedy
S. Wart Remover
S. Zino

Schönlein
  S. disease
  S. purpura
Schönlein-Henoch syndrome
Schopf syndrome
Schridde cancer hair
Schuco 2000 nebulizer
Schüller-Christian syndrome
Schultz-Charlton
  S.-C. phenomenon
  S.-C. reaction
Schultz-Dale reaction
Schultze acroparesthesia
Schultze-type acroparesthesia
Schwann cell
schwannoma
  granular cell s.
Schweninger-Buzzi
  anetoderma of S.-B.
  S.-B. anetoderma
sciatic
  s. nerve
  s. nerve entrapment
SCID
  severe combined immune deficiency
  severe combined immunodeficiency
  severe combined immunodeficiency
    disease
  severe combined immunodeficiency
    disorder
  SCID mice
SCIDA
  Athabascan type of severe combined
    immunodeficiency disease
SCIG
  subcutaneous immunoglobulin
scintigraphy
  salivary s.
  Tc-human serum albumin s.
scintillation counter
scintiscan
scissors
  s. biopsy
  blepharoplasty s.
  dissecting s.
  Gibbs-Gradle s.
  Gorney-Freeman straight facelift s.
  Gorney straight facelift s.
  Gradle s.
  Kaye s.
  LaGrange s.
  Lahey s.

  Laschal s.
  Lister s.
  Littauer s.
  Malis s.
  Matarasso facelift s.
  Metzenbaum s.
  Northbent s.
  O'Brien s.
  Peck-Joseph s.
  Ragnell s.
  Shortbent s.
  Spencer s.
  Stevens tenotomy s.
  utility s.
  Wong-Stall s.
scissura pilorum
sc-kit
  soluble c-kit
Scl-70 antibody
Sclavo serum
SCLE
  subacute cutaneous lupus erythematosus
sclera
  donor s.
scleradenitis
scleral defect
scleredema
  s. adultorum
  Buschke s.
  s. diutinum
  s. neonatorum
sclerema
  s. adiposum
  s. neonatorum
scleriasis
scleritis
  diffuse s.
  nodular s.
  nonrheumatoid s.
  posterior s.
  rheumatoid s.
scleroatrophy, sclerotylosis
  anetoderma s.
  atrophoderma s.
  lichen sclerosus s.
  striae s.
sclerodactylia annularis ainhumoides
sclerodactyly
scleroderma
  adultorum s.
  s. autoantigen CENP-B
  Buchscher s.

S

NOTES

scleroderma *(continued)*
    diffuse s.
    environmental s.
    limited s.
    linear s.
    localized s.
    pediatric s.
    s. renal crisis (SRC)
    scleroderma sine s.
    sclerosis sine s.
    s. septal panniculitis
    systemic sclerosis sine s. (ssSSc)
scleroderma-like
    s.-l. eruption
    s.-l. skin thickening
sclerodermatitis
sclerodermatomyositis
sclerodermatous
sclerodermiformis
    hypodermitis s.
sclerodermitis
sclerodermoid
Sclerodex
ScleroLaser
scleromalacia perforans
scleromyositis
scleromyxedema
scleronychia
ScleroPlus flashlamp-pumped pulsed tunable dye laser
sclerosant
sclerosed
sclerosing
    s. agent
    s. cholangitis
    s. hemangioma
    s. lipogranuloma
    s. lymphangitis
    s. lymphosarcoma
    s. panniculitis
    s. sweat duct carcinoma
sclerosis
    amyotrophic lateral s. (ALS)
    Baló concentric s.
    s. corii
    s. cutanea
    diffuse progressive systemic s.
    drug-induced progressive symptom s.
    environment progressive symptom s.
    limited cutaneous systemic s.
    limited progressive systemic s.
    linear progressive systemic s.
    localized progressive systemic s.
    lupoid s.
    multiple s.
    primary-progressive multiple s. (PPMS)
    progressive symptom s. (PSS)

    progressive systemic s. (PSS)
    relapsing-remitting multiple s. (RRMS)
    s. sine scleroderma
    systemic s. (SSc)
    tuberous s. (TSC)
sclerostenosis
sclerosus
    genital lichen s.
    lichen s.
    s. lichen
sclerotherapy
sclerothrix
sclerotic body
sclerotrichia
sclerotylosis *(var. of* scleroatrophy)
scoliosis
    dolorimeter s.
Scolopendra
    S. heres
    S. heres bite
scombroid
    s. dermatitis
    s. fish poisoning
SCOP
    Structural Classification of Proteins
scopolamine
Scopulariopsis
    S. brevicaulis
    S. brumptii
    S. inflatum
    S. prolificans
SCORAD
    Severity Scoring of Atopic Dermatitis
    SCORAD index
scorbutic
    s. dysentery
    s. purpura
score
    APACHE II s.
    Borg s.
    Brasfield chest radiograph s.
    Child-Pugh s.
    Child-Turcotte-Pugh s.
    damage index s.
    Dreiser functional index s.
    Fitzpatrick wrinkle s.
    Framingham risk s.
    Karnofsky s.
    Kellgren s.
    Leicester s.
    modified Rodman skin thickness s.
    nasal congestion s. (NCS)
    nasal symptom s. (NSS)
    Paulus composite s.
    Quality of Life s.
    rhinitis VS symptom s.
    Rodnan skin thickness s.
    SEI s.

Sharp s.
Shwachman clinical s.
Skin Intensity S. (SIS)
skin thickness s.
SSS s.
t s.
total nasal symptom s. (TNSS)
total nonnasal symptom s.
  (TNNSS)
total skin s.
total symptom s. (TSS)
UNOS 3, 4 s.
vitiligo disease activity s.
WOMAC pain s.
z s.
scorpion
bark s.
common striped s.
s. fish
s. sting
Scotch Tape test
sCR1
soluble complement receptor type 1
scrapie
sheep s.
scraping
fungal s.
KOH s.
nasal s.
Scraple disease
scratch
s. chamber test
s. testing
screen
AlaTOP inhalant allergy s.
drywall sanding s.
medium-grade drywall sanding s.
QuickVue One-Step Allergen S.
s. test
TORCH viral s.
toxoplasmosis, other, rubella,
  cytomegalovirus, and herpes
  viral s.
screening
s. audiometry
S. Patch Test Kit
spirometric s.
systematic polymorphism s.
screw-worm fly
scrofula
scrofuloderma, scrofulodermia
eczema s.

s. gummosa
papular s.
verrucous s.
scrofulosis
scrofulosorum
acne s.
lichen s.
scrotalis
lingua s.
scrotal tongue
scroti
pruritus s.
scrotum
schistosomal granuloma of s.
scrub
Exidine S.
Techni-Care surgical s.
s. typhus
Scrubz
Pocket S.
Travel S.
scruff
SCT
stem cell transplant
Plexion SCT
sculpturatus
Centruroides s.
sculptured nail
scurf
scurfy scalp
scurvy
scute
scutular
scutularis
parakeratosis s.
scutulata
ichthyosis s.
porrigo s.
scutulum
Scytalidium
S. dimidiatum
S. hyalinum
SD
mean
standard deviation
WinRho SD
S/D
Gammagard S/D
Polygam S/D
SDF-1
stromal-cell-derived factor-1

NOTES

SDKT
  simultaneous double kidney
  transplantation
SDS-PAGE
  sodium dodecyl sulfate-polyacrylamide
  gel electrophoresis
SDS-polyacrylamide gel electrophoresis
SE
  surgical excision
SEA
  seronegativity, enthesopathy, arthropathy
sea
  s. anemone
  s. anemone dermatitis
  s. anemone sting
  s. boot foot
  s. cucumber
  s. cucumber dermatitis
  s. cucumber sting
  s. louse dermatitis
  s. nettle dermatitis
  s. snake
  s. snake bite
  s. urchin
  s. urchin dermatitis
  s. urchin granuloma
  s. urchin sting
  s. water boil
seabather's eruption
sea-blue
  s.-b. histiocyte syndrome
  s.-b. histiocytosis
Sea-Clens wound cleanser
sealant
  fibrin s.
  Tisseel fibrin s.
seal finger
seams
  tetracycline s.
Searl ulcer
season
  growing s.
seasonal
  s. allergic conjunctivitis (SAC)
  s. allergic rhinitis (SAR)
  s. allergy
  s. pruritus
SeaSorb
  S. alginate wound cover
  S. alginate wound dressing
seatworm infection
seaweed dermatitis
sebacea
  ichthyosis s.
sebaceoma
  rippled pattern s.
sebaceous, sebaceus
  s. adenocarcinoma
  s. adenoma

  s. carcinoma
  s. cyst
  s. differentiation
  s. epithelioma
  s. gland (SG)
  s. horn
  lupus s.
  s. miliaria
  nevus s.
  s. nevus
  s. nevus of Jadassohn
  s. senile hyperplasia
  s. trichofolliculoma
  s. tubercle
  s. tumor
sebaceum
  adenoma s.
  molluscum s.
  tuberculum s.
sebaceus
  lupus s.
  nevus s.
Seba-Nil
Sebasorb lotion
Sebcur
Sebcur/T
sebolith
sebopsoriasis
seborrhea
  s. adiposa
  s. capitis
  s. cerea
  concrete s.
  s. corporis
  eczematoid s.
  s. faciei
  s. furfuracea
  s. generalis
  s. nigra
  s. oleosa
  s. sicca
  s. squamosa neonatorum
seborrheic
  s. blepharitis
  s. dermatitis
  s. dermatitis-like condition
  s. dermatitis of the scalp
  s. dermatosis
  s. eczema
  s. keratosis
  s. keratosis cluster
  s. keratosis crop
  s. verruca
  s. wart
seborrheica
  acanthoma verrucosa s.
  acanthosis s.
  acne s.
  alopecia s.

corona s.
dermatitis s.
seborrhiasis
seborrhoeicum
eczema s.
Sebulex
Sebulon
sebum
s. cutaneum
s. preputiale
Sebutone
secondary
s. adrenocortical failure
s. agammaglobulinemia
s. amyloid
s. antibody deficiency
s. cataract
s. cutaneous B-cell lymphocytic leukemia
s. cutaneous B-cell lymphoma
s. disease
s. effect
s. encephalitis
s. hyperlipoproteinemia
s. hyperparathyroidism
s. hypogammaglobulinemia
s. immune response
s. immunodeficiency
s. impetiginization
s. infection
s. lesion
s. lymphatic tissue (SLT)
s. lymphedema
s. lymphoid tissue chemokine (SLC)
s. panhypopituitarism
s. psychiatric disorder
s. pyoderma
s. Sjögren syndrome
s. smoke
s. syphilid
s. syphilis
s. systemic amyloidosis
s. telangiectasia
s. tuberculosis
s. tumor-associated cutaneous amyloidosis
second-degree burn
second-line drug (SLD)
second set rejection
Secrétan syndrome
secrete

secreted
regulated on activation, normal T-cell expressed and s. (RANTES)
regulated upon activation, normal T-cell expressed and s. (RANTES)
secretion
C-peptide s.
excessive s.
secretor factor
secretory
s. antibody study
s. coil
s. component
s. component deficiency
s. immunoglobulin
s. immunoglobulin A
s. leukoprotease inhibitor
s. leukoprotease inhibitor protein
s. otitis media
s. PLA$_2$ enzyme
s. vesicle function
section
horizontal s.
snap-frozen s.
vertical s.
SED
spondyloepiphysial dysplasia
sedative therapy
Sedi-Stain
seeberi
Rhinosporidium s.
seed
s. corn
millet s.
psyllium s.
sesame s.
s. tick
s. wart
SEER
Surveillance, Epidemiology and End Results
seglycin CS/DS
segment
apicoposterior s.
N s.
segmental
s. hyalinizing vasculitis
s. neurofibromatosis
s. nevus
s. vitiligo
segmentectomy

S

NOTES

Segond fracture
SEI
     scaling, erythema, and induration
          SEI score
          SEI scoring system
Seidlmayer syndrome
Seip-Lawrence syndrome
seizure
Seldane-D
select
          Coppertone Skin S.'s
selectin
selection
          negative s.
          positive s.
          reflectance-guidance laser s.
          tumor cell negative s.
selective
          s. antipolysaccharide antibody
               deficiency (SPAD)
          s. estrogen receptor modulator
               (SERM)
          s. mesentericography
          s. photothermolysis
          s. sentinel lymph node dissection
               (SSLND)
selenium
          s. deficiency
          s. sulfide
Selestoject
self-administered Psoriasis Area and
     Severity Index (SAPASI)
self-antigen
          muscle s.-a.
Self-Care Assessment Schedule (SCAS)
self-healing reticulohistiocytosis
self-infection
self-injecting epinephrine
self-limited allergic reaction
self-nonself discrimination
Self-Perception Profile for children
Selsun
          S. Blue
          S. Blue Shampoo
          S. Gold
          S. Gold for Women
selvagem
          endemic fogo s.
semelincident
semicircular
          s. lipoatrophy
          s. lipotrophy
semiimpermeable membrane
semimembranosus complex
semipermeable dressing
semiquantitative disease extent index
semisynthetic analog
Semken forceps
Semliki Forest virus

Semmes-Weinstein
          S.-W. test
          S.-W. vibrometry
Semple vaccine
Semprex
Semprex-D
Sendai virus
Senear-Usher
          S.-U. disease
          S.-U. syndrome
Seneca snakeroot
senescence
          replicative s.
senescent arthritis
senile
          s. alopecia
          s. angioma
          s. atrophoderma
          s. ectasia
          s. elastosis
          s. fibroma
          s. gangrene
          s. hemangioma
          s. ichthyosis
          s. keratoderma
          s. keratoma
          s. keratosis
          s. lentigo
          s. melanoderma
          s. pruritus
          s. purpura
          s. sebaceous hyperplasia
          s. skin
          s. wart
senilis
          alopecia s.
          keratosis s.
          lentigo s.
          malum coxae s.
          pruritus s.
          purpura s.
          verruca plana s.
senior synonym
sennetsu
          Ehrlichia s.
sense nucleotide
sensible perspiration
sensitiva
          trichosis s.
sensitive
          temperature s. (TS)
sensitivity
          acquired s.
          allergic s.
          animal dander s.
          antibiotic s.
          aspirin s.
          atopic s.
          autoerythrocyte s.

earlobe sign of nickel s.
idiosyncratic s.
induced s.
multiple chemical s.
nickel s.
peak flow s.
photoallergic s.
phototoxic s.
salt s.
sensitization
active s.
autoerythrocyte s.
cross s.
neuronal s.
photodynamic s.
sensitize
sensitized
s. antigen
s. cell
s. lymphocyte
sensitizer
sensitizing
s. dose
s. injection
s. substance
sensor
ClipTip reusable s.
Cross Top replacement oxygen s.
Infinity s.
SpiroSense flow s.
Sensorcaine-MPF
sensorineural dysfunction
sensory
s. ganglion
s. nerve action potential (SNAP)
s. nerve action potential sleep
recorder
sensu stricto
Sential
sentinel
s. animal
s. lymph node (SLN)
s. tag
sentrin
sentrinization
seositis
seotonin
SEPA dermal absorption enhancer
SEPA/minoxidil
separation
epidermal-dermal s.

eschar s.
hypodermic needle s.
Sephadex Bead
Sepracor
Seprafilm bioresorbable membrane
sepsis, pl. **sepses**
group JK *Corynebacterium* s.
sepsis-induced
s.-i. DIC
s.-i. disseminated intravascular
coagulation
s.-i. thrombocytopenia
septa
interlobular s.
S. Topical Ointment
septal
s. embolus
s. panniculitis
septic
s. arthritis
s. dactylitis
s. embolus
s. shock
s. shock syndrome
SeptiCare wound cleanser
septicemia
Aeromonas s.
bacterial s.
Bruce s.
Candida s.
DF2 s.
gonococcal s.
perinatal s.
streptococcal s.
typhoid s.
Septisol
septoplasty
graft s.
Septra DS
sequela of influenza
sequence
Aertemia Salinas s.
chi s.
complement s.
consensus s.
immunostimulatory DNA s. (ISS)
Kozak s.
long-term repeat s. (LTR)
mitochondrial targeting s. (MTS)
Shine-Dalgarno s.
signal s.

S

NOTES

sequence-specific
    s.-s. oligonucleotide probe
       hybridization (SSOP)
    s.-s. primer (SSP)
sequencing
    direct s.
sequential
    s. determinant
    s. probability ratio test (SPRT)
sequestration
    s. cyst
    s. dermoid
sequestrum, pl. **sequestra**
sequoiosis
sera (*pl. of* serum)
Serax
Seretide
Serevent
Sergent white line
serial
    s. dilutional intradermal skin test
    s. passage
series
    20-allergen Hermal screening s.
serine
    s. esterase
    s. protease
    s. proteinase
serine-threonine kinase
serivumab
SERM
    selective estrogen receptor modulator
sermorelin acetate
seroconversion response
serodiagnosis
seroepidemiology
serofast
serologic test for syphilis (S.T.S.)
serology
seroma
Seromycin Pulvules
seronegative
    s. arthritis
    s. oligoarthritis
    s. rheumatoid arthritis
    s. rheumatoid syndrome
    s. spondyloarthropathy
seronegativity, enthesopathy, arthropathy (SEA)
seropositive
    anti-HCV s.
    antihepatitis C virus s.
    s. disease
    s. rheumatoid arthritis
seroprevalence
seropurulent
serosal fibrosis
serosanguineous
serositis, pl. **serositides**

    adhesive s.
    multiple s.
serotaxis
serotherapy
serotonergic
serotonin
serotype
    heterologous s.
    homologous s.
serotyping
serovaccination
serovar
SERPACWA
    Skin Exposure Reduction Paste Against
      Chemical Warfare
serpentina
    ichthyosis s.
serpentine
serpiginosa
    zona s.
serpiginosum
    angioma s.
    s. angioma
serpiginosus
    lupus s.
serpiginous
    s. pattern
    s. ulcer
serpigo
serpin
Serratia
    S. liquefaciens
    S. marcescens
Serrefine clamp
sertaconazole nitrate
sertraline
    s. HCl
    s. hydrochloride
serum, pl. **sera**
    s. accident
    active s.
    s. agglutinin
    s. alpha-antitrypsin
    s. amyloid A, P component
    antianthrax s.
    antibotulinus s.
    anticholera s.
    anticomplementary s.
    anticrotalus s.
    antiepithelial s.
    s. antiglomerular-basement-membrane
      antibody
    antilymphocyte s. (ALS)
    antimeningococcus s.
    antipneumococcus s.
    antirabies s.
    antireticular cytotoxic s.
    antisnakebite s.
    antitoxic s.

bacteriolytic s.
Behring s.
B fraction s.
blister s.
blood s.
s. C3
s. C4
C fraction s.
s. complement C1–C9
s. complement level
convalescence s.
convalescent s.
Coombs s.
despeciated s.
s. disease
dried human s.
s. eruption
foreign s.
s. hepatitis (SH)
s. hepatitis virus
heterologous s.
homologous s.
horse s.
human measles immune s.
human pertussis immune s.
human scarlet fever immune s.
hyperimmune s.
s. IgA
s. IgM
immune s. (IS)
s. immunofixation electrophoresis
  (SIFE)
inactivated s.
liquid human s.
lymphatolytic s.
s. marker
measles convalescent s.
mouse s.
s. nephritis
s. neutralization
nonimmune s.
normal horse s.
North American antisnakebite s.
polyvalent s.
pooled s.
s. precipitin
s. protein electrophoresis (SPEP)
s. protein electrophoretic finding
s. protein electrophoretogram (SPE)
s. rash
s. reaction
Sclavo s.

s. shock
s. sickness
specific s.
s. therapy
thyrotoxic s.
s. uric acid (SUA)
serumal
serum-fast
serum-free medium (SFM)
serum-opsonized
sesame seed
sesamoid injury
sesquioleate
  sorbitan s. (SS)
sessile
Sessing pressure ulcer assessment scale
set
  s. of idiotopes
  SinoJect puncture s.
seta, pl. **setae**
setosa
  trichosis s.
sevenless
  human son of s. (hSOSI)
Sever disease
severe
  s. acute allergic reaction
  s. adult respiratory syndrome
    (SARS)
  s. aplastic anemia (SAA)
  s. asthma (SA)
  s. chronic allergic condition
  s. combined immune deficiency
    (SCID)
  s. combined immune deficiency
    syndrome
  s. combined immunodeficiency
    (SCID)
  s. combined immunodeficiency
    disease (SCID)
  s. combined immunodeficiency
    disorder (SCID)
  s. combined immunodeficient mice
  s. deforming osteogenesis
    imperfecta
  s. immediate reaction
  s. obstruction
  s. respiratory failure
  s. systemic reaction
severity
  s. of allergy symptoms

S

NOTES

severity *(continued)*
    Dermatology Index of Disease s.
        (DIDS)
    S. Scoring of Atopic Dermatitis
        (SCORAD)
Sevin
sewer fly
sex factor
sexine
sexually
    s. acquired infection
    s. acquired reactive arthritis
        (SARA)
    s. transmitted disease (STD)
Sézary
    S. cell
    S. erythroderma
    S. reticulosis
    S. syndrome (SS)
SF
    stimulating factor
    synovial fluid
sFas
    soluble Fas
SFM
    serum-free medium
SG
    sebaceous gland
    stratum granulosum
SGF
    simulated gastric fluid
SGS
    silicone gel sheeting
SH
    serum hepatitis
    sinus histiocytosis
Shade
    S. UvaGuard sunscreen
    S. UvaGuard sunscreen lotion
shadow
    nodular s.
    s. plaque
    ring s.
shaft
    hair s.
shagbark
    s. hickory
    s. hickory tree
shaggy thick wall
shagreen
    s. patch
    s. skin
shaking of walnuts
Shaklee
    S. Dandruff Control
    S. Sunscreen
Sham
    S. TENS

    S. transcutaneous electrical nerve
        stimulator
shampoo
    A-200 S.
    Anti-Dandruff S.
    Avant Garde S.
    bifonazole s.
    Capex S.
    Carmol S.
    Dandruff Treatment S.
    Dermazine s.
    Exsel S.
    G-well S.
    Head & Shoulders S.
    Keep Clear Anti-Dandruff S.
    Kwell S.
    Lice-Enz S.
    Nizoral A-D S.
    Pronto S.
    P&S S.
    Pyrinex Pediculicide S.
    Pyrinyl Plus S.
    R&C S.
    RID S.
    Scabene S.
    Selsun Blue S.
    tar s.
    Tisit S.
    T/Sal S.
    Zincon S.
Shampooing Anti-Pelliculaire
Shapiro-Wilke W test
shared epitope
sharing
    United Network for Organ S.
        (UNOS)
shark skin
sharp
    s. dissection
    S. score
    s. spoon
**Sharplan SilkTouch flashscan surgical
    laser**
sharply circumscribed nodule
shave
    s. biopsy
    s. technique
shaver
    MicroPlaner soft tissue s.
Shaw hemostatic scalpel
shawl distribution
Shea
    S. pressure ulcer assessment scale
    S. scale (stages I-IV)
sheath
    s. cell
    cuticle of inner root s.
    fibrous s.
    inner root s.

nerve s.
outer root s.
tendon s.
shedding
nail s.
virus s.
Sheehan syndrome
sheep
contagious ecthyma (pustular
dermatitis) virus of s.
s. epithelium
pulmonary adenomatosis of s.
s. scrapie
s. sorrel
s. sorrel weed pollen
s. wool
sheep-pox virus
sheet
AcryDerm hydrogel s.
Aquasorb hydrogel s.
beta-pleated s.
ClearSite hydrogel s.
Conformant contact layer s.
Curagel Hydrogel s.
Derma-Gel hydrogel s.
DermaNet contact layer s.
Elasto-Gel hydrogel s.
Flexderm hydrogel s.
hydrogel s.
keratinous s.
material safety data s. (MSDS)
Mepitel contact layer s.
2nd Skin hydrogel s.
s.'s of nevus cells
N-Terface contact layer s.
Nu-Gel hydrogel s.
patient patch test record s.
Silastic s.
Silk Skin s.
Tegagel hydrogel s.
Tegapore contact-layer s.
Telfa Clear contact layer s.
THINSite hydrogel s.
Transorbent hydrogel s.
Vigilon hydrogel s.
sheeting
Avogel hydrogel s.
Cica-Care topical gel s.
DermaSof gel s.
New Beginnings topical gel s.
occlusive s.

silicone gel s. (SGS)
TopiGel occlusive s.
shellfish
shell nail
shelter foot
shield
Sof-Gel palm s.
shift
antigenic s.
shifting
Raman s.
Shiga-like toxin
Shigella
S. flexneri
S. flexneri dysenteriae
S. infection
S. sonnei
shigelloides
Aeromonas s.
Plesiomonas s.
shigellosis
Shiley tracheostomy tube
shilling scar
Shimada histopathologic classification
shimamushi disease
shin
saber s.
s. splint
s. spot
toasted s.
Shine-Dalgarno sequence
shiner
allergic s.
Shingles Relief Pak
ship fever
shipping
s. fever
s. fever virus
Shiseido Sunblock
shock
anaphylactic s.
anaphylactoid s.
s. antigen
endotoxin s.
gluten s.
histamine s.
hypovolemic s.
osmotic s.
protein s.
pseudoanaphylactic s.
septic s.

S

NOTES

shock (*continued*)
> serum s.
> thermal s.

shocking dose

shoe
> Ambulator s.
> s. dye dermatitis
> Plastizote s.

shoe-leather dermatitis

Shohl solution

Shope
> S. fibroma
> S. fibroma virus
> S. papilloma
> S. papilloma virus

shop typhus

short
> s. anagen telogen effluvium
> s. bowel syndrome
> s. consensus repeats
> s. incubation hepatitis
> s. tau inversion recovery (STIR)

Shortbent scissors

short-chain type X collagen

short-contact
> s.-c. therapy
> s.-c. treatment (SCAT)

shortening
> vegetable s.

short-haired breed

short-term immunotherapy (STI)

shoulder
> cuff-tear arthropathy s.
> frozen s.
> s. girdle
> Milwaukee s.
> s. periarthritis

shoulder-hand syndrome

showerhead infiltrator

SHP
> summer-type hypersensitivity
> pneumonitis

shrimp

shrinking lung syndrome (SLS)

Shuco-Myst nebulizer

Shulman syndrome

shunt
> arteriovenous s.
> distal splenorenal s. (DSRS)
> Gott s.
> hexose monophosphate s. (HMS)
> side-to-side portacaval s.
> ventriculoperitoneal s. (VP)

shunting
> venoarterial s.

Shur-Clens wound cleanser

Shwachman clinical score

Shwachman-Diamond syndrome

Shwartzman
> S. phenomenon
> S. reaction

SI
> stimulation index
> syncytium-inhibiting

SIADH
> syndrome of inappropriate excretion of
> antidiuretic hormone

sialadenitis
> myoepithelial s.

sialectasia

sialidase

sialidosis

sialoglycoprotein antigen

sialography
> parotid s.

sialometaplasia
> necrotizing s.

sialomucin

sialoprotein
> bone s. (BSP)

Sibine
> S. stimulea
> S. stimulea sting

sibling bone marrow transplantation

sicca
> cholera s.
> s. feature
> keratoconjunctivitis s.
> onychia s.
> pityriasis s.
> seborrhea s.
> s. symptom
> s. syndrome

siccation
> electrode s.

siccum
> eczema s.

sick
> s. building syndrome
> s. euthyroid

sickle
> s. cell anemia
> s. cell disease (SCD)
> s. cell trait
> s. cell ulcer

sickle cell intrahepatic cholestasis

sickling
> hepatic s.

sickness
> African horse s.
> S. Impact Profile (SIP)
> motion s.
> serum s.
> spotted s.

side-chain theory

side effect

sideroderma

sideropenic
sideropenica
    canities segmentata s.
side-to-side portacaval shunt
SIDS
    sudden infant death syndrome
Siemens
    ichthyosis bullosa of S. (IBS)
SIF
    simulated intestinal fluid
SIFE
    serum immunofixation electrophoresis
sigmodontine rodent
sign
    ABCD s.
    Albright s.
    Albright dimpling s.
    Asboe-Hansen s.
    Auspitz s.
    Babinski s.
    bandage s.
    Biederman s.
    Biernacki s.
    Blatin s.
    Borsieri s.
    Brunati s.
    bulge s.
    Bunnell s.
    Buschke-Ollendorf s.
    butterfly s.
    clavicular s.
    closed accordion s.
    Comby s.
    contralateral s.
    Crowe s.
    Cullen s.
    cutaneous s.
    Darier s.
    Dawbarn s.
    daylight s.
    Demarquay s.
    Dennie s.
    Dennie-Morgan s.
    Dew s.
    dimple s.
    drawer s.
    Dubois s.
    echo s.
    Elliot s.
    Ewart s.
    Faget s.
    Filipovitch s.

    flag s.
    floating-tooth s.
    Forchheimer s.
    Goggia s.
    Gottron s.
    Grisolle s.
    groove s.
    hair collar s.
    Hamman s.
    Hatchcock s.
    headlight s.
    Hertoghe s.
    Hitzelberger s.
    Hoffman s.
    Hoover s.
    Hoyne s.
    Hutchinson s.
    impingement s.
    Krisovski s.
    Lasgue s.
    Lasègue s.
    Lennhoff s.
    Leser-Trélat s.
    Lhermitte s.
    Lovibond profile s.
    matchbox s.
    McMurray s.
    melanoma warning s.
    Milian s.
    Mirchamp s.
    Muehrcke s.
    Nikolsky s.
    oil drop s.
    Osler s.
    Parrot s.
    Pastia s.
    Popeye s.
    prayer s.
    pseudo-Hutchinson s.
    Remak s.
    Romaña s.
    Romberg s.
    rope s.
    round fingerpad s.
    Rovighi s.
    Rumpel-Leede s.
    Russell s.
    Schick s.
    Silex s.
    Sisto s.
    Spurling s.
    Steinberg thumb s.

NOTES

sign *(continued)*
tail s.
Thomson s.
Tresilian s.
trolley-track s.
Vaughn-Jackson s.
Vierra s.
Waddell s.
Walker-Murdoch s.
Wimberger s.
Winterbottom s.
Yergason supination s.
SignaDress
S. sterile hydrocolloid
S. sterile hydrocolloid dressing
signal
nuclear localization s. (NLS)
s. peptide
punctate area of increased s. (PAIS)
receptors for endogenous danger s.'s (REDS)
s. recognition particle (SRP)
s. sequence
"stop" s.
s. transducer and activator of transcription (STAT)
s. transduction
s. transduction and activator of transcription (STAT)
signet ring lymphoma
significance
granulomatous lesions of unknown s. (GLUS)
McNemar test of s.
monoclonal gammopathy of undetermined s. (MGUS)
monoclonal gammopathy of unknown s. (MGUS)
SIL
squamous intraepithelial lesion
Siladryl oral
Silafed Syrup
Silaminic Expectorant
Silastic
S. sheet
S. tubing
Sildicon-E
silencer of death domain (SODD)
"silent" chest
silent lupus nephritis
Silex sign
Silfedrine
Children's S.
silica
s. dust exposure
s. granuloma
silicone
s. breast augmentation

s. deposition
s. gel
s. gel sheeting (SGS)
s. grease
s. oil
s. particle disease
s. rubber prosthesis
s. sheeting therapy
s. synovitis
silicosis
siliquosa
variola s.
siliquose desquamation
silk
S. Laser
S. Skin sheet
s. suture
SilkLaser
2040 erbium S.
SilkTouch
S. CO_2 Flash Scanner
S. laser
Sillence type II–IV osteogenesis imperfecta
Silon wound dressing
Siloskin dressing
Silphen Cough
sIL-1R
soluble type 1 interleukin-1 receptor
Silvadene
silver
s. and cadexomer iodine-based wound dressing
Grocott methenamine s. (GMS)
s. impregnation
s. nitrate
s. poisoning
s. protein, mild
s. salt
s. stain
s. sulfadiazine
Silverlon wound packing strip
silver-methenamine stain
silver-white-colored scale
silver-white scale
silvery
s. scale
s. scaly lesion
silymarin
SIM
Sandimmune
Simbu virus
simiae
herpesvirus s.
simian vacuolating virus No. 40 (SV40)
Simmond syndrome
Simplastin Excel
simple
s. allotype

s. drug
s. lentigo
s. pulmonary eosinophilia
S. Scoring System (SSS)
s. stitch
simplex
acne s.
angioma s.
Anisakis s.
dermatitis s.
disseminated herpes s.
EB s.
epidermolysis bullosa s.
Epstein-Barr s.
erythema s.
exulceratio s.
generalized epidermolysis bullosa s.
herpes s.
hidroacanthoma s.
hypertrophicum s.
ichthyosis s.
impetigo s.
lentigo s.
lichen chronicus s.
localized epidermolysis bullosa s.
lymphangioma superficium s.
ocular herpes s.
orofacial herpes s.
pityriasis s.
protoporphyria s.
prurigo s.
purpura s.
scarlatina s.
steatocystoma s.
toxoplasmosis, other infections, rubella, cytomegalovirus infection, and herpes s. (TORCH)
s. variant
verruca s.
Simpson dysmorphia syndrome
simulated
s. gastric fluid (SGF)
s. intestinal fluid (SIF)
Simulect
Simulium
simultaneous
s. double kidney transplantation (SDKT)
s. kidney-pancreas transplantation (SKPT)
s. pancreas-kidney transplant (SPK)
simvastatin

Sinarest 12-Hour Nasal solution
Sindbis
S. fever
S. virus
Sine-Aid IB
sinensis
Camellia s.
Cloncorchis s.
Sinequan
Sinex
S. Long-Acting
Vicks S.
Singh index
single
s. gel diffusion precipitin test in one dimension
s. photon emission computed tomography (SPECT)
s. radial immunodiffusion (SRID)
s. spike
single-breath nitrogen washout test
single-cell ion imaging system
single-chain
s.-c. antigen-binding (SCA)
s.-c. antigen-binding protein
single-hit kinetics
single-hook Frazier skin hook
single-lung
s.-l. transplant (SLT)
s.-l. transplant recipient
single-peak pork insulin
single-photon emission computed tomography scan
single-strand conformation polymorphism (SSCP)
single-stranded
s.-s. anti-DNA antibody
s.-s. DNA
Singleton-Merten syndrome
Single-Use Diagnostic System (SUDS)
Singulair
Sin Nombre virus
sinobronchial
SinoJect puncture set
sinopulmonary disease
Sinubid
Sinufed Timecelles
Sinulin
sinus
barber pilonidal s.
cavernous s.
cutaneous s.

S

NOTES

sinus *(continued)*
    dental s.
    s. histiocytosis (SH)
    Motrin IB S.
    pilonidal s.
    Plus S.
    preauricular s.
    Rokitansky-Aschoff s.
    s. tract
    transillumination of s.
sinusitis
    acute paranasal s.
    chronic paranasal s.
    ethmoid s.
sinusoid
    cavernous s.
    hepatic s.
sinusoidal
    s. blood flow
    s. cell
    s. lining cell injury
    s. phagocyte
sinusoidalization
Sinutab
    S. SA
    S. Tablet
sinuvertebral nerve
SIP
    Sickness Impact Profile
Siphonaptera
Siphoviridae
Sippy diet
Sips distribution
SIR
    standardized incidence ratio
siro
    Acarus s.
    Tyroglyphus s.
sirolimus
SIRS
    systemic inflammatory response
        syndrome
SIS
    Skin Intensity Score
sisal
Sister Mary Joseph nodule
Sisto sign
SIT
    specific immunotherapy
    specific injection immunotherapy
site
    antibody combining s.
    antigen-binding s.
    antigen-combining s.
    combining s.
    immune privileged s.
    immunologically privileged s.
    putative oxidative cleavage s.
    receptor s.

SiteGuard
    Centurion S.
    S. MVP transparent adhesive film
        dressing
2-site immunoradiometric assay
sitophila
    Neurospora s.
sitostanol
situ
    carcinoma in s.
    in s.
    malignant melanoma in s.
    melanoma in s.
situs inversus
SITx
    small intestinal transplantation
Six-Area, Six-Sign Atopic Dermatitis
    (SASSAD)
sixth venereal disease
size
    lesion s.
SJ441 antibody
Sjögren
    S. disease
    S. syndrome (SS)
    S. syndrome A (SS-A)
    S. syndrome B (SS-B)
Sjögren-Larsson syndrome
SJS
    Stevens-Johnson syndrome
SkareKare silicon gel-filled cushion
Skeele curette
skeletal abnormality
skiagraphica
    dermatitis s.
skimming
    scalpel s.
skin
    acid s.
    alligator s.
    Apligraf tissue-engineered s.
    artificial s.
    s. atrophy
    s. bends dermatitis
    blistering s.
    bronzed s.
    s. cancer
    citrine s.
    combination s.
    Composite cultured s. (CCS)
    crocodile s.
    deciduous s.
    diamond s.
    s. disease syndrome
    s. dissemination
    dry s.
    elastic s.
    elephant s.
    enamel paint s.

s. eruption
S. Exposure Reduction Paste Against Chemical Warfare (SERPACWA)
farmer's s.
Favre-Racouchot s.
fish s.
for s. (FS)
freeze-dried s.
glabrous s.
glossy s.
golfer's s.
granulomatous slack s.
hanging s.
hidden nail s.
s. hook
s. hydration
hyperextensible s. type I–VIII
hyperirritable s.
India rubber s.
infantile acute hemorrhagic edema of the s.
Integra artificial s.
S. Intensity Score (SIS)
s. involvement
knobby s.
lackluster s.
lax s.
leopard s.
s. lesion
s. lipid
lizard s.
loose s.
s. lubrication
s. lubrication therapy
lymphocytic infiltration of the s.
marble s.
Milian citrine s.
mixed tumor of s.
monoclonal protein, s.
mosaic s.
nail s.
non-fish-sensitive Prausnitz s.
oily s.
Oxy-5 Advanced Formula for Sensitive S.
Oxy-10 Advanced Formula for Sensitive S.
parchment s.
s. peel
piebald s.
pig s.

plucked chicken s.
porcupine s.
s. prick test (SPT)
primary macular atrophy of s.
primary neuroendocrine carcinoma of s. (PNCS)
s. punch
s. purpura
s. rash
s. reaction
s. rubor
sailor's s.
senile s.
shagreen s.
shark s.
2nd S. hydrogel sheet
slack s.
s. stone
striate atrophy of s.
sulci of s.
s. tag
S. Temp collagen
s. test antigens, multiple
s. testing
s. test unit (STU)
thickened s.
s. thickness score
toad s.
s. trephine
true s.
tuberculosis of s.
s. type
s. typing I–VI
s. ulcer
volar s.
waxy s.
s. wheal
white spots of s.
s. window technique
s. writing
yellow s.
skin-associated lymphoid tissue (SALT)
skin-based assay
skinbound disease
Skin-Cap spray
skin-colored lesion
Skindex questionnaire
skin-dominated
s.-d. epidermolysis bullosa acquisita
s.-d. linear IgA bullous dermatosis
SkinLaser system

NOTES

S

Skinlight
  S. erbium:YAG laser
  S. erbium:YAG laser system for
    skin resurfacing
skin-limited histiocytosis
skin-puncture test
Skinscan device
skin-sensitizing antibody
Skin-So-Soft
  Avon S.-S.-S.
skin-specific histocompatibility antigen
SkinTech medical tattooing device
SkinTegrity
  S. hydrogel dressing
  S. impregnated gauze
  S. wound cleanser
Skinvisible lotion
Sklowsky symptom
SKPT
  simultaneous kidney-pancreas
    transplantation
SK-SD
  streptokinase-streptodornase
skull
  hot-cross-bun s.
  natiform s.
sky-blue spot
SLA
  soluble liver antigen
slack skin
SLAM
  Systemic Lupus Activity Measure
SLAP
  superior labrum anterior and posterior
slapped-cheek
  s.-c. appearance
  s.-c. rash
slapped-face appearance
slash
  s. pine
  s. pine tree
SLC
  secondary lymphoid tissue chemokine
  synovial lining cell
SLD
  second-line drug
SLE
  systemic lupus erythematosus
  ACR diagnostic criteria for SLE
  SLE Disease Activity Index
    (SLEDAI)
SLEDAI
  SLE Disease Activity Index
sleep
  S. Aid
  alpha-nonrapid eye movement s.
  alpha-NREM s.
  s. anomaly
  s. apnea

  s. apnea/hypopnea syndrome
  s. apnea syndrome
  delta s.
  desynchronized s.
  s. disturbance
  s. efficiency
  nonREM s.
  nonrestorative s.
  paradoxical s.
  s. physiology
  rapid eye movement s.
  REM s.
  restorative s.
  slow wave s.
  stage 1, 4 s.
  s. study
sleep-disordered breathing
Sleep-Eze
  S.-E. D
  S.-E. 3 Oral
Sleepinal
Sleepwell 2-nite
SLE-like syndrome
  systemic lupus erythematosus-like
    syndrome
slender ragweed
Sleuth
  CO S.
  ETO S.
  HBT S.
SLICC
  Systemic Lupus International
    Collaborating Clinics
sliding-bucket mucosal flap
slippery
  s. elm
  s. elm tree
SLIT
  sublingual immunotherapy
SLJM
  syndrome of limited joint mobility
SLN
  sentinel lymph node
Sloan liniment
Slo-bid
Slo-Niacin
slooffiae
  Malassezia s.
slope-shouldered lesion
Slo-Phyllin GG
slough
sloughed bronchial epithelium
sloughing
  mucosal s.
  s. phagedena
  s. ulcer
slow
  s. fever
  s. virus

s. virus disease
s. vital capacity (SVC)
s. wave sleep

slow-acting antirheumatic drug (SAARD)

slow-reacting
s.-r. factor of anaphylaxis (SRF-A)
s.-r. substance (SRS)
s.-r. substance of anaphylaxis (SRS-A)

slow-twitch morphology of muscle fiber

SLP
super long-pulse

SLP1000 diode laser system

SLS
shrinking lung syndrome

SLT
secondary lymphatic tissue
single-lung transplant
split-liver transplantation
SLT recipient

slurry
talc s.

slush
dry-ice s.

sly
S. mucopolysaccharidosis
S. syndrome

SMAD
Sma- and Mad-related protein

small
s. airways dysfunction
s. bowel transplantation (SBTx)
s. intestinal transplantation (SITx)
s. noncleaved cell (SNC)
s. nuclear ribonucleoprotein (snRNP)
s. tonsil
s. vessel vasculitis

small-plaque
s.-p. parapsoriasis (SPP)
parapsoriasis s.-p.

smallpox
fulminating s.
hemorrhagic s.
malignant s.
modified s.
s. vaccine
s. virus
West Indian s.

smallpox-handler's lung

Sma- and Mad-related protein (SMAD)

Sm antigen

SMART
S. anti-CD3
S. anti-IFN-gamma

Smart Trigger

SMAS
superficial musculoaponeurotic system

smear
darkfield examination of tissue s.
nasal s.
Tzanck s.
wet s.
Ziehl-Neelsen s.

smegmatis
Mycobacterium s.

Smith antigen

Smith-Pedersen mold

Smith-Riley syndrome

smog
industrial s.
photochemical s.

smoke
cigarette s.
environmental tobacco s. (ETS)
s. inhalation
secondary s.
tobacco s.

smoker
s. keratosis
s. patch

smooth
s. jawed needle holder
s. leprosy
s. muscle hamartoma
s. muscle relaxation
s. skin-colored lesion
s. stinger

Smoothbeam nonablative diode laser technology

smotherweed

SMR
standardized mortality ratio
Standard Morbidity Ratio

SMS
stiff-man syndrome

smut
Bermuda s.
corn s.
cultivated barley s.
cultivated corn s.
cultivated oat s.
cultivated rye s.

S

NOTES

smut (*continued*)
    cultivated wheat s.
    Johnson s.
snail-track ulcer
snake
    Arizona coral s.
    s. bite
    copperhead s.
    coral s.
    cottonmouth s.
    Eastern coral s.
    pit viper s.
    sea s.
    terrestrial s.
    Texas coral s.
    s. venom
    venomous s.
    water moccasin s.
snakebite
snakeroot
    Seneca s.
SNAP
    sensory nerve action potential
    SNAP sleep recorder
snap-frozen section
Snaplets-EX
Snaplets-FR granule
snapping
    s. finger
    s. hip
SNC
    small noncleaved cell
Sneddon syndrome
Sneddon-Wilkinson disease
sneezeweed
sneezing
    paroxysmal s.
SnET2
    tin ethyl
snowball aggregate
snowbank aggregate
snowshoe hare virus
snRNP
    small nuclear ribonucleoprotein
    U3 snRNP
snuffles
SNV
    systemic necrotizing vasculitis
SO₂
    sulfur dioxide
soak therapy
soap
    Alpha-Keri s.
    antibacterial s.
    Ayndet moisturizing s.
    Baby Magic s.
    Basis s.
    Cetaphil s.
    Clinique Antiacne S.

    Clinique antibacterial s.
    deodorized mineral spirits,
      propylene glycol, fatty acid s.
    Derma S.
    s. dermatitis
    Derm-Vi S.
    Dial s.
    Dove s.
    hard-milled s.
    Lever 2000 moisture response s.
    Mazon Medicated S.
    Oil of Olay s.
    s. photoallergy
    syndet-based bar s.
soapfish dermatitis
soap-free cleanser
sobria
    Aeromonas s.
soccer toe
SODD
    silencer of death domain
sodium
    actinoquinol s.
    alendronate s.
    aminosalicylate s.
    Ampicin S.
    s. aurothioglucose
    s. aurothiomalate
    s. bicarbonate
    Brequinar s.
    carboxymethylcellulose s.
    cefazolin s.
    cefmetazole s.
    cefonicid s.
    cefoperazone s.
    cefotaxime s.
    cefoxitin s.
    ceftizoxime s.
    ceftriaxone s.
    cephalothin s.
    cephapirin s.
    s. citrate and citric acid
    cloxacillin s.
    colistimethate s.
    s. cromoglycate
    cromolyn s.
    diclofenac s.
    dicloxacillin s.
    Diphenylan S.
    s. dodecyl sulfate-polyacrylamide
      gel electrophoresis (SDS-PAGE)
    s. dodecyl sulfate-polyacrylamide
      gradient slab gel
    ertapenem s.
    s. etidronate
    s. fluoride
    foscarnet s.
    s. hyaluronate
    s. hydroxide

s. hypochlorite solution
s. hyposulfite
intravesical oxychlorosene s.
s. lauryl sulfate
Lescol fluvastatin s.
levothyroxine s.
meclofenamate s.
2-mercaptoethane sulfonate s.
  (mesna)
methicillin s.
mezlocillin s.
s. morrhuate
nafcillin s.
naproxen s.
nedocromil s.
olsalazine s.
oxacillin s.
oxychlorosene s.
pantoprazole s.
paraaminosalicylate s.
S. P.A.S.
s. pentosan
pentosan polysulfate s.
Photofrin porfimer s.
piperacillin sodium and
  tazobactam s.
s. salt
stibogluconate s.
S. Sulamyd Ophthalmic
s. sulfacetamide
s. sulfacetamide and
  fluorometholone
s. sulfacetamide lotion
s. sulfacetamide and phenylephrine
s. sulfacetamide and prednisolone
s. sulfacetamide and sulfur
s. tetradecyl sulfate
s. thiosulfate
tolmetin s.
s. versenate solution
warfarin s.
sodium-PCA
  lactic acid and s.-P.
sodium-potassium (Na⁺-K⁺)
  s.-p. ATPase pump
Sofban orthopedic padding wool
Sof-Cil
Sof-Gel palm shield
SofPulse
SofSorb absorptive dressing
soft
  s. chancre

s. corn
s. keratin
s. lesion
S. N Dry Merocel sponge
s. nevus
s. papilloma
s. sore
s. tick
s. tissue
s. tissue calcification
s. ulcer
s. wart
SoftCloth absorptive dressing
Softech endotracheal tube
SoftForm facial implant
softgel
  Sotret s.
  Vita-Plus E S.'s
SoftLight
  S. laser hair removal system
  S. laser/skin resurfacing process
Softscan laser scanner
soft-tissue
  s.-t. injection
  s.-t. injury syndrome
software
  Preview treatment planning s.
Sof-Wick dressing
Solage Topical solution
solani
  Fusarium s.
  Stemphylium s.
Solaquin
  S. Forte
  S. Forte cream
solar
  s. cheilitis
  s. comedo
  s. dermatitis
  s. elastosis
  s. fever
  s. ink-spot lentigo
  s. keratosis
  s. lentigines
  s. purpura
  s. urticaria
Solaraze gel
solare
  eczema s.
  erythema s.
solaris
  dermatitis s.

NOTES

S

solaris *(continued)*
    macula s.
    s. urticaria
Solatene
Solbar sunscreen
soldering
    s. flux
    s. fumes
soldier patch
sole
    diffuse hyperkeratosis of palms
      and s.'s
    s. dyshidrosis
    symmetric lividity of the s.'s
solenonychia
Solenopsis
    S. geminata
    S. invecta
    S. invecta sting
    S. richteri sting
    S. saevissima richteria
Solganal
solid
    s. carbon dioxide
    s. carbon dioxide pencil
    s. hidradenoma
    s. organ transplantation (SOT)
    s. phase immunoassay (SPIA)
solid-phase C1q-binding assay
solid-state dye laser
solid-tumor marker
solitary
    s. angiokeratoma
    s. keratoacanthoma
    s. mastocytoma
    s. pancreatic islet cell
      transplantation
    s. simple lymphangioma
solium
    Taenia s.
SoloSite
    S. hydrogel dressing
    S. wound gel
Soltara
soluble
    s. cell adhesion molecule
    s. c-kit (sc-kit)
    s. complement receptor type 1
      (sCR1)
    s. co-stimulatory factor
    s. Fas (sFas)
    s. liver antigen (SLA)
    s. receptor
    s. specific substance (SSS)
    S. T4
    s. tumor necrosis factor-a receptor
      (sTNFR, sTNF-RI)
    s. type 1 interleukin-1 receptor
      (sIL-1R)

Solu-Cortef
Solugel
Solumbra sunscreen clothing
Solu-Medrol Injection
solum unguis
Solurex L.A.
Soluspan
    Celestone S.
solution
    Adsorbotear Ophthalmic s.
    Afrin Nasal S.
    AK-Dilate Ophthalmic s.
    AK-Nefrin Ophthalmic s.
    Akwa Tears s.
    Alibour s.
    Allerest 12-Hour Nasal S.
    aluminum chloride s.
    Anti-Sept bactericidal scrub s.
    AquaSite Ophthalmic s.
    aqueous s.
    Atrovent Inhalation S.
    azelastine hydrochloride
      ophthalmic s.
    B5 s.
    Belzer s.
    Bion Tears s.
    Bluboro s.
    Bouin s.
    Burow s.
    carbol-fuchsin s.
    Carolina rinse s.
    Chloresium s.
    Chlorphed-LA Nasal S.
    ciclopirox topical s.
    Collins s.
    Comfort Tears s.
    Crolom Ophthalmic s.
    Custodiol HTK s.
    Dakrina Ophthalmic s.
    Dey-Drop Ophthalmic s.
    Dristan Long Lasting Nasal s.
    Dry Eye Therapy s.
    DuoFilm S.
    Duration Nasal s.
    Dwelle Ophthalmic s.
    EC s.
    elastoviscous s.
    Euro-Collins s.
    Exidine s.
    extracellular crystalloid s.
    Eye-Lube-A s.
    flunisolide nasal s.
    Fowler s.
    Fungoid AF Topical s.
    hairdressing s.
    Hanks balanced salt s. (HBSS)
    HypoTears PF s.
    hypotonic s.
    Intal Nebulizer s.

intracellular crystalloid s.
I-Phrine Ophthalmic s.
Isopto Frin Ophthalmic s.
Isopto Plain s.
Isopto Tears s.
Just Tears s.
Kaletra oral s.
Lacril Ophthalmic s.
Liquifilm Forte s.
Liquifilm Tears s.
lopinavir/ritonavir oral s.
Lotrimin AF S.
LubriTears s.
Melanex s.
Mercuroclear s.
methoxsalen sterile s.
Michel s.
Monsel s.
Murine s.
Murocel Ophthalmic s.
Mydfrin Ophthalmic s.
NasalCrom nasal s.
Nature's Tears s.
Neosporin Ophthalmic S.
Neosporin scar s.
Neo-Synephrine 12-Hour Nasal s.
Neo-Synephrine Ophthalmic s.
NTZ Long Acting Nasal S.
Nu-Tears II s.
OcuCoat PF Ophthalmic s.
POL sclerosing s.
potassium permanganate s.
precipitate in s.
Prefrin Ophthalmic s.
Procuven s.
Puralube Tears s.
Refinity skin care s.
Refresh Plus Ophthalmic s.
Relief Ophthalmic s.
Resectisol Irrigation s.
Saint Thomas s.
salt s.
SangCya oral s.
Shohl s.
Sinarest 12-Hour Nasal s.
sodium hypochlorite s.
sodium versenate s.
Solage Topical s.
STS sclerosing s.
Tear Drop s.
TearGard Ophthalmic s.
Teargen Ophthalmic s.

Tearisol s.
Tears Naturale Free s.
Tears Naturale II s.
Tears Plus s.
Tears Renewed s.
Travatan s.
travoprost s.
tris-buffered saline s. (TBS)
trivalent oral poliovirus s.
Tween-TRIS-buffered saline s.
 (TTBS)
Twice-A-Day Nasal s.
Ultra Tears s.
University of Wisconsin s.
UV s.
UW s.
Verukan s.
Vicks Sinex Long-Acting Nasal s.
vinegar s.
Viva-Drops s.
Vleminckx s.
4-Way Long Acting Nasal S.

Soluver plus
solvent-based mascara
somaliensis
    Streptomyces s.
somatic
    s. agglutinin
    s. antigen
    s. hypermutation
    s. mutation
SomatoKine
somatomedin C
somatosensory evoked response
somatotype
    body s.
somatropin
Somavert
Sominex Oral
sommeil
    maladie du s.
SomnoStar apnea testing device
soni
    Moniliformis s.
sonicate
Sonne dysentery
sonnei
    Shigella s.
sonometer
    UBIS 500 ultrasound bone s.
Sony VHS HQ Digital Picture video
Soothe-N-Seal

NOTES

soot wart
SorbaView
    Centurion S.
    S. wound dressing
sorbitan sesquioleate (SS)
Sorbsan
    S. alginate dressing
    S. alginate wound cover
    S. wound dressing
sordes
sore
    bay s.
    bed s.
    canker s.
    chrome s.
    Cochin s.
    cold s.
    Delhi s.
    desert s.
    diphtheric desert s.
    fever s.
    fungating s.
    Gallipoli s.
    hard s.
    Kandahar s.
    Lahore s.
    mixed s.
    s. mouth
    Naga s.
    Oriental s.
    pressure s.
    primary s.
    soft s.
    summer s.
    tropical s.
    Umballa s.
    veldt s.
    venereal s.
    water s.
soremouth virus
soremuzzle
soreness
sor gene
sorghum grass
Soriatane
sorivudine
sorrel
    sheep s.
sorter
sorting
    automated magnetic cell s.
      (autoMACS)
    fluorescent-activated cell s. (FACS)
SOT
    solid organ transplantation
Soto syndrome
Sotradecol
Sotret softgel
souffle

sound
    coarse breath s.'s
    diminished breath s.'s
    pulmonic valve closure s.
source
    intense pulsed light s. (IPLS)
    monochromatic light s.
    PhotoDerm filtered, flashlamp-
      pumped light s.
    PhotoDerm VL light s.
south
    S. African genetic porphyria
    S. African hemorrhagic fever
    S. African tick fever
    S. American blastomycosis
    S. American trypanosomiasis
Southeast Asian fever
Southern blot
sowdah
soy
    s. milk
    s. protein allergy
Soyalac
soybean
    s. flour
    s. grain dust mite
    s. meal
    s. trypsin inhibitor (STI)
SP
    Cordran SP
Sp-100
SP-10 spirometer
SP90 miniblade
SpA
  spondyloarthropathy
space
    blood-filled slit-like s.
    intercellular s.
    marrow s.
    medial hemijoint articular s.
    physiological dead s.
    subgaleal s.
    Tenon s.
space-occupying lesion
spacer
    Ellipse compact s.
SPAD
    selective antipolysaccharide antibody
      deficiency
spade finger
spaghetti and meatballs appearance of
  spores and hyphae
Spanish
    S. fly
    S. fly sting
    S. influenza
    S. toxic oil syndrome
Spanlang-Tappeiner syndrome

spanner
  multimembrane s.
sparfloxacin
sparganosis
sparing
  island of s.
spark-gap apparatus
SPART analyzer
spasm
  epidemic transient diaphragmatic s.
spasmogen
spatiotemporal gait parameters
SpaTouch PhotoEpilation system
spatula
  Roux s.
SPE
  serum protein electrophoretogram
  streptococcal pyrogenic exotoxin
Spearman rank test
spearmint
specialized transduction
special lesion
species
  Phoma s.
  reactive oxygen s. (ROS)
species-specific antigen
specific
  s. active immunity
  s. allergy vaccination (SAV)
  s. alteration in immunologic
    reactivity
  s. anergy
  s. antibody deficiency (SAD)
  s. antigen
  s. antiserum
  s. bactericide
  s. capsular substance
  s. disease
  s. hemolysin
  s. IgE antibody level
  s. immune globulin (human)
  s. immunotherapy (SIT)
  s. injection immunotherapy (SIT)
  s. opsonin
  s. passive immunity
  s. reaction
  s. serum
  s. soluble polysaccharide
  s. soluble sugar
  s. transduction
specificity
speck finger

speckled
  s. lentiginous nevus
  s. staining
speckled-pattern
  s.-p. ANA
  s.-p. antinuclear antibody
SPECT
  single photon emission computed
  tomography
  SPECT scan
Spectam injection
Spectazole topical
spectinomycin hydrochloride
spectra (*pl. of* spectrum)
spectral analysis
spectratyping
Spectrobid
spectrofluorometer
spectrofluorometry
spectrophotometer
spectrophotometry
spectroscopy
  diffuse reflectance s. (DRS)
Spectro Tar
spectrum, pl. **spectra**
  antimicrobial s.
  broad s.
  S. Designs facial implant
  radiation s.
  S. ruby laser
  toxin s.
  wide s.
speech apraxia
Spencer scissors
Spengler fragment
SPEP
  serum protein electrophoresis
  SPEP test
spermatolysin
spermatolysis
spermatolytic
spermatoxin
spermine
spermolysis
spermotoxin
Spexil
SPF
  sun protection factor
sphacelation
sphaceloderma
sphaericus
  Bacillus s.

S

NOTES

sphenoethmoidectomy
sphenoid dysplasia
spherocytosis
> hereditary s.

Spherulin
sphigosine kinase
Sphingobacterium
sphingolipid
sphingolipidosis
Sphingomonas paucimobilis
sphingomyelinase-D
SPI
> Standards for Pediatric Immunization

SPIA
> solid phase immunoassay

spica cast
spicata
> *Mentha s.*

spicule
> hyperkeratotic s.

spider
> s. angioma
> arterial s.
> s. bite
> black widow s.
> brown recluse s.
> s. ectasia
> fiddle-back s.
> s. hemangioma
> s. mole
> s. nevus
> s. telangiectasia
> s. telangiectasis
> s. venom
> violin-back s.

spider-burst
Spiegler-Fendt
> S.-F. pseudolymphoma
> S.-F. sarcoid

Spiegler tumor
spike
> s. formation
> single s.

spiloma
spiloplaxia
spilus
> nevus s.

spina
> s. bifida-associated latex allergy
> s. pedis

spinach
spinal
> s. accessory nerve palsy
> s. dysraphism
> s. fluid test

spinale
> tache s.

spindle
> s. cell

s. cell carcinoma (SC)
s. cell hemangioendothelioma
s. cell lipoma
s. cell melanoma
s. and epithelioid cell nevus
spindle-shaped cell
spine
> bamboo s.
> horny s.
> lumbar s.
> Rugger-jersey s.
> venom-bearing s.

spin-echo pulse
Spinhaler inhaler
spinigerum
> *Gnathostoma s.*

spinipalpis
> *Ixodes s.*

spinosa
> ichthyosis s.

spinosum
> stratum s.

spinous layer
spinulosa
> trichostasis s.

spinulosus
> folliculitis decalvans et lichen s.
> lichen pilaris seu s.

spiny
> s. pigweed
> s. structure

spiradenitis
spiradenoma
> eccrine s.
> malignant eccrine s.

spiral
> Curschmann s.
> Herxheimer s.

spiralis
> *Trichinella s.*

spiramycin
spirillar
> s. abscess
> s. dysentery

Spirillum minus
Spirochaeta pallida
spirochetal
> s. disease
> s. isolate

spirochete
> corkscrew s.
> s. infection

spirochetemia
spirochetolysis
spirochetosis
spirogram
spirometer
> Flash portable s.
> MicroPlus s.

Pulmonet s.
SP-10 s.
Spirovit SP-1 portable s.
spirometric screening
spirometry
incentive s.
Tri-Flow incentive s.
spironolactone
Spiroplasma apis
SpiroSense flow sensor
Spirovit SP-1 portable spirometer
spiruroid larva migrans
Spitz
S. nevus
S. tumor
spitzoid malignant melanoma
SPK
simultaneous pancreas-kidney transplant
SPK transplant
splash
rain s.
wave s.
splatter
fountain-spray s.
spleen
synergic s.
splendens
lamina s.
Splendore-Hoeppli phenomenon
splenectomy (Splx)
splenic index
splenomegaly
splenotoxin
spliceosomal component
splicing
phosphorylated serine/arginine s.
splint
hindfoot s.
resting s.
shin s.
splinter
s. forceps
s. hemorrhage
split
s. adjuvant technique
s. papule
s. tolerance
split-liver transplantation (SLT)
split-thickness skin graft (STSG)
splitting nail
split-virus vaccine

Splx
splenectomy
spodogenous
spodophorous
Spondweni virus
spondylitica
psoriasis s.
spondylitis
ankylosing s. (AS)
Bekhterev-Strümpell s.
juvenile ankylosing s. (JAS)
s. ossificans ligamentosa
predominant s.
psoriatic s.
Schober test for s.
spondyloarthropathy (SpA)
seronegative s.
undifferentiated s.
spondylodiscitis
spondylodiscitis, spondylodiskitis
spondyloepiphysial, spondyloepiphyseal
s. dysplasia (SED)
spondylolisthesis
isthmic s.
spondylolysis
spondylometry
spondylosis
s. deformans
s. hyperostotica
ochronotic s.
sponge
chondrocyte s.
s. diver disease
s. fisherman disease
Helistat collagen matrix s.
Instat collagen matrix s.
Soft N Dry Merocel s.
s. spicule dermatitis
spongiform
s. pustule
s. pustule of Kogoj
spongiosis
eosinophilic s.
spongiotic vesicle
spontanea
dactylolysis s.
spontaneous
s. agglutination
s. allergy
s. gangrene of newborn
s. phagocytosis
s. pseudoscar

S

NOTES

spontaneous *(continued)*
  s. regression
  s. spinal epidural hematoma
    (SSEH)
spoon
  s. nail
  sharp s.
spora
  air s.
sporadic
  s. atypical mole-melanoma
    syndrome
  s. dysentery
  s. typhus
sporangiospore
sporangium
Sporanox oral
spore
  airborne s.
  mold s.
Sporidin-G
sporoagglutination
Sporobolomyces salmonicolor
Sporothrix schenckii
sporotrichosis
  cutaneous s.
  disseminated s.
  fixed cutaneous s.
  mucocutaneous s.
  visceral s.
sporotrichositic chancre
sporotrichotic chancre
Sporotrichum schenckii
sporotricoid pattern
sporotriquin test
sporozoite
sporozooid
sport
  Coppertone S.
  Fruit of the Earth Moisturizing
    Aloe S.
  London Drugs S.
  s.'s medicine
  S. Wipes
sports-related pain syndrome
SPO₂T
  Pocket SPO₂T
spot
  antimony s.
  ash leaf s.
  Bier s.
  Bitot s.
  blue s.
  café-au-lait s.
  Campbell-De Morgan s.
  cayenne pepper s.
  cherry s.
  Christopher s.
  cinnabar red s.

cotton-wool s.
De Morgan s.
Filatov s.
Forchheimer s.
Fordyce s.
gift s.
Horder s.
Koplik s.
liver s.
mongolian s.
mulberry s.
pain s.
pink s.
rose s.
Roth s.
ruby s.
sacral s.
shin s.
sky-blue s.
temperature s.
s. test
Trousseau s.
typhoid s.
warm s.
s. weld
SpotCheck+ handheld pulse oximeter
spotted
  s. fever
  s. leprosy
  s. lunula
  s. sickness
spotted-fever tick
SPP
  small-plaque parapsoriasis
spray
  aerosol s.
  Astelin Nasal S.
  azelastine hydrochloride nasal s.
  CaldeCort Anti-Itch Topical S.
  Clear Caladryl S.
  Decongestant nasal s.
  Eucerin itch-relief moisturizing dry
    skin therapy s.
  Fluori-Methane Topical S.
  fluticasone propionate aqueous
    nasal s. (FPANS)
  Nasarel Nasal S.
  Ony-Clear S.
  Skin-Cap s.
  triamcinolone acetonide s.
  Tri-Nasal S.
  vapocoolant s.
spreading
  epitope s.
  s. phenomenon
spring
  s. dermatosis
  s. ophthalmia
spring-assisted knee extension orthosis

Spritz
    Itch Relief Gel S.
sprout
    Brussels s.
SPRT
    sequential probability ratio test
spruce
    s. pollen
    s. tree
sprue
    celiac s.
    nontropical s.
SPS
    Proteque SPS
SPT
    skin prick test
SPTL
    subcutaneous panniculitis-like T-cell leukemia
    subcutaneous panniculitis-like T-cell lymphoma
Spumavirinae
Spumavirus
spun-glass hair
spur
    bony s.
    calcaneal s.
    heel s.
Spurling sign
sputum, pl. **sputa**
    copious s.
    purulent s.
    s. viscosity and elasticity
SpyroDerm
SQ
    subcutaneous
squama, squame
squamate
squamosum
    eczema s.
    erythroderma s.
squamous
    s. cell
    s. cell carcinoma (SCC)
    s. cell epithelioma
    s. cell layer
    s. cell lung tumor
    s. intraepithelial lesion (SIL)
square-shouldered lesion
squaric acid dibutylester (SADBE)
squarrose
squash

squeeze effect
Squirt wound irrigation system
SR
    sustained release
      Aerolate SR
      Deconamine SR
      Respaire-120 SR
      Respaire-60 SR
      Surgam SR
Sr
    Congess Sr
SRC
    scleroderma renal crisis
SRF-A
    slow-reacting factor of anaphylaxis
SRID
    single radial immunodiffusion
SRM
    standardized response mean
SRP
    signal recognition particle
SRS
    slow-reacting substance
SRS-A
    slow-reacting substance of anaphylaxis
SS
    Sézary syndrome
    Sjögren syndrome
    sorbitan sesquioleate
      SS hemoglobin disease
      Uroplus SS
S.S.
    Argyrol S.S.
SS-A
    Sjögren syndrome A
SS-B
    Sjögren syndrome B
SSC
    saline sodium citrate
    suprascapular nerve compression
SSc
    systemic sclerosis
SSCP
    single-strand conformation polymorphism
SSD
      SSD AF
      SSD Cream
SSEH
    spontaneous spinal epidural hematoma
S-shaped closure
SSKI
    saturated solution of potassium iodide

NOTES

SSLND
  selective sentinel lymph node dissection
SSM
  superficial spreading melanoma
SSOP
  sequence-specific oligonucleotide probe
    hybridization
SSP
  sequence-specific primer
SSPE
  subacute sclerosing panencephalitis
SSS
  Simple Scoring System
  soluble specific substance
    SSS score
SSSS
  staphylococcal scalded skin syndrome
ssSSc
  systemic sclerosis sine scleroderma
SSZ
  sulfasalazine
S-T
  S-T Cort
  S-T Cort topical
ST
  surrogate tolerogenesis
St. (*var. of* Saint)
stabilate
stable
  s. fly
  s. fly bite
  s. knob trimer
  microsatellite s.
  s. vitiligo
stacking
  epidermal s.
stadiometry
stadium, pl. **stadia**
  s. acmes
  s. augmenti
  s. caloris
  s. decrementi
  s. defervescentiae
  s. fluorescentiae
  s. frigoris
  s. incrementi
  s. invasionis
  s. sudoris
stage
  algid s.
  cold s.
  convalescent s.
  defervescent s.
  IAET s.'s
  incubative s.
  s. of invasion
  Kellgren-Lawrence s.
  latent s.
  meningeal s.

  patch s.
  plaque s.
  prodromal s.
  s. 1, 4 sleep
  Tanner pubertal s.
  tumor s.
staged abdominal repair (STAR)
2-stage reaction
staging
  Ann Arbor s.
  Breslow thickness in melanoma s.
  s. classification for Hodgkin
    disease
  TNM s.
stain
  acid Schiff s.
  ACIS immunohistochemical s.
  Alcian blue s.
  aldehyde-fuchsin s. (AFS)
  alizarin red S s.
  Automated Cellular Imaging System
    immunohistochemical s.
  Bodian s.
  bovine rotavirus s.
  Brown-Brenn s.
  Brown and Brenn s.
  calcofluor s.
  Clay-Adams s.
  Congo red s.
  cytotoxin-positive s.
  Dieterle s.
  Diff-Quik s.
  dopa s.
  elastic fiber s.
  eosin s.
  Evans blue s.
  Fite s.
  Giemsa s.
  Gram s.
  hematoxylin and eosin s. (H&E)
  Hotchkiss-McManus s.
  immunofluorescent s.
  Kinyoun s.
  levodopa s.
  Masson trichrome s.
  MPO bone marrow s.
  mucicarmine s.
  myeloperoxidase bone marrow s.
  neuron-specific enolase s.
  nonspecific esterase s.
  NSE s.
  PAS s.
  periodic acid-Schiff s.
  phloxine-tartrazine s.
  pneumococcal s.
  port-wine s. (PWS)
  potassium chloride s. (KOH)
  rose-bengal s.
  Safranin O s.

silver s.
silver-methenamine s.
Swartz-Lamkins s.
Swartz-Medrik s.
Verhoeff-van Gieson s.
walnut-juice s.
Warthin-Starry s.
Wright s.
Ziehl-Neelsen s.
staining
avidin-biotin-peroxidase s.
diffuse s.
hematoxylin-eosin s.
Hoechst s.
nucleolar s.
oil s.
pattern of s.
peripheral s.
phalloidin s.
Safranin O/Fast-Green s.
speckled s.
Stallerkit
Stallerpointe needle
staminate
standard
s. deviation (SD)
S. Morbidity Ratio (SMR)
National Committee for Clinical
Laboratory S.'s (NCCLS)
S.'s for Pediatric Immunization
(SPI)
Uranyl Standard fluorescence s.
standardized
s. incidence ratio (SIR)
s. mortality ratio (SMR)
s. response mean (SRM)
standing cutaneous cone defect
**Stanford Health Assessment
Questionnaire (HAQ)**
stanozolol
Stanton disease
Staphcillin
StaphVAX
staphylococcal
s. abscess
s. blepharitis
s. enterotoxin
s. protein A binding assay
s. scalded skin syndrome (SSSS)
s. toxic shock syndrome
staphylococcal-binding assay

staphylococcolysin
staphylococcolysis
Staphylococcus
S. *albus*
S. antitoxin
S. *aureus*
S. *aureus* arthritis
S. *aureus* vaccine
S. *epidermidis*
S. *hominis*
S. *lugdunensis*
S. protein A column therapy
staphyloderma
staphylodermatitis
staphylogenes
impetigo s.
sycosis s.
staphylohemolysin
staphylolysin
staphylotoxin
stapler
Auto Suture SFS s.
Precise s.
Premium s.
Proximate II, III s.
Proximate RH s.
USSC s.
stapling
bleb s.
STAR
staged abdominal repair
star
S. Sync
venous s.
**Starcam large field of view gamma
camera**
starch bath
starch-iodine test
starfish
s. dermatitis
s. sting
starry-sky pattern
startle disease
starvation syndrome
stasis
dermatitis s.
s. dermatitis
eczema s.
s. eczema
s. purpura
s. vascular ulcer

S

NOTES

STAT
    signal transducer and activator of transcription
    signal transduction and activator of transcription
state
    anaphylactic s.
    carrier s.
    excited s.
    hypercoagulable s.
    hyperimmune s.
static gangrene
Staticin topical
stationary phase
statistical analysis system (SAS)
statistics
    National Center for Health S. (NCHS)
stature
    brittle hair, intellectual impairment, decreased fertility, short s. (BIDS)
    decreased fertility, short s.
    ichthyosis plus brittle hair, intellectual impairment, decreased fertility, short s. (IBIDS)
    photosensitivity, ichthyosis, brittle hair, impaired intelligence, decreased fertility, and short s.
    photosensitivity, ichthyosis, brittle hair, intellectual impairment, decreased fertility, and short s.
status
    s. asthmaticus
    s. cosmeticus
    s. criticus
    s. epilepticus
staurosporine
stavudine
STD
    sexually transmitted disease
STD-E Pads
steal effect
stealthing gene
Stealth virus
stearalkonium ammonium chloride
stearic acid
stearothermophilus
    Bacillus s.
steatocystoma
    multiplex s.
    s. multiplex
    s. simplex
steatohepatitis
steatoides
    pityriasis s.
steatoma
steatorrhea
    postinfectious s.

steatosis
    macrovesicular s.
    microvesicular s.
steel
    S. Bars high protein nutrition bar
    s. factor
Steen and Medsger study
Stegman-Tromovitch bandage
Steinberg
    S. test
    S. thumb sign
Steinbrocker
    S. classification
    S. criteria
Stein-Leventhal syndrome
stellar nevus
stellate
    s. abscess
    s. angioma
    s. ganglion block
    s. ganglion blockade
    s. hair
    s. morphology
    s. pattern
    s. patterned disease
    s. pseudoscar
    s. telangiectasis
stem
    s. cell
    s. cell factor (SCF)
    s. cell transplant (SCT)
    s. cell transplantation
Stemex
Stemphylium
    S. botryosum
    S. solani
stenosing tenosynovitis
stenosis, pl. stenoses
    bronchial s.
    cicatricial s.
    lumbar spinal s.
    subglottic tracheal s.
    tracheal s.
stenothermal
Stenotrophomonas maltophilia
stent
    T-Y s.
stenting
    ureteric s.
Stephania tetranda
Stephanurus dentatus
Sterapred oral
stercoralis
    Strongyloides s.
stereomicroscope
sterile
    s. abscess
    s. eosinophilic pustulosis

s. pustule
s. technique
sterilisans
therapia magna s.
sterility
sterilization
discontinuous s.
fractional s.
intermittent s.
sterilize
sterilizer
Steri-Strips
Sterneedle tuberculin test
sternoclavicular
s. articulation
s. disease
s. hyperostosis
s. joint
s. joint degeneration
sternocleidomastoid muscle
sternocostal joint
sternocostoclavicular hyperostosis
sternomastoid
steroid
s. acne
anabolic s.
s. burst
s. chalk
s. fever
group 5 topical s.
s. myopathy
Psorcon topical s.
s. pulse
s. purpura
s. sulfatase deficiency
systemic s.
s. taper
topical s.
s. ulcer
steroid-dependent asthma
steroidogenic enzyme
steroid-resistant acute rejection
steroid-sparing
s.-s. regimen
s.-s. treatment
sterol
stethoscope dermatitis
Stevens-Johnson syndrome (SJS)
Stevens tenotomy scissors
Stewart-Treves syndrome

STI
short-term immunotherapy
soybean trypsin inhibitor
stibogluconate sodium
Sticker disease
Stickler
S. syndrome
S. syndrome, type I, II, III
Stieva-A Forte
Stifcore
stiff-hand syndrome
stiff-man syndrome (SMS)
stiffness
morning s.
stiff-person syndrome
stiff-skin syndrome
stigma, pl. **stigmata**
stigmatic
stilbestrol
Still disease
stimulating factor (SF)
stimulation
alpha adrenergic s.
beta-adrenergic s.
s. index (SI)
juxtacrine s.
transcutaneous electrical nerve s. (TENS)
stimulator
long-acting thyroid s. (LATS)
photonic s.
Sham transcutaneous electrical nerve s.
transcutaneous electrical neuromuscular s. (TENS)
stimulea
Sibine s.
stimulus, pl. **stimuli**
chemical s.
extrauterine environmental s.
physical s.
psychological s.
sting
Africanized honeybee s.
ant s.
Apis mellifera s.
arthropod s.
ashgray blister beetle s.
bark scorpion s.
bee s.
blister beetle s.
blue bottle s.

NOTES

S

sting *(continued)*
  Bombus s.
  box jellyfish s.
  brown moth larvae s.
  brown-tail moth s.
  bumblebee s.
  caterpillar s.
  catfish s.
  Centruroides exilicauda s.
  Centruroides sculpturatus s.
  Centruroides vittatus s.
  Chironex fleckeri s.
  coelenterate s.
  common striped scorpion s.
  Dolichorespula s.
  Epicauta fabricii s.
  Epicauta vitlata s.
  Euproctis chrysorrhoea s.
  European blister beetle s.
  fire ant s.
  fire coral s.
  gypsy moth larva s.
  honeybee s.
  hornet s.
  Hymenoptera s.
  insect s.
  Io moth larva s.
  jellyfish s.
  Lymantria dispar s.
  Lytta vesicata s.
  marine animal s.
  Megabombus s.
  Megalopyge opercularis s.
  millipede s.
  Paederus gemellus s.
  Paederus limnophilus s.
  Paravespula s.
  Polistes s.
  Portuguese man-of-war s.
  puss caterpillar s.
  Pyrobombus s.
  red imported fire ant s.
  saddleback caterpillar s.
  scorpion s.
  sea anemone s.
  sea cucumber s.
  sea urchin s.
  Sibine stimulea s.
  Solenopsis invecta s.
  Solenopsis richteri s.
  Spanish fly s.
  starfish s.
  sting ray s.
  striped blister beetle s.
  Vespula s.
  wasp s.
  yellow jacket s.
stinger
  barbed s.

embedded s.
smooth s.
stinging
  s. caterpillar
  s. coral dermatitis
  s. water dermatitis
stingray hickey
stink gland
stinkweed
stippled nail
STIR
  short tau inversion recovery
stitch
  buried subcutaneous s.
  corner s.
  half-buried mattress s.
  horizontal mattress s.
  running intradermal s.
  running simple s.
  simple s.
  tip s.
  vertical mattress s.
STM
  streptomycin
sTNFR
  soluble tumor necrosis factor-a receptor
  sTNFR gene
sTNF-RI
  soluble tumor necrosis factor-a receptor
Stobo antigen
stochastic methylation
stock
  s. strain
  s. vaccine
stocking
  s. nevus
  Venodyne compression s.
  Zipzoc s.
Stockman nodule
stoichiometry
Stokoguard outdoor cream
stomach
  watermelon s.
stomal dermatitis
stomatitis
  allergic contact s.
  angular s.
  aphthous s.
  bovine papular s.
  cotton roll s.
  denture s.
  fusospirochetal s.
  gangrenous s.
  gonococcal s.
  herpetiform aphthous s.
  lead s.
  s. medicamentosa
  mercurial s.
  nicotine s.

s. papulosa
primary herpetic s.
ulcerative s.
vesicular s. (VS)
stomatodynia
stomatomalacia
stomatomycosis
stomatonecrosis
stomatonoma
stomatopyrosis
Stomoxys **bite**
stone
pumice s.
renal s.
skin s.
uric acid s.
stool
s. culture
mucous s.
stool-step maneuver
stop bath
"stop" signal
storage
cold s. (CS)
ex vivo organ s.
neutral lipid s.
phytanic acid s.
store and forward images
stork-bite lesion
Stoxil
straight hair nevus
straight-leg
s.-l. duration maneuver
s.-l. lift maneuver
s.-l. raising test
strain
BORSA s.
carrier s.
cell s.
0157-H7 s.
hypothetical mean s. (HMS)
lysogenic s.
modified vaccinia virus Ankara s.
musculoligamentous s.
pseudolysogenic s.
rabies virus, Flury s.
rabies virus, Kelev s.
recombinant s.
stock s.
type s.
strand
AcryDerm S.'s

complementary s.
homology of s.
plus s.
viral s.
S-transferase
strata (*pl. of* stratum)
StrataSorb composite wound dressing
strategy
prime-boost s.
sawtooth s.
stratification
stratum, pl. **strata**
s. basale
central s.
s. compactum
s. corneum (SC)
s. corneum epidermidis
s. corneum hydration device
s. corneum unguis
s. disjunctum
s. germinativum
s. granulosum (SG)
s. lucidum
s. malpighii
s. mucosum
s. spinosum
straw
s. itch
oat s.
strawberry
s. angioma
s. birthmark
s. hemangioma
s. hypertrophicum
s. mark
s. nevus
s. tongue
streak
angioid s.
meningitic s.
streaking
s. leukocyte factor
linear s.
street virus
strength
Allerest Maximum S.
Aspirin Free Anacin Maximum S.
Bayer Low Adult S.
Clearasil Maximum S.
Clocort Maximum S.
Cortaid Maximum S.
Vanceril Double S.

S

NOTES

streptavidin-biotinperoxidase procedure
streptobacillary fever
Streptobacillus moniliformis
streptocerca
    Dipetalonema s.
    Mansonella s.
streptococcal
    s. balanoposthitis
    s. cellulitis
    s. M1
    s. M3
    s. M antigen
    s. nephritis
    s. pharyngitis
    s. pyrogenic exotoxin (SPE)
    s. septicemia
    s. tonsillitis
    s. toxic shock syndrome
streptococci
Streptococcus
    S. agalactiae
    beta-hemolytic *S.*
    S. erythrogenic toxin
    S. faecalis
    group A *S.* (GAS)
    group A beta-hemolytic *S.*
      (GABHS)
    group B *S.* (GBS)
    hemolytic *S.*
    S. infection
    S. intermedius
    S. M antigen
    S. pyogenes
    S. viridans
streptoderma
streptodermatitis
streptogenes
    erythema s.
streptogramin
streptokinase-streptodornase (SK-SD)
streptolysin O
Streptomyces
    S. somaliensis
    S. toyocaensis
    S. tsukubaensis
streptomycin (STM)
    G unit of s.
    L unit of s.
    s. sulfate
    S unit of s.
    s. unit
streptozyme
    s. agglutination test
    s. titer
stress
    emotional s.
    s. fracture
    intrapsychic s.

    oxidative s. (OS)
    redox s.
stress-activated protein 1 (SAP-1)
stress-generated electric potential
stretch
    s. mark
    s. reflex
stria, pl. **striae**
    s. alba
    s. albicans
    atrophic s.
    s. atrophica
    striae cutis distensae
    elastotic s.
    striae gravidarum
    s. nasi transversa
    s. rubra
    s. scleroatrophy
    Wickham s.
striaelike epidermal distention
striata
    dermatitis pratensis s.
    leukonychia s.
    melanonychia s.
striatal
striate atrophy of skin
striatum
    atrophoderma s.
striatus
    lichen s.
stricto
    sensu s.
stridor
string
    s. bean
    s. of pearls configuration
strip
    Breathe Right nasal s.
    Cover-Strip wound closure s.
    Hansamed s.
    Nu-Hope skin barrier s.
    Silverlon wound packing s.
stripe
    Mees s.
    s. technique
striped
    s. blister beetle
    s. blister beetle sting
stripper
    Fischer s.
    Oesch perforation invagination s.
stroke volume (SV)
stromal cell
stromal-cell-derived factor-1 (SDF-1)
stromatolysis
stromelysin
Strongyloides
    S. stercoralis
    S. venezuelensis

strongyloidiasis
disseminated s.
Strongylus
strontium sulfide
strophulosus
lichen s.
strophulus
s. candidus
s. intertinctus
s. pruriginosus
Strother acrochordonectomy
Structural Classification of Proteins (SCOP)
structure
amyloid s.
fibril s.
gene s.
hair-like s.
osmiophilic crystal s.
pilosebaceous s.
spiny s.
tertiary s.
struma, pl. strumae
Riedel s.
strumosa
dactylitis s.
strumous
s. abscess
s. bubo
Strümpell disease
Struthers
ligament of S.
strychnine poisoning
Stryker
S. arthroscope
S. microshaver
Stryker-Halbeisen syndrome
S.T.S.
serologic test for syphilis
STSG
split-thickness skin graft
STS sclerosing solution
STU
skin test unit
stucco keratosis
stuck-on appearance
study
aerometric s.
case control s.
cohort s.
Collaboration Transplant S.

European Anti-ICAM Renal Transplant S. (EARTS)
S. of Left Ventricular Dysfunction
meglumine diatrizoate enema s.
metabolic s.
NASTRA s.
nerve conduction s. (NCS)
North American Pediatric Rental Transplant Cooperative S. (NAPRTCS)
North American Study of Treatment for Refractory Ascites s.
Pepscan s.
QUEST s.
Rodriguez-Castellanos s.
secretory antibody s.
sleep s.
Steen and Medsger s.
tagged white blood cell s.
T1-weighted s.
T2-weighted s.
UFC s.
urinary free cortisol s.
stupe
Sturge-Weber
S.-W. encephalotrigeminal angiomatosis
S.-W. syndrome
stutzeri
Pseudomonas s.
sty, stye
Styloviridae
styptic
s. collodion
s. pencil
STZ titer
SUA
serum uric acid
Su antigen
subacromial bursitis
subacuta
prurigo simplex s.
subacute
s. bacterial endocarditis (SBE)
s. cutaneous lupus erythematosus (SCLE)
s. inclusion body encephalitis
s. nodular migratory panniculitis
s. phase shoulder impairment
s. sclerosing leukoencephalitis

S

NOTES

subacute *(continued)*
   s. sclerosing panencephalitis (SSPE)
   s. spongiform encephalopathy
subaponeurotic hemorrhage
subaxial
   s. involvement
   s. listhesis
subbasement
   s. membrane (SBM)
   s. membrane thickening
subcalcaneal pain syndrome
subchondral
   s. bone pain
   s. cyst
   s. erosion
   s. fracture
subclass
   immunoglobulin s.
subclinical
   s. asthma
   s. leprosy
subconfluent keratinocyte
subcorneal
   s. blister
   s. pustular dermatitis
   s. pustular dermatosis
subcutanea
   lipogranulomatosis s.
   urticaria s.
subcutaneous (sc, SQ)
   s. calcification
   s. dirofilariasis
   s. emphysema
   s. epinephrine
   s. fat necrosis
   s. fat necrosis of newborn
   s. felon
   s. fungal infection
   s. fungus
   s. granuloma annulare
   s. granulomatous nodule
   s. immunoglobulin (SCIG)
   s. injection
   s. morphea
   s. mycosis
   s. myiasis
   s. necrotizing infection
   s. nevus
   s. panniculitis-like T-cell lymphoma (SPTL)
   s. phycomycosis
   s. pseudosarcomatous fibromatosis
   s. rheumatoid nodule
   s. T-cell lymphoma
subcuticular felon
subcutis
subdeltoid bursitis
subdermal
subdermic

subepidermal
   s. abscess
   s. calcified nodule
   s. nodular fibrosis
   s. vesiculation
subepithelia
subepithelial
   s. basement membrane (SBM)
   s. fibrosis
subepithelium
suberosis
subfecundity
subgaleal space
subgallate
   bismuth s.
subglottic tracheal stenosis
subglottis
subinfection
subinhibitory
subintegumental
subitum
   exanthema s.
subjective synonym
sublamina densa
sublingual immunotherapy (SLIT)
sublingual-swallow immunotherapy
subluxation
   atlantoaxial s.
   dorsoradial s.
   metacarpophalangeal joint s.
   palmar s.
   rheumatoid atlantoaxial s.
submersion reflex
submitogenic
submucosa
submucosal
   s. gland hypertrophy
   s. plaque
subpapular
subperiosteal felon
subplasmalemmal F-actin
subpolar lepromatous leprosy
subsalicylate
   bismuth s.
subscale
   WOMAC Physical Function s.
subsegmental bronchus
subsensitivity
   bronchoprotective s.
subset
   CD4 T cell s.
   CD4+ T cell s.
   CD8 T cell s.
substance
   amorphous s.
   bacteriotropic s.
   blood group s.
   bone-seeking s.
   exogenous s.

ground s.
nonirritating test s.
s. P
s. P peptide
reducing s.
sensitizing s.
slow-reacting s. (SRS)
soluble specific s. (SSS)
specific capsular s.
thiobarbituric acid-reactive s.
substitute
Apligraf skin s.
bilayered skin s. (BSS)
Biobrane/HF skin s.
Biobrane synthetic skin s.
Dermagraft dermal s.
Dermagraft skin s.
Dermagraft-TC skin s.
Platelin, phospholipid platelet s.
saliva s.
TransCyte skin s.
substrate solution additive
subsulfate
ferric s.
subsynovium
subtalar joint
subtegumental
subtilis
Bacillus s.
subtraction
differential gene s.
subtrochanteric
subtropical
subtype
Reston s.
Russian spring-summer encephalitis Eastern s.
Russian spring-summer encephalitis Western s.
Sudan s.
tickborne encephalitis Central European s.
tickborne encephalitis Eastern s.
Zaire s.
subungual
s. abscess
s. debris
s. exostosis
s. hematoma
s. hyperkeratosis
s. melanoma
s. wart

subungualis
hyperkeratosis s.
subunit vaccine
succinate
hydrocortisone sodium s.
lithium s.
sumatriptan s.
succinyl
succinylcholine
succulence
sucking
s. blister
s. louse
Sucquet-Hoyer canal
sucralfate
suction
Bowins s.
s. loose body forceps
s. sampler
suction-socket prosthetic dermatitis
Sudafed
S. 12 Hour
S. Plus Liquid
S. Plus Tablet
sudamen
sudamina
sudaminal
Sudan
S. black
S. cell marker
S. subtype
sudation
sudden
s. infant death syndrome (SIDS)
s. unexpected death in infants (SUDI)
s. unexplained death in infants (SUDI)
Sudex
SUDI
sudden unexpected death in infants
sudden unexplained death in infants
Sudodrin
sudomotor
sudor
s. sanguineus
s. urinosus
sudoral
sudoresis
sudoriferous
s. abscess
nevus s.

NOTES

529

sudorific
sudorikeratosis
sudoriparous
    s. abscess
    s. angioma
sudoris
    stadium s.
sudorometer
sudorrhea
SUDS
    Single-Use Diagnostic System
Suds
    Murex s.
SUDS HIV-1 diagnostic testing
Sufedrin
sufentanil
suffodiens
    folliculitis et perifolliculitis
      abscedens et s.
    perifolliculitis capitis abscedens
      et s.
sugar
    s. beet
    s. maple
    s. maple tree
    specific soluble s.
sugarcane ear
suggillation
suicide
    s. cell
    s. gene
    procollagen s.
suid herpesvirus
suis
    Actinobacillus s.
    Haemophilus s.
suit
    sauna s.
sukhapakla
sulbactam
    ampicillin and s.
sulcatum
    keratoderma plantare s.
    keratolysis plantare s.
    keratoma plantare s.
sulci
    s. cutis
    s. of skin
sulconazole nitrate
Sulcosyn topical
sulcus
    s. chancre
    s. of matrix of nail
Sulf-10 Ophthalmic
sulfacetamide
    sodium s.
    s. sodium scalp treatment lotion
    sulfur and sodium s.
Sulfacet-R topical

sulfadiazine
    silver s.
    s., sulfamethazine, and
      sulfamerazine
sulfadoxine and pyrimethamine
sulfa drug
Sulfair Ophthalmic
sulfamerazine
    sulfadiazine, sulfamethazine, and s.
Sulfamethoprim
sulfamethoxazole
Sulfamylon topical
sulfapyridine
sulfasalazine (SSZ)
sulfate
    albuterol s.
    amikacin s.
    aminosidine s.
    atropine s.
    bleomycin s.
    Capastat s.
    capreomycin s.
    chondroitin s.
    chondroitin sulfate/dermatan s.
     (CS/DS)
    colistin s.
    dehydroepiandrosterone s. (DHEAS)
    ephedrine s.
    gentamicin s.
    glucosamine s.
    heparin s.
    hydroxychloroquine s.
    hydroxyquinoline s.
    indinavir s.
    kanamycin s.
    magnesium s.
    metaproterenol s.
    morphine s.
    neomycin s.
    netilmicin s.
    nickel s.
    paromomycin s.
    polymyxin b s.
    quinine s.
    sodium lauryl s.
    sodium tetradecyl s.
    streptomycin s.
    terbutaline s.
    trospectomycin s.
    vinblastine s.
    zinc s.
sulfation
Sulfatrim DS
sulfhydryl compound
sulfide
    barium s.
    selenium s.
    strontium s.
Sulfimycin

sulfinpyrazone
sulfisoxazole
> erythromycin and s.
> s. and phenazopyridine

sulfite
sulfonamide
> alpha-amino-p-toluene s.
> toluene s.

sulfonate
sulfonylurea
sulfosalicylate
> meclocycline s.

sulfoxide
> albendazole s.

Sulfoxyl
sulfur
> s. dioxide (SO_2)
> s. flake
> s. granule
> s. and salicylic acid
> sodium sulfacetamide and s.
> s. and sodium sulfacetamide

sulfureum
> *Trichophyton s.*

sulfuric acid
sulindac
Sulsal
Sulzberger-Bloch syndrome
Sulzberger-Chase phenomenon
Sulzberger-Garbe
> S.-G. disease
> S.-G. syndrome

sumac, sumach
> poison s.
> swamp s.

sumatriptan succinate
summer
> s. acne
> s. asthma
> s. dermatosis
> s. eruption
> s. itch
> s. pneumonitis
> s. prurigo
> s. rash
> s. sore

summer-type hypersensitivity pneumonitis (SHP)
sump
> van Sonnenberg s.

Sumycin Oral

sun
> s. and chemical combination damage
> S. Defense Lip Block
> S. Defense Sunscreen
> s. exposure
> s. lamp
> S. Management Lip Protection
> S. Management Sensible Protection
> s. protection factor (SPF)

sunblock
> Coppertone Waterproof S.
> London Drugs S.
> Marcelle S.
> Shiseido S.

sunburn-like rash
sunburn reactivation
Sundown Extra Protection
sunflower
sunscreen
> chemical s.
> s. clothing
> Coppertone S.
> DuraScreen s.
> Esoterica S.
> London Drugs S.
> NO-AD S.
> Ombrelle s.
> Parsol 1789 s.
> physical s.
> Porcelana S.
> Shade UvaGuard s.
> Shaklee S.
> Solbar s.
> Sun Defense S.
> Umbrelle S.

Sunseekers
sunset glow
Supartz
> S. injection
> S. joint fluid therapy

Supasa
super
> s. long-pulse (SLP)
> s. long-pulse diode laser system

superantigen syndrome
superaspirin
superciliorum
> heterotrichosis s.

superfamily
> immunoglobulin s.

superfatted synthetic detergent

S

NOTES

531

superficial
>s. angioma
>s. basal cell carcinoma
>s. basal cell epithelioma
>s. burn
>s. corium
>s. follicular pyoderma
>s. folliculitis
>s. granulomatous pyoderma
>s. hemangioma
>s. infection
>s. malignant melanoma
>s. migratory thrombophlebitis
>s. musculoaponeurotic system (SMAS)
>s. peroneal nerve entrapment
>s. pustular
>s. pustular perifolliculitis
>s. radial nerve entrapment
>s. spreading melanoma (SSM)

superficialis
>esophagitis dissecans s.
>lupus s.
>nevus lipomatodes s.
>nevus lipomatosus cutaneus s.

superinduce
superinfection
superior labrum anterior and posterior (SLAP)
supernatant
>concanavalin A-stimulated T^H cell line s.

supernate
supernumerary digit
superoxide anion
superpigmentation
supine-to-prone maneuver
supine-to-sit maneuver
supisotype
suppedanium
supplement
>SAM-e nutritional s.

supplemental oxygen
support
>s. group
>volume-assured pressure s. (VAPS)

supporter
>lumbosacral s.

supportive
>s. device
>s. therapy

suppository
>Anucort HC s.
>Anuprep HC s.
>Anusol-HC s.
>AVC s.
>Truphylline s.

suppression
>allotype s.

>linked s.
>T-cell s.
>transferable T-cell s.

suppressor
>s. cell
>immune s. (Is)

suppressor-sensitive mutant
suppuration
suppurativa
>genital hidradenitis s.
>hidradenitis s.

suppurative arthritis
suprabasal clefting
suprabasilar acantholysis
supracondylar nonunion
suprafollicularis
>keratosis s.

supragaleal plexus
supramalleolaris
>erythrocyanosis s.

Supramid suture
suprascapular
>s. nerve compression (SSC)
>s. nerve entrapment
>s. nerve palsy

supraspinatus tendon
suprasternal reaction
Suprax
suprofen
sural nerve entrapment
suramin keratosis
SureCell Strep A test
Sure-Closure skin stretching system
SurePress leg compression dressing
SureSite transparent film
surface
>s. antigen
>coarse s.
>dorsal s.
>dry s.
>extensor s.
>flexor s.
>s. freezing
>greasy s.
>hepatitis B s. (HB$_s$)
>s. Ig-expressing B cell
>keratotic s.
>s. microscopy
>pebbly s.
>s. proteoglycan
>RBC s.
>s. receptor
>red blood cell s.
>velvety s.
>verrucous s.
>waxy s.

surface-targeted plasmin inhibitor

surfactant
  hydrolysis of s.
  pulmonary s.
surfer's knot
Surgam SR
surgeon
  American Society of
    Transplant S.'s
  cutaneous s.
surgery
  acne s.
  collimated bema handpiece (CBH-1)
    for laser s.
  continuous-wave dye laser s.
  laser s.
  microscopically controlled s.
  Mohs micrographic s. (MMS)
  video-assisted thoracic s. (VATS)
surgical
  s. erysipelas
  s. excision (SE)
  s. therapy
  s. thrombectomy
  s. tuberculosis
Surgifoam absorbable powder
Surgilene suture
SurgiPulse XJ laser
Surgitron
  Ellman S.
Surgitube tubing
surrogate
  s. marker
  s. tolerogenesis (ST)
sursanure
surveillance
  S., Epidemiology and End Results
    (SEER)
  immune s.
  immunological s.
survey
  Curious Experiences S.
  environmental s.
  Health and Activity Limitation S.
    (HALS)
  human immune status s. (HISS)
  Medical Outcomes Study 36-Item
    Short Form Health S.'s
  Papworth heart donor s.
  reduced joint s. (RJS)
survival
  failure-free s. (FFS)
susceptibility cassette

suspectum
  Heloderma s.
suspension
  AK-Spore H.C. Ophthalmic s.
  amoxicillin/clavulnate s.
  AMX/CL s.
  Aristocort Intralesional s.
  Atuss-12DX extended release
    oral s.
  betamethasone sodium phosphate
    and acetate s.
  Children's Advil S.
  Children's Motrin S.
  Cortisporin Ophthalmic S.
  FML-S Ophthalmic s.
  penicillin V s.
  polymyxin b-hydrocortisone s.
  Poly-Pred Ophthalmic s.
  Terra-Cortril Ophthalmic S.
  Tussi-12D S oral s.
  Vexol Ophthalmic s.
  Viravan-DM oral s.
Sus-Phrine
Sustacal Plus
sustained release (SR)
Sustaire
Sustiva
sutilains
Sutton
  S. disease
  S. nevus
  S. ulcer
suture
  chromic gut s.
  Dexon s.
  Ethicon s.
  Ethilon s.
  Maxon s.
  Novafil s.
  nylon s.
  PDS s.
  plain gut s.
  poliglecaprone s.
  polydioxanone s.
  polyglactin 910 s.
  polyglycolic acid s.
  polyglyconate s.
  polypropylene s.
  Prolene s.
  silk s.
  Supramid s.

S

NOTES

suture *(continued)*
    Surgilene s.
    Vicryl s.
SV
    stroke volume
SV40
    simian vacuolating virus No. 40
SV40-adenovirus hybrid
SVC
    slow vital capacity
swamp
    s. fever
    s. fever virus
    s. itch
    s. sumac
Swann antigen
swan-neck deformity
Sw^a antigen
swarming
Swartz-Lamkins stain
Swartz-Medrik stain
sweat
    s. bee
    black s.
    s. chloride
    s. chloride elimination
    colliquative s.
    fetid s.
    s. gland
    s. gland carcinoma
    insensitive s.
    malodorous s.
    red s.
sweating
    excessive s.
sweat-retention syndrome
sweaty
    s. feet syndrome
    s. sock dermatitis
    s. sock syndrome
Swedish old tuberculin
Sween Cream
sweet
    s. clover
    S. disease
    s. potato
    S. syndrome
    s. vernal
    s. vernal grass
    s. vernal grass pollen
sweetgum tree
swelling
    boggy s.
    Calabar s.
    cervical lymph node s.
    fugitive s.
    joint s.
    Neufeld capsular s.

    nodules, eosinophilia, rheumatism,
        dermatitis, and s. (NERDS)
    rhomboid s.
    tropical s.
Swift disease
Swim-Ear Otic
swimmer's
    s. dermatitis
    s. itch
swimming pool granuloma
swine
    atrophic rhinitis of s.
    s. encephalitis virus
    s. epithelium
    s. fever
    s. fever virus
    s. influenza
    s. influenza virus
    s. pest
    transmissible gastroenteritis virus
        of s.
    s. vesicular disease
swinepox virus
Swiss
    S. chard
    S. cheese appearance
    S. mouse leukemia virus
    S. 3T3 fibroblast
    S. Therapy eye mask
    S. type agammaglobulinemia
switch
    class s.
    s. region
switching
    immunoglobulin class s.
sycamore tree
sycoma
sycosiforme
    ulerythema s.
sycosiform fungous infection
sycosis
    bacillogenic s.
    s. barbae
    Brocq lupoid s.
    coccogenic s.
    s. contagiosa
    s. frambesiformis
    s. framboesia
    s. framboesiaeformis
    herpetic s.
    hyphomycotic s.
    lupoid s.
    nonparasitic s.
    s. nuchae
    s. nuchae necrotisans
    parasitic s.
    s. staphylogenes
    tinea s.
    s. vulgaris

Sydenham chorea
sydowi
    Aspergillus s.
Syllamalt
Sylvest disease
Symadine
Symmers pipe-stem fibrosis
Symmetrel
symmetric
    s. keratoderma
    s. lividity of the soles
    s. progressive leukopathy
    s. reticulonodular x-ray change
symmetrica
    dyschromatosis s.
    erythrokeratodermia progressive s.
    keratoderma s.
    leukopathia punctata reticularis s.
symmetrical gangrene
symmetricum faciei
symmetry
    axis of s.
sympathectomy
    digital s.
sympathetic
    s. nervous system
    s. ophthalmia
    s. synovitis
sympathica
    meningitis s.
sympathomimetic
sympathoneural response
symphalangism
Symphony patient monitoring system
symphysis
sympodialis
    Malassezia s.
symptom
    asthma-like s.
    classic allergy s.
    coincidental s.
    drug rash with eosinophil and
      systemic s. (DRESS)
    frequency of allergy s.
    gastrointestinal s.
    Haenel s.
    lower respiratory tract s.'s (LRSx)
    McLean Limbic Somatic S.
    neuropsychiatric s.
    prodromal s.
    Roger s.
    severity of allergy s.'s

    sicca s.
    Sklowsky s.
    upper respiratory tract s.'s (URSx)
    Wartenberg s.
symptomatic
    s. erythema
    s. fever
    s. porphyria
    s. pruritus
    s. reaction
    s. therapy
    s. ulcer
symptomatica
    alopecia s.
    livedo reticularis s.
    purpura s.
Synacort topical
Synagis
Synalar-HP Topical
Synalar Topical
synanthem
synapsin I
synaptophysin
Synarel
synarthrosis
Sync
    Star S.
synchronized intermittent mechanical
  ventilation
synchronous
    s. intermittent mandatory ventilation
    s. tissue lesion
syncopal attack
syncope
syncytia
syncytial virus
syncytioblast
syncytiotrophoblast
    placental s.
syncytium-inhibiting (SI)
syndactylia
syndactyly
syndecan
syndesmophyte formation
syndesmophytosis
syndesmosis, pl. **syndesmoses**
syndet
    synthetic detergent
syndet-based bar soap
syndrome
    Aarskog-Scott s.
    Achard-Thiers s.

S

NOTES

syndrome *(continued)*
Achenbach s.
actinic reticuloid s.
acute retroviral s.
acute seroconversion s.
Adamantiades-Behçet s.
Adams-Oliver s.
addicted scrotum s.
adulterated rapeseed oil-associated
  toxic oil s.
AEC s.
Alagille s.
Albright s.
Alcock s.
Aldrich s.
Alezzandrini s.
Alibert-Bazin s.
Alström s.
aminopterin s.
amyloid s.
anaphylactic s.
androgen-dependent s.
Angelman s.
angioedema-urticaria-eosinophilia s.
angry back s.
ANOTHER s.
anterior interosseous nerve s.
anterior spinal artery s.
anterior tarsal tunnel s.
antibody-deficient s. (ADS)
anticardiolipin antibody s.
antiphospholipid antibody s. (APS)
antisynthetase s.
aortic arch s.
APECED s.
Apert s.
Arndt-Gottron s.
arterial-ecchymotic type Ehlers-
  Danlos s.
arthrochalasia-type Ehlers-Danlos s.
arthrogryposis congenita, distal,
  type I, II s.
Ascher s.
ataxia telangiectasia s.
atypical mole s.
auriculotemporal s.
autoerythrocyte sensitization s.
autoimmune lymphoproliferative s.
  (ALPS)
autoimmune paraneoplastic s.
autoimmune polyglandular s. (APS)
autonomic imbalance s.
autosomal dominant periodic
  fever s.
Babinski s.
Babinski-Vaquez s.
baboon s.
Bäfverstedt s.
Baló concentric s.

Bannayan-Riley-Ruvalcaba s.
Bannwarth s.
Banti s.
Bardet-Biedl 1–5 s.
bare lymphocyte s.
Barraquer-Simons s.
Bart s.
Barth s.
Bart-Pumphrey s.
basal cell nevus s.
Basan s.
Basex s.
Bateman s.
Bazex s.
Bearn-Kunkel s.
Bearn-Kunkel-Slater s.
Bechterew s.
Behçet s.
Beradinelli-Seip s.
Bernard-Soulier s.
bicipital s.
BIDS s.
bird egg s.
Björnstad s.
Blatin s.
Blau s.
bleached rubber s.
blind loop s.
Blizzard s.
Bloch-Siemens-Sulzberger s.
Bloch-Sulzberger s.
Bloom s.
Bloom-Torre-Machacek s.
blue rubber-bleb nevus s.
blue-toe s.
Bockenheimer s.
bone marrow edema s.
Böök s.
Bourneville s.
Bourneville-Pringle s.
bowel bypass s.
brachio-oto-renal s.
brachydactyly, mental retardation s.
brachydactyly, type B1, C, E s.
Brett s.
brittle hair, intellectual impairment,
  decreased fertility, short stature s.
brittle nail s.
Brooke-Spiegler s.
brown-spot s.
Bruck s.
Brugsch s.
Bruns s.
B-thalassemia s.
Buckley s.
Budd-Chiari s.
burning mouth s.
burning vulva s.
Buschke-Ollendorf s.

bypass arthritis-dermatitis s.
C s.
cachexia s.
café coronary s.
Cairns s.
calcinosis cutis, Raynaud
  phenomenon, esophageal motility
  disorder, sclerodactyly, and
  telangiectasia s.
Caldwell s.
Canada-Cronkhite s.
Canale-Smith s.
Caner-Decker s.
Caplan s.
carcinoid s.
cardiocutaneous s.
cardio-facio-cutaneous s.
Carney s.
cauda equina s.
cellular immune deficiency s.
  (CIDS)
cellular immunity deficiency s.
cervical acceleration-deceleration s.
Chanarin-Dorfman s.
chancriform s.
Charlin s.
Chauffard s.
Chauffard-Still s.
chemical hypersensitivity s.
CHILD s.
CHIME s.
Chinese restaurant s.
chondrodysplasia punctata s.
chorda tympani s.
Christ-Siemens-Touraine s.
chronic fatigue s.
chronic infantile neurological,
  cutaneous and auricular s.
chronic mucocutaneous
  candidiasis s.
chronic pain s.
CINCA s.
classic type Ehlers-Danlos s.
Clouston s.
CMC s.
Cobb s.
Cockayne s.
Coffin-Lowry s.
Coffin-Siris s.
Cogan s.

coloboma, heart anomaly,
  ichthyosis, mental retardation, and
  ear abnormality s.
combined immunodeficiency s.
complex regional pain s. (CRPS)
congenital hemidysplasia with
  ichthyosiform erythroderma and
  limb defects s.
congenital rubella s.
Conradi-Hünermann s.
COPS s.
cosmetic intolerance s.
Costello s.
Crandall s.
craniocarpotarsal s.
cranio-carpo-tarsal s.
craniosynostosis Adelaide type s.
craniosynostosis type (1, 2) s.
CREST s.
Crigler-Najjar s.
Cronkhite-Canada s.
Cross-McKusick-Breen s.
Crouzon s.
Crowe-Dickermann s.
Crow-Fukase s.
crowned dens s.
cubital tunnel s.
Cushing s.
DaCosta s.
Danbolt-Closs s.
defibrination s.
Degos s.
Degos-Delort-Tricot s.
dengue shock s.
Dennie-Marfan s.
denture-sore-mouth s.
de Quervain s.
dermatitis-arthritis-tenosynovitis s.
De Sanctis-Cacchione s.
Desbuquois s.
Devic s.
diabetic hand s.
diabetic stiff-hand s.
diffuse infiltrative lymphocytosis s.
DiGeorge s.
disease s.
distal intestinal obstruction s.
Donath-Landsteiner s.
Dorfman-Chanarin s.
double-crush s.
Down s.

S

NOTES

syndrome *(continued)*

drug-induced delayed multiorgan
hypersensitivity s. (DIDMOS)
drug-induced SLE s.
Duncan s.
Dunnigan s.
dysfunctional gut s.
dyskinetic cilia s.
dysplastic nevus s.
easy bruising s.
Eaton-Lambert s.
EEC s.
effort s.
Ehlers-Danlos s.
Ellis-van Creveld s.
empty sella s.
eosinophilia-myalgia s. (EMS)
eosinophilic fasciitis s.
eosinophilic myalgia s.
eosinophilic pulmonary s.
erythrodysesthesia s.
euthyroid sick s.
excited skin s. (ESS)
Fabry s.
familial amyloidotic
polyneuropathy s.
familial articular hypermobility s.
familial cholestasis s.
familial dysplastic nevus s.
familial hypermobility s.
familial nephropathic amyloidosis s.
Fanconi s.
fasciitis-panniculitis s.
favid Favre-Racouchot s.
Favre-Racouchot s.
Fegeler s.
Felty s.
female pseudo-Turner s.
fetal alcohol s.
fetal hydantoin s.
fibronectin-deficient type Ehlers-
Danlos s.
fibrosing s.
Fiessinger-Leroy s.
Fiessinger-Leroy-Reiter s.
Fiessinger-Rendu s.
Fisher s.
Fitz-Hugh and Curtis s.
Fleischner s.
Flynn-Aird s.
follicular degeneration s.
Fong s.
food protein-induced enterocolitis s.
(FPIES)
Franceschetti-Jadassohn s.
Franceschetti-Klein s.
Franschetti-Klein s.
Freeman-Sheldon s.
Frey s.

Gardner s.
Gardner-Diamond s.
genital Reiter s.
Gerstmann-Straussler-Scheinker s.
Gianotti-Crosti s.
giant cell arteritis s.
Gilbert s.
Giroux-Barbeau s.
glucagonoma s.
glucocorticoid withdrawal s.
GLUS s.
Gold Schnapps s.
Goltz s.
Goltz-Gorlin s.
Goodpasture s.
Gopalan s.
Gorlin s.
Gorlin-Chaudhry-Moss s.
Gorlin-Goltz s.
Gorman s.
Gottron s.
Gougerot s.
Gougerot-Blum s.
Gougerot-Carteaud s.
Graham Little s.
Graham-Little-Piccardi-Lasseur s.
gravis-type Ehlers-Danlos s.
green nail s.
Greither s.
Griscelli s. (GS)
Grönblad-Strandberg s.
Guillain-Barré s.
Gulf War s. (GWS)
Günther s.
Haber s.
HAIR-AN s.
Hallermann-Streiff s.
Hallopeau-Siemens s.
Hamman-Rich s.
hand-and-foot s.
1-hand 2-foot s.
Happle s.
Harada s.
Harter s.
Hawes-Pallister-Landor s.
Hay-Wells s.
Heck s.
Heerfordt s.
Heiner s.
HELLP s.
Helweg-Larssen s.
hemangioma-thrombocytopenia s.
hematopoietic failure s.
hemolytic uremic s. (HUS)
hemophagocytic s.
hemorrhagic fever with renal s.
(HFRS)
Henoch-Schönlein s. (HSS)
hepatopulmonary s. (HPS)

hereditary periodic fever s.
Herlitz s.
Hermansky-Pudlak s. type IV, VI
Hirschowitz s.
Hitzig s.
Holmes-Adie s.
Holt-Oram s.
Horner s.
Howell-Evans s.
human dermatosparaxis type Ehlers-
  Danlos s.
Hunt s.
Hunter s.
Hunter-Thompson s.
Huriez s.
Hurler s.
Hurler-Scheie s.
Hutchinson-Gilford s.
hydralazine s.
hydralazine-associated lupus-like s.
hypereosinophilic s. (HES)
hyper-IgE s.
hyper-IgM s. (HIM)
hyperimmunoglobulinemia s. (HID)
hyperimmunoglobulinemia D, E s.
hypermobile-type Ehlers-Danlos s.
hypermobility s.
hyperostotic s.
hyperventilation s. (HVS)
hyperviscosity s.
hypocomplementemic urticarial
  vasculitis s. (HUVS)
hypocomplementemic vasculitis
  urticarial s.
iatrogenic Cushing s.
IBIDS s.
ichthyosis plus brittle hair,
  intellectual impairment, decreased
  fertility, short stature s.
idiopathic hypereosinophilic s.
  (IHES)
idiopathic nephrotic s.
iliotibial band s.
immunodeficiency s.
impingement s.
s. of inappropriate excretion of
  antidiuretic hormone (SIADH)
inflammatory bowel s. (IBS)
inherited complement deficiency s.
IPEX s.
irritable bowel s. (IBS)
Isaacs s.

Jackson-Lawler s.
Jackson-Sertoli s.
Jackson-Weiss s.
Jacobsen s.
Jadassohn-Lewandowsky s.
Jaffe-Campanacci s.
Jessner s.
Job s.
junctional epidermolysis bullosa-
  pyloric atresia s. (JEB-PA)
Kabuki s.
Kartagener s.
Kasabach-Merritt s.
Kawasaki s.
Kelley-Seegmiller s.
keratitis-ichthyosis-deafness s.
Kettle s.
Keutel s.
KID s.
Kindler s.
kinky-hair s.
Klauder s.
Klein-Waardenburg s.
Klinefelter s.
Klippel-Feil s.
Klippel-Trenaunay s.
Klippel-Trenaunay-Parkes-Weber s.
Klippel-Trenaunay-Weber s.
Kobberling-Dunnigan s.
Kostmann s.
Kuru s.
kyphoscoliosis type Ehlers-Danlos s.
LAMB s.
Lambert-Eaton s.
Lambert-Eaton myasthenic s.
  (LEMS)
Landry s.
Landry-Guillain-Barré s.
Langer-Giedion s.
Larsen s.
late respiratory systemic s. (LRSS)
latex-fruit s.
Laugier-Hunziger s.
Lawrence-Seip s.
lazy leukocyte s. (LLS)
Ledderhose s.
lentigines, atrial myxoma, and blue
  nevi s.
Lenz-Majewski s.
LEOPARD s.
Lépine-Froin s.
Leredde s.

NOTES

syndrome *(continued)*

Leri-Weill s.
Lesch-Nyhan s.
Lewis-Summer s.
Libman-Sacks s.
lichen planus overlap s.
Liddle s.
limb-mammary s.
s. of limited joint mobility (SLJM)
limited joint mobility s.
Löffler s.
Lofgren s.
loose anagen hair s.
Louis-Bar s.
lupus s.
lupus-like s.
lupus-scleroderma overlap s.
Lyell s.
lymphedema-distichiasis s.
lymphocytosis s.
Maffucci s.
malignant mole s.
malignant neuroleptic s.
Marfan s.
Marie-Bamberger s.
Marinesco-Sjögren s.
Maroteaux-Lamy s.
marrow failure s.
Marshall s.
Marshall-White s.
MASS s.
mastocytosis s.
Mauriac s.
May-Thurner s.
McCune-Albright s.
McKusick s.
McKusick-Kaufman s.
Meadow s.
megacystic microcolon s.
Meischer s.
Melkersson s.
Melkersson-Rosenthal s.
Melnick-Fraser s.
MEN s.
Mendelson s.
Menkes kinky hair s.
Mibelli s.
Milian s.
Milwaukee knee s.
Milwaukee shoulder s.
Mitis-type Ehlers-Danlos s.
mitochondrial DNA s.
mitral valve prolapse, aortic
  anomalies, skeletal changes, and
  skin changes s.
modified varicella-like s. (MVLS)
MORFAN s.
Morquio s.
Moynahan s.

Mucha-Habermann s.
Muckle-Wells s.
mucocutaneous lymph node s.
  (MLNS)
Muir-Torre s.
multiple drug allergy s.
multiple endocrine neoplasm s.
multiple hamartoma s.
multiple lentigines s.
multiple mucosal neuroma s.
multiple sulfatase deficiency s.
Munchausen s.
Muscle-Wells s.
musician's overuse s.
myasthenia gravis s.
myelodysplastic s. (MDS)
myofascial pain s. (MPS)
myonecrosis s.
Naegeli s.
Naegeli-Franceschetti-Jadassohn s.
nail-patella s.
nail-patella-elbow s.
NAME s.
Nelson s.
nephrotic s.
NERDS s.
nerve compression-degeneration s.
nerve entrapment s.
Netherton s. (NS)
neurocutaneous s.
neurofibromatosis, type 1 s.
nevi, atrial myxoma, myxoid
  neurofibroma, and ephelides s.
nevoid basal cell carcinoma s.
  (NBCCS)
Nezelof s.
Nicolau s.
Nieden s.
Nijmegen breakage s.
nodules, eosinophilia, rheumatism,
  dermatitis, and swelling s.
nonallergic rhinitis with
  eosinophilia s. (NARES)
nonarticular s.
Nonne-Milroy-Meige s.
Noonan s.
occipital horn s.
occuloglandular s.
occupation-related s.
ocular-mucous membrane s.
ocular-scoliotic type Ehlers-
  Danlos s.
oculo-oral-genital s.
odonto-tricho-ungual-digital-palmar s.
Ollendorf s.
Olmsted s.
Omenn s.
oral allergy s. (OAS)
oral-ocular-genital s.

organic dust toxic s. (ODTS)
Osler s. II
Osler-Weber-Rendu s.
OSMED s.
osteogenesis imperfecta s.
overlap s.
overuse s.
4-p s.
Paget abscess s.
painful-bruising s.
Pallister-Hall s.
Pallister mosaic aneuploid s.
palmar fasciitis and polyarthritis s.
palmoplantar erythrodysesthesia s.
pants paresthesia s.
PAPA s.
Papillon-Lèfevre s.
papular-purpuric gloves and
  socks s.
papular-purpuric stocking and
  glove s.
papulovesicular acrolocated s.
paraneoplastic s.
Parinaud oculoglandular s.
Parrot s.
Parry-Romberg s.
Pasini-Pierini s.
patellofemoral pain s.
peeling-skin s.
periarticular s.
periodic fever s.
periodontitis-type Ehlers-Danlos s.
Persian Gulf s.
Peutz-Jeghers s.
Pfeiffer s.
pharyngeal pouch s.
photosensitivity, ichthyosis, brittle
  hair, impaired intelligence,
  decreased fertility, and short
  stature s.
photosensitivity, ichthyosis, brittle
  hair, intellectual impairment,
  decreased fertility, and short
  stature s. (PIBIDS syndrome)
PIBIDS s.
PIE s.
piriformis s.
placental sulfatase deficiency s.
plantar nerve s.
plica s.
Plummer-Vinson s.
POEMS s.

polyangiitis overlap s.
polyarteritis nodosa s.
polycystic ovary s.
polymyalgia rheumatica s.
popliteal pterygium s.
postcardiotomy s.
posterior interosseous nerve s.
posterior tarsal tunnel s.
postinfectious encephalomyelitis s.
postphlebitic s.
Prader-Willi s.
Prausnitz-Kustner s.
Prieur-Griscelli s.
primary Sjögren s.
progeroid Ehlers-Danlos s.
pronator teres s.
Proteus s.
pseudoradicular s.
pseudo-Turner s.
psychogenic pain s.
psychological irritable
  bowel/migraine s. (PIMS)
pulmonary disease anemia s.
pulmonary sling s.
pyriformis s.
quadrilateral space s.
Quincke I s.
Rabson-Mendenhall s.
Ramsay Hunt s.
Raynaud s.
reactive airways dysfunction s.
  (RADS)
rectus abdominis s.
red man s.
reflex sympathetic dystrophy s.
Refsum s.
Reiter s.
REM s.
Rendu-Osler-Weber s.
respiratory distress s. (RDS)
restaurant s.
reticular erythematous mucinosis s.
Reye s.
rhabdomyolysis s.
rheumatoid s.
Richner-Hanhart s.
Richter s.
Riley-Day s.
Riley-Smith s.
Romberg s.
Rombo s.
Rosai-Dorfman s.

S

NOTES

syndrome *(continued)*
Rothmann-Makai s.
Rothmund s.
Rothmund-Thomson s.
Rowell s.
RSD s.
rubber man s.
Rubinstein-Taybi s.
Rud s.
runting s.
Rust s.
Ruvalcaba-Myhre-Smith s.
sacral agenesis s.
sacral agenesis type 1 s.
Samter s.
Sanfilippo s.
SAPHO s.
scalded skin s.
scapulocostal s.
scapulothoracic s.
Schäfer s.
Schafer-Branauer s.
Scheie s.
Schimmelpenning s.
Schmidt s.
Schnitzler s.
Schönlein-Henoch s.
Schopf s.
Schüller-Christian s.
sea-blue histiocyte s.
secondary Sjögren s.
Secrétan s.
Seidlmayer s.
Seip-Lawrence s.
Senear-Usher s.
septic shock s.
seronegative rheumatoid s.
severe adult respiratory s. (SARS)
severe combined immune
   deficiency s.
Sézary s. (SS)
Sheehan s.
short bowel s.
shoulder-hand s.
shrinking lung s. (SLS)
Shulman s.
Shwachman-Diamond s.
sicca s.
sick building s.
Simmond s.
Simpson dysmorphia s.
Singleton-Merten s.
Sjögren s. (SS)
Sjögren-Larsson s.
skin disease s.
sleep apnea s.
sleep apnea/hypopnea s.
SLE-like s.
Sly s.

Smith-Riley s.
Sneddon s.
soft-tissue injury s.
Soto s.
Spanish toxic oil s.
Spanlang-Tappeiner s.
sporadic atypical mole-melanoma s.
sports-related pain s.
staphylococcal scalded skin s.
   (SSSS)
staphylococcal toxic shock s.
starvation s.
Stein-Leventhal s.
Stevens-Johnson s. (SJS)
Stewart-Treves s.
Stickler s.
Stickler s., type I, II, III
stiff-hand s.
stiff-man s. (SMS)
stiff-person s.
stiff-skin s.
streptococcal toxic shock s.
Stryker-Halbeisen s.
Sturge-Weber s.
subcalcaneal pain s.
sudden infant death s. (SIDS)
Sulzberger-Bloch s.
Sulzberger-Garbe s.
superantigen s.
sweat-retention s.
sweaty feet s.
sweaty sock s.
Sweet s.
synostosis s.
systemic inflammatory response s.
   (SIRS)
systemic lupus erythematosus-like s.
   (SLE-like syndrome)
TAR s.
tarsal tunnel s.
TASS s.
Tay s.
tendonitis-fascitis s.
thalassemia s.
Thibierge-Weissenbach s.
third and fourth pharyngeal
   pouch s.
Thompson s.
thoracic outlet s.
thrombocytopenic purpura/hemolytic
   uremic s. (TTP-HUS)
Tietze s.
tight building s.
TINU s.
toasted skin s.
TORCH s.
Torre s.
total allergy s.
Touraine s.

Touraine-Solente-Golé s.
Townes-Brock s.
toxic oil s. (TOS)
toxic shock s. (TSS)
toxic shock-like s. (TSLS)
toxoplasmosis, other infections,
  rubella, cytomegalovirus infection,
  and herpes simplex s.
Treacher Collins s.
tricho-rhino-phalangeal s.
trichothiodystrophy s.
trigeminal trophic s.
trisomy 20 s.
trophic s.
Trousseau s.
tumor lysis s.
tumor necrosis factor receptor-
  associated periodic s. (TRAPS)
Turner s.
Turner-Kieser s.
two feet-one hand s.
Ullrich-Turner s.
uncombable hair s.
undifferentiated autoimmune s.
  (UAS)
undifferentiated connective tissue s.
  (UCTS)
Unna-Thost s.
unusual lupus erythematosus-like s.
Urbach-Wiethe s.
Van Lohuizen s.
vascular type Ehlers-Danlos s.
velocardiofacial s.
Verner s.
Vogt-Koyanagi s.
Vogt-Koyanagi-Harada s. (VKHS)
Vohwinkel s.
von Hippel-Landau s.
vulvar vestibulitis s.
Waardenburg s.
Waardenburg-Shah s.
Waldenström s.
wasting s.
Waterhouse-Friderichsen s.
Weber-Cockayne s.
Wegener granulomatosis s.
Weill-Marchesani s.
Weissenbach s.
Weissenbacher-Zweymuller s.
Well s.
Wells s.
Werner s.

Wernicke-Korsakoff s.
whistling face s.
Widal s.
Windmill-Vane-Hand s.
Wiskott-Aldrich s. (WAS)
Wissler s.
Wissler-Fanconi s.
Wyburn-Mason s.
X-linked Ehlers-Danlos s.
X-linked lymphoproliferative s.
XYY s.
yellow nail s.
Young s.
Yunis-Varon s.
Zimmerman-Laband s.
Zinsser-Cole-Engman s.
Zinsser-Engman-Cole s.
syndromic
Synemol topical
Synercid IV
synergic spleen
synergistic gangrene
synergy
  Esteem s.
Synflex
Syn-Flunisolide
Syngamus trachea
syngeneic
  s. cell
  s. graft
  s. heart transplant
  s. transplantation
syngenesioplasty
syngenesiotransplantation
syngenic
syngraft
Syn-Minocycline
synonym
  objective s.
  senior s.
  subjective s.
synophrys
synostosis syndrome
synovectomy
synovial
  s. antigenic peptide
  s. biopsy
  s. capillary
  s. cyst
  s. fibroblast
  s. fluid (SF)
  s. fluid change

S

NOTES

synovial *(continued)*
   s. hemangioma
   s. hemosiderosis
   s. hyperplasia
   s. hypoxia
   s. lining
   s. lining cell (SLC)
   s. lining cell type A
   s. lipoma
   s. membrane
   s. membrane tophus
   s. mesenchyme
   s. tissue
synovia T cell
synoviocyte
   fibroblast lineage s.
   fibroblast-shaped s.
   macrophage-like s.
   type A s.
synovioma
   benign giant cell s.
synoviorthosis
synovitis
   s., acne, pustulosis, hyperostosis,
      osteitis (SAPHO)
   asymptomatic cricoarytenoid s.
   discrete s.
   eosinophilic s.
   glenohumeral s.
   nodular s.
   pigmented villonodular s. (PVNS)
   polyarticular s.
   proliferative s.
   reactive postinfectious s.
   remitting seronegative
      symmetrical s.
   silicone s.
   sympathetic s.
   tuberculous s.
   villonodular s.
synovium
   hyperplastic s. (HS)
   proliferative s.
Syn-Rx
syntenic group
Synthaderm wound dressing
synthase
   brain PGD_2 s.
   citrate s. (CS)
   endoperoxide s.
   hematopoietic PGD_2 s.
   inducible nitric oxide s.
   LTC4 s.
   oligoadenylate s.
   PGE_2 s.
   PGF_2 s.
   PGI_2 s.
   prostacyclin s.

prostaglandin H s.-1, -2 (PGHS-1, -
   2)
thromboxane s.
synthesis, pl. **syntheses**
   cellular immunodeficiency with
      abnormal immunoglobulin s.
   chondrocyte proteoglycan s.
   citrate s. (CS)
   de novo pyrimidine s.
   s. inhibitor
   matrix s.
   melanin s.
   vitamin D s.
synthetase
   adenylosuccinic acid s.
   alanyl-transfer ribonucleic acid s.
   alanyl-tRNA s.
   aminoacyl-tRNA s.
   glycyl-transfer ribonucleic acid s.
   glycyl-tRNA s.
   histidyl-tRNA s.
   isoleucyl-tRNA s.
   threonyl-tRNA s.
   tRNA s.
synthetic
   s. antigen
   s. depot corticosteroid
   s. detergent (syndet)
   s. pyrethroid
Synvisc
syphilid
   acneform s.
   acuminate papular s.
   anular s.
   bullous s.
   corymbose s.
   ecthymatous s.
   erythematous s.
   flat papular s.
   follicular s.
   frambesiform s.
   gummatous s.
   impetiginous s.
   lenticular s.
   macular s.
   miliary papular s.
   nodular s.
   nummular s.
   palmar s.
   papular s.
   papulosquamous s.
   pemphigoid s.
   pigmentary s.
   plantar s.
   pustular s.
   rupial s.
   secondary s.
   tertiary s.
   varioliform s.

syphilide
syphilionthus
syphilis
    Captia test for s.
    s. chancre
    congenital s.
    s. d'emblée
    early congenital s.
    early latent s.
    endemic s.
    gumma of tertiary s.
    gummatous s.
    s. hereditaria tarda
    s. of iris
    late benign s.
    late cardiovascular s.
    late congenital s.
    late latent s.
    latent s.
    late osseous s.
    noduloulcerative s.
    noduloulcerative tertiary s.
    nonvenereal s.
    osseous s.
    parenchymatous s.
    ping-pong s.
    primary s.
    quaternary s.
    secondary s.
    serologic test for s. (S.T.S.)
    tertiary cutaneous s.
    tertiary noduloulcerative s.
    tubercular tertiary s.
    visceral s.
syphilitic
    s. alopecia
    s. dactylitis
    s. fever
    s. inguinal adenitis
    s. leukoderma
    s. onychia
    s. roseola
    s. spastic spinal paralysis
    s. spinal muscular atrophy
    s. ulcer
syphilitica
    acne s.
    alopecia s.
    impetigo s.
syphiliticum
    erythema nodosum s.
    tuberculum s.

syphiliticus
    clavus s.
    lichen s.
    pemphigus s.
    tophus s.
syphiloderm
syphiloderma
    papular s.
syphilologist
syphilology
syphiloma
    Fournier s.
syphilomatous
syphilophobia
syringadenoma
syringe
    Luer-Lok s.
syringe-assisted liposuction
syringoacanthoma
syringoadenoma papilliferum
syringocystadenoma papilliferum
syringofibroadenoma
    eccrine s.
syringoid carcinoma
syringoma
    chondroid s.
    clear cell s.
    eruptive s.
    malignant chondroid s.
syringometaplasia
    eccrine squamous s.
syringomyelia
syrup
    AccuHist PDX S.
    Actagen S.
    AeroKid S.
    albuterol sulfate S.
    Allerfrin S.
    Allerphed S.
    Anamine S.
    Aprodine S.
    S. of Aristocort
    Benylin Cough S.
    Bromfed S.
    Bydramine Cough S.
    Carbodec S.
    Carbodex DM S.
    Cardec-S S.
    Decofed S.
    Deconamine S.
    DMax S.
    Drixoral S.

S

NOTES

syrup *(continued)*
    Histalet S.
    Hydramyn S.
    Kenacort S.
    Naldecon-EX Children's S.
    Rondec S.
    Silafed S.
    Triofed S.
    Triposed S.
    Tusstat S.
    Uni-Bent Cough S.

Sysmex SE-9500 machine

system
    Aastrom Replicell S.
    Accents s.
    AccuProbe s.
    Accu-set S.
    Acusyst-Xcell monoclonal antibody culturing s.
    Aladdin infant flow s.
    AlaSTAT allergy immunoassay s.
    Allerderm Protective Glove S.
    APACHE II s.
    arch-loop-whorl s.
    Aria CPAP s.
    Aura Laser s.
    Automated Cellular Imaging S. (ACIS)
    automated cytochemical s.
    autonomic nervous s.
    BacT/Alert Microbial Detection S.
    BACTEC s.
    Basic Clinical Scoring S.
    BClear s.
    Bionicare 1000 stimulator s.
    blood group s.
    Brasfield scoring s.
    carbon dioxide laser scanner s.
    Cardiovit AT-10 ECG/spirometry combination s.
    Carolon multi-layer stocking s.
    Circulaire aerosol drug delivery s.
    CMS AccuProbe 450 s.
    Coleman microinfiltration s.
    common mucosal immune s. (CMIS)
    Companion 314 nasal CPAP s.
    complement s.
    CoolGlide aesthetic laser s.
    CoolTouch 1320nm laser s.
    Costa Simple Scoring S.
    DAR breathing s.
    da Vinci Surgical s.
    DELM imaging s.
    dermal s.
    Derma 20 laser s.
    Dermaphot s.
    DermMaster s.
    Digital Medical S.'s

    DNA-anti-DNA s.
    DPAP interactive airway management s.
    drug-induced depression of immune s.
    Dyna-Care pressure pad s.
    Dyonics Dyosite office arthroscopy s.
    Dyonics InteliJet fluid management s.
    ELISA-Light Chemiluminescent Detection s.
    ENTec Coblator plasma s.
    EpiLaser laser-based hair removal s.
    EpiLight hair removal s.
    EpiStar diode laser s.
    EsteLux s.
    Finger Phantom pulse oximeter testing s.
    FL3095 fluorescence spectrometer s.
    Gell and Coombs classification s.
    genetic depression of immune s.
    GentleLASE Plus laser s.
    GentlePeel skin exfoliation s.
    Haversian s.
    hematopoietic s.
    Hunstad tumescent liposuction s.
    hypothalamic-pituitary-adrenal s.
    HY-TEC automated allergy diagnostic s.
    immune s.
    indicator s.
    integumentary s.
    Kaplan PenduLaser 115 laser s.
    kinin s.
    Larsen grading s.
    Levulin PDT s.
    LightSheer SC laser hair removal s.
    Litx s.
    LPI excimer laser s.
    lymphoreticular s. (LRS)
    Lyra laser s.
    s. of macrophage
    masticatory s.
    Medi-Facts s.
    metric s.
    monocyte-macrophage s.
    mononuclear phagocyte s. (MPS)
    MultiLight s.
    MultiPulse laser s.
    MW 2000 microwave delivery s.
    myeloperoxidase-hydrogen peroxide halide s.
    NADPH oxidase s.
    nervous s.
    Norwood classification s.
    Nu-Derm S.

Nu-Trake Weiss emergency
  airway s.
Nuvolase 660 laser s.
Orbasone s.
organ transplantation s.
Ortho-Ice Multipaks s.
Oxyfil oxygen refilling s.
Palomar SLP1000 diode laser s.
Panasol II home phototherapy s.
Para-Pak Ultra Ecofix s.
Perimed PeriFlux Doppler probe s.
peripheral nervous s. (PNS)
peripheral vascular s.
PhotoDerm MultiLight s.
PhotoGenica laser s.
Plast-O-Fit thermoplastic bandage s.
PodoSpray nail drill s.
primary angiitis of the central
  nervous s.
properdin s.
Quanti-Test S.
radiometric resin s.
Rajka and Langeland scoring s.
Refinity Coblation s.
ReLume s.
reticuloendothelial s. (RES)
RinoFlow nasal wash and sinus s.
scaling, erythema, and induration
  scoring s.
SEI scoring s.
Simple Scoring S. (SSS)
single-cell ion imaging s.
Single-Use Diagnostic S. (SUDS)
SkinLaser s.
SLP1000 diode laser s.
SoftLight laser hair removal s.
SpaTouch PhotoEpilation s.
Squirt wound irrigation s.
statistical analysis s. (SAS)
superficial musculoaponeurotic s.
  (SMAS)
super long-pulse diode laser s.
Sure-Closure skin stretching s.
sympathetic nervous s.
Symphony patient monitoring s.
TenderWet s.
Tewameter TM 210 open loop s.
ThAIRapy vest airway clearance s.
Therakos UVAR S.
TheraPEP positive expiratory
  pressure therapy s.
transdermal therapeutic s. (TTS)

TruPulse CO2 laser s.
Uganda Cancer Institute staging s.
UlcerJet high-pressure fluid jet s.
UltraFine erbium laser s.
United States Renal Data S.
  (USRDS)
UVAR photophoresis s.
Vaccine Adverse Events
  Reporting S. (VAERS)
VAC Freedom s.
Vbeam pulse dye laser s.
Visage Cosmetic Surgery s.
Vornado Air Quality S.
Wound Stick measuring s.
XTRAC laser s.
YagLazr s.
Zassi Bowel Management s.
Zimmer Pulsavac wound
  debridement s.
systematic polymorphism screening
systematized nevus
systemic
  s. acne
  s. amyloid
  s. anaphylaxis
  s. antibacterial therapy
  s. antifungal therapy
  s. autoaggression
  s. autoimmune disease
  s. candidiasis
  s. contact dermatitis
  s. corticosteroid
  s. febrile disease
  s. fungal infection
  s. hyalinosis
  s. hypersensitivity angiitis
  s. inflammatory response syndrome
    (SIRS)
  s. juvenile rheumatoid arthritis
  S. Lupus Activity Measure
    (SLAM)
  s. lupus erythematosus (SLE)
  s. lupus erythematosus-like
    syndrome
  s. malignancy
  s. mastocytosis
  s. necrotizing vasculitis (SNV)
  s. poisoning
  s. polyarteritis nodosa
  s. polyarthralgia
  s. proliferating
    angioendotheliomatosis

NOTES

S

systemic *(continued)*
  s. reaction
  s. sclerosis (SSc)
  s. sclerosis sine scleroderma (ssSSc)
  s. steroid
  s. visceral amyloidosis
Syzygium cumini

T
    time
        T agglutinogen
        T antigen
        T cell
        T cell-B cell collaboration
        T cell fibroblast
        chloramine T
        Cleocin T
        T cytotoxic cell (Tc)
        Dalacin T
        T gel
        T locus
        T lymphocyte
        Ortho-Kung T (OKT)
        T tubule
        T zone
        T zone complexion
T3
    triiodothyronine
T4
    thyroxine
        Soluble T4
T1-weighted study
T2-weighted study
T4N5 liposome lotion
TA
    treatment adherence
TAA
    triamcinolone acetonide
TA-AIDS
    transfusion-associated AIDS
TAB
    temporal artery biopsy
T.A.B.
    typhoid A&B
        T.A.B. vaccine
Tabanidae
tabes dorsalis
tabetic
    t. facies
    t. neurosyphilis
    t. osteoarthropathy
tablet
    Actagen T.
    Actifed Allergy T.
    Actonel t.
    Adoxa t.
    Afrin T.
    Allercon T.
    Allerfrin T.
    allergy t.
    Aprodine T.
    Aristocort T.
    Avelox t.

    Benadryl Decongestant Allergy T.
    BQ T.
    Bromfed T.
    Bromphen T.
    Carbiset T.
    Carbiset-TR T.
    Cenafed Plus T.
    Chlor-Trimeton 4 Hour Relief T.
    Coldec D extended release t.
    Deconamine T.
    decongestant t.
    desloratadine t.
    Dimaphen T.
    Dimetapp T.
    Ditropan XL oxybutynin chloride
      extended-release t.
    doxycycline hyclate t.
    Dynacin t.
    Elidel t.
    Fedahist T.
    Genac T.
    headache t.
    Histalet Forte T.
    Hista-Vadrin T.
    Kenacort T.
    Klerist-D T.
    Lamisil T.
    meloxicam t.
    Mobic t.
    moxifloxacin HCl t.
    Mylocel 1000 mg t.
    Periostat t.
    Phyllocontin T.
    PSE CPM chewable t.
    Pseudo-Gest Plus T.
    Sinutab T.
    Sudafed Plus T.
    terbinafine hydrochloride t.
    Triposed T.
    Tylenol Cold Effervescent
      Medication t.
    Veltane T.
    Vicks DayQuil Allergy Relief 4
      Hour t.
    zolmitriptan disintegrating t.
    Zomig-ZMT disintegrating t.
    Zyrtec-D 12-hour extended-
      release t.
Tabs
    Apo-Doxy T.
    Travel T.
tabulated
    Quality, Utilization, Effectiveness,
      Statistically T. (QUEST)

TAC
    tacrolimus
    transiently amplifying cell
    triamcinolone cream
Tac-3, -40 Injection
Tacalciol
Tacalcitol
Tac antigen
Tacaribe complex of virus
Tacaryl
TACE
    transarterial chemoembolization
tache
    t. bleuâtres
    t. cérébrale
    t. méningéale
    t. noire
    t. spinale
tachetic
tachyarrhythmia
tachycardia
tachyphylaxis
tachypnea
tacrolimus (FK506, TAC)
    t. capsule
    t. hydrate
    t. injection
    t. ointment
    t. ointment
    t. ointment
tacrolimus-associated
    t.-a. diabetes
    t.-a. mutism
tacrolimus-based immunosuppression
tactile
    t. cell of Merkel-Ranvier
    toruli t.'s
TAD
    transient acantholytic dermatosis
TAE
    total abdominal evisceration
Taenia
    T. saginata
    T. solium
taeniacide
tag
    cutaneous t.
    identification t.
    pleural t.
    sentinel t.
    skin t.
Tagamet
Tagamet-HB
tagged white blood cell study
Tahyna virus
TAI
    thoracoabdominal irradiation
tailor bunion
tail sign

Takahara disease
Takayasu
    T. arteriopathy
    T. arteritis
    T. disease
TAL
    triamcinolone lotion
talalgia
    plantar t.
talc
    t. lotion
    purified t.
    t. slurry
    zinc oxide, cod liver oil, and t.
talcum
tall dock
talon noir
talus
Tamine
Tamm-Horsfall protein
tamoxifen
Tanafed
T-and B-cell severe combined immunodeficiency disease
tangential
    t. biopsy
    t. excision
tangent-to-circle excision
Tangier disease
tannate
    dextromethorphan tannate, phenylephrine tannate, pyrilamine t.
tanned red cell
Tanner
    T. mesher
    T. mesher device
    T. pubertal stage
tanner's ulcer
Tanner-Vandeput mesh dermatome
tannin
tanning
    t. bed
    delayed t.
    immediate t.
    t. lotion
Tantafed
TAO
    thromboangiitis obliterans
    thyroid-associated ophthalmopathy
    triamcinolone ointment
TAP1, TAP2 protein
tapasin
tape
    Cath-Secure t.
    ColorZone t.
    Cordran t.
    Deknatel wound t.
    Dermicel t.

Elastikon elastic t.
Micropore t.
Scanpor t.
taper
prednisone t.
steroid t.
tapeworm
dog t.
TaqMan assay
Taq polymerase
TAR
thrombocytopenia-absent-radius
TAR syndrome
tar
t. acne
t. bath
coal t.
DHS T.
T. Distillate
T. Doak
juniper t.
t. keratosis
t. melanosis
ointment of t.
t. preparation
t. shampoo
Spectro T.
wood t.
Tarabine PFS
Taractan
TARC
thymus and activation-regulated
chemokine
tarda
familial spondyloepiphyseal
dysplasia t.
lues t.
osteogenesis imperfecta t.
porphyria cutanea t. (PCT)
syphilis hereditaria t.
Tardan
Tardieu petechia
tardus
nevus spilus t.
Targel SA
target
t. cell
t. lesion
t. of rapamycin inhibitor
**targetoid hemosiderotic hemangioma
(THH)**
Targretin

Taro-Desoximetasone
Taro-Sone
Tarpley scale
tarsal tunnel syndrome
tarsi
acne t.
tinea t.
tartaric acid
Tart cell
tartrate
belladonna, phenobarbital, and
ergotamine t.
phenindamine t.
trimeprazine t.
tartrate-resistant
t.-r. acid phosphatase (TRAP)
t.-r. acid phosphatase positive cell
tartrazine
Tarui disease
TASS
thyroiditis, Addison disease, Sjögren
syndrome, sarcoidosis
TASS syndrome
TAT
thrombin-antithrombin III
TATA
tumor-associated transplantation antigen
TATA-binding protein
tat gene
tattoo
amalgam t.
eyeline t.
oral t.
tattooing effect
Tau-Cl
tau-globulin
taurine chloramine
tautology
Tavist Allergy/Sinus/Headache
Tavist-1, -D
tax
viral protein t.
taxa
Taxol
taxon
taxonomic
taxonomy
numerical t.
Taxoprexin DHA-paclitaxel
Taylor disease
Tay-Sachs disease
Tay syndrome

T

NOTES

tazarotene
>t. cream
>t. topical gel

Tazicef

Tazidime

tazobactam

Tazorac cream

TB
>tuberculosis
>>TB test by PCR

TBAB
>thyroid-blocking antibody

TBE
>tris-boric acid-ethylenediaminetetraacetic acid

TBI
>total body irradiation
>tumor burden index

TBII
>thyroid-binding inhibitory immunoglobulin
>thyrotropin-binding inhibitory immunoglobulin

TBS
>tris-buffered saline
>tris-buffered saline solution

TBSA
>total body surface area

3TC
>lamivudine triphosphate

Tc
>T cytotoxic cell
>technetium
>>Tc polyphosphate scan

Tc1, Tc2 cell

TCA
>trichloroacetic acid

TCB
>total counts bound

Tc-dimercaptosuccinic acid (DMSA)

T-cell
>T-c. antibody labeling
>T-c. antigen receptor
>T-c. clonality
>T-c. counter-receptor interaction
>T-c. defect
>T-c. erythroderma
>T-c. growth factor (TCGF)
>T-c. growth factor-1
>T-c. growth factor-2
>T-c. involvement
>T-c. large granuloma lymphocyte leukemia
>T-c. leukemia virus type 1
>T-c. lymphocytic leukemia
>T-c. lymphocytoma cutis
>T-c. lymphoma
>T-c. marker
>T-c. pseudolymphoma

>T-c. replacing factor
>T-c. rosette
>T-c. suppression
>T-c. xenorecognition

T-cell-mediated
>T.-c.-m. autoimmune disease
>T.-c.-m. delayed type hypersensitivity dermatitis

TCGF
>T-cell growth factor

^{99m}Tc-HMPAO

TCHT
>traditional Chinese herbal therapy

Tc-human serum albumin scintigraphy

TCN
>tetracycline

TCR

TD
>trichodiscoma

T.D.
>Diamine T.D.

Td
>tetanus-diphtheria

TDD
>thoracic duct drainage

T-dependent
>T-d. antigen
>T-d. response

T/Derm
>Neutrogena T/D.

TDI
>isocyanate TDI

T1DM
>type 1 diabetes mellitus

T2DM
>type 2 diabetes mellitus

TDT
>transmission disequilibrium testing

TDTH cell

TdT-positive

TDX analyzer

TE
>trichoepithelioma

tea
>Mexican t.
>t. tree oil

tear
>artificial t.'s
>T. Drop solution
>Liquifilm T.'s
>T.'s Naturale
>T.'s Naturale Free solution
>T.'s Naturale II solution
>T.'s Plus solution
>T.'s Renewed solution

TearGard Ophthalmic solution

Teargen Ophthalmic solution

Tearisol solution

tebutate
    prednisolone t.
tecastemizole
Tec family of cytoplasmic protein tyrosine kinase
technetium (Tc)
    t. diphosphonate
    t. pertechnetate
    t. scan
technetium-99m hexamethylpropylene amine oxime-single-photon-emission computed tomography (HMPAO-SPECT)
Techni-Care
    T.-C. surgical scrub
    T.-C. wound cleanser
technician
    nail t.
technique
    aseptic t.
    Blenderm patch t.
    Boyden chamber t.
    cognitive-behavioral t.
    cytogenic t.
    dipstick t.
    enzyme-multiplied immunoassay t. (EMIT)
    Fegan t.
    fluorescent antibody t.
    freehand t.
    gene array t.
    Hotchkiss-McManus t.
    immunodiffusion t.
    immunofluorescence t.
    immunology laboratory t.
    immunometric t.
    Ingram t.
    interval mapping t.
    Jerne t.
    joint protection t.
    laser-assisted internal fabrication t.
    Lich t.
    LIFT t.
    lifting t.
    light scatter t.
    lymphoablative t.
    Mancini t.
    Mohs fresh-tissue t.
    Nambudripad allergy elimination t. (NAET)
    Ouchterlony double diffusion t.
    PAS t.

    P-E t.
    percutaneous conchotome biopsy t.
    periodic acid-Schiff t.
    polka-dot t.
    portal venous and enteric drainage t.
    problem elicitation t. (PET)
    Rebuck skin window t.
    saucerization t.
    shave t.
    skin window t.
    split adjuvant t.
    sterile t.
    stripe t.
    thermal quenching t.
    trichloroacetic acid-tape t.
    tumescent t.
    volumetric t.
    whole-body antibody t. (IMX)
technology
    gene-knockout t.
    PulseDose oxygen delivery t.
    Smoothbeam nonablative diode laser t.
Tecnu Outdoor Skin Cleanser lotion
tecogalan
tectate
Tectiviridae
Tedral
Teejel
teeth (*pl. of* tooth)
Tegaderm
    T. HP
    T. HP transparent film
    T. semipermeable dressing
    T. transparent dressing
    T. transparent dressing with absorbent pad
Tegagel
    T. dressing/sheet
    T. hydrogel
    T. hydrogel dressing
    T. hydrogel sheet
Tegagen
    T. HG alginate wound dressing
    T. HG, HI alginate wound cover
    T. HI alginate dressing
Tegapore
    T. contact-layer sheet
    T. contact-layer wound dressing
Tegasorb
    T. hydrocolloid

T

NOTES

Tegasorb *(continued)*
    T. synthetic dressing
    T. Thin hydrocolloid
    T. Thin hydrocolloid dressing
Tega-Vert Oral
Tegison
Tegopen
Tegretol
Tegrin
Tegrin-HC topical
tegument
tegumentary epithelium
tegumentum
TEH
    theophylline, ephedrine, and hydroxyzine
teicoplanin
Telachlor Oral
Teladar topical
telangiectasia
    ataxia t.
    calcinosis cutis, Raynaud
      phenomenon, esophageal motility
      disorder, sclerodactyly, and t.
      (CREST)
    cephalooculocutaneous t.
    dermatomal superficial t.
    essential t.
    hemorrhagic t.
    hereditary hemorrhagic t. (HHT)
    t. macularis eruptiva perstans
      (TMEP)
    nevoid t.
    oculocutaneous t.
    periungual t.
    primary t.
    secondary t.
    spider t.
    unilateral dermatomal superficial t.
    unilateral nevoid t.
    t. verrucosa
    wire-loop shaped t.
telangiectasis, pl. **telangiectases**
    hereditary hemorrhagic t.
    linear t.
    multiple hereditary hemorrhagic t.
    spider t.
    stellate t.
    tortuous t.
telangiectatic
    t. erythema
    t. mat
    t. matting (TM)
    t. systemic mastocytosis
    t. wart
telangiectatica
    livedo t.
telangiectaticum
    granuloma t.

telangiectodes
    acne t.
    elephantiasis t.
    purpura annularis t.
Telangitron device
telar
Teldrin Oral
telemetry
    home-based t. (HBT)
    multiple parameter t. (MPT)
telepathology
teletactor
teleutospore
Telfa
    T. Clear contact layer sheet
    T. composite dressing
Telfamax absorptive dressing
Teline oral
teliospore
telmisartan
telogen
    t. effluvium
    t. hair
    t. phase
telomerase reverse transcriptase (TERT)
telomeric
telopeptide
TEM
    transmission electron microscopy
    triethylenemelamine
temafloxacin
Temaril
Temovate topical
temperate
    t. bacteriophage
    t. virus
temperature
    maximum t.
    minimum t.
    optimum t.
    room t.
    t. sensitive (TS)
    t. spot
temperature-controlled electrophoresis
temperature-dependent dermatosis
temperature-sensitive
    t.-s. mutant
    t.-s. oculocutaneous albinism
template
    Dermal Regeneration T.
    t. theory
temporal
    t. artery biopsy (TAB)
    t. canthus
    t. giant cell arteritis
    t. relationship
temporary auxiliary liver transplantation

temporomandibular
    t. dysfunction (TMD)
    t. joint (TMJ)
Tempra
TEN
    toxic epidermal necrolysis
tenascin
tender point
Tendersorb ABD absorptive dressing
TenderWet system
Tenderwrap leg compression dressing
tendinitis
    Achilles t.
    bicipital t.
    t. bursitis
    calcific t.
    flexor hallucis longus t.
    patellar t.
    peroneal t.
    rotator cuff t.
tendinopathy
    degenerative t.
tendinosis
tendinosum
    xanthoma t.
tendinous xanthoma
tendon
    Achilles t.
    t. friction rub
    peroneal t.
    t. sheath
    supraspinatus t.
    t. xanthoma
tendonesis effect
tendonitis-fascitis syndrome
tenesmus
teniposide
tennis
    t. elbow
    t. shoe foot
    t. toe
Tenon
    T. capsule
    T. space
TENOR
    The Epidemiology and Natural History of
    Asthma: Outcome and Treatment
    Regimens
    The Epidemiology and Natural History of
    Asthma: Outcome and Treatment
    Regimens
Ten-O-Six

tenosynovectomy
tenosynovitis
    de Quervain stenosing t.
    dorsal wrist t.
    flexed t.
    gonococcic t.
    gonorrheal t.
    proliferative t.
    stenosing t.
    tenosynovium t.
tenosynovium tenosynovitis
tenoxicam acid
TENS
    transcutaneous electrical nerve
    stimulation
    transcutaneous electrical neuromuscular
    stimulator
    Sham TENS
tensile strength of osteoarthritic
  cartilage
tension-time index
tentacle print
tenuifolia
    Schizonepeta t.
tenuis
    Alternaria t.
    Nocardia t.
Tequin
Terak Ophthalmic Ointment
teratogenic effect on pregnant women
Terazol
terbinafine
    t. hydrochloride
    t. hydrochloride cream
    t. hydrochloride tablet
terbutaline sulfate
terconazole
terebrans
    basiloma t.
terfenadine and pseudoephedrine
Terfonyl
Terinacei
terminal
    t. cascade
    t. hair
    postsynaptic t.
    presynaptic t.
    visual display t. (VDT)
terminator
    DNA-chain t.
terpine anhydride
Terra-Cortril Ophthalmic Suspension

T

NOTES

Terramycin
    T. IM injection
    T. oral
    T. w/Polymyxin B Ophthalmic
      Ointment
terrestrial snake
terrestris
    Tribulus t.
terreus
    Aspergillus t.
Terry nail
Tersa-Tar
TERT
    telomerase reverse transcriptase
tertiary
    t. cutaneous syphilis
    t. follicle
    t. granule
    t. noduloulcerative syphilis
    t. structure
    t. syphilid
    t. yaw
tertile
Teschen
    T. disease
    T. disease virus
Tessalon Perles
TEST
    T.R.U.E. TEST
test
    A1 t.
    Acaderm patch t.
    acid-Schiff t.
    adhesion t.
    Adson t.
    AlaSTAT latex allergy t.
    alkali patch t.
    allergen inhalation challenge t.
    allergy skin t.
    Amplicor viral load t.
    Amplified Mycobacterium
      Tuberculosis Direct T.
    analysis of variance t.
    Ana-Sal HIV t.
    ANOVA t.
    antibiotic sensitivity t.
    antigenemia t.
    antigen leukocyte cellular
      antibody t. (ALCAT)
    antiglobulin t.
    antihuman globulin t.
    antinuclear antibody screening t.
    Apley grind t.
    Ascoli t.
    ASLO t.
    augmented histamine t.
    bacterial phagocytosis t.
    basophil degranulation t.
    BCR/abl gene re-arrangement t.

bentonite flocculation t.
Bioclot t.
blood coagulation t.
Bonferroni t t.
bronchial inhalation challenge t.
bronchial provocation t.
broth t.
Brucella card t.
Buhler t.
C3 t.
C4 t.
Calmette t.
Candida skin t.
capillary fragility t.
capillary resistance t.
Captia t.
Casoni intradermal t.
Casoni skin t.
cellular antigen stimulation t.
  (CAST)
CF t.
challenge t.
chamber-scarification t.
Chiron bDNA viral load t.
chi-square t.
chloride sweat t.
Christmas tree t.
chrome patch t.
closed patch t.
Clostridium difficile t. (CLOtest)
Coamatic protein C t.
Cobas Amplicor CMV Monitor t.
coccidioidin skin t.
Cochran-Mantel-Haenszel t.
COLAP t.
collagen vascular serologic t.
colonoscopic allergen provocation t.
Combi t.
combion t.
complement t.
complement-fixation t.
Confide HIV t.
Coombs t.
cosmetic allergy t.
Coulter ICD-Prep t.
Cox-Mantel t.
CSD skin t.
cutaneous tuberculin t.
cutireaction t.
cystic fibrosis t.
cytotoxic t.
cytotropic antibody t.
DA pregnancy t.
Davidsohn differential t.
dexamethasone suppression t. (DST)
DFA t.
diagnostic t.
Dick t.
dimethylgloxime nickel spot t.

direct agglutination t.
direct amplification t.
direct Coombs t.
direct fluorescent antibody t.
DNA-binding t.
DNA hybridization t.
DNA probe t.
double immunodiffusion in agarose gels t.
Draize Repeat Insult patch t.
Ducrey t.
Dunnett multiple comparison t.
EBNA IgG ELISA t.
EB nuclear antigen t.
EB-specific IgM t.
EB viral capsid antigen t.
electrotransfer t.
ELISA t.
ELISPOT t.
Envacor t.
enzyme-linked immunosorbent assay t.
epicutaneous t.
epsilometric t.
Epstein-Barr nuclear antigen t.
Epstein-Barr-specific immunoglobulin M t.
Epstein-Barr virus t.
erythrocyte adherence t.
false-negative patch t.
false-positive patch t.
false-positive syphilis t.
Farr t.
Finkelstein t.
First Check rapid diagnostic t.
Fisher two-tailed exact t.
flocculation t.
fluorescein-conjugated monoclonal antibody immunofluorescent t.
fluorescein-tagged monoclonal antibody immunofluorescent t.
fluorescent treponemal antibody-absorption t.
forearm ischemic exercise t.
Formo-Test t.
Foshay t.
Frei t.
Freund complete adjuvant t.
FTA-ABS t.
gel diffusion precipitin t.
Gen-Probe rapid tuberculosis t.
Gerhardt t.

glove-powder inhalation t.
glove-use t.
goodness-of-fit chi-square t.
Göthlin t.
grind t.
guinea pig maximization t. (GPMT)
Hair dressing screening tray t.
Ham t.
Hamilton t.
HBV DNA probe t.
head compression t.
head distraction t.
Heaf t.
Helisal rapid blood t.
hemadsorption virus t.
hemagglutination t.
Hess t.
Hinton t.
histoplasmin-latex t.
HIV DNA PCR t.
H-SLAP t.
human basophil degranulation t. (HBDT)
human stromelysin aggregated proteoglycan t.
hybridization t.
Hycor rheumatoid factor IgA ELISA autoimmune t.
hydrogen breath t.
hyperventilation provocation t. (HVPT)
ice cube t.
IgE radioallergosorbent t.
IgG avidity t.
immune adhesion t.
ImmunoCard STAT! Rotavirus t.
immunologic pregnancy t.
indirect agglutination t.
indirect Coombs t.
indirect fluorescent antibody t.
indirect hemagglutination t.
INR clotting t.
insulin skin t.
international normalized ratio clotting t.
intracutaneous t.
intradermal skin t.
intraperitoneal glucose tolerance t. (IPGTT)
intravenous glucose tolerance t. (IVGTT)

NOTES

test *(continued)*

Ito-Reenstierna t.
Jadassohn-Bloch t.
Keller ultraviolet t.
killing t.
k82 ImmunoCap t.
Kolmer t.
Kolmogorov-Smirnov t.
Kruskal-Wallis t.
Kveim t.
Lachman t.
latex agglutination t.
latex allergy t.
latex fixation t.
leishmania t.
leishmanin t.
Leishman-Montenegro-Donovan
  intradermal t.
lepromin t.
leukocyte esterase t. (LET)
leukocyte histamine release t.
Liatest C4b-BP t.
lignocaine monoethylgylycine
  xylidine excretion t.
lupus erythematosus cell t.
macrophage migration inhibition t.
macroscopic agglutination t.
Mann-Whitney U t.
Mantel-Haenszel t.
Mantoux t.
mast cell degranulation t.
t. material
Maurer optimization t.
Mazzotti t.
McKenzie t.
McNemar t.
McNemar t. of significance
Mecholyl skin t.
Meinicke t.
methacholine chloride skin t.
MHA-TP t.
microimmunofluorescence t. (MIF)
microlymphocytotoxicity t.
microscopic agglutination t.
MicroTrak t.
midpoint skin t.
migration inhibition t.
migration inhibitory factor t.
Minor iodine-starch t.
Mitsuda t.
mixed agglutination t.
mixed lymphocyte culture t.
MLC t.
modified Draize t.
Moloney t.
monolisa t.
Mono-Vac t.
Montenegro t.
MTD T.

mucin clot t.
multiple puncture t. (MPT)
multiple puncture tuberculin t.
Multitest t.
mumps sensitivity t.
Murray t.
Mycobacterium tuberculosis
  Direct T.
nasal antigen challenge t.
nasal provocation t.
negative control t.
negative patch t.
negative Schick t.
neutralization t.
Newman-Keuls t.
nitroblue tetrazolium t.
nontreponemal flocculation t.
N-telopeptide urine t.
occlusive patch t.
t. for O&P
open application t.
open epicutaneous t. (OET)
open patch t.
OsteoGram bone density t.
Osteomark urine-based t.
Ouchterlony t.
OX-2, -19 t.
oxacillin disk diffusion t.
Pap t.
Papanicolaou t.
paper radioimmunosorbent t.
  (PRIST)
paracoccidioidin skin t.
passive cutaneous anaphylaxis t.
passive transfer t.
patch t.
Paul t.
Paul-Bunnell t.
PCA t.
Pearson chi square t.
pediatric infectious disease
  developmental screening t.
  (PIDDST)
percutaneous t.
pertussis agglutination t.
photo-patch t.
physiologic t.
pilocarpine iontophoresis sweat t.
Pirquet t.
P-K t.
platelet neutralization t.
POCkit herpes t.
Porges-Meier t.
positive patch t.
PPD t.
PPL skin t.
PRA t.
Prausnitz-Kustner t. (P-K test)
precipitation t.

precipitin t.
predictive patch t.
prick-prick t.
prick puncture t.
prick-to-prick t.
protection t.
provocation-neutralization t.
provocative dose t. (PDT)
provocative use t. (PUT)
pulmonary function t. (PFT)
pulse t.
purified protein derivative t.
Quality of Upper Extremities T. (QUEST)
quellung t.
radioallergosorbent t. (RAST)
radioimmunosorbent t. (RIST)
rapid whole blood t. (RWBT)
reagin screen t. (RST)
red cell adherence t.
Reiter t.
repeat open reaction application t.
RF t.
Rh blocking t.
Rheumatex t.
rheumatoid factor t.
Rheumaton t.
rhinovirus challenge t.
ring precipitin t.
Rinne t.
Römer t.
rosette t.
Rose-Waaler t.
RoSSA/RoSSB antibody t.
RPR circle card t.
rub t.
rubella HI t.
rubella IgG ELISA t.
Rumpel-Leede t.
Sabin-Feldman dye t.
Sachs-Georgi t.
scarification t.
Schick t.
Schirmer t.
Schober t.
Scotch Tape t.
scratch chamber t.
screen t.
Semmes-Weinstein t.
sequential probability ratio t. (SPRT)
serial dilutional intradermal skin t.

Shapiro-Wilke W t.
single-breath nitrogen washout t.
skin prick t. (SPT)
skin-puncture t.
Spearman rank t.
SPEP t.
spinal fluid t.
sporotriquin t.
spot t.
starch-iodine t.
Steinberg t.
Sterneedle tuberculin t.
straight-leg raising t.
streptozyme agglutination t.
SureCell Strep A t.
TheoFAST t.
thermostable opsonin t.
Third Heir Avidin Biotin Enzyme System T. (THABEST)
tine t.
tourniquet t.
TPHA t.
TPI t.
transfer t.
Trendelenburg t.
treponemal t.
Trichophyton skin t.
Trolab wool alcohol t.
T.R.U.E. allergy patch t.
tube precipitin t.
tuberculin skin t.
tuberculin tine t.
tuberculin titer t.
Tukey standardized range t.
Tzanck t.
urea breath t. (UBT)
use t.
VDRL t.
Vega t.
virus neutralization t.
vitamin C t.
in vitro t.
Vollmer t.
volume t.
Wassermann fast t.
Weber t.
Weil-Felix t.
Western blot electrotransfer t.
Whiff t.
Widal serum t.
Wilcoxon rank sum t.
Winn t.

NOTES

test *(continued)*
    x-square t.
    Yates corrected chi square t.
testacea
    cutis t.
testerma
    Jadassohn t.
testing
    antimicrobiology susceptibility t.
    battery patch t.
    cold air t.
    conjunctival t.
    delayed hypersensitivity skin t.
    drug challenge t.
    electrodermal t.
    epidermal t.
    exercise challenge t.
    genotypic antiretroviral resistance t. (GART)
    histocompatibility t.
    human immunodeficiency virus antigen t.
    hypersensitivity skin t.
    John Dory fish prick t.
    methacholine challenge t.
    panel-reactive antibody t.
    p24 antigen t.
    patch t.
    PCR t.
    placebo-controlled oral challenge t. (DPOC)
    polymerase chain reaction t.
    population-based t.
    PRA t.
    predictive t.
    prick t.
    provocative dose t.
    RCR t.
    repeat open-application t. (ROAT)
    RIBA II antibody t.
    Rinkel t.
    scratch t.
    skin t.
    SUDS HIV-1 diagnostic t.
    transmission disequilibrium t. (TDT)
    venom t.
testis-specific binding protein (TSBP)
Testoderm patch
testosterone
test/score
    MEGX t./s.
TET
    tetracycline
tetanolysin
tetanospasmin
tetanotoxin
tetanus
    t. antitoxin
    t. antitoxin unit

    t. immune globulin
    t. immune globulin, human
    t. immunoglobulin
    t. toxin
    t. toxoid
    t. toxoid, adsorbed
    t. toxoid, fluid
    t. vaccine
tetanus-diphtheria (Td)
tetanus-perfringens antitoxin
Tete virus
tetra-acetate
tetracaine
    t. hydrochloride
    t. with dextrose
Tetracap oral
tetracycline (TCN, TET)
    t. seams
    t. transactivator
tetracycline-resistant *Neisseria gonorrhoeae* **(TRNG)**
Tetracyn
tetrad
    acne t.
tetrahydrozoline hydrochloride
Tetralan oral
tetralin
    acetyl ethyl tetramethyl t. (AETT)
tetramethylthiuram dermatitis
Tetram oral
Tetramune fish food
tetranda
    Stephania t.
Tetrasine Extra Ophthalmic
tetratricopeptide
    t. repeat
    ubiquitously transcribed t. (UTY)
tetrazolium
    nitroblue t. (NBT)
tetrodotoxin
tetter
    branny t.
    brawny t.
    crusted t.
    dry t.
    foot t.
    honeycomb t.
    humid t.
    milk t.
    moist t.
    scaly t.
    wet t.
Tewameter TM 210 open loop system
TEWL
    transepidermal water loss
Texacort topical
Texas
    T. coral snake
    T. coral snake bite

textile
    t. dermatitis
    t. finish
texture
    coarse t.
textus, pl. **textus**
TF
    tissue factor
TFCC
    triangular fibrocartilage complex
TFI
    tumor of the follicular infundibulum
TFPI
    tissue factor pathway inhibitor
TG
    thyroglobulin
6-TG
Tg cell
TGE
    transmissible gastroenteritis virus
        TGE virus
T/Gel
    Neutrogena T/G.
    T/G. Neutrogena
TGF
    transforming growth factor
    trypanosome growth factor
TGF-alpha
    transforming growth factor-alpha
TGF-B
    transforming growth factor-beta
TGF-induced immunosuppression
TH2
    T-helper-2 lymphocyte
Th
    T-helper cell
    thyroid
Th1
    T-helper type 1
        Th1 cell
        Th1 cytokine
Th2
    T-helper type 2 cell
        Th2 cell
Th3
    T-helper type 3 cell
Th-1 mediated immune response
THABEST
    Third Heir Avidin Biotin Enzyme System Test
ThAIRapy vest airway clearance system

thalassemia
    alpha t.
    Bart t.
    t. major
    t. syndrome
thalidomide
thallus
Thalomid
thanatophobic
thanatophoric diastrophic chondrodysplasia
thapsigargin pool
Thayer-Martin medium
thecal felon
Theiler
    T. disease
    T. mouse encephalomyelitis virus
    T. original strain of mouse encephalomyelitis virus (TO)
Thelazia
thelerethism
thelium, pl. **thelia**
T-helper
    T-h. cell (Th)
    T-h. type 1 (Th1)
    T-h. type 2 cell (Th2)
    T-h. type 3 cell (Th3)
T-helper-2 lymphocyte (TH2)
Theo-24
Theobald Smith phenomenon
Theobid
Theochron
Theoclear L.A.
Theo-Dur
TheoFAST test
Theo-G
Theolair
Theolate
theophylline
    anhydrous t.
    dihydroxypropyl t.
    t., ephedrine, and hydroxyzine (TEH)
    t., ephedrine, and phenobarbital
    t. and guaifenesin
    t. salt
theophylline-induced convulsion
theorem
    binomial t.
theory, pl. **theories**
    Arrhenius-Madsen t.
    cellular immune t.

NOTES

theory *(continued)*
    clonal deletion t.
    clonal selection t.
    Ehrlich side-chain t.
    Fisher-Race t.
    forbidden-clone t.
    germ t.
    immune t.
    instructive t.
    Metchnikoff t.
    neural t.
    side-chain t.
    template t.
Theospan-SR
Theovent
Theo-X
thèque
Thera-Boot leg compression dressing
theraccine
    melanoma t.
TheraCys
Therafectin
TheraFlu
Therakos UVAR system
Theramin Expectorant
TheraPEP positive expiratory pressure therapy system
therapeutic
    t. immunology
    t. interferon
    t. irradiation
    t. malaria
    t. ratio
therapia magna sterilisans
therapist
Theraplex Z
TheraPress
    T. DUO
    T. DUO Lite
therapy
    ACTH t.
    ActiPatch t.
    adrenocorticosteroid t.
    adrenocorticotropic hormone t.
    alkylating t.
    alternate-day t.
    antibacterial t.
    antibody-directed enzyme prodrug t. (ADEPT)
    antifungal t.
    anti-IIb-IIIA mAB t.
    antiinflammatory t.
    antipruritic t.
    antirheumatic t.
    antituberculous t.
    antiviral t.
    around-the-clock oral maintenance bronchodilator t.
    5 ATGAM antilymphocyte t.

    augmentation t.
    autoserum t.
    BAL t.
    biologic t.
    biomagnetic t.
    blood transfusion t.
    calcipotriene t.
    Candida t.
    chloroquine t.
    cognitive-behavior t. (CBT)
    coherence t.
    conventional asthma t. (CAT)
    cyclosporine maintenance t.
    cytotoxic immunosuppressive t.
    depigmentation t.
    Diabetic Skin T.
    diagnostic surgical t.
    dressing t.
    empiric t.
    estrogen replacement t. (ERT)
    Excimer laser t.
    factor replacement t.
    fever t.
    fluid t.
    fluorinated corticosteroid-occlusive t.
    foreign protein t.
    gene t.
    genetic t.
    gold t.
    grenz ray t.
    heat t.
    heparinoid t.
    herbal t.
    heterovaccine t.
    high-dose immunosuppressive t. (HDIT)
    highly active antiretroviral t. (HAART)
    HSV-thymidine kinase ex-vivo cell t.
    hydroxychloroquine t.
    hyperbaric oxygen t.
    immunocompetent tissue t.
    immunoglobulin replacement t.
    immunosuppressive t. (IST)
    interferon t.
    International Association of Enterostomal T. (IAET)
    intraarticular t.
    intralesional corticosteroid t.
    laser t.
    leukaphersis-based immunomodulatory t.
    Levulan photodynamic t.
    MAb t.
    maggot t.
    malarial t.
    medical t.
    monoclonal antibody t.

multidrug t. (MDT)
negative pressure wound t.
Neova Eye T.
nonspecific t.
NTBC t.
occlusal appliance t.
occlusive t.
occupational t. (OT)
5 OKT3 antilymphocyte t.
oral iron t.
orthomolecular t.
penicillin t.
pharmacologic t.
photodynamic t. (PDT)
physical t.
plasma t.
postnatal t.
preemptive t.
prenatal t.
protective t.
protein shock t.
psychotropic agent t.
pulsed-dye laser t.
radiation t.
replacement t.
repository t.
retinoid t.
salvage t.
Saran Wrap t.
sedative t.
serum t.
short-contact t.
silicone sheeting t.
skin lubrication t.
soak t.
Staphylococcus protein A column t.
Supartz joint fluid t.
supportive t.
surgical t.
symptomatic t.
systemic antibacterial t.
systemic antifungal t.
toothpaste swish t.
topical antibacterial t.
topical antifungal t.
topical cytotoxic t.
topical photodynamic t.
traditional Chinese herbal t. (TCHT)
triple t.
vaccine t.

Vaseline Lip T.
VIMRxyn light-activated t.
vitamin B t.
vitamin K t.
TheraSnore oral appliance
Theratope-STn vaccine
ThermaCool TC radiofrequency device
thermal
   t. anhidrosis
   t. burn
   t. cycler
   t. elastosis
   t. flushing
   t. hyperalgia
   t. quenching technique
   t. relaxation time
   t. shock
Thermazene
thermescent Skin Treatment
***Thermoactinomyces* vulgaris**
thermoduric
ThermoFlow ETC unit
thermogenic anhidrosis
thermolabile opsonin
thermolamp
thermophile
thermophilic
thermophylic
thermoplastic elastomer (TPE)
thermoregulation
thermoresistable
   Mycobacterium t.
thermosetting resin
thermostabile
thermostable
   t. opsonin
   t. opsonin test
thermotolerant
Theroxide Wash
thesaurismosis
thesaurosis
theta, θ
   t. antigen
The VAC Vacuum Assisted Closure
THH
   targetoid hemosiderotic hemangioma
thiabendazole
thiacetazone
thiamine deficiency
thiazide
Thibierge-Weissenbach syndrome

NOTES

thick
    t. and sticky mucus
    t. tongue
thickened skin
thickening
    disciform t.
    scleroderma-like skin t.
    subbasement membrane t.
thickness
    Breslow t.
    carotid intima-media wall t.
Thiemann disease
thienamycin
Thiersch graft
thimerosal
Thin
    Hydrocol T.
thin-layer immunoassay
thin-section CT
THINSite
    T. hydrogel sheet
    T. with BioFilm hydrogel topical
      wound dressing
thiobarbituric acid-reactive substance
thioglucose
Thioglycollate
thioguanine
thiol protease
thiomalate
Thiomersal
thiopronine
thiopropanolsulphonate
    gold t.
thioredoxin reductase (TR)
thioridazine
thiosulfate
    sodium t.
thiosulphate
    gold t.
thiourea
third
    t. disease
    t. and fourth pharyngeal pouch
      syndrome
    T. Heir Avidin Biotin Enzyme
      System Test (THABEST)
third-degree burn
third-generation cephalosporin
thistle
    Russian t.
thiuram-alcohol reaction
thiuram mix
Thomas needle
Thompson
    T. dermatoplasty
    T. syndrome
Thomsen antibody
Thomson
    T. poikiloderma congenitale

    T. scattering
    T. sign
thoracentesis
thoracic
    t. duct drainage (TDD)
    t. organ transplant
    t. outlet syndrome
thoracoabdominal
    t. dyssynchrony
    t. irradiation (TAI)
    t. paradox
thoracocardiography
thoraco-lumbar-sacral orthosis
thoracoplasty
thoracoscope
    rigid t.
thoracoscopy
thoracostomy
    tube t.
Thoratec ventricular assist device
Thorazine
threonyl-tRNA synthetase
thresher's lung
threshold
    acoustic reflex t.
    t. audiometry
    erythema t.
    t. limit value (TLV)
    minimum elicitation t. (MET)
thrive
    failure to t.
thrix annulata
throat
    itchy t.
thrombasthenia
    Glanzmann t.
thrombectomy
    surgical t.
thrombi (*pl. of* thrombus)
thrombin-antithrombin III (TAT)
thromboangiitis obliterans (TAO)
thrombocytopenia
    amegakaryocytic t. (AT)
    autoimmune neonatal t.
    drug-induced t.
    familial t.
    immune t.
    isoimmune neonatal t.
    multifocal
      lymphangioendotheliomatosis
      with t.
    sepsis-induced t.
thrombocytopenia-absent-radius (TAR)
thrombocytopenic
    t. hemangiomatosis
    t. purpura
    t. purpura/hemolytic uremic
      syndrome (TTP-HUS)
thrombogenesis

thrombolytic
thrombomodulin
thrombophilia
    lupus t.
thrombophlebitis
    retinal t.
    superficial migratory t.
thrombopoietin (TPO)
thrombosis, pl. thromboses
    dural sinus t.
    graft t.
thrombospondin (TSP)
thrombotic
    t. gangrene
    t. thrombocytopenic purpura (TTP)
thromboxane
    t. A_2 (TXA_2)
    t. synthase
thrombus, pl. thrombi
    intramural t.
    phagocytic t.
throwing act
thrush
    oral t.
thumb
    t. forceps
    gamekeeper's t.
Thunder God vine
thylacitis
thymectomy
thymi (*pl. of* thymus)
thymic
    t. alymphoplasia
    t. dysplasia
    t. epithelial cell
    t. hormone
    t. hypoplasia
    t. irradiation (TI)
    t. lymphopoietic factor
    t. peptide
    t. transplantation
thymidine
    hypoxanthine, aminopterin and t. (HAT)
thymin
thymine
thymocyte
Thymoglobulin
Thymol
thymoma
    murine t.
thymopathy

thymopentin
thymopoietin
thymosin
thymus, pl. thymi, thymuses
    t. and activation-regulated chemokine (TARC)
    congenital aplasia of t.
    t. nurse cell
thymus-derived leukemia
thymus-independent antigen
thymus-replacing factor
Thyro-Block
thyroglobulin (TG)
thyroglossal cyst
thyroid (Th)
    t. acropachy
    t. disorder
    t. gland
    t. peroxidase (TPO)
thyroid-associated ophthalmopathy (TAO)
thyroid-binding inhibitory immunoglobulin (TBII)
thyroid-blocking antibody (TBAB)
thyroiditis
    t., Addison disease, Sjögren syndrome, sarcoidosis (TASS)
    chronic autoimmune t.
    Hashimoto t.
    immune-mediated t.
    painless t.
    postpartum t. (PPT)
thyroid-stimulating
    t.-s. antibody
    t.-s. hormone (TSH)
    t.-s. hormone-displacing antibody
    t.-s. hormone receptor (TSH-R)
    t.-s. hormone receptor antibody
thyroperoxidase antibody
thyrotoxic
    t. complement-fixation factor
    t. serum
thyrotoxicosis
thyrotoxin
thyrotropin-binding inhibitory immunoglobulin (TBII)
thyroxine (T4)
Thysanosoma actinoides
thysanotrichica
    ichthyosis t.
TI
    thymic irradiation

T

NOTES

TI-23 cytomegalovirus monoclonal antibody
Tiacid
Tiamol
tiaprofenic acid
tibial nerve
Ticar
ticarcillin
- t. and clavulanic acid
- t. disodium

tic-Douloureux
tic douloureux
TICE BCG
tick
- t. bite
- t. bite alopecia
- black-legged t.
- California black-legged t.
- deer t.
- t. fever
- hard t.
- *Ixodes dammini* t.
- *Ixodes pacificus* t.
- *Ixodes ricinus* wood t.
- Lone Star t.
- Pacific t.
- t. paralysis
- t. pyrexia
- Rocky Mountain t.
- seed t.
- soft t.
- spotted-fever t.
- t. typhus
- t. vector
- western black-legged t.
- wood t.

tickborne
- t. encephalitis Central European subtype
- t. encephalitis Eastern subtype
- t. encephalitis virus
- t. relapsing fever

TI-CMV
- tissue-invasive cytomegalovirus
- TI-CMV disease

tidal
- t. irrigation
- t. volume

Tièche nevus
Tielle absorptive dressing
tie-over bolster dressing
Tietze syndrome
TIF
- tropic immersion foot

tiger snake antivenom
tight
- t. asthmatic
- t. building syndrome
- t. skin mouse

tightness
- Bunnell intrinsic t.

TIL
- tumor-infiltrating lymphocyte
  - TIL cell
  - TIL cell assay

Tilade Inhalation Aerosol
Tilcotil
tilorone
tiludronate
TIM
- topical immunomodulator
  - TIM drug classification
  - TIM therapeutic category

time (T)
- activated partial thromboplastin t. (APTT)
- cold ischemia t.
- dilute Russell viper venom t.
- epidermal transit t.
- generation t.
- germinative t.
- kaolin clotting t.
- lead t.
- median survival t. (MST)
- partial thromboplastin t. (PTT)
- reduced cold ischemic t.
- Russell viper venom t.
- thermal relaxation t.
- transit t.

Timecelles
- Sinufed T.

timed intermittent rotation
Timentin
timolol
Timoptic Ophthalmic
Timoptic-XE Ophthalmic
timori
- *Brugia t.*

timorian filariasis
timothy grass
TIMP
- tissue inhibitor of metalloproteinase

TIN
- tubulointerstitial nephritis

Tinactin
Tinamed
- T. plantar patch
- T. wart remover

TINA monitor
TinBen
TinCoBen
tinctorial change
tincture
- Arning t.
- Fungoid t.
- Green soap t.

Tindall effect
T-independent response

tinea
> t. amiantacea
> t. axillaris
> t. barbae
> black dot t.
> t. capitis
> t. ciliorum
> t. circinata
> t. conus
> t. corporis
> t. cruris
> t. decalvans
> t. dermatitis
> t. faciei
> t. favosa
> t. furfuracea
> t. glabrosa
> t. imbricata
> t. incognito
> t. infection
> t. inguinalis
> t. kerion
> t. manuum
> t. nigra
> t. nodosa
> t. pedis
> t. pedis et manus
> t. profunda
> t. rubrum
> t. sycosis
> t. tarsi
> t. tonsurans
> t. tropicalis
> t. unguium
> t. versicolor

tine test
tin ethyl (SnET2)
tingible body
Tinidazole
Tinted
> Oxy-5 T.

TINU
> tubulointerstitial nephritis with uveitis
> TINU syndrome

Tinver Lotion
tinzaparin sodium injectable
tip stitch
tire-patch appearance
Ti-Screen
Tisit
> T. Blue Gel

> T. Liquid
> T. Shampoo

Tisseel fibrin sealant
tissue
> acellular pannus t.
> autodigestion of connective t.
> t. confirmation
> connective t.
> cynomolgus macaque t.
> decidual t.
> t. detritus
> elastic t.
> extraarticular t.
> t. factor (TF)
> t. factor pathway inhibitor (TFPI)
> fibroblastic t.
> t. fluke
> granulation t.
> gut-associated lymphoid t. (GALT)
> hemangiomatous t.
> t. inhibitor of metalloproteinase (TIMP)
> mesenchymal t.
> t. metalloproteinase
> mucosa-associated lymphoid t. (MALT)
> necrotic t.
> neural t.
> nose-associated lymphoid t. (NALT)
> organ-cultured corneal t.
> t. remodeling
> t. repair
> secondary lymphatic t. (SLT)
> skin-associated lymphoid t. (SALT)
> soft t.
> synovial t.
> t. transglutaminase (Ttg)

tissue-activated fibroblast
tissue-engineered polymer device
tissue-invasive cytomegalovirus (TI-CMV)
tissue-specific antigen
Tissue-Tek OCT medium
titanium dioxide
titanium:sapphire laser
titer
> antinuclear antibody t.
> antirotavirus IgA t.
> ASLO t.
> C-ANCA t.
> IgG t.
> indirect Coombs t.
> mycoplasma IgM t.

T

NOTES

titer *(continued)*
    P-ANCA t.
    rheumatoid factor t.
    streptozyme t.
    STZ t.
titin
titration
    Rinkel serial endpoint t.
Ti-U-Lac HC
Ti-UVA-B
tixocortol-21-pivalate
Tj antigen
TL-01 UV-B regimen
TLC
    total lung capacity
TLI
    total lymphoid irradiation
TLV
    threshold limit value
T-lymphocyte
TM
    telangiectatic matting
    tympanic membrane
Tm cell
TMD
    temporomandibular dysfunction
TMEP
    telangiectasia macularis eruptiva perstans
TMJ
    temporomandibular joint
TMP
    trimethyl psoralen
TMP-SMX
    trimethoprim-sulfamethoxazole
TN
    tree nut allergy
TNF
    tumor necrosis factor
        TNF inhibitor
        TNF mRNA cytokine
        TNF receptor II gene
TNF-alpha
    tumor necrosis factor-alpha
TNF-beta
    tumor necrosis factor-beta
TNF-R
    pegylated p55 TNF-R
TNM
    tumor, nodes, metastasis
        TNM staging
TNNSS
    total nonnasal symptom score
TNSS
    total nasal symptom score
TO
    Theiler original strain of mouse
      encephalomyelitis virus
        TO virus
toad skin

toasted
    t. shin
    t. skin syndrome
tobacco
    t. leaf extract
    t. smoke
    wild t.
TobraDex Ophthalmic
tobramycin and dexamethasone
Tobrex Ophthalmic
tocopherol deficiency
Todd-Hewitt broth
toe
    black t.
    hammer t.
    Hong Kong t.
    t. itch
    jogger's t.
    mallet t.
    sausage t.
    soccer t.
    tennis t.
toeweb
Tofranil
Togaviridae virus
togavirus
toilet
    bronchial t.
    pulmonary t.
Tokelau ringworm
tolbutamide
Tolectin DS
tolerance
    acquired intrathymic t.
    donor-specific t.
    high dose t.
    immune t.
    immunological t.
    immunologic high dose t.
    impaired glucose t. (IGT)
    nonresponder t.
    oral t.
    organ-specific t.
    split t.
    t. through deletion
    t. through regulation
tolerization
tolerize
tolerogen
tolerogenesis
    surrogate t. (ST)
tolerogenic
tolerogenicity
Toll receptor
tolmetin sodium
tolnaftate
tolu
    balsam of t.
toluene sulfonamide

tomato tumor
tombstoning
tomodensitometry
    computerized t.
tomography
    cine computed t.
    computed t. (CT)
    high-resolution computed t. (HRCT)
    optical coherent t.
    positron emission t. (PET)
    quantitative computed t. (QCT)
    single photon emission computed t.
      (SPECT)
    technetium-99m hexamethylpropylene
      amine oxime-single-photon-emission
      computed t. (HMPAO-SPECT)
tone
    Ambi Skin T.
    bronchial smooth muscle t.
tongue
    baked t.
    black hairy t.
    burning t.
    caviar t.
    claudication of t.
    coated t.
    fissured t.
    furrowed t.
    geographic t.
    glossy t.
    grooved t.
    hobnail t.
    osseous choristoma of the t.
    painful t.
    raspberry t.
    scrotal t.
    strawberry t.
    thick t.
    transitory benign plaque of t.
    white strawberry t.
tonofibril
tonofilament
tonofilament-cytoplasmic plaque linker
tonsil
    absent t.
    hypertrophic t.
    small t.
tonsillectomy
tonsillitis
    streptococcal t.
tonsillopharyngitis

tonsurans
    herpes t.
    tinea t.
    Trichophyton t.
tool
    Bates-Jensen pressure ulcer status t.
    Pressure Ulcer Scale for Healing t.
    PUSH t.
tooth, pl. teeth
    Hutchinson teeth
    Micro-Adson forceps with teeth
    t. pit
    t. rash
toothpaste swish therapy
top
    red t.
Topactin
Top-Count microplate scintillation
  counter
tophaceous gout
tophus, pl. tophi
    intraarticular t.
    synovial membrane t.
    t. syphiliticus
topical
    Achromycin t.
    Aclovate t.
    Acticort t.
    Actinex t.
    Aeroseb-HC t.
    Akne-Mycin t.
    Ala-Cort t.
    Ala-Quin t.
    Ala-Scalp t.
    Alphatrex t.
    t. anesthetic
    t. antibacterial therapy
    t. antifungal therapy
    t. antipruritic
    Anusol-HC1 t.
    Aquacare t.
    Aquaphor Antibiotic t.
    Aristocort A t.
    A/T/S t.
    Baciguent t.
    BactoShield t.
    Bactroban t.
    t. BCNU
    Benadryl t.
    Betalene t.
    Betatrex t.
    Beta-Val t.

T

NOTES

topical *(continued)*
　　Borofax t.
　　CaldeCort t.
　　Caldesene t.
　　Carmol t.
　　Carmol-HC t.
　　Cetacort t.
　　Cleocin T t.
　　Clinda-Derm t.
　　Cloderm t.
　　Cordran SP t.
　　Corque t.
　　CortaGel t.
　　Cortaid Maximum Strength t.
　　Cortaid with Aloe t.
　　Cort-Dome t.
　　Cortef Feminine Itch t.
　　t. corticosteroid
　　Cortin t.
　　Cortizone-10 t.
　　Cruex t.
　　Cutivate t.
　　Cyclocort t.
　　t. cytotoxic therapy
　　Debrisan t.
　　t. decongestant
　　Delcort t.
　　Del-Mycin t.
　　Delta-Tritex t.
　　Dermacomb t.
　　Dermacort t.
　　Dermarest Dricort t.
　　Derma-Smoothe/FS t.
　　Dermolate t.
　　Dermtex HC with Aloe t.
　　Desitin t.
　　DesOwen t.
　　Diprolene AF t.
　　Diprosone t.
　　Dyna-Hex t.
　　t. eczema
　　Efudex t.
　　Elase t.
　　Elase-Chloromycetin t.
　　Eldecort t.
　　Elocon t.
　　Emgel t.
　　EMLA t.
　　t. emollient
　　Erycette t.
　　EryDerm T.
　　Erygel T.
　　Erymax t.
　　erythromycin t.
　　E-Solve-2 t.
　　ETS-2% t.
　　Eurax t.
　　Exelderm t.
　　Florone E t.

Fluonex t.
Fluonid t.
Fluoroplex t.
Flurosyn t.
Flutex t.
FS Shampoo t.
Furacin t.
Garamycin T.
G-myticin t.
Gynecort t.
Halog t.
Halog-E t.
Halotex t.
t. hemostatic agent
Hibiclens t.
Hibistat t.
Hi-Cort.
Hycort t.
Hydrocort t.
Hydro-Tex t.
Hysone t.
Hytone t.
t. immunomodulator (TIM)
t. immunomodulator drug
　classification
t. immunomodulator therapeutic
　category
Kenalog t.
Kenonel t.
t. khellin
LactiCare-HC t.
Lamisil t.
Lanaphilic T.
Lanvisone t.
LidaMantle HC t.
Lidex t.
Lidex-E t.
Locoid t.
Maxiflor t.
Maxivate t.
Meclan t.
Merlenate t.
t. methyl aminolevulinate
MetroGel t.
Micatin T.
t. moisturizer
Monistat-Derm t.
Mycifradin Sulfate T.
Mycitracin T.
Mycogen II T.
Mycolog-II T.
Myconel T.
Mycostatin t.
Mytrex F t.
Naftin t.
Neo-Cortef T.
Neomixin t.
N.G.T. T.
Nilstat t.

t. nitrogen mustard (NH2)
Nizoral T.
Novacet t.
Nutracort t.
Nutraplus T.
Nystex t.
Nyst-Olone II t.
t. ophthalmic vasoconstrictor
Orabasc HCA t.
Ovide t.
Oxistat t.
Oxsoralen t.
Pedi-Cort V t.
Pedi-Pro t.
Penecort t.
t. photodynamic therapy
Polysporin T.
Pontocaine t.
Psorcon t.
Psorion t.
t. PUVA
Quinsana Plus t.
Racet T.
Retin-A Micro t.
Rogaine t.
Scalpicin t.
t. skin protection (TSP)
Spectazole t.
Staticin t.
S-T Cort t.
t. steroid
Sulcosyn t.
Sulfacet-R t.
Sulfamylon t.
Synacort t.
Synalar T.
Synalar-HP T.
Synemol t.
Tegrin-HC t.
Teladar t.
Temovate t.
Texacort t.
Topicycline t.
Travase t.
Triacet t.
Tridesilon t.
Triple Antibiotic t.
Tri-Statin II t.
T-Stat t.
UAD t.
U-Cort t.
Ultra Mide t.

Ultravate t.
Undoguent t.
Ureacin-20, -40 t.
Valisone t.
Vioform t.
Vitec t.
Vytone t.
Westcort t.
Zovirax t.
topical-BCNU
Topicort-LP
Topicycline topical
TopiGel occlusive sheeting
Topilene
Topisone
Topo I
topoisomerase
DNA t. I
Toposar injection
Topsyn
TOR
toremifene
TOR inhibitor
Toradol injection
TORCH
toxoplasmosis, other infections, rubella, cytomegalovirus infection, and herpes simplex
TORCH syndrome
TORCH viral screen
toremifene (TOR)
tori (*pl. of* torus)
Tornalate
Torpedo californica
Torre syndrome
torti
pili t.
torticollis
dermatogenic t.
tortuous telangiectasis
tortus
pilus t.
Torula
T. *histolytica*
T. meningitis
torular meningitis
toruli tactiles
toruloidea
Hendersonula t.
Torulopsis glabrata
torulosis
torus, pl. **tori**

T

NOTES

torus *(continued)*
  t. mandibulae
  mandibular t.
  t. palatinus
TOS
  toxic oil syndrome
Totacillin-N
total
  t. abdominal evisceration (TAE)
  t. allergy syndrome
  t. biopsy
  t. body bone mineral content
  t. body irradiation (TBI)
  t. body surface area (TBSA)
  t. contact cast
  t. counts bound (TCB)
  t. hemolytic complement
  t. lipodystrophy
  t. lung capacity (TLC)
  t. lymphoid irradiation (TLI)
  t. nasal symptom score (TNSS)
  t. nonnasal symptom score
    (TNNSS)
  t. serum IgE
  t. serum IgE level
  t. skin electron beam (TSEB)
  t. skin score
  t. symptom score (TSS)
  t. water gradient across the nose
    (TWG)
totalis
  alopecia capitis t.
total-lymphoid irradiation
toto
  in t.
touch
  t. object maneuver
  t. prep
Toulon typhus
Touraine
  T. aphthosis
  T. centrofacial lentigo
  T. syndrome
Touraine-Solente-Golé syndrome
tourniquet
  Löfqvist t.
  t. test
Touro LA
Touton giant cell
Townes-Brock syndrome
toxemia
toxemic
toxic
  t. alopecia
  t. appearance
  t. bullous epidermolysis
  t. epidermal necrolysis (TEN)
  t. erythema
  t. inhalant

  t. nephrosis
  t. oil syndrome (TOS)
  t. organ damage
  t. shock-like syndrome (TSLS)
  t. shock syndrome (TSS)
  T. Substance Control Act
  t. systemic reaction
  t. unit (TU)
toxica
  alopecia t.
toxicemia
toxicity
  bladder t.
  cumulative t.
  ocular t.
  transplant-related t.
toxicodendron
  T. diversilobum
  T. radicans
  Rhus t.
  T. dermatitis
  T. verniciferum
toxicoderma
toxicodermatitis
toxicodermatosis
toxicogenic conjunctivitis
toxicopathic
toxicosis
toxicum
  erythema neonatorum t.
toxigenic
toxigenicity
toxin
  adenylate cyclase t.
  animal t.
  anthrax t.
  antitetanus t.
  Bacillus anthracis t.
  bacterial t.
  botulinus t.
  cholera t.
  Coley t.
  detoxified t.
  diagnostic diphtheria t.
  Dick test t.
  dinoflagellate t.
  diphtheria t.
  edema t. (ET)
  erythrogenic t.
  extracellular t.
  fusion t.
  intracellular t.
  lethal t. (LT)
  normal t.
  plant t.
  RNA glycosidase t.
  scarlet fever erythrogenic t.
  Schick test t.
  Shiga-like t.

t. spectrum
streptococcus erythrogenic t.
tetanus t.
toxinic
toxinogenic
toxinogenicity
toxinology
toxinosis
toxipathic
toxipathy
Toxocara
T. canis
T. cati
toxocariasis
toxoid
diphtheria and tetanus t.
tetanus t.
toxon
toxonosis
toxophil
toxophore
toxophorous
Toxoplasma gondii
toxoplasmosis
congenital t.
cutaneous t.
epidermotropic cutaneous t.
t., other infections, rubella,
cytomegalovirus infection, and
herpes simplex (TORCH)
t., other infections, rubella,
cytomegalovirus infection, and
herpes simplex syndrome
ToxR protein
toyocaensis
Streptomyces t.
TP10
TPE
thermoplastic elastomer
TPHA
Treponema pallidum hemagglutination
assay
TPHA test
TPI
Treponema pallidum immobilization
TPI reaction
TPI test
TPO
thrombopoietin
thyroid peroxidase
TR
thioredoxin reductase

TRAb
TSH receptor antibody
trabecular carcinoma
trace element
trachea
extrinsic compression of t.
Syngamus t.
tracheal
t. stenosis
t. tumor
t. vascular ring
tracheitis
tracheobronchial amyloidosis
Tracheolife HME
tracheomalacia
tracheostomy
trachoma
t. body
t. virus
trachomatis
Chlamydia t.
trachyonychia
track
tram t.'s
tracking
railroad t.
tract
central polypurine t. (cPPT)
dental sinus t.
sinus t.
traction
t. alopecia
t. atrophy
trade acne
**traditional Chinese herbal therapy
(TCHT)**
tragacanth
Gum t.
tragal
tragomaschalia
tragus, pl. **tragi**
accessory t.
TRAIL
tumor necrosis factor-related apoptosis-
inducing ligand
training
AsthmaCare Education:
Intensive T. (ACE IT)
joint protection t.
trait
autosomal recessive t.
beta thalassemia t.

NOTES

T

trait *(continued)*
    recessive t.
    sickle cell t.
TRALI
    transfusion-related acute lung injury
tram
    t. line
    t. tracks
tramadol
tranexamic acid
Tranquility Quest
tranquilizer
transactivator
    reverse tetracycline t.
    tetracycline t.
transaldolase
transaminase
transarterial chemoembolization (TACE)
transaxillary apical bullectomy
transcapsidation
transcellular metabolism
transcervical infection
transchondral fracture
transcript
    bcr-abl chimeric t.
transcriptase
    t. inhibitor
    reverse t.
    telomerase reverse t. (TERT)
transcription
    calcium-dependent t.
    t. factor
    gene t.
    germline t.
    signal transducer and activator
      of t. (STAT)
    signal transduction and activator
      of t. (STAT)
transcutaneous
    t. electrical nerve stimulation
      (TENS)
    t. electrical neuromuscular
      stimulator (TENS)
TransCyte skin substitute
transdermal therapeutic system (TTS)
transdermic
Transderm Scōp Patch
transdiaphragmatic pressure (Pdi)
transduce
transducer
    fluid-filled pressure t.
    force t.
transductant
transduction
    abortive t.
    complete t.
    general t.
    high frequency t.

    low frequency t.
    signal t.
    specialized t.
    specific t.
Transeal transparent film
transection
transendothelial neutrophil migration
transepidermal water loss (TEWL)
transfection
    adenoviral gene t.
    ex vivo adenoviral t.
transfer
    adenovirus-mediated gene t.
    t. factor
    t. gene
    melanin t.
    passive t.
    t. ribonucleic acid (tRNA)
    t. test
transferable T-cell suppression
transferase
    catechol-*O*-methyl t. (COMT)
transference
    passive t.
transferred immune response
transformant
transformation
    blast t.
    Box-Cox t.
    cell t.
    logit t.
    lymphocyte t.
    malignant t.
    refractory anemia with excess
      blasts in t. (RAEB-t)
    von Krogh t.
transformation-sensitive
    large external t.-s. (LETS)
transformed lymphocyte
transforming
    t. agent
    t. gene
    t. growth factor (TGF)
    t. growth factor-alpha (TGF-alpha)
    t. growth factor-beta (TGF-B)
    t. growth factor-induced
      immunosuppression
    t. infection
transfusion
    blood t.
    donor-specific t. (DST)
    exchange t.
    granulocyte t.
    haplotype-shared t.
    t. hepatitis
    t. nephritis
    packed red cell t.
    pretransplant donor blood t.

t. reaction
reciprocal t.
transfusion-associated AIDS (TA-AIDS)
transfusion-related acute lung injury
  (TRALI)
transgene
transgenic
t. mice
t. organism
transglutaminase
tissue t. (Ttg)
transglutamination
protein t.
transient
t. acantholytic dermatosis (TAD)
t. acantholytic dyskeratosis
t. agammaglobulinemia
t. bullous dermolysis of the
  newborn
t. cerebral ischemia
t. erythroporphyria of infancy
t. hypogammaglobulinemia of
  infancy
t. macrochimerism
t. migratory infiltrate
t. neonatal pustular melanosis
t. neonatal systemic lupus
  erythematosus
t. pulmonary infiltrate
transiently amplifying cell (TAC)
TransiGel impregnated gauze
transillumination of sinus
transin
transition mutation
transitory
t. benign plaque of tongue
t. palsy
transit time
transjugular hepatic biopsy
translation
translocation
bacterial t.
chromosomal t.
unbalanced t.
transmembrane
t. connector
t. linker
t. receptor
transmissible
t. dementia
t. enteritis
t. gastroenteritis virus (TGE)

t. gastroenteritis virus of swine
t. mink encephalopathy
t. plasmid
t. spongiform encephalopathy (TSE)
t. turkey enteritis virus
transmission
airborne t.
bedbug disease t.
t. disequilibrium testing (TDT)
t. electron microscopy (TEM)
horizontal t.
transovarian t.
vertical t.
Transorbent hydrogel sheet
transovarian transmission
transparent facial powder
transpeptidase
transphosphorylation
transplacental infection
transplant
allogenic t.
autologous bone marrow t.
auxiliary partial orthotopic liver t.
  (APOLT)
bone marrow t. (BMT)
dual kidney t.
t. elbow
en bloc t.
hair t.
hematopoietic stem cell t.
International Society for Heart and
  Lung T. (ISHLT)
islet cell t.
matched unrelated donor stem
  cell t. (mini-MUD)
PAK t.
pancreas after kidney t. (PAK)
reduced liver t. (RLT)
reduced-size liver t. (RSLT)
t. rejection classification
related t.
renal t.
simultaneous pancreas-kidney t.
  (SPK)
single-lung t. (SLT)
SPK t.
stem cell t. (SCT)
syngeneic heart t.
thoracic organ t.
Trans-Plantar Transdermal Patch
transplantation (Tx)
ABO-incompatible kidney t.

T

NOTES

transplantation *(continued)*
    allogenic bone marrow t.
    allogenic hematopoietic stem cell t.
      (allo-HSCT)
    t. antigen
    arthroscopic autologous
      chondrocyte t.
    autologous t.
    auxiliary partial heterotopic liver t.
      (APHLT)
    auxiliary partial orthotopic liver t.
      (APOLT)
    Bethesda Conference on Cardiac T.
    bone marrow t. (BMT)
    cadaver donor t.
    cardiomyocyte t.
    combined liver and kidney t.
      (CLKTx)
    corneal t.
    domino heart t. (DHT)
    en bloc t.
    European Group for Bone
      Marrow T. (EBMT)
    fetal liver t.
    fetal pig cell t.
    fetal thymus t.
    fetal ventral mesencephalic tissue t.
    FISH protocol in bone marrow t.
    fluorescence in situ hybridization
      protocol in bone marrow t.
    heart t. (HTX)
    heart-lung t. (HLT)
    hematopoietic progenitor t.
    hematopoietic progenitor cell t.
    hematopoietic stem cell t. (HCT,
      HSCT)
    heterotopic heart t. (HHT)
    International Society of Heart and
      Lung T. (ISHLT)
    intestinal t.
    intrasplenic t. (isp-Tx)
    islet t.
    isolated pancreatic islet t. (IPITx)
    kidney t. (KTx)
    living donor liver t. (LDLT)
    NHBD t.
    nonheart-beating donor liver t.
    nude bone graft t.
    orthotopic heart t.
    orthotopic liver t. (OLT)
    pancreas t.
    pancreaticoduodenal t.
    peripheral blood stem cell t.
      (PBSCT)
    pigment cell t.
    porcine bone marrow t. (PBMTx)
    reduced-size liver t. (RSLT)
    Registry of the International
      Society for Heart and Lung T.

    renal t. (RTx)
    sibling bone marrow t.
    simultaneous double kidney t.
      (SDKT)
    simultaneous kidney-pancreas t.
      (SKPT)
    small bowel t. (SBTx)
    small intestinal t. (SITx)
    solid organ t. (SOT)
    solitary pancreatic islet cell t.
    split-liver t. (SLT)
    stem cell t.
    syngeneic t.
    temporary auxiliary liver t.
    thymic t.
    vascularized bone marrow t.
      (VBMT)
    xenogeneic t.
    xenograft t.
    xenoislet t.
transplantin
transplant-related toxicity
transport
    active t.
    basolateral t.
transpose
transposition flap
transposon
Trans-Sal
transthyretin
    amyloidogenic t. (ATTR)
    t. amyloidosis
    t. Val30Met variant
transthyretin-origin amyloid deposit
transtracheal
transubstantiation
transvalensis
    Nocardia t.
transvector
transvenous endoluminal radiofrequency
    ablation
transversa
    stria nasi t.
Trans-Ver-Sal Transdermal Patch
    Verukan solution
transverse
    t. furrow
    t. ligament
    t. myelitis
    t. nasal groove
transversion mutation
Trantas dots
Tra **antigen**
Tranxene
TRAP
    tartrate-resistant acid phosphatase
trap
    Allergenco MK-3 spore t.
    Burkard spore t.

Hirst spore t.
Kramer-Collins Spore t.
trap-door deformity
trapping
air t.
TRAP-positive cell
TRAPS
tumor necrosis factor receptor-associated
periodic syndrome
trastuzumab
trauma
inadvertent t.
Parkland formula for fluid
resuscitation for burn t.
traumatic
t. alopecia
t. anserine folliculosis
t. arthritis
t. bursitis
t. calcinosis
t. dermatitis
t. fat necrosis
t. fever
t. herpes
t. lesion
t. neuroma
t. panniculitis
t. purpura
traumatica
alopecia t.
t. dermatitis
**traumatically induced inflammatory
disease**
traumaticum
chloasma t.
erythema t.
Travamine
Travase topical
Travatan solution
travel
T. Aid
T. Scrubz
T. Tabs
traveler
Pulmo-Aide T.
Travelmate
travoprost solution
Treacher Collins syndrome
treatment
t. adherence (TA)
Anti-Acne Spot T.
Artecoll permanent wrinkle t.

Ascoli t.
AuTolo Cure Process wound t.
Brehmer t.
Carmol Scalp T.
Castellani t.
Clear Pore T.
cold laser t.
complementary and alternative
medicine t.
double drug t.
duration of t.
emergency t.
etretinate t.
Fine Line wrinkle t.
FotoFacial t.
Gennerich t.
Goeckerman t.
grenz ray t.
Histofreezer cryosurgical wart t.
Hylaform Plus wrinkle t.
isoserum t.
light t.
Mother2Be skin t.
No-Name Dandruff T.
nonpharmacologic measure of t.
oatmeal t.
Perlane wrinkle t.
preventive t.
prophylactic t.
t. of psoriasis
PVAC t.
Restylane Fine Lines wrinkle t.
Reviderm wrinkle t.
short-contact t. (SCAT)
steroid-sparing t.
thermescent Skin T.
triple drug t.
Wartner over-the-counter wart
removal t.
Trecator-SC
tree
acacia t.
alder t.
American elm t.
arbor vitae t.
Arizona ash t.
Arizona cypress t.
Arizona/Fremont cottonwood t.
ash t.
aspen t.
Australian pine t.
bald cypress t.

T

NOTES

tree *(continued)*
    bayberry t.
    beech t.
    birch t.
    black locust t.
    box elder maple t.
    Brazilian rubber t.
    California peppertree t.
    Chinese elm t.
    cottonwood t.
    Douglas fir t.
    elm t.
    eucalyptus t.
    fall elm t.
    Gambel oak t.
    green ash t.
    groundsel t.
    hackberry t.
    hazelnut t.
    hickory t.
    Italian cypress t.
    Japanese cedar t.
    Japanese lacquer t.
    juniper mix t.
    lilac t.
    live oak t.
    loblolly pine t.
    lodgepole pine t.
    malaleuca t.
    maple t.
    mesquite t.
    Monterey cypress t.
    mountain cedar t.
    t. nut allergy (TN)
    oak t.
    olive t.
    palm t.
    paper mulberry t.
    pecan t.
    t. pollen
    ponderosa pine t.
    poplar t.
    privet t.
    queen palm t.
    red alder t.
    red cedar t.
    red maple t.
    red mulberry t.
    redwood t.
    Russian olive t.
    salt cedar t.
    shagbark hickory t.
    slash pine t.
    slippery elm t.
    spruce t.
    sugar maple t.
    sweetgum t.
    sycamore t.
    walnut t.
    wax myrtle t.
    weeping fig t.
    Western juniper t.
    white ash t.
    white mulberry t.
    white oak t.
    white pine t.
    white poplar t.
    willow t.
    yew t.

trefoil
    t. dermatitis
    t. family peptides

Treg development

Trematoda

trematode

tremor
    epidemic t.

trench
    t. fever
    t. foot
    t. hand
    t. mouth

Trendar

Trendelenburg test

Trental

trephine
    skin t.

Treponema
    T. carateum
    T. denticola
    T. endemicum
    T. pallidum
    T. pallidum hemagglutination assay (TPHA)
    T. pallidum immobilization (TPI)
    T. paraluis-cuniculi
    T. pertenue
    T. phagedenis

treponema-immobilizing antibody

treponemal
    t. antibody
    t. test

treponemata

treponematosis
    bejel t.
    nonsyphilitic t.
    nonvenereal t.
    pinta t.

treponeme

treponemiasis

Tresilian sign

tresperimus

tretinoin
    t. cream
    t. gel
    mequinol and t.

tretoin
>fluocinolone acetonide, hydroquinone, t.

Trexall
triacetin
Triacet topical
triad
>aspirin t.
>follicular occlusion t.
>Gougerot t.
>Hutchinson t.
>T. hydrocolloid
>T. hydrocolloid dressing
>Osler t.
>Phemister t.
>retention t.

Triaderm
trial
>Fracture Intervention T.
>GESICA t.
>Hy-C t.
>Metoprolol in Dilated Cardiomyopathy T.
>Outcome Measures in Rheumatology Clinical T.
>randomized controlled t. (RCT)
>Veterans' Administrative Cooperative T.

Triam
>T. Forte
>T. Forte Injection

Triam-A Injection
Triamcine-A
>Scheinpharm T.-A

triamcinolone
>t. acetonide (TAA)
>t. acetonide spray
>t. cream (TAC)
>t. hexacetonide
>t. lotion (TAL)
>nystatin and t.
>t. ointment (TAO)

Triaminic
>T. AM Decongestant Formula
>T. Expectorant
>T. Oral Infant drops

Triamolone
Triamonide Injection
triangle
>Burow t.

triangular fibrocartilage complex (TFCC)

triangularis
>alopecia t.

Triatoma
>*T. gerstaeckeri*
>*T. gerstaeckeri* bite
>*T. protracta*
>*T. sanguisuga*
>*T. sanguisuga* bite

Triatominae
Triaz gel
triazolam
triazole
Tribulus terrestris
trichatrophia
trichatrophy
trichauxis
trichiasis
trichilemmal
>t. carcinoma
>t. cyst
>t. differentiation

trichilemmoma
>benign t.
>desmoplastic t.

Trichinella spiralis
trichinelliasis
trichinellosis
trichiniasis
trichinosis
trichitis
trichiura
>*Trichuris* t.

Tri-Chlor
trichloroacetic
>t. acid (TCA)
>t. acid-tape technique

trichloroethylene
trichloromonofluoromethane
>dichlorodifluoromethane and t.

trichoadenoma
trichobezoar
trichoblastoma
trichoclasia
trichoclasis
trichocryptomania
trichocryptosis
trichocryptotillomania
Trichoderma
>*T. harzianum*
>*T. longibrachiatum*
>*T. viride*

T

NOTES

trichoderma
trichodiscoma (TD)
trichodystrophy
trichoepithelioma (TE)
    acquired t.
    desmoplastic t.
    hereditary multiple t.
    multiple t.
    t. papillosum multiplex
trichofolliculoma
    sebaceous t.
trichogen
trichogenous
trichoglossia
trichogram
trichokinesis
trichokleptomania
trichokryptomania
tricholemmal differentiation
tricholemmoma
tricholith
trichologia
trichology
trichoma
trichomatose
trichomatosis
trichomatous
trichomatrioma
trichomegaly
Trichomonas vaginalis
trichomoniasis
trichomycetosis
trichomycosis
    t. axillaris
    t. axillaris nodosa
    t. axillaris nodularis
    t. chromatica
    t. favosa
    t. nigra
    t. palmellina
    t. pustulosa
    t. rubra
trichonocardiosis axillaris
trichonodosis
trichonosis
trichonosus versicolor
trichopathic
trichopathophobia
trichopathy
trichophagy
trichophobia
trichophytic
    t. dyshidrosis
    t. granuloma
trichophytica
trichophyticum
    granuloma t.
trichophyticus
    lichen t.

trichophytid
trichophytin
trichophytina
    dermatomycosis t.
Trichophyton, Trichophytum
    T. concentricum
    T. erinacei
    T. gypseum
    T. mentagrophytes
    T. purpureum
    T. rubrum
    T. schoenleinii
    T. skin test
    T. sulfureum
    T. tonsurans
    T. tonsurans fungus
    T. verrucosum
    T. violaceum
Trichophyton-**induced asthma**
trichophytosis
    t. barbae
    t. capitis
    t. corporis
    t. cruris
    t. unguium
Trichophytum (*var. of* *Trichophyton*)
trichopoliodystrophy
trichopoliosis
trichoptilosis
tricho-rhino-phalangeal syndrome
trichorrhea
trichorrhexis
    t. invaginata
    t. nodosa
trichorrhexomania
trichoschisia
trichoschisis
trichoscopy
trichosis
    t. carunculae
    t. sensitiva
    t. setosa
Trichosporon beigelii
trichosporonosis
trichosporosis
trichostasis spinulosa
Trichostrongylus
trichothiodystrophy syndrome
trichotillomania
trichotoxin
trichotrophy
trichrome
    Masson t.
Trichuris trichiura
Tri-Clear Expectorant
triclocarban
triclosan
tricolor
    Viola t.

Tricomin
tricone defect
Tricoplast adhesive elastic bandage
Tricosal
tricuspid valvular leaflet
tricyclic antidepressant
Triderm
Tridesilon topical
Tridione
triethylenemelamine (TEM)
trifida
    Ambrosia t.
Tri-Flow incentive spirometry
trifluridine
trigeminal
    t. ganglion
    t. trophic syndrome
TriGem vaccine
trigger
    t. factor
    t. finger
    Smart T.
triglyceride
Trigonella foenum-gaecum
trihexoside
Tri-Immunol
triiodothyronine (T3)
Trikacide
Tri-Kort Injection
Trilafon
trilete
Trilisate
Trilog Injection
Trilone Injection
Tri-Luma cream
trimellitic anhydride
trimeprazine tartrate
trimer
    stable knob t.
trimethadione
trimethoprim and polymyxin b
trimethoprim-sulfamethoxazole (TMP-SMX)
trimethyl psoralen (TMP)
trimetrexate glucuronate
Trimox
Trimpex
Trinalin
Tri-Nasal Spray
trinucleotide
Triofed Syrup

trioxide
    arsenic t.
trioxsalen
Tripedia
tripelennamine
tripe palm
Tri-Phen-Chlor
Triphenyl Expectorant
triphosphatase
    adenosine t. (ATPase)
triphosphate
    guanosine t. (GTP)
    inositol t.
    lamivudine t. (3TC)
    purine nucleotide adenosine t.
    uridine t.
triple
    T. Antibiotic topical
    t. drug treatment
    t. helix
    t. palm
    T. Paste
    t. response
    t. response of Lewis
    t. therapy
    T. X liquid
triple-drug therapy immunosuppression protocol
triple-jawed pedicellaria
triplet
    nonsense t.
Tri-P Oral Infant drops
Triposed
    T. Syrup
    T. Tablet
Triprofed
triprolidine and pseudoephedrine
TripTone Caplets
triradius
trisalicylate
    choline magnesium t.
tris-boric acid-ethylenediaminetetraacetic acid (TBE)
tris-buffered
    t.-b. saline (TBS)
    t.-b. saline solution (TBS)
trisodium phosphonoformate
Trisoject Injection
trisomy
    t. 21, 22

NOTES

T

trisomy *(continued)*
    t. of chromosome II, dup(1) (q23q31)
    t. 20 syndrome
Trisoralen oral
Tri-Statin II topical
Tristoject
Tritin
    Dr. Scholl's Maximum Strength T.
Trivagizole 3
trivalent oral poliovirus solution
TriZol reagent
tRNA
    transfer ribonucleic acid
    tRNA synthetase
TRNG
    tetracycline-resistant *Neisseria gonorrhoeae*
Trobicin injection
trochanteric bursitis
troche
    Mycelex t.
trochleo-ginglymoid joint
Trolab wool alcohol test
trolamine salicylate
troleandomycin
trolley-track sign
Trombicula
    T. akamushi
    T. deliensis
    T. irritans
Trombiculidae
trombidiasis
trombidiosis
tromethamine
    fosfomycin t.
    ketorolac t.
    lodoxamide t.
Tronothane ointment
Trophermyma whippleii
trophic
    t. syndrome
    t. ulcer
trophodermatoneurosis
trophoneurotic leprosy
tropica
    acrodermatitis vesiculosa t.
    elephantiasis t.
    frambesia t.
    Leishmania t.
    leishmaniasis t.
    phagedena t.
    pyosis t.
tropicae
    aphtha t.
tropical
    t. acne
    t. anhidrotic asthenia
    t. boil

    t. disease
    t. eczema
    t. eosinophilia
    t. immersion foot
    t. lichen
    t. mask
    t. measles
    t. phagedena
    t. phagedenic ulcer
    t. pyomyositis
    t. sloughing phagedena
    t. sore
    t. spastic paraparesis (TSP)
    t. swelling
    t. typhus
tropicalis
    acne t.
    Blomia t.
    Candida t.
    tinea t.
tropicalum
    pyoderma ulcerosum t.
tropic immersion foot (TIF)
tropicum
    acanthoma t.
    angiofibroma contagiosum t.
    granuloma inguinale t.
    papilloma inguinale t.
    ulcus t.
tropicus
    lichen t.
tropism
    viral t.
tropomyosin
troponin
trospectomycin sulfate
trough
    peak and t.
Trousseau
    T. spot
    T. syndrome
Tru-Area Determination measuring device
T.R.U.E.
    T.R.U.E. allergy patch test
    T.R.U.E. TEST
true
    t. progeria
    t. skin
trumpeter wart
trumpet nail
truncated
trunk dermatitis
Truphylline suppository
TruPulse
    T. CO2 laser system
    T. laser
Truxcillin
TruZone peak flow meter

trypan blue
trypanid
Trypanosoma
    T. brucei
    T. cruzi
trypanosome growth factor (TGF)
trypanosomiasis
    African t.
    American t.
    South American t.
trypanosomid
tryparsamide organic arsenic
trypsin, balsam Peru, and castor oil
trypsinization
tryptase
tryptophan dysmetabolism
TS
    temperature sensitive
T/Sal
    T/Sal Neutrogena
    T/Sal Shampoo
TSBP
    testis-specific binding protein
TSC
    tuberous sclerosis
    tuberous sclerosis complex
t score
TSE
    transmissible spongiform encephalopathy
TSE-424
TSEB
    total skin electron beam
tsetse
    t. fly
    t. fly bite
TSH
    thyroid-stimulating hormone
    TSH receptor (TSH-R)
    TSH receptor antibody (TRAb)
TSH-displacing antibody
TSH-R
    thyroid-stimulating hormone receptor
    TSH receptor
TSK mouse
TSLS
    toxic shock-like syndrome
TSP
    thrombospondin
    topical skin protection
    tropical spastic paraparesis

TSS
    total symptom score
    toxic shock syndrome
TSTA
    tumor-specific transplantation antigen
T-Stat topical
Tsukamurella paurometabolum
tsukubaensis
    Streptomyces t.
T-suppressor cell
tsutsugamushi
    t. disease
    t. fever
    Rickettsia t.
TTBS
    Tween-TRIS-buffered saline solution
t-test
Ttg
    tissue transglutaminase
TTP
    thrombotic thrombocytopenic purpura
TTP-HUS
    thrombocytopenic purpura/hemolytic
      uremic syndrome
TTS
    transdermal therapeutic system
TU
    toxic unit
    tuberculin unit
tubba
tube
    Chaoul t.
    Eppendorf t.
    eustachian t.
    Lymphoprep T.
    t. precipitin test
    pus t.
    Shiley tracheostomy t.
    Softech endotracheal t.
    t. thoracostomy
tubercle
    anatomical t.
    butcher's t.
    dissection t.
    Lister t.
    naked t.
    necrogenic t.
    postmortem t.
    prosector's t.
    sebaceous t.
tubercula dolorosa

T

NOTES

tubercular
  t. eruption
  t. tertiary syphilis
tuberculation
tuberculatum
  erythema t.
tuberculid
  bacillary-barren t.'s
  micronodular t.
  micropapular t.
  nodular t.
  papular t.
  papulonecrotic t.
  rosacea-like t.
tuberculin
  Koch old t.
  old t. (OT)
  purified protein derivative of t.
  t. skin test
  Swedish old t.
  t. tine test
  t. titer test
  t. unit (TU)
tuberculin-type hypersensitivity
tuberculitis
tuberculization
tuberculochemotherapeutic
tuberculocidal
tuberculocide
tuberculoderma
tuberculoid
  t. leprosy
  t. rosacea
tuberculoides
  lepra t.
tuberculoprotein
tuberculosa
  dactylitis t.
tuberculosis (TB)
  adult t.
  aerogenic t.
  appendicular t.
  arthritic t.
  attenuated t.
  cestodic t.
  childhood-type t.
  chronic fibroid t.
  cutaneous t.
  t. cutis colliquativa
  t. cutis follicularis disseminata
  t. cutis indurata
  t. cutis indurativa
  t. cutis lichenoid
  t. cutis lichenoides
  t. cutis luposa
  t. cutis miliaris
  t. cutis miliaris disseminata
  t. cutis orificialis
  t. cutis papulonecrotica

  t. cutis verrucosa
  dermal t.
  disseminated t.
  extrapulmonary t.
  t. fungosa cutis
  hepatosplenic t.
  hilus t.
  t. lymphadenitis
  miliary t.
  multidrug-resistant t. (MDR-TB)
  mycobacteria other than t. (MOTT)
  Mycobacterium t. (MBT)
  open t.
  oral t.
  orificial t.
  orofacial t.
  osteoarticular t.
  postprimary t.
  primary inoculation t.
  reinfection t.
  rifampin-isoniazid-streptomycin-
    ethambutol-resistant t.
  RISE-resistant t.
  secondary t.
  t. of serous membrane
  t. of skin
  surgical t.
  t. ulcerosa
  t. vaccine
  t. verrucosa cutis
  vertebral t.
  warty t.
tuberculostat
tuberculostatic
tuberculosus
  lupus t.
tuberculotic
tuberculous
  t. abscess
  t. arthritis
  t. chancre
  t. dactylitis
  t. nephritis
  t. phlyctenulosis
  t. pleurisy
  t. polyserositis
  t. rheumatism
  t. synovitis
  t. wart
tuberculum
  t. sebaceum
  t. syphiliticum
tuberoeruptive xanthoma
tuberosa
  urticaria t.
tuberosis
tuberositas, pl. **tuberositates**
tuberosum
  xanthoma t.

tuberous
    t. angioma
    t. sclerosis (TSC)
    t. sclerosis complex (TSC)
    t. xanthoma
Tubersol
TubiFast bandage
tubing
    Silastic t.
    Surgitube t.
    X-span t.
tubocurarine
tubular venectasia
tubule
    T t.
tubulitis
tubulointerstitial
    t. nephritis (TIN)
    t. nephritis with uveitis (TINU)
tuft
    t. of hair
    ungual t.
tufted angioma
tuftsin
Tukey
    T. post-hoc correction
    T. standardized range test
tularemia
tularemic chancre
tularensis
    Francisella t.
    Pasteurella t.
tulip bulb dermatitis
tumbleweed weed pollen
tumbu
    t. fly
    t. fly myiasis
tumefaciens
    Agrobacterium t.
tumefacient
tumefaction
tumentia
tumescent technique
tumid lupus erythematosus
tumidus
    lupus erythematosus t.
tumor
    Abrikosov t.
    adnexal t.
    amyloid t.
    ANGEL t.
    t. antigen

Bednar t.
benign t.
Brooke t.
brown t.
t. burden index (TBI)
Buschke-Löwenstein t.
carcinoid t.
t. cell negative selection
t. cell purging
cutaneous t.
Dabska t.
dermal duct t.
desmoid t.
eccrine t.
epithelial t.
Ewing t.
filiform t.
t. of the follicular infundibulum
  (TFI)
genital t.
giant cell t.
glomus t.
granular cell t.
haarscheibe t.
insulin t.
Koenen t.
Landschutz t.
Leydig cell t.
t. lysis factor
t. lysis syndrome
Malherbe t.
malignant glomus t. (MGT)
malignant peripheral nerve sheath t.
t. marker
Merkel cell t.
mixed t.
t. necrosis factor (TNF)
t. necrosis factor-alpha (TNF-alpha)
t. necrosis factor-beta (TNF-beta)
t. necrosis factor inhibitor
t. necrosis factor receptor
t. necrosis factor receptor-associated
  periodic syndrome (TRAPS)
t. necrosis factor-related apoptosis-
  inducing ligand (TRAIL)
neuroendocrine t.
t. node, metastasis
t. node, metastasis staging
t., nodes, metastasis (TNM)
osseous t.
papillary t.
peripheral nerve sheath t.

T

NOTES

tumor *(continued)*
>phantom t.
>Pinkus t.
>Pott puffy t.
>precancerous t.
>premalignant t.
>primary neuroendocrine t.
>Rous t.
>sebaceous t.
>Spiegler t.
>Spitz t.
>squamous cell lung t.
>t. stage
>t. suppressor gene
>tomato t.
>tracheal t.
>turban t.
>vertical growth of t.
>villous t.
>t. virus
>Wilms t.
>Yaba t.

tumoral calcinosis
tumor-associated transplantation antigen (TATA)
tumoriform
tumorigenic
tumorigenicity
tumor-infiltrating
>t.-i. lymphocyte (TIL)
>t.-i. lymphocyte cell

tumor-specific transplantation antigen (TSTA)
tumor/stromal interaction
tuna fish
TUNEL method
Tunga
>*T. penetrans*
>*T. penetrans* bite

tungiasis
>pulicosis t.

tunica dartos
tuning fork
tunnel of Guyon
turban tumor
turbidimetry
Turbinaire
>Decadron Phosphate T.
>Dexacort Phosphate T.

turbinate
>nasal t.

turbo nebulizer
turbot
Turbuhaler
>T. inhaler
>Pulmicort T.

turgometer
turkey
>bluecomb disease of t.

>t. feather
>t. meningoencephalitis virus

Turlock virus
Turner
>T. phenotype
>T. syndrome

Turner-Kieser syndrome
turnover
>inositol phospholipid t.

Turpentine oil
turtleback nail
Tusibron-DM
Tussi-12D S oral suspension
Tussin
>Safe T.

Tussionex
Tussi-Organidin NR
Tuss-LA
Tusstat Syrup
Tween
Tween-TRIS-buffered saline solution (TTBS)
twentieth century disease
TWG
>total water gradient across the nose

Twice-A-Day Nasal solution
Twilite oral
Twin Jet nebulizer
twisted
>t. chondrodysplasia
>t. hair

two feet-one hand syndrome
Twort-d'Herelle phenomenon
Twort phenomenon
Tx
>transplantation

TXA$_2$
>thromboxane A$_2$

Ty21a vaccine
tyle
Tylenol
>T. Cold Effervescent Medication tablet
>T. Sinus Severe Congestion

tyloma
Tylophora asthmatica
tylosis, pl. **tyloses**
>t. ciliaris
>t. lingua
>t. palmaris et plantaris

tylotic
tyloticum
>eczema t.

tympanic membrane (TM)
tympanocentesis
tympanometry
tympanosclerosis
tyndallization

type
t. 68–72
t. A, B, C acanthosis nigricans
t. (1, 1A, 1B, 2) diabetes
APS t. 1, 2
t. A synoviocyte
axial t.
t. B fibroblast
blood t.
t. 1-24 cornification
dermatosparaxis t.
t. 1 diabetes mellitus (T1DM)
t. 2 diabetes mellitus (T2DM)
Duffy blood antibody t.
Ehlers-Danlos syndrome, arterial-ecchymotic t.
Ehlers-Danlos syndrome, arthrochalasia t.
Ehlers-Danlos syndrome, classic t.
Ehlers-Danlos syndrome, fibronectin-deficient t.
Ehlers-Danlos syndrome, Gravis t.
Ehlers-Danlos syndrome, human dermatosparaxis t.
Ehlers-Danlos syndrome, hypermobile t.
Ehlers-Danlos syndrome, kyphoscoliosis t.
Ehlers-Danlos syndrome, Mitis t.
Ehlers-Danlos syndrome, ocular-scoliotic t.
Ehlers-Danlos syndrome, periodontitis t.
Ehlers-Danlos syndrome, vascular t.
epidermolysis bullosa, dermal t.
epidermolysis bullosa, epidermal t.
epidermolysis bullosa, Gravis t.
epidermolysis bullosa, junctional t.
epidermolysis bullosa, Mitis t.
Fitzpatrick classification of skin t.
t. I glycogen storage disease
t. (I, IA, IB, II) oculocutaneous albinism
t. II alveolar cell
t. (I, IIb) antineuronal antibody
t. I–III hypersensitivity reaction
t. III immune complex drug reaction
t. (I, II) ocular albinism
t. (I, II) osteoporosis
t. (I, II) tyrosinemia
t. II pachyonychia congenita
t. II pneumocyte
t. I–IV immunologic drug reaction
t. (I-MP, I-TS) oculocutaneous albinism
t. IV collagenase
t. IV delayed hypersensitivity reaction
t. I–VII mucopolysaccharidosis
t. (I–XI, XIV) collagen
Kell blood antibody t.
keratosis palmaris et plantaris of the Meleda t.
Kidd blood antibody t.
kyphoscoliotic t.
Lewis blood antibody t.
peripheral t.
skin t.
t. strain
T-helper t. 1 (Th1)
t. V collagenase

typhi
Rickettsia t.
Salmonella t.

Typhim
T. Vi
T. Vi vaccine

typhimurium
Salmonella t.

typhoid
t. A&B (T.A.B.)
t. bacteriophage
t. cholera
t. fever
t. osteomyelitis
provocation t.
t. septicemia
t. spot

typhoid-paratyphoid A&B vaccine
typholysin
typhosepsis
typhous
typhus
African tick t.
t. degenerativus amstelodamensis
endemic t.
epidemic t.
t. exanthematique
exanthematous t.
flea-borne t.
Gubler-Robin t.
Hildenbrand t.
Indian tick t.

NOTES

typhus *(continued)*
    Kenya tick t.
    louse-borne t.
    Manchurian t.
    mite t.
    mite-borne t.
    t. mitior
    Moscow t.
    murine t.
    North Asian tick t.
    North Queensland tick t.
    petechial t.
    Queensland tick t.
    recrudescent t.
    scrub t.
    shop t.
    sporadic t.
    tick t.
    Toulon t.
    tropical t.
    urban t.
    t. vaccine
typing
    bacteriophage t.
    HLA t.
    HLA-DRB and HLA-DRQ DNA t.
    LCR-based HLA t.
    skin t. I–VI
tyramine

Tyrell skin hook
Tyrocidine
Tyroglyphus
    T. longior
    T. siro
Tyrophagus putrescentiae
tyrosinase inhibitor
tyrosinase-negative oculocutaneous
  albinism
tyrosinase-positive oculocutaneous
  albinism
tyrosinase-related oculocutaneous
  albinism
tyrosine
    t. aminotransferase deficiency
    t. kinase
    t. kinase inhibitor
    t. metabolism
    t. phosphorylation
tyrosinemia
    neonatal t.
    type (I, II) t.
Tyrothricin
T-Y stent
Tyzine Nasal
Tzanck
    T. preparation
    T. smear
    T. test

U3
    U3 small nuclear ribonucleoprotein
    U3 snRNP
UAD
  upper airway disorder
    UAD topical
UAS
  undifferentiated autoimmune syndrome
ubiquitin
ubiquitin-conjugating enzyme
ubiquitinization
ubiquitously transcribed tetratricopeptide
  (UTY)
UBIS 500 ultrasound bone sonometer
UBT
  urea breath test
UCB
  umbilical cord blood
U-cell
  undefined-cell
    U-cell lymphoma
U-Cort topical
UCTD
  undifferentiated connective tissue disease
UCTS
  undifferentiated connective tissue
    syndrome
Udder Butter lubricant/emollient
UFC
  urinary free cortisol
    UFC study
Uganda Cancer Institute staging system
UIFE
  urine immunofixation electrophoresis
UIP
  usual interstitial pneumonia
ulcer
    acute decubitus u.
    Aden u.
    amebic u.
    amputating u.
    aphthous genital u.
    aphthous oral u.
    arterial u.
    atonic u.
    Bairnsdale u.
    Bazin u.
    Buruli u.
    chiclero u.
    chrome u.
    chronic undermining burrowing u.
    cockscomb u.
    cold u.
    constitutional u.
    corneal u.

    corrosive u.
    crateriform u.
    creeping u.
    Curling u.
    cutaneous u.
    decubitus u.
    diabetic foot u.
    diphtheritic u.
    Gaboon u.
    genital aphthous u.
    gravitational u.
    groin u.
    gummatous u.
    hard u.
    healed u.
    herpetic u.
    idiopathic giant esophageal u.
    indolent u.
    inflamed u.
    inflammatory u.
    ischemic u.
    Jacob u.
    Kurunegala u.
    u. lesion
    Lipschütz u.
    lupoid u.
    Malabar u.
    Marjolin u.
    Meleney chronic undermining u.
    nasopharyngeal u.
    necrotic u.
    neurotrophic u.
    in noma u.
    oral aphthous u.
    Oriental u.
    Parrot u.
    perambulating u.
    phagedenic u.
    phlegmonous u.
    postencephalitic trophic u.
    pressure u.
    pudendal u.
    recurrent u.
    ring u.
    rodent u.
    Searl u.
    serpiginous u.
    sickle cell u.
    skin u.
    sloughing u.
    snail-track u.
    soft u.
    stasis vascular u.
    steroid u.
    Sutton u.

U

ulcer *(continued)*
    symptomatic u.
    syphilitic u.
    tanner's u.
    trophic u.
    tropical phagedenic u.
    undermining u.
    varicose u.
    vascular u.
    venereal u.
    venous stasis u.
    Zambesi u.
ulcera
ulcerans
    Mycobacterium u.
ulcerate
ulcerated hemangioma
ulcerating granuloma of pudendum
ulceration
    gastrointestinal u.
    intertrigo with u.
    intestinal u.
    mucous membrane u.
    nasal mucosal u.
    oral u.
    u. of oral mucosa
    rectal u.
ulcerative
    u. colitis
    u. dermatosis
    u. gingivitis
    u. lichen planus
    u. proctocolitis
    u. stomatitis
UlcerJet high-pressure fluid jet system
ulcerogenicity
ulceroglandular
ulceronecrotic lesion
ulcerosa
    tuberculosis u.
ulcerous
ulcerovegetating plaque
Ulcosan unna boot with inelastic zinc plaster bandage
ulcus
    u. ambulans
    u. ambustiforme
    u. durum
    u. hypostaticum
    u. migrans
    u. tropicum
    u. venereum
    u. vulvae acutum
ULE
    unilateral laterothoracic exanthem
ulerythema
    u. acneiforma
    u. centrifugum

    u. ophryogenes
    u. sycosiforme
ulerythematosa
    atrophoderma u.
Ulex europaeus
Ullrich-Turner syndrome
ulmoides
    Eucommia u.
ulnar
    u. deviation
    u. nerve
ulnaris
ulodermatitis
ulotrichous
ULR
ULR-LA
Ultec
    U. hydrocolloid
    U. hydrocolloid dressing
Ultra
    Grisactin U.
    U. Mide topical
    U. Tears solution
Ultracef
ultracentrifugation
Ultracet
Ultracortinol
UltraFine erbium laser system
ultrahigh frequency ventilation
UltraKlenz wound cleanser
Ultram
ultramicrosize griseofulvin
Ultramop
UltraPulse CO_2 laser
Ultraquin Plain
ultrasonic nebulizer
ultrasonography
    Power Doppler u.
ultrasonometer
    QUS-2 calcaneal u.
ultrasound
    Acuson 128XT u.
    A-mode u.
    B-mode u.
    Diasonic u.
    Doppler u.
    intravascular u. (IVUS)
ultrasound-guided bronchoscopy
ultrastructural
    u. analysis
    u. component
UltraThon insect repellent
Ultravate topical
ultraviolet (UV)
    u. A (UVA)
    u. actinotherapy
    u. A lamp
    u. B (UVB)
    u. B lamp

u. B-range (UVB)
u. C (UVC)
u. light
u. light index
u. radiation
u. recall
ultravirus
Umballa sore
umbilical
    u. cord
    u. cord blood (UCB)
    u. fungus
umbilicated
umbilication
Umbrelle sunscreen
Umbre virus
Unasyn
unbalanced translocation
uncharacteristic leprosy
Uncinaria
uncinarial dermatitis
uncinariasis
unclassified
    u. air cleaner
    u. erythema multiforme majus
uncombable hair syndrome
uncomplemented
uncovertebral arthrosis
unction
unctuosa
    cutis u.
undecamer
undecapeptide
undecylenic
    u. acid
    u. acid and derivatives
undefined-cell (U-cell)
    u.-c. lymphoma
undercover cosmetic
underexcretion-type gout
undermining ulcer
Underwood disease
undifferentiated
    u. autoimmune syndrome (UAS)
    u. connective tissue disease
      (UCTD)
    u. connective tissue syndrome
      (UCTS)
    u. somatoform IA anaphylaxis
    u. spondyloarthropathy
    u. type fever
Undoguent topical

undulant fever
undulin
unexpected phenotype
ungual tuft
unguent
    Lasan U.
unguentum, pl. **unguenta**
unguinal
unguis
    u. incarnatus
    leukopathia u.
    lunula u.
    matrix u.
    pterygium inversum u.
    solum u.
    stratum corneum u.
    vallum u.
unguium
    achromia u.
    albedo u.
    canities u.
    defluvium u.
    dystrophia u.
    fragilitas u.
    gryposis u.
    scabrities u.
    tinea u.
    trichophytosis u.
unheated serum reagin (USR)
Uni-Ace
Unibase cream
Uni-Bent Cough Syrup
unicameral cyst
unicellular protozoa
unicondylar arthritis
Unicort
Uni-Decon
Uni-Dur
Uniflex polyurethane adhesive surgical
    dressing
unifocal Langerhans cell
unilateral
    u. dermatomal superficial
      telangiectasia
    u. hemangiomatosis
    u. hemidysplasia
    u. hemidysplasia cornification
      disorder
    u. hyperhidrosis
    u. laterothoracic exanthem (ULE)
    u. macular degeneration
    u. nevoid telangiectasia

U

NOTES

unilateralis
nevus acneiformis u.
unilocular cyst
uninflamed
Unipen
U. injection
U. oral
Uniphyl
Uni-Pro
Uniserts
Hemril-HC U.
Unisom
Unisom-C
unit
Å u.
alexin u.
allercoat enzyme allergosorbent u.
(AEU)
amboceptor u.
Angström u.
antigen u.
antitoxin u.
antivenene u.
Asepticator u.
Bell international u.
biological standard u.
Brymill CryAc cryosurgical u.
Brymill 30 cryosurgical u.
complement u.
Cryo-Surg liquid nitrogen spray u.
dermal microvascular u.
diphtheria antitoxin u.
ELISA u. (EI.U)
environmental exposure u. (EEU)
epidermal-melanin u.
fingertip u. (FTU)
Flexercell Strain U.
Florey u.
follicular melanin u.
Geiger electrocautery u.
GPL u.
hemolysin u.
immunologic contact u. (ICU)
inhalation breath u.
iontophoretic u.
LAD-01 ER:YAG lightweight
portable laser u.
Lf u.
musculotendinous u.
nectary of floral u.
noon u.
Noon pollen u.
ostiomeatal u. (OMU)
Oxford u.
u. of penicillin
pilosebaceous u.
plaque-forming u. (PFU)
priming renal dialysis u.
protein nitrogen u. (PNU)

skin test u. (STU)
streptomycin u.
tetanus antitoxin u.
ThermoFlow ETC u.
toxic u. (TU)
tuberculin u. (TU)
Wood u.
unitarian hypothesis
United
U. Network for Organ Sharing
(UNOS)
U. States Renal Data System
(USRDS)
Unithroid
Unitrol
unius
univalent antibody
univariant
univariate
u. Cox proportional hazard
u. regression analysis
Uni-Vent
universal
u. acquired melanosis
u. allergy
u. angiomatosis
u. donor
universale
angiokeratoma corporis diffusum u.
melasma u.
universalis
albinismus u.
alopecia u.
calcinosis u.
hypertrichosis u.
protoporphyria u.
psoriasis u.
vitiligo u.
University
U. of Wisconsin (UW)
U. of Wisconsin solution
unmethylated oligodeoxynucleotide
Unna
U. boot
U. cell
U. comedo extractor
U. dermatosis
U. disease
U. expressor
U. mark
U. nevus
U. paste
UNNA-FLEX
Unna-Flex leg compression dressing
Unna-Pak leg compression dressing
Unna-Thost
U.-T. disease
U.-T. keratoderma

keratosis palmaris et plantaris
of U.-T.
U.-T. syndrome
unopsonized zymosan
UNOS
United Network for Organ Sharing
UNOS 3, 4 score
UNOS transplant listing
unroofed vesicle
unsaponifiable
avocado soybean u.
unusual
u. lupus erythematosus-like
syndrome
u. opportunistic infection
upcurved punch
UPEP
urine protein electrophoresis
upper
u. airway disorder (UAD)
u. airway obstruction
u. dermis
U. Hands self-retaining retractor
u. respiratory tract infection
(URTI)
u. respiratory tract mucosa
u. respiratory tract symptoms
(URSx)
up-regulation
upstream
u. enzyme
u. regulatory region (URR)
uralensis
Glycyrrhiza u.
Uranyl Standard fluorescence standard
urate
u. deposition
monosodium u. (MSU)
u. nephropathy
u. oxidase
urate-associated inflammation
Urbach-Oppenheim disease
Urbach-Wiethe
U.-W. disease
U.-W. syndrome
urban
u. cutaneous leishmaniasis
u. typhus
urchin
sea u.
urea
u. breath test (UBT)

u. frost
u. and hydrocortisone
imidazolidinyl u.
Ureacin
Ureacin-20, -40 topical
ureae
Actinobacillus u.
urealyticum
Ureaplasma u.
Ureaphil Injection
Ureaplasma urealyticum
urediospore, uredinospore, ureidospore
uredo
Uree
ureidospore (*var. of* urediospore)
uremia
perforating disorder of u.
uremic
u. pneumonitis
u. pruritus
Uremol
Uremol-HC
ureteric stenting
ureteroneocystostomy
Lich-Gregoire u.
urethritis
chlamydial u.
gonorrheal u.
nongonococcal u.
urhidrosis
uric
u. acid
u. acid stone
uricase
uricemia
uricosuria
uricosuric drug
uridine
u. diphosphoglucose dehydrogenase
u. triphosphate
uridrosis crystallina
urinary
u. alkalinizer
u. electrophoresis
u. free cortisol (UFC)
u. free cortisol study
u. tract infection (UTI)
urine
cellular casts in u.
u. immunofixation electrophoresis
(UIFE)
mouse u.

U

NOTES

urine *(continued)*
  u. myoglobin immunoassay
  u. protein electrophoresis (UPEP)
  u. pyridinoline collagen cross-link
urinosus
  sudor u.
Urisec
Uri-Tet oral
uritis
U1 RNP antibody
Urobak
urolithiasis
Uroplus
  U. DS
  U. SS
uroporphyrin
urostomy dermatitis
URR
  upstream regulatory region
ursodiol
URSx
  upper respiratory tract symptoms
URTI
  upper respiratory tract infection
urtica
urticans
  erythema u.
  purpura u.
urticant
urticaria
  u. acuta
  acute allergic u.
  adrenergic u.
  allergic u.
  angioedema-induced u.
  aquagenic u.
  autonomic u.
  u. bullosa
  cholinergic u.
  chronic u.
  u. chronica
  chronic familial giant u.
  cold-induced u.
  cold reflex u.
  u. conferta
  congelation u.
  contact u.
  cyclic u.
  delayed pressure u.
  endemic u.
  u. epidemica
  exercise-induced cholinergic u.
  u. factitia
  factitious u.
  familial cold u.
  febrile u.
  u. febrilis
  generalized heat u.
  giant u.

  u. gigantea
  heat u.
  heat-induced u.
  u. hemorrhagica
  heredofamilial u.
  idiopathic cold u.
  idiopathic solar u.
  immediate contact u.
  immunological contact u. (ICU)
  immunologic contact u.
  irritant contact u.
  light u.
  u. maculosa
  u. medicamentosa
  Milton u.
  u. multiformis endemica
  nonconimmunological contact u.
   (NICU)
  papular u.
  u. papulosa
  u. perstans
  u. photogenica
  physical u.
  u. pigmentosa
  u. pigmentosum
  pressure u.
  pressure-induced u.
  recall u. (RU)
  recurrent u.
  solar u.
  solaris u.
  u. subcutanea
  u. tuberosa
  u. vesiculosa
  vibratory u.
urticarial
  u. dermatographia
  u. plaque
  u. vasculitis
  u. xanthoma
urticariogenic
urticarioides
  acarodermatitis u.
urticata
  acne u.
urticate
urtication
urticatus
  lichen u.
urushiol
use
  injecting-drug u. (IDU)
  u. test
usitatissimum
  Linum u.
USR
  unheated serum reagin
USRDS
  United States Renal Data System

USSC stapler
ustilaginism
Ustilago
ustus
    Aspergillus u.
usual interstitial pneumonia (UIP)
uta
uterine leiomyoma
uterus, pl. **uteri**
    ichthyosis uteri
UTI
    urinary tract infection
Uticort
utility
    Asthma Symptom U. (ASU)
    u. scissors
utilization
UTY
    ubiquitously transcribed tetratricopeptide
UV
    ultraviolet
    UV biometer
    UV solution
UVA
    ultraviolet A
    UVA lamp
    photochemotherapy with oral
      methoxypsoralen therapy followed
      by UVA (PUVA)

Uvadex
UVAR photophoresis system
UVB
    midrange-wavelength ultraviolet light
    ultraviolet B
    ultraviolet B-range
    UVB lamp
    narrowband UVB (NBUVB)
    UVB phototherapy
UVC
    ultraviolet C
uveitis
    anterior u.
    idiopathic posterior u.
    lens-induced u.
    phacoanaphylactic u.
    tubulointerstitial nephritis with u.
      (TINU)
uveomeningoencephalitis
uviofast
uviol lamp
uvioresistant
uviosensitive
UW
    University of Wisconsin
    Belzer UW
    UW solution

NOTES

U

V

V antigen
Big V
V gene

V-2 carcinoma

Va

coagulation factor Va

vaccae

Mycobacterium v.

vaccina

vaccinal areola

vaccinate

vaccination

cancer v.
DNA v.
specific allergy v. (SAV)

vaccinator

vaccinatum

eczema v.

vaccine

ActHIB v.
adjuvant v.
V. Adverse Events Reporting
 System (VAERS)
AIDS v.
allergy v.
antiidiotype v.
aqueous v.
attenuated live mumps virus v.
autogenous v.
Avicine v.
Bacille Calmette-Guérin v.
bacterial v.
BCG v.
Biken-CAM v.
brucella strain 19 v.
Calmette-Guérin v.
chickenpox v.
cholera v.
crystal violet v.
diphtheria, tetanus toxoid, and
 whole-cell pertussis vaccine and
 Haemophilus b conjugate v.
diphtheria toxoid, tetanus toxoid,
 and pertussis v. (DTP)
DNA v.
duck embryo origin v. (DEV)
Edmonston-Zagreb v.
Flury strain v.
foot-and-mouth disease virus v.
gene-based v.
Haffkine v.
Havrix v.
HbOC v.
HbOC/DTP v.

heat-phenol inactivated v.
hepatitis A v.
hepatitis B v.
heterogenous v.
HGP-30W v.
Hib-TT v.
high-egg-passage v.
hog cholera v.
human diploid cell rabies v.
 (HDCV)
Imovax Rabies intradermal v.
Imovax Rabies intramuscular v.
ImuLyme v.
inactivated poliovirus v. (IPV)
Infanrix v.
influenza virus v.
IR502 psoriasis v.
Japanese encephalitis virus v. (JE-
 VAX)
killed-virus v.
Lipomel melanoma v.
lipopolysaccharide v.
live oral polio v.
live oral poliovirus v.
low-egg-passage v.
low virulence v.
v. lymph
measles and rubella virus v. (MR-
 VAX)
measles virus v.
Melacine v.
melanoma cell lysate v.
meningococcal v.
MMR v.
multivalent v.
mumps virus v.
M-Vax v.
oil v.
Oka v.
oral polio v. (OPV)
Pasteur v.
pertussis v.
plague v.
PncCRM v.
pneumococcal polysaccharide v.
pneumococcal polysaccharide/protein
 conjugate v.
poliomyelitis v.
poliovirus v.
polyvalent v.
rabies virus v.
rheumatoid arthritis v.
Rocky Mountain spotted fever v.
Rotamune v.
RotaShield v.

V

vaccine *(continued)*
  Sabin v.
  Salk v.
  Semple v.
  smallpox v.
  split-virus v.
  Staphylococcus aureus v.
  stock v.
  subunit v.
  T.A.B. v.
  tetanus v.
  v. therapy
  Theratope-STn v.
  TriGem v.
  tuberculosis v.
  Ty21a v.
  Typhim Vi v.
  typhoid-paratyphoid A&B v.
  typhus v.
  varicella virus v.
  variola v.
  viral v.
  v. virus
  vital v.
  whooping-cough v.
  yellow fever v. (YF-VAX)
vaccinia
  disseminated v.
  v. gangrenosa
  generalized v.
  v. immune globulin
  v. infection
  v. necrosum
  Orthopoxvirus v.
  progressive v.
  roseola v.
  variola v.
  v. virus
vaccinial
vacciniform
  estival v.
vacciniforme
  hydroa v.
vaccinist
vaccinization
vaccinogen
vaccinogenous
vaccinoid reaction
vaccinostyle
vaccinum
VAC Freedom system
Vacu-Aide portable suction device
vacuolar
  v. change
  v. myelopathy
  v. myopathy
vacuolated
vacuolating virus
vacuole

vacuolization
  basket-weave v.
vacutome
vacuum
  v. phenomenon
  Rainbow v.
  v. tube apparatus
  v. tube cutting current
VAERS
  Vaccine Adverse Events Reporting
  System
vagabond's disease
vaginal
  Cleocin V.
  Dalacin V.
vaginalis
  Trichomonas v.
Vaginex
vaginitis
  Gardnerella v.
  granular v.
vaginosis
vagrant's disease
vagus nerve
valacyclovir HCl
Valcyte
valdecoxib
valency
valerate
  betamethasone v.
  hydrocortisone v.
valganciclovir
valgum
  genu v.
valgus
  forefoot v.
  hallux v.
  rearfoot v.
Valisone topical
Valium
  V. injection
  V. oral
vallum unguis
Val30Met
  ATTR V.
valproic acid and derivatives
Valrelease oral
Valsalva maneuver
Valtrex
value
  negative predictive v. (NPV)
  positive predictive v. (PPV)
  threshold limit v. (TLV)
valve
  Passy-Muir tracheostomy
  speaking v.
valvulae conniventes
valvular disease
Vamate

van
- v. Buchem disease
- V. der Bend chamber
- v. der Heijde modification of Sharp method
- v. der Waals force
- V. Lohuizen syndrome
- v. Sonnenberg sump

VanA phenotype
vanA, vanH, vanS gene
Vancenase
- V. AQ
- V. AQ Inhaler
- V. Nasal Inhaler
- V. Pockethaler

Vanceril
- V. Double Strength
- V. Oral Inhaler

Vancocin
- V. injection
- V. oral

Vancoled injection
vancomycin
- v. hydrochloride
- kanamycin and v. (KV)

vancomycin-resistant
- v.-r. enterococci (VRE)
- v.-r. *Enterococcus* (VRE)
- v.-r. *Enterococcus faecium* (VREF)
- v.-r. *Enterococcus faecium* bacteremia

Vanex-LA
Vanicream
vanilla-fudge cyst
vanillism
Vaniqa cream
Vanoxide
Vanoxide-HC
Vansil
Vantin
vapocoolant spray
Vaponefrin
VAPS
- volume-assured pressure support

Varady phlebectomy hook
variabilis
- *Dermacentor v.*
- erythrokeratoderma v. (EKV)
- erythrokeratodermia figurata v.

variable
- v. numbers of tandem repeats (VNTR)
- v. region

variance
- analysis of v. (ANOVA)
- multivariate analysis of v. (MANOVA)

variance-covariance matrix
variant
- v. amyloidogenic protein
- v. asthma
- dystrophic epidermolysis bullosa, albopapuloid v.
- generalized morphea v.
- junctional v.
- linear scleroderma v.
- Miller-Fisher v.
- morphea v.
- v. neurofibromatosis
- simplex v.
- transthyretin Val30Met v.

variation
- antigenic v.
- coefficient of v. (CV)

varicella
- congenital v.
- v. disease
- v. encephalitis
- v. gangrenosa
- v. inoculata pustulosa
- v. virus vaccine
- v. virus vaccine live

varicellation
varicella-zoster (VZ)
- v.-z. immune globulin
- v.-z. immunoglobulin (VZIG)
- v.-z. infection
- v.-z. virus (VZV)
- v.-z. virus retinitis

varicelliform lesion
varicelloid
varicellosus
- herpes zoster v.

varices (*pl. of* varix)
varicography
varicose
- v. eczema
- v. ulcer

varicosis
varicosity
- venous v.

V

NOTES

varicosum
    lymphangioma capillare v.
variegata
    parakeratosis v.
    parapsoriasis v.
    porphyria v.
variegated color
variegate porphyria (VP)
variegatum
    Hyalomma v.
Vari/Moist wound dressing
variola
    v. benigna
    v. crystallina
    v. hemorrhagica
    v. inserta
    v. major
    v. maligna
    v. miliaris
    v. minor
    v. mitigata
    v. pemphigosa
    v. siliquosa
    v. sine eruptione
    v. vaccine
    v. vaccinia
    v. vera
    v. verrucosa
    v. virus
variolar
variolate
variolation
variolic
varioliformis
    acne v.
    folliculitis v.
    molluscum v.
    parapsoriasis acuta et v.
varioliform syphilid
variolization
varioloid
variolosa
    impetigo v.
    osteomyelitis v.
    purpura v.
variolous
variolovaccine
variotii
    Paecilomyces v.
Varivax
varix, pl. **varices**
    lymph v.
    v. lymphaticus
    venous v.
VariZIG
varus
    forefoot v.
    hallux v.

    hindfoot v.
    v. intertrochanteric
VAS
    visual analog scale
    VAS 972
VasaMed
vasa nervorum
vascular
    v. arcade
    v. cell adhesion molecule (VCAM)
    v. cell adhesion molecule-1 (VCAM-1)
    v. claudication
    v. dermatosis
    v. disorder
    v. dysfunction
    v. endothelial growth factor (VEGF)
    v. endothelial growth factor-2
    endothelium v.
    v. FLPD
    v. malformation birthmark
    v. nevus
    v. permeability
    v. permeability factor/vascular endothelial cell growth factor (VPF/VEGF)
    v. reaction
    v. type Ehlers-Danlos syndrome
    v. ulcer
vasculare
    poikiloderma atrophicans v.
vascularis
    nevus v.
vascularized
    v. bone marrow transplantation (VBMT)
    v. xenograft
vasculature
vasculitic lesion
vasculitis, pl. **vasculitides**
    allergic v.
    ANCA-associated v. (AAV)
      antineutrophil cytoplasmic antibody-associated vasculitis
    ANCA-positive v. (APV)
      antineutrophil cytoplasmic antibody-positive vasculitis
    antineutrophil cytoplasmic antibody-associated v. (ANCA-associated vasculitis)
    antineutrophil cytoplasmic antibody-positive v. (ANCA-positive vasculitis)
    Churg-Strauss v.
    coronary v.
    cutaneous leukocytoclastic v.
    cutaneous necrotizing v.
    granulomatous v.

Henoch-Schönlein v.
hypersensitivity v.
hypocomplementemic urticarial v.
immune complex v.
large vessel v.
leukocytoclastic v. (LCV)
livedo v.
livedoid v.
lymphocytic v.
mesenteric v.
necrotizing v.
nodular granulomatous v.
primary systemic v. (PSV)
pustular v.
rheumatoid rheumatic v.
segmental hyalinizing v.
small vessel v.
systemic necrotizing v. (SNV)
urticarial v.
vasculopathy
basilar v.
Churg-Strauss v.
livedoid v.
pulmonary occlusive v.
vasculosus
nevus v.
Vaseline
V. Intensive Care moisturizer
V. Lip Therapy
V. petroleum jelly
Vaselinoderma
vasoactive
v. intestinal peptide (VIP)
v. mediator
Vasocidin Ophthalmic
Vasocon
vasoconstriction
hypoxic v.
vasoconstrictor
topical ophthalmic v.
Vasodilan
vasodilatation
vasodilation
Vasofrinic
vasomotor
v. reaction
v. rhinitis (VMR)
vasoocclusive disease
vasopressor
vasospasm
cold-induced v.

Vasosulf Ophthalmic
vasovagal reaction
Vater-Pacini corpuscle
VATS
video-assisted thoracic surgery
Vaughn-Jackson
V.-J. lesion
V.-J. sign
Vav/Rac pathway
VaxGen
VaxSyn
Vbeam pulse dye laser system
VBMT
vascularized bone marrow transplantation
VC
vital capacity
VC25
Gravicon VC25
VCAM
vascular cell adhesion molecule
VCAM-1
vascular cell adhesion molecule-1
V-Cillin K oral
V-Dec-M
V-D-J
V.-D.-J. gene
V.-D.-J. gene arrangement
VDRL
Venereal Disease Research Laboratory
VDRL test
VDS
venereal disease-syphilis
VDT
visual display terminal
vection
vector
attenuated poxvirus v.
biological v.
gene-based v.
mechanical v.
pBlueScript v.
v. of plague
recombinant v.
retroviral v.
tick v.
viral v.
vector-borne disease
vectorial
vector-transfected cell clone
Vectrin
vecuronium

NOTES

V

VEE
Venezuelan equine encephalomyelitis
VEE virus
Veetids oral
Vega test
vegetable
v. gum
raw v.'s
v. shortening
vegetans
benign pemphigus v.
dermatitis v.
herpes v.
hyperkeratosis follicularis v.
keratosis v.
pemphigus v.
pyoderma v.
pyostomatitis v.
vegetating
v. bromidism
v. halogenosis
vegetative bacteriophage
VEGF
vascular endothelial growth factor
Veiel paste
veiled cell
vein
Linton procedure for varicose v.'s
modified Linton procedure for
varicose v.'s
right renal v. (RRV)
Veingard dressing
Vel antigen
Velban
Velband orthopedic padding wool
Velbe
Velcade
Velcro
V. closure
V. crackle
Veldona
veldt sore
Velella velella **dermatitis**
vellus
v. hair
v. olivae
velocardiofacial syndrome
velocimetry
laser Doppler v.
velocity
nerve conduction v.
velogenic
Velosef
Veltane Tablet
Velvelan
velvet grass
velvety surface
Ven antigen
vena satia

venectasia
tubular v.
venenata
acne v.
cheilitis mycotic v.
dermatitis v.
Rhus v.
venenatum
erythema v.
venerea
lues v.
venereal
v. bubo
v. disease
V. Disease Research Laboratory
(VDRL)
v. disease-syphilis (VDS)
v. sore
v. ulcer
v. wart
venereal-associated arthritis
venereum
granuloma v.
lymphopathia v.
papilloma v.
ulcus v.
veneris
corona v.
Venezuelan
V. equine encephalomyelitis (VEE)
V. equine encephalomyelitis virus
venezuelensis
Strongyloides v.
venoarterial shunting
Venodyne compression stocking
Venoglobulin-I, -S
venom
bee v.
v. extract
flea v.
v. hemolysis
Hymenoptera v.
v. immunotherapy (VIT)
v. sac
snake v.
spider v.
v. testing
venom-bathed nematocyst
venom-bearing spine
venomous snake
venoocclusive (VOD)
venoocclusive disease
venoplasty
venoscope
venosus
nevus v.
venous
v. gangrene
v. lake

v. malformation
v. nevus
v. star
v. stasis ulcer
v. varicosity
v. varix
Ventex composite dressing
ventilated alveolus
ventilation
airway pressure release v. (APRV)
alveolar v.
high-frequency jet v.
high-frequency positive pressure v.
intermittent mandatory v.
inverse ratio v. (IRV)
maximal v. (MV)
maximal voluntary v. (MVV)
mechanical v. (MV)
minute v.
pressure-controlled inverse ratio v.
pressure-regulated volume control v.
pressure support v. (PSV)
proportional assist v.
synchronized intermittent
    mechanical v.
synchronous intermittent
    mandatory v.
ultrahigh frequency v.
volume-cycled decelerating-flow v.
ventilation/perfusion (V/Q)
v./p. lung scan
v./p. ratio
ventilator
high frequency oscillatory v.
mechanical v.
volume-limited v.
ventilator-associated pneumonia
ventilatory failure
Ventolin
V. nebules
V. Rotacaps
VenTrak respiratory mechanics monitor
ventral
ventricosus
dermatitis pediculoides v.
Pediculoides v.
Pyemotes v.
ventricular pseudoaneurysm (VPA)
ventriculography
radionuclide v.
ventriculoperitoneal shunt (VP)
Venture demand oxygen delivery device

venular lesion
venule
dilated v.
high endothelial v. (HEV)
venulitis
cutaneous necrotizing v.
Venus
collar of V.
crown of V.
necklace of V.
VePesid
V. injection
V. oral
vera
cutis v.
polycythemia v.
variola v.
verdoperoxidase
verge
nasal v.
vergeture
Vergogel Gel
Vergon
Verhoeff-van Gieson stain
Veriderm
Medrol V.
vermicular
vermicularis
atrophoderma v.
Enterobius v.
Oxyuris v.
vermiculate atrophoderma
vermiculation
vermiculatum
atrophoderma v.
vermiculous
vermifugal
vermifuges
vermilion border
verminous abscess
Vermizine
Vermox
vernal
v. conjunctivitis
v. encephalitis
v. grass
v. keratoconjunctivitis
sweet v.
Verner syndrome
Verneuil
hidradenitis axillaris of V.
V. neuroma

V

NOTES

verniciferum
  Toxicodendron v.
vernix
  Rhus v.
Vero cell
veronii
  Aeromonas v.
Verrex-C&M
verruca, pl. **verrucae**
  v. acuminata
  v. digitata
  v. filiformis
  v. glabra
  v. mollusciformis
  v. necrogenica
  v. palmaris et plantaris
  v. peruana
  v. peruviana
  Phialophora v.
  v. plana
  v. plana juvenilis
  v. plana senilis
  v. planta
  seborrheic v.
  v. simplex
  v. vulgaris
Verruca-Freeze
verruciformis
  acrokeratosis v.
  dermatodysplasia v.
  epidermodysplasia v. (EV)
verruciforms
verruciform xanthoma
verrucosa
  Betula v.
  v. cutis
  dermatitis v.
  elephantiasis nostra v.
  pachyderma v.
  Phialophora v.
  telangiectasia v.
  tuberculosis cutis v.
  variola v.
verrucose dermatitis
verrucosis
  lymphostatic v.
verrucosum
  eczema v.
  erysipelas v.
  molluscum v.
  pyoderma v.
  Trichophyton v.
verrucosus
  lichen planus v.
  lichen ruber v.
  lupus v.
  nevus v.
verrucous
  v. angiokeratoma

  v. carcinoma
  v. hemangioma
  v. hypertrophicum
  v. nevus
  v. scrofuloderma
  v. surface
  v. xanthoma
verruga peruana
Versacaps
VersaLight laser
VersaPulse laser
Versed
Versel
versican CS/DS
Versiclear
versicolor
  Aspergillus v.
  pityriasis v.
  tinea v.
  trichonosus v.
vertebra, pl. **vertebrae**
  cervical v.
  codfish v.
vertebral
  v. artery compression
  v. tuberculosis
vertex
vertical
  v. growth phase
  v. growth of tumor
  v. mattress stitch
  v. section
  v. transmission
Verticillium alboatrum
Verukan solution
very
  v. late activation antigen
  v. late antigen-4 (VLA-4)
very-low-density
  v.-l.-d. lipoprotein (VLDL)
  v.-l.-d. lipoprotein cholesterol
vesica, pl. **vesicae**
  pachyderma v.
vesicant
vesicate
vesication
vesicatoria
  Lytta v.
vesicatory
vesicle
  deep-seated v.
  minute v.
  pustular v.
  spongiotic v.
  unroofed v.
vesicobullous lesion
vesicopustular eruption
vesicopustule

vesicular
    v. dermatitis
    v. eruption
    v. exanthem
    v. exanthema
    v. exanthema of swine virus
    v. stomatitis (VS)
    v. viral infection
vesiculate
vesiculated
vesiculation
    creeping v.
    intraepidermal v.
    subepidermal v.
vesiculiform
vesiculobullous disease
vesiculopapular
vesiculopustular lesion
vesiculosa
    miliaria v.
    urticaria v.
vesiculose
vesiculosum
    eczema v.
    erysipelas v.
    hydroa v.
vesiculotomy
vesiculous
Vesiculovirus
vespid
    v. antigen
    hymenopterous v.
Vespula
    V. crabro
    V. sting
vessel-based lobular panniculitis
vessel blockage
vest
    halo v.
vestibular
    v. adenitis
    v. cyst
    v. papilla
vestibulum nasi
vestimenti
    pediculosis v.
vestimentorum
    pediculosis corporis vel v.
Veterans' Administrative Cooperative Trial
veto effect
Vexol Ophthalmic suspension

V-Gan injection
VH
    viral hepatitis
    VH gene
VHF
    viral hemorrhagic fever
VHL
    von Hippel-Lindau gene
Vi
    Vi antibody
    Vi antigen
    Typhim Vi
Viasorb
    V. composite dressing
    V. wound dressing
ViaSpan
vibesate
vibex, pl. **vibices**
Vibramycin
    V. injection
    V. oral
Vibra-Tabs
vibration
    chest percussion and v.
vibration-induced white finger (VWF)
vibratory
    v. angioedema
    v. urticaria
vibrio
    v. cholerae
    Nasik v.
    v. vulnificus
vibriocidal
vibrometry
    Semmes-Weinstein v.
vicious cicatrix
Vicks
    V. DayQuil Allergy Relief 4 Hour tablet
    V. DayQuil Sinus Pressure & Congestion Relief
    V. 44D Cough & Head Congestion
    V. 44 Non-Drowsy Cold & Cough Liqui-Caps
    V. Sinex
    V. Sinex Long-Acting Nasal solution
Vicryl suture
VIDA
    vitiligo disease activity
Vidal disease

V

NOTES

vidarabine
video
    Sony VHS HQ Digital Picture v.
video-assisted thoracic surgery (VATS)
videomicroscopic imaging
Videx oral
Vierra sign
view
    coronal v.
    Waters v.
Vif
vigabatrin
Vigilon
    V. dressing
    V. hydrogel sheet
vigorous hydration
VIIIa
villi (*pl. of* villus)
villoma
villonodular synovitis
villous
    v. atrophy
    v. fold
    v. frond
    v. tumor
villus, pl. **villi**
    blunted v.
vimentin
VIMRxyn
    V. light-activated therapy
vinblastine sulfate
Vinca **alkaloid**
Vincasar PFS
Vincent
    V. angina
    V. disease
    V. infection
    V. white mycetoma
vincristine
vine
    Thunder God v.
vinegar solution
vinosus
    nevus v.
vinyl
    v. chloride
    v. chloride disease
    v. chloride exposure
    v. gloves
vinyl-alternating air mattress
Vioform topical
violaceous
    v. plaque
    v. shawl pattern rash
    v. V-neck pattern rash
violaceum
    Trichophyton v.
Viola tricolor

violet
    crystal v.
    gentian v.
    hexamethyl v.
    Hofmann v.
    Lauth v.
violet-blue erythema
violin-back
    v.-b. spider
    v.-b. spider bite
violin deformity
Vioxx
VIP
    vasoactive intestinal peptide
Vira-A Ophthalmic
Viracept
viral
    v. arthritis
    v. capsid antigen
    v. conjunctivitis
    v. disease
    v. dysenteriae
    v. encephalomyelitis
    v. envelope
    v. exanthema
    v. gastroenteritis
    v. genome
    v. hemagglutination
    v. hemorrhagic fever (VHF)
    v. hemorrhagic fever virus
    v. hepatitis (VH)
    v. hepatitis type A–E
    v. immunization
    v. neurolabyrinthitis
    v. neutralization
    v. pneumonia
    v. probe
    v. protein gag
    v. protein tax
    v. respiratory infection
    v. sandfly fever
    v. strand
    v. tropism
    v. vaccine
    v. vector
    v. wart
Viramune
Viravan-DM oral suspension
Virazole Aerosol
virchowian leprosy
viremia
Virend
virginiana
    Hamamelis v.
virginium
    chloasma periorale v.
viricidal
viricide

viridans
    v. hemolysis
    Streptococcus v.
viride
    Trichoderma v.
Viridis pulsed laser
virilization
    frank v.
virion
Virivac
viroceptor
viroid
virokine
virologist
virology
viropexis
Viroptic Ophthalmic
virosis, pl. viroses
virostatic effect
virucidal
virucide
virucopria
virulence
virulent bacteriophage
viruliferous
viruria
    BK v.
virus
    2060 v.
    Abelson murine leukemia v.
    acquired immunodeficiency
      syndrome-related v. (ARV)
    adeno-associated v. (AAV)
    adenoidal-pharyngeal-conjunctival v.
    adenosatellite v.
    African horse sickness v.
    African swine fever v. (ASFV)
    African tick v.
    v. A hepatitis
    Akabane v.
    Aleutian mink disease v.
    Amapari v.
    amphotropic v.
    Andes v.
    animal v.
    anti-Epstein-Barr v. (anti-EBV)
    antihepatitis A v.
    A-P-C v.
    Arenaviridae v.
    Argentine hemorrhagic fever v.
    arthropod-borne v.
    Astroviridae v.

    attenuated v.
    attenuate vaccinia v.
    Aujeszky disease v.
    Australian X disease v.
    avian encephalomyelitis v.
    avian erythroblastosis v.
    avian infectious laryngotracheitis v.
    avian influenza v.
    avian leukosis-sarcoma v.
    avian lymphomatosis v.
    avian myeloblastosis v.
    avian neurolymphomatosis v.
    avian pneumoencephalitis v.
    avian sarcoma v.
    avian viral arthritis v.
    B v.
    B19 v.
    bacterial v.
    Barmah Forest v.
    Bayou v.
    Bittner v.
    BK v.
    Black Creek Canal v.
    Black Lagoon v.
    v. blockade
    bluecomb v.
    bluetongue v.
    Borna disease v.
    Bornholm disease v.
    bovine leukosis v.
    bovine papular stomatitis v.
    bovine virus diarrhea v.
    Bunyamwera v.
    Bwamba v.
    CA v.
    Caliciviridae v.
    California v.
    canarypox v.
    canine distemper v.
    Capim v.
    Caraparu v.
    cat distemper v.
    cattle plague v.
    Catu v.
    CELO v.
    Central European tick-borne
      encephalitis v.
    C group v.
    Chagres v.
    chicken embryo lethal orphan v.
    chickenpox v.
    chikungunya v.

NOTES

V

virus *(continued)*
Coe v.
cold v.
Columbia S. K. v.
common cold v.
contagious pustular stomatitis v.
Coronaviridae v.
cowpox v.
Coxsackie B v.
Crimean-Congo hemorrhagic
  fever v.
croup-associated v.
CTF v.
cytopathogenic v.
Dakar bat v.
defective v.
delta v.
dengue v.
distemper v.
DNA v.
dog distemper v.
duck hepatitis v.
duck influenza v.
duck plague v.
Duvenhaga v.
EB v.
Ebola v.
ECBO v.
ECHO v.
ECMO v.
ecotropic v.
ECSO v.
ectromelia v.
EEE v.
EMC v.
emerging v.
encephalitis v.
v. encephalomyelitis
encephalomyocarditis v.
enteric cytopathogenic bovine
  orphan v.
enteric cytopathogenic human
  orphan v.
enteric cytopathogenic monkey
  orphan v.
enteric cytopathogenic swine
  orphan v.
enzootic encephalomyelitis v.
ephemeral fever v.
epidemic gastroenteritis v.
epidemic keratoconjunctivitis v.
epidemic myalgia v.
epidemic parotitis v.
epidemic pleurodynia v.
Epstein-Barr v. (EBV)
equine abortion v.
equine arteritis v.
equine coital exanthema v.
equine infectious anemia v.

equine influenza v.
equine rhinopneumonitis v.
FA v.
feline rhinotracheitis v.
fibrous bacterial v.
filamentous bacterial v.
Filoviridae v.
filtrable v.
fixed v.
Flury strain rabies v.
FMD v.
foamy v.
foot-and-mouth disease v.
fowl erythroblastosis v.
fowl lymphomatosis v.
fowl myeloblastosis v.
fowl neurolymphomatosis v.
fowl plague v.
fowlpox v.
fox encephalitis v.
Friend leukemia v.
GAL v.
gallus adeno-like v.
gastroenteritis v. type A, B
genital herpes simplex v.
German measles v.
Germiston v.
goatpox v.
Graffi v.
green monkey v.
Gross leukemia v.
Guama v.
Guaroa v.
HA1, HA2 v.
hand-foot-and-mouth disease v.
Hantaan v.
hard pad v.
Harvey murine sarcoma v.
helper v.
hemadsorption v. type 1, 2
Hendra v.
hepatitis A v. (HAV)
hepatitis B v. (HBV)
hepatitis C v. (HCV)
hepatitis D v. (HDV)
hepatitis E v. (HEV)
hepatitis G v. (HGV)
herpes simplex v. (HSV)
herpes simplex v. type I, II
herpes zoster v.
HIV-1E v.
H5N1 v.
hog cholera v.
horsepox v.
human immunodeficiency v. (HIV)
human mammary tumor v.
human T-cell leukemia v. (HTLV)
human T-cell leukemia v. I
  (HTLV-I)

human T-cell leukemia v. III
  (HTLV-III)
human T-cell
  leukemia/lymphoma v.
human T-cell lymphotrophic v.
human T-cell lymphotrophic v.
  type I (HTLV-I)
human T-cell lymphotrophic v.
  type II (HTLV-II)
human T-cell lymphotrophic v.
  type III
Ibaraki v.
IBR v.
v. III of rabbit
Ilhéus v.
inclusion conjunctivitis v.
infantile gastroenteritis v.
infectious bovine rhinotracheitis v.
infectious bronchitis v. (IBV)
infectious ectromelia v.
infectious hepatitis v.
infectious papilloma v.
infectious porcine
  encephalomyelitis v.
influenza v.
insect v.
iridescent v.
Jamestown Canyon v. (JCV)
Japanese B encephalitis v.
JC v.
JH v.
Junin v.
Juquitiba v.
K v.
Kelev strain rabies v.
v. keratoconjunctivitis
Kilham rat v.
Kisenyi sheep disease v.
Koongol v.
Korean hemorrhagic fever v.
Kotonkan v.
Kyasanur Forest disease v.
labial herpes simplex v.
La Crosse v.
lactate dehydrogenase v.
Laguna Negra v.
Lassa v.
latent rat v.
LCM v.
Lipovnik v.
louping ill v.
Lucké v.

Lunyo v.
lymphadenopathy-associated v.
  (LAV)
lymphogranuloma venereum v.
lytic Epstein-Barr v.
Machupo v.
maedi v.
malignant catarrhal fever v.
Maloney leukemia v.
Marburg v.
Marek disease v.
marmoset v.
masked v.
Mason-Pfizer v.
Mayaro v.
measles v.
medi v.
Mengo v.
milker's nodule v.
mink enteritis v.
MM v.
Mokola v.
molluscum contagiosum v. (MCV)
Moloney murine leukemia v.
monkey B v.
monkeypox v.
mouse encephalomyelitis v.
mouse hepatitis v.
mouse leukemia v.
mouse mammary tumor v.
mouse parotid tumor v.
mouse poliomyelitis v.
mousepox v.
mouse thymic v.
mucosal disease v.
Muerto Canyon v.
mumps v.
murine sarcoma v.
Murray Valley encephalitis v.
Murutucu v.
MVE v.
myxomatosis v.
Nairobi sheep disease v.
naked v.
ND v.
Nebraska calf scours v.
Neethling v.
negative strand v.
Negishi v.
neonatal calf diarrhea v.
neonatal herpes simplex v.
neurotrophic v.

NOTES

virus *(continued)*
  neurotropic v.
  v. neutralization test
  Newcastle disease v.
  Nipah v.
  non-A non-B hepatitis v.
  nonoccluded v.
  nonsyncytium-inducing variant of
   the AIDS v.
  Norwalk v.
  occluded v.
  Omsk hemorrhagic fever v.
  oncogenic v.
  o'nyong-nyong v.
  Oriboca v.
  ornithosis v.
  orphan v.
  Orthomyxoviridae v.
  Oscar v.
  Pacheco parrot disease v.
  pantropic v.
  papilloma v.
  pappataci fever v.
  parainfluenza v.
  Paramyxoviridae v.
  paravaccinia v.
  parrot v.
  Patois v.
  pharyngoconjunctival fever v.
  Phlebotomus fever v.
  Picornaviridae v.
  Pirital v.
  plant v.
  v. pneumonia of pig
  poliomyelitis v.
  polymerase chain reaction-based
   detection of hepatitis G v.
  porcine hemagglutinating
   encephalomyelitis v.
  Powassan v.
  primary genital herpes simplex v.
  progressive pneumonia v.
  pseudocowpox v.
  pseudolymphocytic
   choriomeningitis v.
  pseudorabies v.
  psittacosis v.
  Puumala v.
  PV v.
  quail bronchitis v.
  Quaranfil v.
  rabbit fibroma v.
  rabbit myxoma v.
  rabbitpox v.
  rabies v.
  Rauscher leukemia v.
  recurrent genital herpes simplex v.
  recurrent intraoral herpes
   simplex v.

  recurrent labial herpes simplex v.
  REO v.
  respiratory enteric orphan v. (REO
   virus)
  respiratory syncytial v. (RSV)
  Rida v.
  Rift Valley fever v.
  rinderpest v.
  RNA tumor v.
  Ross River v.
  Rous-associated v. (RAV)
  Rous sarcoma v. (RSV)
  Rs v.
  Rubarth disease v.
  rubella vaccine v.
  rubeola v.
  Russian autumn encephalitis v.
  Russian spring-summer
   encephalitis v.
  Saint Louis encephalitis v.
  Salisbury common cold v.
  salivary gland v.
  sandfly fever v.
  San Miguel sea lion v.
  Semliki Forest v.
  Sendai v.
  serum hepatitis v.
  v. shedding
  sheep-pox v.
  shipping fever v.
  Shope fibroma v.
  Shope papilloma v.
  Simbu v.
  simian vacuolating v. No. 40
   (SV40)
  Sindbis v.
  Sin Nombre v.
  slow v.
  smallpox v.
  snowshoe hare v.
  soremouth v.
  Spondweni v.
  Stealth v.
  street v.
  swamp fever v.
  swine encephalitis v.
  swine fever v.
  swine influenza v.
  swinepox v.
  Swiss mouse leukemia v.
  syncytial v.
  Tacaribe complex of v.
  Tahyna v.
  temperate v.
  Teschen disease v.
  Tete v.
  TGE v.
  Theiler mouse encephalomyelitis v.

Theiler original strain of mouse encephalomyelitis v. (TO)
tickborne encephalitis v.
TO v.
Togaviridae v.
trachoma v.
transmissible gastroenteritis v. (TGE)
transmissible turkey enteritis v.
tumor v.
turkey meningoencephalitis v.
Turlock v.
Umbre v.
vaccine v.
vaccinia v.
vacuolating v.
varicella-zoster v. (VZV)
variola v.
VEE v.
Venezuelan equine encephalomyelitis v.
vesicular exanthema of swine v.
viral hemorrhagic fever v.
visceral disease v.
visna v.
VS v.
WEE v.
Wesselsbron disease v.
western equine encephalitis v.
western equine encephalomyelitis v.
West Nile encephalitis v.
v. X disease
xenotropic v.
Yaba monkey v.
yellow fever v.
Zika v.
virus-1
human immunodeficiency v.-1 (HIV-1)
virus-2
human immunodeficiency v.-2 (HIV-2)
virus-inactivating agent
virus-induced
v.-i. asthma
v.-i. wheezing
virus-infected cell
virusoid
virus-transformed cell
visage
V. Cosmetic Surgery system
Hippocratic v.

viscera
visceral
v. disease virus
v. hemangiomatosis
v. larva migrans
v. leishmaniasis (VL)
v. lymphomatosis
v. schistosomiasis
v. sporotrichosis
v. syphilis
viscerocutaneous loxoscelism
viscerotropic leishmaniasis (VTL)
viscosity
Visine
V. L.R. Ophthalmic
V. Workplace
vision, right eye (VOD)
Visiport
visna virus
Vistacrom
Vistaquel
Vistaril
V. Injection
V. oral
Vistazine Injection
Vistide
visual
v. analog scale (VAS)
v. display terminal (VDT)
VIT
venom immunotherapy
VitaCuff
Vitadye makeup by Elder
Vita-E
vitae
arbor v.
vital
v. capacity (VC)
v. vaccine
vitamin
v. A
v. A deficiency
antioxidant v.
v. A and vitamin D
v. B_6
v. B_1 deficiency
v. B_5 deficiency
v. B_6 deficiency
v. B_{12} deficiency
v. B deficiency
v. B therapy
v. C

V

NOTES

vitamin *(continued)*
    v. C deficiency
    v. C test
    v. D deficiency
    v. D synthesis
    v. E
    v. E deficiency
    v. K deficiency
    v. K therapy
    microbial v.
vitamin-related obesity
Vita-Plus E Softgels
viteae
    Acanthocheilonema v.
Vitec topical
Vite E creme
Vitex agnus-castus
vitiligines
vitiliginous
vitiligo
    acral v.
    acrofacial v.
    v. antibody
    v. capitis
    Cazenave v.
    Celsus v.
    v. disease activity (VIDA)
    v. disease activity score
    facial v.
    generalized v.
    lip-tip v.
    localized v.
    occupational v.
    perinevic v.
    perinevoid v.
    segmental v.
    stable v.
    v. universalis
vitiligoidea
vitlata
    Epicauta v.
Vitrasert intraocular device
Vitrax
    AMO V.
vitreitis
vitreous body
vitro
    in v.
vitronectin
vittatus
    Centruroides v.
Viva-Drops solution
vivax
    Plasmodium v.
Vivelle
Vivelle-Dot
viviparus
    Dictyocaulus v.

vivo
    in v.
Vivonex
    V. formula
    V. Plus
Vivotif Berna oral
VK
    Apo-Pen VK
VKH
    Vogt-Koyanagi-Harada
VKHS
    Vogt-Koyanagi-Harada syndrome
VL
    visceral leishmaniasis
VLA-4
    very late antigen-4
VLA-1 antigen
VLDL
    very-low-density lipoprotein
Vlemasque
Vleminckx solution
VM-301
Vmax
VMR
    vasomotor rhinitis
VNTR
    variable numbers of tandem repeats
VO$_2$
    oxygen consumption per minute
        VO$_2$ max
vocational intervention
voces (*pl. of* vox)
VOD
    venoocclusive
    vision, right eye
        VOD disease
Voerner disease
Vofenal
Vogt-Koyanagi-Harada (VKH)
    V.-K.-H. syndrome (VKHS)
Vogt-Koyanagi syndrome
Vohwinkel
    mutilating keratoderma of V.
    V. syndrome
Voigt line
volar
    v. psoriasis
    v. skin
volatile odor
volcanic border
vole bacillus
Volkmann cheilitis
Vollmer test
Volmax
voltage-gated potassium channel
voltametry
    adsorptive v.

Voltaren
  V. oral
  V. Rapide
Voltaren-XR oral
volume
  erosion v.
  high lung v.
  intrathoracic blood v. (ITBV)
  pulmonary blood v. (PBV)
  residual v.
  stroke v. (SV)
  v. test
  v. thickness index (VTI)
  tidal v.
volume-assured pressure support
  (VAPS)
volume-cycled decelerating-flow
  ventilation
volume-limited ventilator
volumetric
  v. magnetization transfer imaging
  v. method
  v. technique
volutrauma
volvae
volvulosis
volvulus
  Onchocerca v.
vomiting
  epidemic v.
  explosive v.
von
  v. Behring law
  v. Economo disease
  v. Economo encephalitis
  v. Gierke glycogen storage disease
  v. Hippel-Landau syndrome
  v. Hippel-Lindau gene (VHL)
  v. Krogh transformation
  v. Recklinghausen disease
  v. Willebrand disease (vWD)
  v. Willebrand factor (vWF)
  v. Zumbusch disease
  v. Zumbusch pustular psoriasis
Vontrol
vorax
  lupus v.
Vornado Air Quality System
Vorner variant of Unna-Thost
  keratoderma
vortices pilorum

VoSol HC Otic
vox, pl. **voces**
  v. cholerica
VP
  variegate porphyria
  ventriculoperitoneal shunt
VPA
  ventricular pseudoaneurysm
VPF/VEGF
  vascular permeability factor/vascular
    endothelial cell growth factor
V-plasty to Y-plasty
Vpr
Vpu
V/Q
  ventilation/perfusion
V/Q lung scan
VRE
  vancomycin-resistant enterococci
  vancomycin-resistant *Enterococcus*
VREF
  vancomycin-resistant *Enterococcus*
    faecium
    VREF bacteremia
VS
  vesicular stomatitis
    VS virus
VTI
  volume thickness index
VTL
  viscerotropic leishmaniasis
V-type microtiter plate
vulgaris
  acne v.
  apple jelly papule of lupus v.
  Artemis v.
  Artemisia v.
  Faba v.
  ichthyosis v.
  impetigo v.
  lupus v.
  pemphigus v. (PV)
  Proteus v.
  refractory pemphigus v.
  sycosis v.
  Thermoactinomyces v.
  verruca v.
  xerosis v.
vulnificus
  Vibrio v.
vulva, pl. **vulvae**
  kraurosis vulvae

V

NOTES

vulva *(continued)*
    leukoplakia v.
    pruritus v.
vulvar
    v. dermatosis
    v. intraepithelial neoplasia
    v. itch
    v. lesion
    v. nevus
    v. vestibulitis syndrome
    v. wart
vulvitis
    chronic atrophic v.
    follicular v.
    leukoplakic v.
    plasma cell v.
vulvodynia
vulvovaginal candidiasis (VVC)
vulvovaginitis
    herpetic v.
Vumon injection

VVC
    vulvovaginal candidiasis
Vw antigen
vWD
    von Willebrand disease
VWF
    vibration-induced white finger
vWF
    von Willebrand factor
VX-497
VX-740
VX-745
Vytone topical
VZ
    varicella-zoster
VZIG
    varicella-zoster immunoglobulin
VZV
    varicella-zoster virus
        VZV retinitis

W
Benzac W
Compound W
W-135
meningococcal polysaccharide
vaccine, groups A, C, Y, W-135
Waardenburg-Shah syndrome
Waardenburg syndrome
Waddell sign
Wagner-Meissner tactile corpuscle
Wagner potion
Waldenström
hypergammaglobulinemia of W.
W. macroglobulinemia (WM)
W. purpura
W. syndrome
Waldmann UV5000 cabinet
walk cycle phase
Walker-Murdoch sign
walking
chromosome w.
wall
nail w.
w. pellitory
shaggy thick w.
Wallgren aseptic meningitis
walnut
black w.
shaking of w.'s
w. tree
walnut-juice stain
Walsh pressure ring
Walter
W. Reed classification
W. splinter forceps
Walton
W. expressor
W. extractor
wandering
w. erysipelas
w. rash
waning
waxing and w.
warble
Wardrop disease
warehouseman's itch
warfare
Skin Exposure Reduction Paste
Against Chemical W.
(SERPACWA)
warfarin sodium
warm
w. agglutinin
w. autoantibody

w. spot
w. water immersion foot (WWIF)
warm-cold hemolysin
warm-reactive antibody
wart
acuminate w.
anatomical w.
anogenital w.
asbestos w.
black seeds in w.
cattle w.
common w.
digitate w.
doughnut w.
fig w.
filiform w.
flat w.
fugitive w.
genital w.
infectious w.
moist w.
mosaic w.
myrmecia w.
nail w.
necrogenic w.
palmar w.
paronychial w.
periungual w.
Peruvian w.
pitch w.
plane w.
plantar w.
pointed w.
postmortem w.
prosector's w.
recalcitrant w.
W. Remover
ridged w.
seborrheic w.
seed w.
senile w.
soft w.
soot w.
subungual w.
telangiectatic w.
trumpeter w.
tuberculous w.
venereal w.
viral w.
vulvar w.
water w.
Wart-Away
Wartenberg symptom
Warthin-Finkeldey cell
Warthin-Starry stain

W

Warthin-Starry-staining bacillus
wart-like excrescence
Wartner over-the-counter wart removal
  treatment
wartpox
warty
> w. dyskeratoma
> w. horn
> w. keratotic plaque
> w. tuberculosis

WAS
> Wiskott-Aldrich syndrome

wash
> Benzac AC W.
> Benzac W W.
> Desquam-X W.
> Dryox W.
> Fostex W.
> Neutrogena Oil-Free acne W.
> Oil-Free Acne W.
> Oxy 10 W.
> OxyBalance Facial Cleansing W.
> SAStid Plain Therapeutic Shampoo
>   and Acne w.
> Theroxide W.

washed maternal platelet
washerman's mark
washerwoman's itch
WASP
> Wiskott-Aldrich syndrome protein

wasp
> paper w.
> w. sting

Wassermann
> W. antibody
> W. fast test
> W. reaction (W.r.)

Wassilieff disease
wasting
> w. disease
> w. syndrome

watch
> Oxy Night W.

water
> W. Babies
> w. blister
> w. canker
> w. itch
> w. moccasin snake
> w. sore
> w. wart

water-based
> w.-b. facial foundation
> w.-b. mascara

water-buffalo leprosy
water-free facial foundation
Waterhouse-Friderichsen syndrome
water-impermeable, nonsilicone-based
  occlusive dressing

water-in-oil ointment
watermelon stomach
waterpox
water-repellent ointment
water-soluble ointment
Waters view
water-washable cream
waveform
> high-energy, pulse-doublet w.

wave splash
wax
> w. epilation
> w. myrtle
> w. myrtle tree

waxing and waning
waxy
> w. contracture
> w. finger
> w. skin
> w. surface

4-Way Long Acting Nasal Solution
Ways of Coping Scale
WB
> wheezy bronchitis

WBC
> white blood cell
> white blood count
>   WBC count

WBI
> whole-body irradiation

WCD
> Weber-Christian disease

WCS-90
> Clorpactin WCS-90

WDE
> wound dressing emulsion
>   Biafine WDE

WDEIA
> wheat-dependent, exercise-induced
> anaphylaxis

weakness
> generalized w.
> motor neuron w.
> muscle w.

weal
weanling diarrhea
Webb antigen
webbed pattern
Weber-Christian disease (WCD)
Weber-Cockayne
> W.-C. disease
> W.-C. syndrome

Weber test
web formation
Webril
Webster needle holder
wedge renal biopsy

WEE
western equine encephalomyelitis
WEE virus
weed
careless w.
poverty w.
weekly
Prozac W.
weeping
w. dermatitis
w. eczema
w. fig
w. fig tree
w. lesion
w. willow
Wegener
W. granulomatosis (WG)
W. granulomatosis syndrome
Weibull regression model
Weichselbaum lacunar resorption
weight
high molecular w. (HMW)
w. loss
weight-bearing exercise
Weil disease
Weil-Felix
W.-F. reaction
W.-F. test
Weill-Marchesani syndrome
Weinberg reaction
Weissenbacher-Zweymuller syndrome
Weissenbach syndrome
weld
spot w.
Well
W. disease
W. syndrome
Wellcovorin
W. injection
W. oral
well-demarcated skin reaction
Wells
W. Johnson pump
W. syndrome
welt
indurated w.
wen
Werlhof
W. disease
W. purpura

werneckii
Cladosporium w.
Exophiala w.
Werner syndrome
Wernicke-Korsakoff syndrome
Werther
W. disease
W. nevus
Wesselsbron
W. disease
W. disease virus
W. fever
Wessely ring
west
W. African fever
W. Indian smallpox
W. Nile encephalitis virus
W. Nile fever
Westcort topical
Westergren sedimentation rate
westermani
Paragonimus w.
western
w. black-legged tick
W. blot
W. blot electrotransfer test
W. blot infection
W. blot vaccine profile
w. equine encephalitis virus
w. equine encephalomyelitis (WEE)
w. equine encephalomyelitis virus
W. juniper
W. juniper tree
W. Ontario and McMaster
Universities Osteoarthritis Index
(WOMAC)
W. Ontario and McMaster
Universities Osteoarthritis Index
Physical Functioning subscale and
chair-stand performance
(WOMAC-PF)
w. poison oak
W. ragweed
W. ragweed weed pollen
W. red cedar
w. water hemp
Westrim LA
wet
w. cutaneous leishmaniasis
w. dressing
w. flush
w. gangrene

W

NOTES

617

wet *(continued)*
    w. pellagra
    w. smear
    w. tetter
WG
    Wegener granulomatosis
whale finger
Whatman 3MM
wheal
    w. and erythema radiation
    w. and erythema reaction
    erythematous w.
    w. and flare
    w. and flare reaction
    skin w.
whealing
wheat
    w. flour
    w. grain dust mite
    whole w.
wheat-dependent, exercise-induced anaphylaxis (WDEIA)
wheeze
    monophonic w.
wheezing
    intractable w.
    nocturnal w.
    virus-induced w.
wheezy bronchitis (WB)
Whiff test
whiplash injury
Whipple
    W. bacillus
    W. disease
whippleii
    Trophermyma w.
whisker hair
whistling face syndrome
white
    w. ash
    w. ash tree
    w. blood cell (WBC)
    w. blood count
    w. burrobrush
    w. dermatographia
    w. dermographism
    w. finger
    w. frontal forelock
    w. gangrene
    w. graft
    w. lesion
    w. line
    w. line response
    w. melanin
    w. mulberry
    w. mulberry tree
    w. oak
    w. oak tree
    w. petrolatum
    w. piedra
    w. pine
    w. pine tree
    w. poplar tree
    w. scar
    w. sponge nevus
    w. spot disease
    w. spots of the nail plate
    w. spots of skin
    w. strawberry tongue
white-faced hornet
whitegraft reaction
whitehead
whitepox
Whitewater Arroyo
Whitfield ointment
whitlow
    herpes w.
    herpetic w.
    melanotic w.
Whitmore
    W. disease
    W. fever
    W. melioidosis
WHO
    World Health Organization
    WHO Class IV
    WHO criteria
WHO/ILAR
    World Health Organization/International League of Associations for Rheumatology
whole
    w. blood
    w. ragweed extract (WRE)
    w. wheat
whole-body
    w.-b. antibody technique (IMX)
    w.-b. extract
    w.-b. irradiation (WBI)
whooping cough
whooping-cough vaccine
whorl
    digital w.
whorled
Whytt disease
wick
wickerhamii
    Prototheca w.
Wickham stria
Widal
    W. reaction
    W. serum test
    W. syndrome
wide
    w. excision
    w. spectrum
widow's peak
Wigraine

Wilcoxon rank sum test
wild
> w. oat grass pollen
> w. rye
> w. rye grass
> w. tobacco

wildfire rash
Willan
> W. disease
> W. lepra

Willebrand factor
willow
> w. tree
> w. tree pollen
> weeping w.

Wilms tumor
Wilson
> W. disease
> W. lichen

Wilson-Brocq erythroderma
Wimberger sign
Win
> wound-induced

windborne pollen
windburn
Windmill-Vane-Hand syndrome
window
> core w.
> nasoantral w.
> Rebuck skin w.

wind-pollinated plant
wine-induced asthma
Winer
> dilated pore of W.
> pore of W.

wingscale
Winkler disease
Winks
Winn test
Winpred
WinRho
> W. SD
> W. SD antibody

Winstrol
winter
> w. dysentery of cattle
> w. eczema
> w. itch
> w. protoporphyria
> w. pruritus
> w. vomiting disease

Winterbottom sign

wipe
> Ivy Cleanse medicated w.
> Sport w.'s

wire-loop
> w.-l. lesion
> w.-l. shaped telangiectasia

Wisconsin
> University of W. (UW)

Wiskott-Aldrich
> W.-A. syndrome (WAS)
> W.-A. syndrome protein (WASP)

Wissler-Fanconi syndrome
Wissler syndrome
Wistar rat
witch hazel
witkop
Witkop-Von Sallman disease
WM
> Waldenström macroglobulinemia

Wohlfahrtia
wolf-biter habit
WOMAC
> Western Ontario and McMaster Universities Osteoarthritis Index
> WOMAC pain score
> WOMAC Physical Function subscale
> WOMAC stiffness scale

WOMAC-PF
> Western Ontario and McMaster Universities Osteoarthritis Index Physical Functioning subscale and chair-stand performance

women
> Selsun Gold for W.
> teratogenic effect on pregnant w.

Wong-Stall scissors
wood
> W. glass
> W. lamp
> W. light
> W. light examination
> pao ferro w.
> w. tar
> w. tick
> W. unit

woodcutter's encephalitis
wood-pulp worker's disease
wool
> sheep w.
> Sofban orthopedic padding w.

NOTES

W

wool *(continued)*
Velband orthopedic padding w.
w. wax alcohol
woolly hair
woolly-hair nevus
Wor Ditchling agent
Woringer-Kolopp disease
work disability
workplace
Visine W.
work-setting factor
Work-Station Sun-Sparcs 20
World
W. Health Organization (WHO)
W. Health Organization
classification of lupus nephritis (I,
IIA, IIB, III, IV, V)
W. Health Organization criteria
W. Health Organization/International
League of Associations for
Rheumatology (WHO/ILAR)
worm
biting reef w.
blood w.
guinea w.
medina w.
worm-like
wormwood
Woronoff ring
wort
Saint John's w.
wortmannin
wound
abraded w.
w. botulism
w. contraction
w. dressing emulsion (WDE)
w. fever
fish-mouth w.
w. grading 1-6
w. healing
w. myiasis
puncture w.
W. Span Bridge II dressing
W. Stick measuring system
wound-induced (Win)

Woun'Dres
W. collagen
W. hydrogel dressing
Wound-Span Bridge II
W-plasty
W.r.
Wassermann reaction
Wr^a
Wright antigen
Wr^a antigen
wrap
body w.
Coban w.
Coflex flexible w.
Comprilan w.
elastic w.
plastic occlusive w.
WRE
whole ragweed extract
wreath
Hippocratic w.
wrestler herpes
Wright
W. antigen (Wr^a)
W. nebulizer
W. stain
wrinkle
wrinkling
cigarette-paper w.
writing
skin w.
wt gene
wucher atrophy
Wuchereria bancrofti
wuchereriasis
Wu-Kabat plot
WWIF
warm water immersion foot
Wyamycin S
Wyburn-Mason syndrome
Wycillin injection
Wydase
Wyeth bifurcated needle
Wymox

X
    X chromosome
    X factor
    Histalet X
    histiocytosis X
XAb
  xenoantibody
Xanar 20 Ambulase CO$_2$ laser
Xanax
xanchromatic
Xanelim
xanthelasma
    generalized x.
    x. palpebrarum
xanthelasmoidea
xanthelasmoideum
    lymphangioma x.
xanthine
    x. crystal
    x. inhibition
    x. stone excretion
xanthinuria
xanthism
xanthochroia
xanthochromatic
xanthochromia striata palmaris
xanthochromic
xanthochrous
xanthoderma
xanthoerythrodermia perstans
xanthogranuloma (XG)
    juvenile x. (JXG)
    necrobiotic x.
xanthoma, pl. xanthomata
    x. diabeticorum
    diffuse plane x.
    x. dissemination
    x. disseminatum (XD)
    eruptive x.
    fibrous x.
    generalized plane x.
    hypercholesteremic x.
    hyperlipemic x.
    juvenile x.
    x. multiplex striatum palmare
    nodular x.
    normocholesteremic x.
    palmar x.
    palpebrarum x.
    x. palpebrarum
    papular x.
    planar x.
    plane x.
    x. planum
    x. striata palmaris

    x. tendinosum
    tendinous x.
    tendon x.
    tuberoeruptive x.
    x. tuberosum
    x. tuberosum multiplex
    tuberous x.
    urticarial x.
    verruciform x.
    verrucous x.
xanthomatosis
    cerebrotendinous x.
    generalized plane x.
    normolipemic x.
    normolipoproteinemic x.
xanthomatous biliary cirrhosis
Xanthomonas maltophilia
xanthopathy
xanthopsydracia
xanthosis diabeticorum
Xcellerate T-cell product
XD
  xanthoma disseminatum
Xe
  xenon
XeCl excimer laser
Xenaderm ointment
X-encoded immune system gene
xenoantibody (XAb)
XenoDerm graft
xenogeneic
    x. cellular immune response
    x. graft
    x. transplantation
xenogenic
xenogenous
xenograft
    discordant cellular x.
    discordant organ x.
    free-tissue x.
    organ x.
    porcine x.
    x. rejection
    x. transplantation
    vascularized x.
xenoislet transplantation
xenon (Xe)
    x. arc lamp
xenoparasite
xenopi
    Mycobacterium x.
Xenopsylla
    X. cheopis
    X. cheopis bite
xenoreactive natural antibody (XNA)

X

xenorecognition
T-cell x.
xenosis
xenotransplant
xenotransplantation
cellular x.
pig-to-primate model of x.
xenotropic virus
xenozoonoses
Xerac AC
xerasia
xerochilia
xeroderma, xerodermia
Kaposi x.
x. pigmentosum
Xeroform
Xero-Lube
xeronosus
xerophthalmia
xerosis vulgaris
xerostomia
xerotes
xerotica
xerotic eczema
xerotripsis
XG
xanthogranuloma
Xg antigen
X-inactivation
xinafoate
salmeterol x.
XL
Biaxin XL
X-linked
X-l. agammaglobulinemia
X-l. Ehlers-Danlos syndrome
X-l. hypogammaglobulinemia
X-l. ichthyosis
immune dysregulation,
polyendocrinopathy,
enteropathy, X-l. (IPEX)
X-l. immunodeficiency with hyper
IgM
X-l. lymphoproliferative disease
(XLP)

X-l. lymphoproliferative syndrome
X-l. mucopolysaccharidosis
X-l. ocular albinism (XOAN)
X-l. recessive inheritance
X-l. severe combined
immunodeficiency (XSCID)
XLP
X-linked lymphoproliferative disease
XMMEN-OE5 monoclonal antibody
XNA
xenoreactive natural antibody
XOAN
X-linked ocular albinism
Xolair
Xopenex
Xosten
x-radiation
x-ray
x-r. alopecia
x-r. crystallographic data
x-r. dermatitis
x-r. finding
XSCID
X-linked severe combined
immunodeficiency
X-Seb T
X-span tubing
x-square test
XT
Contuss XT
XTRAC laser system
XXMEN-OE5 antiendotoxin
XXYY genotype
xylene
Xylocaine with epinephrine
Xylol prep
xylometazoline
xylose
xylosoxidans
Achromobacter x.
Alcaligenes x.
XYY syndrome

Y
>histiocytosis Y

Y12 monoclonal antibody

Yaba
>Y. monkey virus
>Y. tumor

YAC
>yeast artificial chromosome

YAG
>yttrium-aluminum-garnet
>YAG laser

YagLazr system

Yangtze edema

Yates corrected chi square test

yaw
>bosch y.
>bush y.
>crab y.
>early y.
>foot y.
>forest y.
>guinea corn y.
>late y.
>mother y.
>osseous y.
>ringworm y.
>tertiary y.

7-year itch

yeast
>y. artificial chromosome (YAC)
>brewer's y.
>y. form
>y. infection
>lipophilic y.
>y. meningitis

Yeast-Gard Medicated Douche

yellow
>y. disease
>y. dock
>y. fever
>y. fever vaccine (YF-VAX)

>y. fever virus
>y. hornet
>y. jacket
>y. jacket sting
>y. lesion
>y. mecuric oxide
>y. mustard
>y. mutant albinism
>y. nail
>y. nail syndrome
>y. oculocutaneous albinism
>y. papule
>y. skin

Yergason supination sign

Yersinia
>*Y.* antigen
>*Y.* arthritis
>*Y. enterocolitica*
>*Y. pestis*
>*Y. pestis* bite
>*Y. pseudotuberculosis*

yew tree

YF-VAX
>yellow fever vaccine

ying-yang fashion

YKL-40 antigen

ylang-ylang oil

Yodoxin

young
>maturity-onset diabetes of the y. (MODY)
>Y. syndrome

Y-plasty
>V-plasty to Y.-p.

Yt^a antigen

Yttrium-90

yttrium-aluminum-garnet (YAG)
>y.-a.-g. laser

yucca

Yunis-Varon syndrome

YXXZ motif

Zaditen
Zaditor
zafirlukast
Zagam
Zahorsky disease
Zaire subtype
zalcitabine (ddC)
Zambesi ulcer
Zambusch (*See* Zumbusch)
Zanfel cream
Zantac
 Z. injection
 Z. oral
ZAP-70 deficiency
Zartan
Zassi Bowel Management system
ZDV
 zidovudine
Zeasorb-AF superabsorbent antifungal
 powder
zebra body
zebra-like hyperpigmentation
ZEEP
 zero end-expiratory pressure
Zefazone
Zeis gland
Zenapax
Zen macrobiotic diet
Zephiran mouthwash
Zephrex LA
Zerit (d4T)
zero end-expiratory pressure (ZEEP)
zeta, ζ
 z. potential
 z. sedimentation rate
Zetar
Zetone cream
Zetran injection
Ziagen
zidovudine (ZDV)
 z. and lamivudine
Ziehl-Neelsen
 Z.-N. smear
 Z.-N. stain
zigzag
 z. approximation
 zigzag deformity
Zika
 Z. fever
 Z. virus
zileuton
Zimmerman-Laband syndrome
Zimmerman-Walton expressor
Zimmer Pulsavac wound debridement
 system

Zinacef injection
Zinaderm
zinc
 z. chloride paste
 z. deficiency
 DHS z.
 z. finger protein
 z. gluconate lozenge
 z. oxide
 z. oxide, cod liver oil, and talc
 z. oxide microfine
 z. oxide, talc, carbolic acid, boric
  acid
 z. pox
 z. protoporphyrin (ZPP)
 z. protoporphyrin:heme ratio
 pyrithione z.
 z. pyrithione
 z. sulfate
Zincoderm
Zincofax
Zincon Shampoo
Zindaclin
Zino
 Scholl Z.
Zinsser-Cole-Engman syndrome
Zinsser-Engman-Cole syndrome
ZIP
 zoster immune plasma
ziprasidone
 Z. capsule
 ziprasidone hydrochloride
Zipzoc
 Z. stocking
 Z. Stocking leg compression
  dressing
zirconium granuloma
zit
Zithromax
ZLN
 zosteriform lentiginous nevus
Zn-dependent endopeptidase
ZNP bar
zoacanthosis
Zoderm
 Z. cleanser
 Z. cream
 Z. gel
zoledronic acid for injection
Zolicef
zolmitriptan disintegrating tablet
Zoloft
Zometa
Zomig-ZMT disintegrating tablet
zona, pl. zonae

Z

zona *(continued)*
- z. corona
- z. dermatica
- z. epithelioserosa
- z. facialis
- z. fasciculata
- z. glomerulosa
- z. ignea
- z. ophthalmica
- z. reticularis
- z. serpiginosa

Zonalon Topical cream
zonal type reaction
zonary
zone
- barrier z.
- basement membrane z. (BMZ)
- equivalence z.
- floristic z.
- Head z.
- z. of hyperalgesia
- z. of hyperemia
- hyperesthetic z.
- keratogenous z.
- perinuclear z.
- T z.

zonesthesia
zoniform nevus
zonula occludens
zoograft
zoom endoscopy
Zoon
- balanitis of Z.
- Z. disease
- Z. erythroplasia

zoonosis
zoonotic
- z. cutaneous leishmaniasis
- z. erysipelas
- z. infection
- z. potential
- z. retrovirus

zoophilic fungus
zootoxin
ZORprin
zoster
- acute herpes z.
- dermatomal z.
- disseminated herpes z.
- z. encephalomyelitis

- herpes z. (HZ)
- z. immune globulin
- z. immune plasma (ZIP)
- ophthalmic z.
- z. sine herpetic

zosteriform
- z. distribution of lesion
- z. lentiginous nevus (ZLN)
- z. lichen planus
- z. pattern

zosteroid
Zostrix
Zostrix-HP
Zosyn
Zovirax
- Z. injection
- Z. oral
- Z. topical

Zoysia
ZP 11
Z-plasty
- O-plasty to Z-p.
- Z-p. procedure

ZPP
- zinc protoporphyrin

z score
Zumbusch
- Z. disease

Zyderm
- Z. collagen implant
- Z. II collagen

zygapophysial, zygapophyseal
- z. joint

Zygomycetes
zygomycosis
zygospore
Zyloprim
Zyloric
zymographic analysis
zymography
- gelatin z.

zymosan
- unopsonized z.

zymotic papilloma
Zyplast
- Z. collagen
- Z. collagen implant

Zyrtec
Zyrtec-D 12-hour extended-release tablet

Appendix 1
Anatomical Illustrations

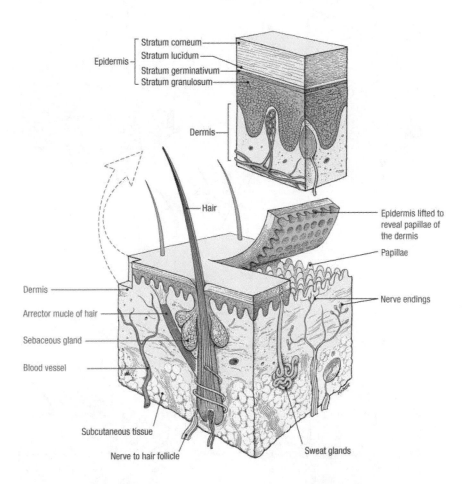

Figure 1. Skin components and layers.

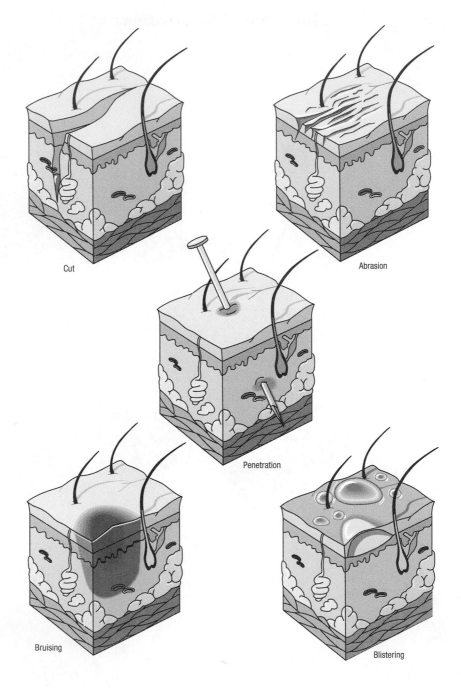

Figure 2. Types of skin injuries.

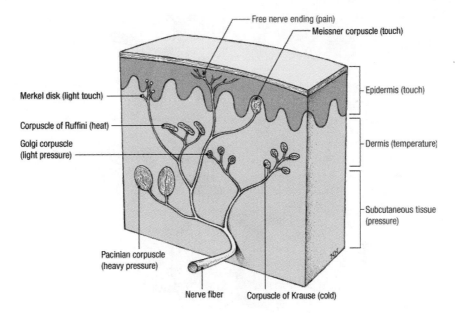

Figure 3. Sensory corpuscles.

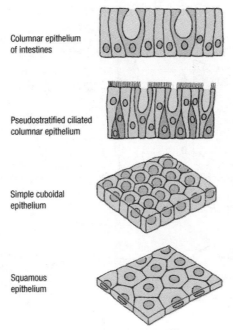

Figure 4. Types of epithelium (simplified schematic).

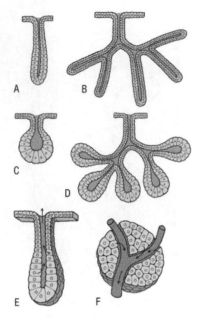

Figure 5. Types of glands: tubular (A), compound tubular (B), acinous (C), compound acinous (D), exocrine (E), endocrine (F).

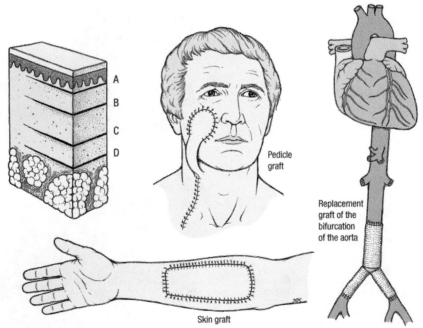

Figure 6. Graft types: split-thickness grafts (A, B, C), full-thickness graft (D).

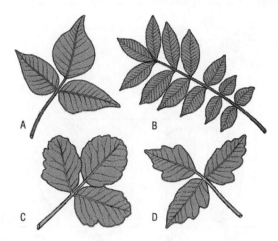

Figure 7. *Toxicodendron*: poison ivy (A), poison sumac (B), Western poison oak (C), Eastern poison oak (D).

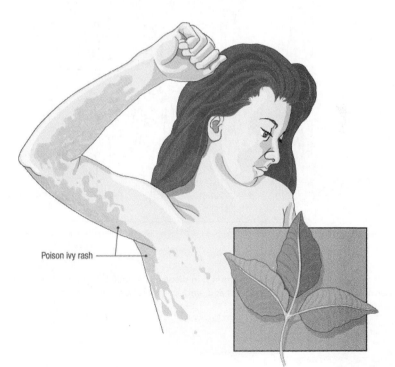

Poison ivy rash

Figure 8. Young girl with arm lifted to show typical poison ivy rash with weepy blisters on underside of arm and wrist; inset shows poison ivy leaflet of three.

A5

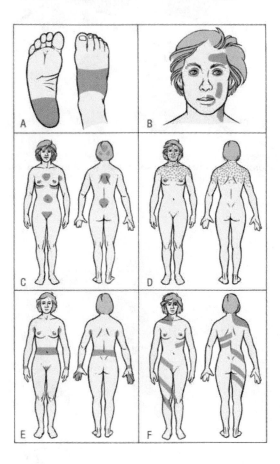

Figure 9. Anatomic distribution of common skin disorders: contact dermatitis from shoes (A), contact dermatitis from cosmetics, perfumes and earrings (B), seborrheic dermatitis (C), acne (D), scabies (E), and herpes zoster (shingles) (F).

Primary lesions

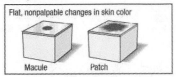

Flat, nonpalpable changes in skin color

Macule Patch

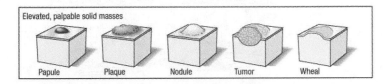

Elevated, palpable solid masses

Papule Plaque Nodule Tumor Wheal

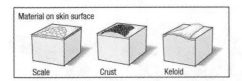

Elevation formed by fluid in a cavity

Vesicle Bulla Pustule

Secondary lesions

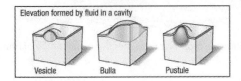

Loss of skin surface

Erosion Ulcer Excoriation Fissure

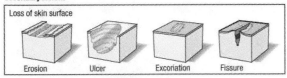

Material on skin surface

Scale Crust Keloid

Vascular lesions

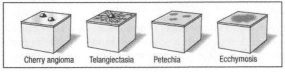

Cherry angioma Telangiectasia Petechia Ecchymosis

Figure 10. Lesions. Types of primary, secondary and vascular lesions.

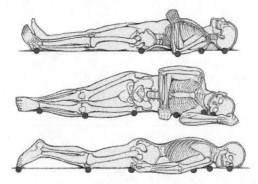

Figure 11. Decubitus ulcer. Dots indicate most common sites due to proximity of bone to skin.

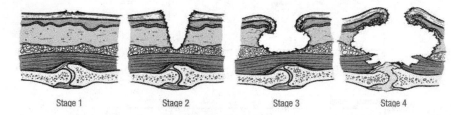

Figure 12. Cross-section of skin showing 4 stages of pressure sore and ulcer classification. Stage 1: inflammation, redness of epidermis. Stage 2: loss of epidermis, damage to dermis. Stage 3: involvement of subcutaneous tissue. Stage 4: damage to tendon, muscle and bone.

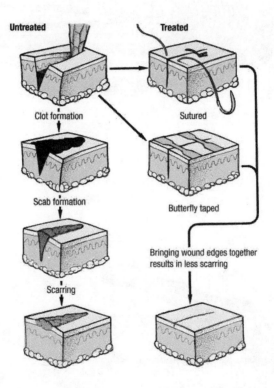

Figure 13. Wound healing.

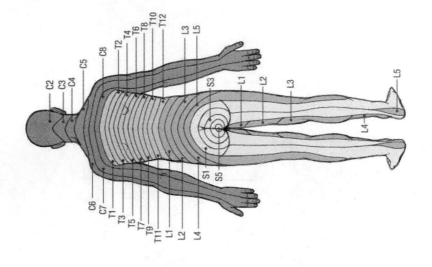

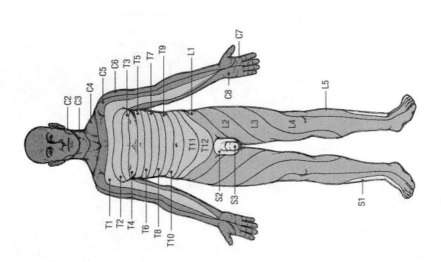

Figure 14 Dermatomes. Areas of skin supplied by cutaneous branches of spinal nerves.

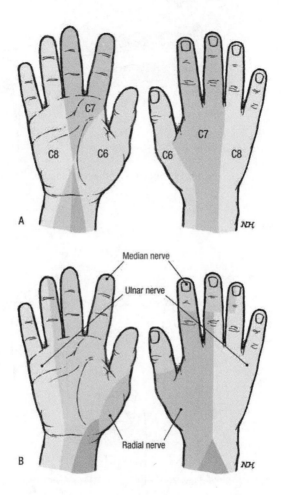

Figure 15. Innervation of the hand and wrist: segmental dermatomes (A), and cutaneous nerve distribution (B).

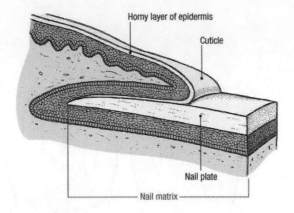

Figure 16. Structure of the nail (unguis).

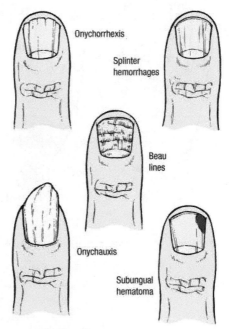

Figure 17. Nail abnormalities.

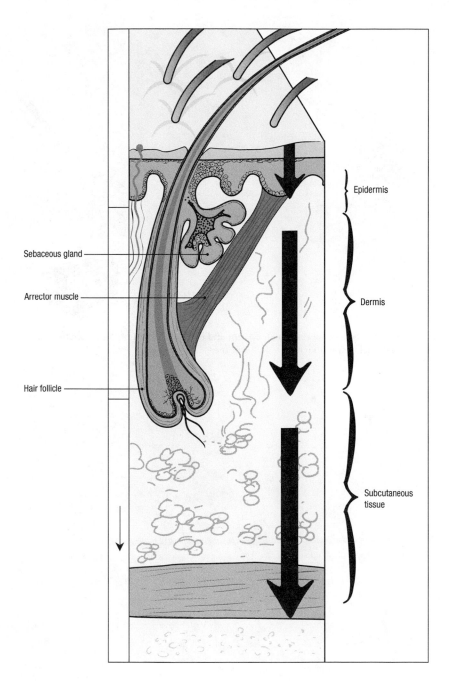

Sebaceous gland

Arrector muscle

Hair follicle

Epidermis

Dermis

Subcutaneous
tissue

Figure 18. Cross-section of skin layers, muscle and bone, with corresponding classification of burn depths.

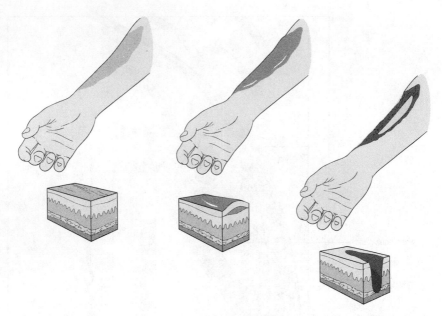

Figure 19. Three types of burns shown on arm and in cross-section of skin. Superficial burn (left). Partial-thickness burn (center). Full-thickness burn (right).

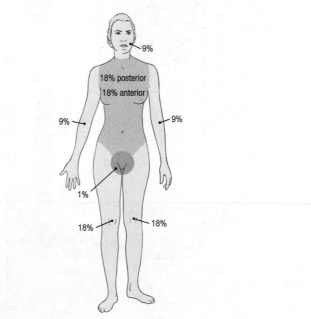

Figure 20. Adult female illustrating the rule of nines used when assessing burn damage to various body parts

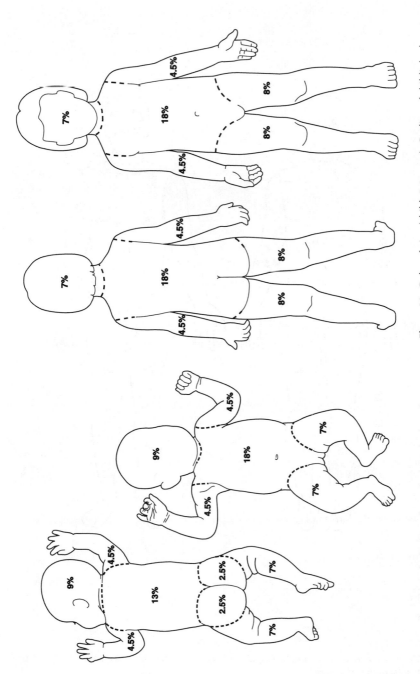

Figure 21. Rules of nine (infant). Outline of infant's body with areas and percentages indicated to calculate total burn surface area.

Figure 22. Rules of nine (child, 5-9 years). Outline of child's body with areas and percentages indicated to calculate total burn surface area.

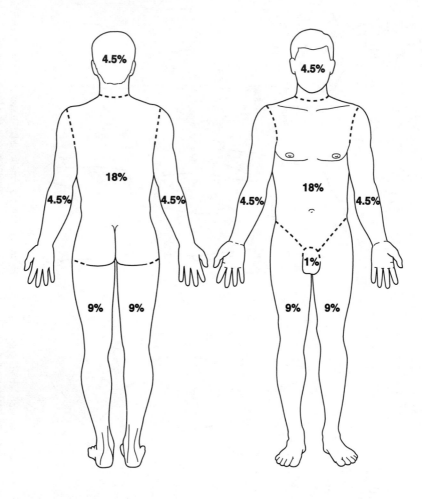

Figure 23. Rules of nine (adult). Outline of adult's body with areas and percentages indicated to calculate total burn surface area.

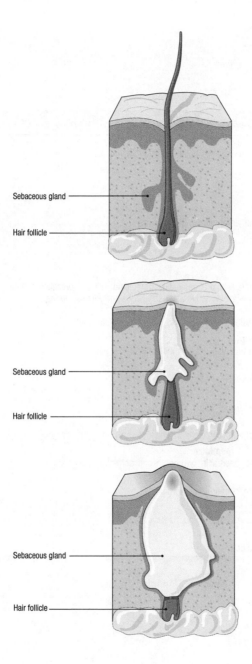

Sebaceous gland

Hair follicle

Sebaceous gland

Hair follicle

Sebaceous gland

Hair follicle

Figure 24. Cross-section of sebaceous gland of the skin showing three stages in the development of acne.

Antibiotic groups
Aminoglycosides (e.g., streptomycin, gentamicin, sisomicin, tobramycin, amicacin)
Ansamycins (e.g., rifamycin)
Antimycotics *Polyenes* (e.g., nystatin, pimaricin, amphotericin B, pecilocin) *Benzofuran derivatives* (Griseofulvin)
β–lactam antibiotics *Penicillins* (Penicillin G and its derivatives, oral penicillins, penicillinase-fixed penicillins, broad--spectrum penicillins, penicillins active against *Proteus* and *Pseudomonas*) *Cephalosporins* (e.g., cephalothin, cephaloridine, cephalexin, cefazolin, cefotaxime)
Chloramphenicol group (Chloramphenicol, thiamphenicol, azidamphenicol)
Imidazole Fluconazole, itraconazole
Linosamides (Lincomycin, clindamycin)
Macrolides (e.g., azithromycin, erythromycin, oleandomycin, spiramycin, clarithromycin)
Peptides, peptolides, polypeptides (e.g., polymyxin B and E, bacitracin, tyrothricin, capreomycin, vancomycin)
Quinolones (Nalidixic acid, ofloxacin, ciprofloxacin, norfloxin)
Tetracyclines (e.g., tetracycline, oxytetracycline, minocycline, doxycycline)
Other antibiotics (Phosphomycin, fusidic acid)

Figure 25. Antibiotic groups.

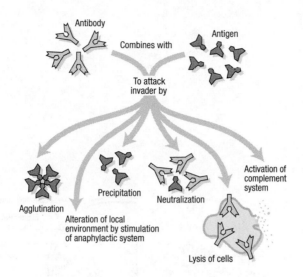

Figure 26. Humoral immunity.

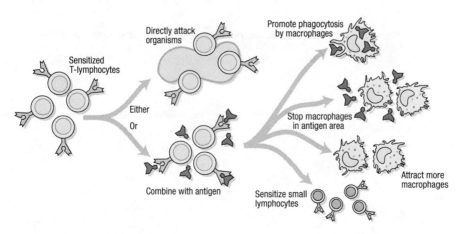

Figure 27. Cell-mediated immunity.

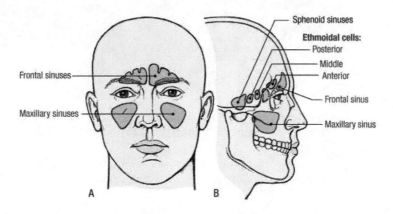

Figure 28. Paranasal sinuses: anterior (A) and lateral (B) views of the head.

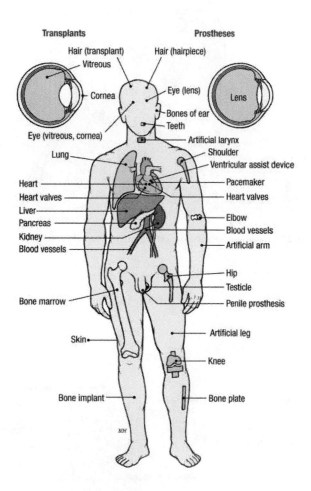

Figure 29. Transplants and prostheses.

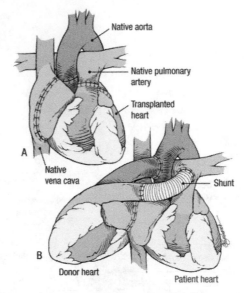

Figure 30. Heart transplantation: orthotopic method (A), heterotopic method (B).

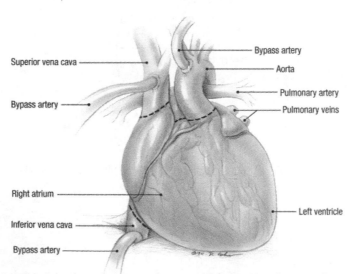

Figure 31. Anterior view of recipient heart prior to removal. Resection lines are shown dashed.

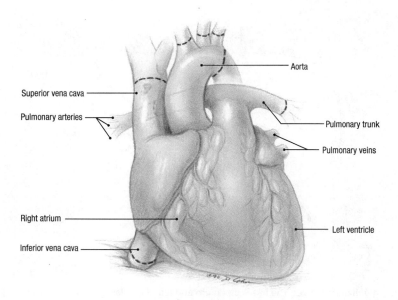

Figure 32. Anterior view of donor heart prior to transplantation showing dissection lines.

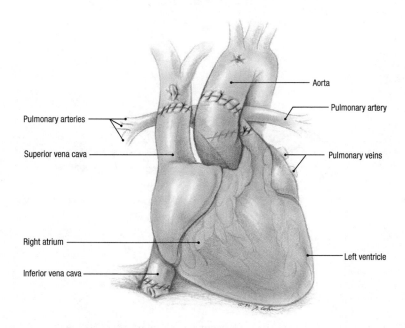

Figure 33. Anterior view of transplanted heart showing sutured areas.

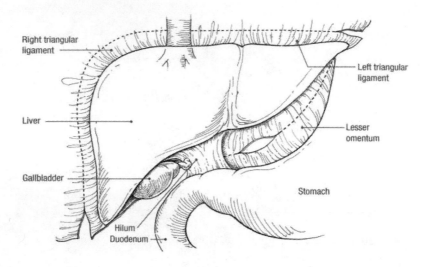

Figure 34. Mobilizing the liver. The lesser omentum and left triangular ligament are divided. The right triangular ligament and peritoneal reflections on the bare area are divided. The mobilization of the right lobe of the liver may be reserved until venovenous bypass has been initiated, and the liver has been devascularized.

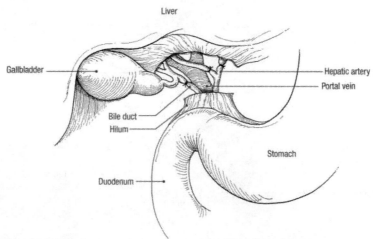

Figure 35. Dissection of the hilum. The peritoneum and adventitial structures are divided. Nerve, lymphatics, and particularly large venous collaterals are dissected. The hepatic artery is ligated and divided, and the bile duct is divided.

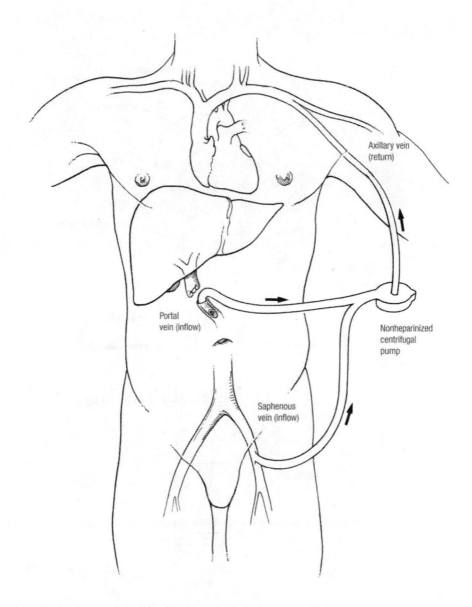

Figure 36. Venous bypass. The portal vein is divided and cannulated, and a second cannula is placed into the inferior vena cava. The blood is pumped in a nonheparinized system and returned to the patient via cannula in the axillary vein.

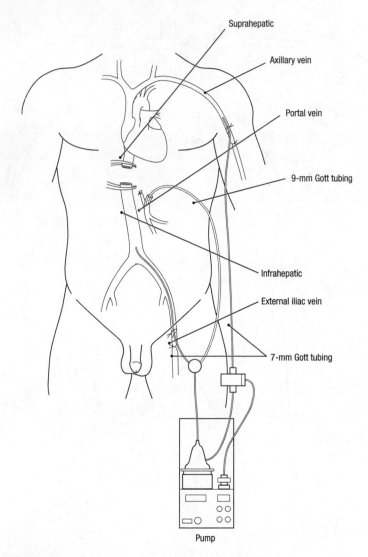

Suprahepatic

Axillary vein

Portal vein

9-mm Gott tubing

Infrahepatic

External iliac vein

7-mm Gott tubing

Pump

Figure 37. During the "anaphetic" phase of the transplant the blood from the portal vein and iliac vein are pumped back to the heart through the pump. This is the venoveneous bypass used during liver transplant surgery.

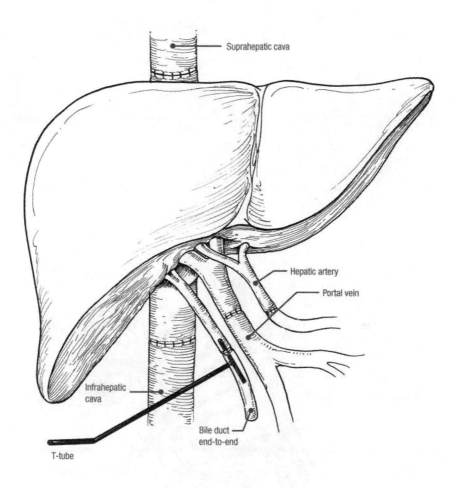

Suprahepatic cava

Hepatic artery

Portal vein

Infrahepatic
cava

Bile duct
end-to-end

T-tube

Figure 38. Completed transplant of the liver. Vascular anastomoses include the suprahepatic vena cava, the infrahepatic vena cava, the portal vein, and the hepatic artery. A choledochocholedochostomy biliary reconstruction is depicted.

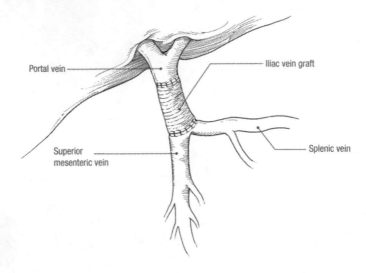

Figure 39. Iliac vein graft to the portal vein confluence.

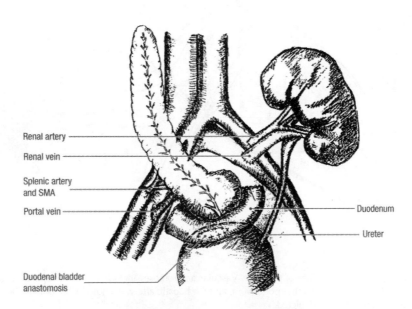

Figure 40. Simultaneous pancreas-kidney transplant with bladder drainage.

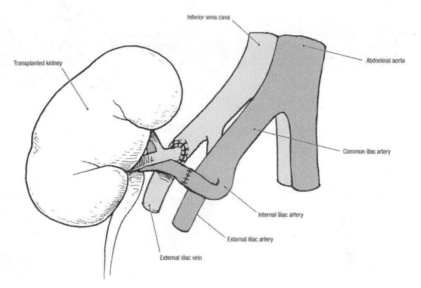

Inferior vena cava

Abdominal aorta

Transplanted kidney

Common iliac artery

Internal iliac artery

External iliac artery

External iliac vein

Figure 41. The transplanted kidney.

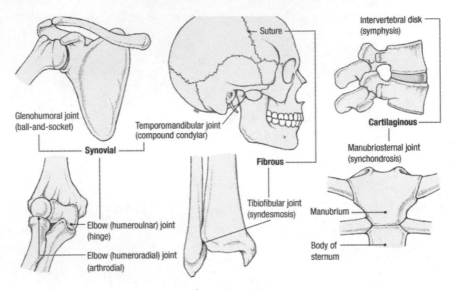

Figure 42. Joints.

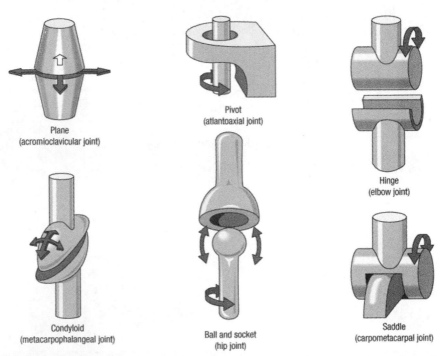

Figure 43. Illustration of different types of movements of joints as demonstrated by mechanical models.

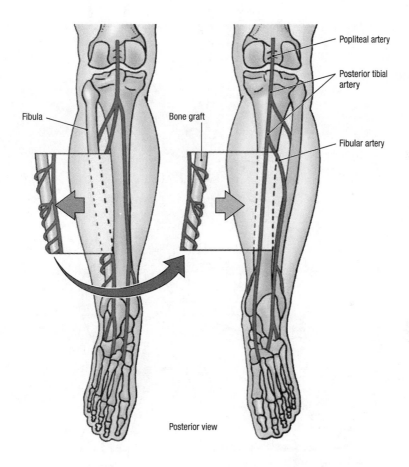

Figure 44. Bone grafts. The fibula is a common source of bone for grafting.

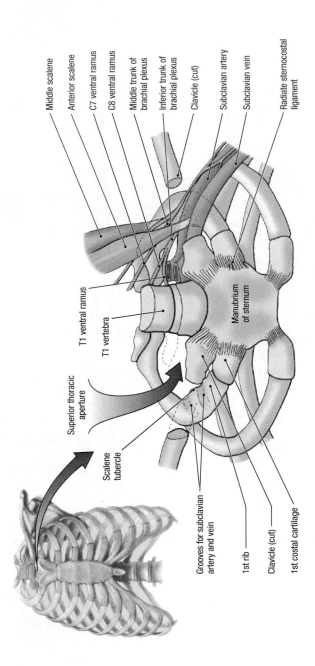

Middle scalene

Anterior scalene

C7 ventral ramus

C8 ventral ramus

Middle trunk of brachial plexus

Inferior trunk of brachial plexus

Clavicle (cut)

Subclavian artery

Subclavian vein

Radiate sternocostal ligament

T1 ventral ramus

T1 vertebra

Superior thoracic aperture

Scalene tubercle

Manubrium of sternum

Grooves for subclavian artery and vein

1st rib

Clavicle (cut)

1st costal cartilage

Figure 45. Thoracotomy and bone grafting.

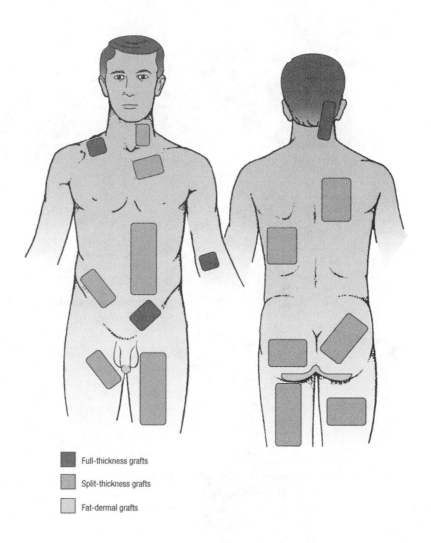

Full-thickness grafts

Split-thickness grafts

Fat-dermal grafts

Figure 46. Common donor skin graft sites. Dark gray skin areas are appropriate for full-thickness grafts; medium gray areas are used for split-thickness grafts and light gray sites are used for fat-dermal grafts.

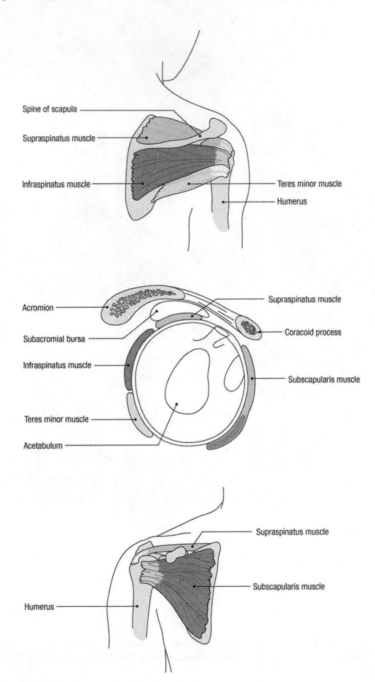

Figure 47. Three images showing the anatomy of the rotator cuff area. Posterior view (top), lateral view (middle) and anterior view (bottom).

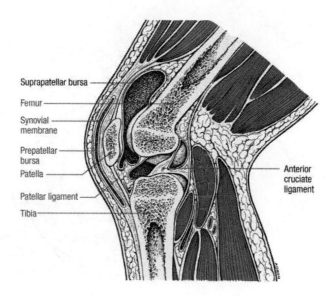

Suprapatellar bursa

Femur

Synovial membrane

Prepatellar bursa

Patella

Patellar ligament

Tibia

Anterior cruciate ligament

Figure 48. Knee joint. Sagittal section showing prepatellar and suprapatellar bursae.

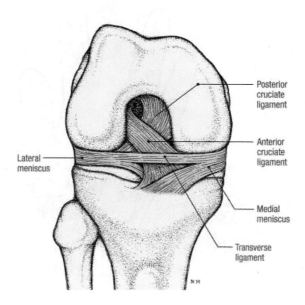

Posterior cruciate ligament

Anterior cruciate ligament

Lateral meniscus

Medial meniscus

Transverse ligament

Figure 49. Cruciate ligaments of the knee.

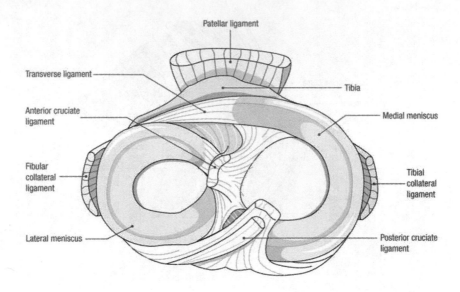

Figure 50. Knee joint viewed from above showing the crescent-shaped menisci that serve as cushions between the bones of the joint.

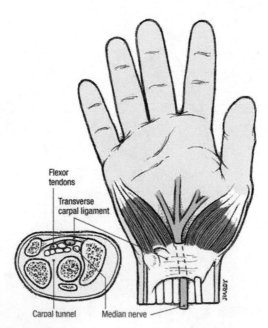

Figure 51. The carpal tunnel contains the median nerve and the flexor tendons of the fingers and thumb.

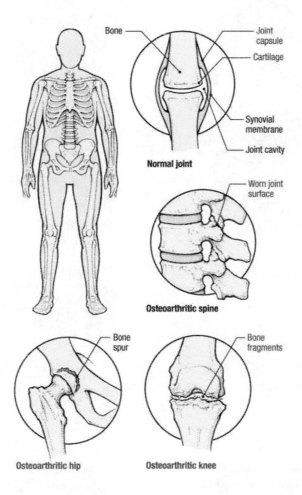

Figure 52. Osteoarthritis. Problems associated with osteoarthritis and some sites where they commonly occur.

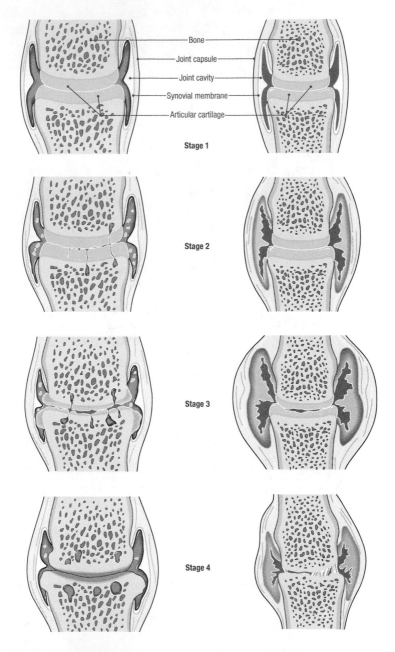

Bone

Joint capsule

Joint cavity

Synovial membrane

Articular cartilage

Stage 1

Stage 2

Stage 3

Stage 4

Figure 53. Cross-sections of synovial joints showing the progression of osteoarthritis (left) and rheumatoid arthritis (right) in four stages.

Normal Lab Values

Tests	Conventional Units	SI Units
Alanine aminotransferase (ALT, SGPT), serum		
Male	13-40 U/L (37°C)	0.22-0.68 μkat/L (37°C)
Female	10-28 U/L (37°C)	0.17-0.48 μkat/L (37°C)
Aldolase, serum	1.0-7.5 U/L (30°C)	0.02-0.13 μkat/L (30°C)
Ammonia		
Plasma (Hep)	9-33 μmol/L	9-33 μmol/L
Aspartate aminotransferase (AST, SGOT), serum	10-59 U/L (37°C)	0.17-1.00 -2 to +3 kat/L (37oC)
Bilirubin		
Serum		
Adult		
Conjugated	0.0-0.3 mg/dL	0-5 μmol/L
Unconjugated	0.1-1.1 mg/dL	1.7-19 μmol/L
Delta	0-0.2 mg/dL	0-3 μmol/L
Total	0.2-1.3 mg/L	3-22 μmol/L
Neonate		
Conjugated	0-0.6 mg/dL	0-10 μmol/L
Unconjugated	0.6-10.5 mg/dL	10-180 μmol/L
Total	1.5-12 mg/dL	1.7-180 μmol/L
Urine, qualitative	Negative	Negative
Ceruloplasmin, serum	20-60 mg/dL	0.2-6.0 g/L
Coagulation tests		
Antithrombin III (synthetic substrate)	80-120% of normal	0.8-1.2 of normal
Bleeding time (Duke)	0-6 min	0-6 min
Bleeding time (Ivy)	1-6 min	1-6 min
Bleeding time (template)	2.3-9.5 min	2.3-9.5 min
Clot retraction, qualitative	50-100% in 2 h	0.5-1.0/2 h
Coagulation time (Lee-White)	5-15 min (glass tubes) 19-60 min (siliconized tubes)	5-15 min (glass tubes) 19-60 min (siliconized tubes)
Cold hemolysin test (Donath-Landsteiner)	No hemolysis	No hemolysis
Complement components		
Total hemolytic complement activity, plasma (EDTA)	75-160 U/mL	75-160 kU/L
Total complement decay rate (functional), plasma (EDTA)	10-20% Deficiency >50%	Fraction decay rate: 0.10-0.20 >0.50
C1q, serum	14.9-22.1 mg/dL	149-221 mg/L
C1r, serum	2.5-10.0 mg/dL	25-100 mg/L
C1s(C1 esterase), serum	5.0-10.0 mg/dL	50-100 mg/L
C2, serum	1.6-3.6 mg/dL	16-36 mg/L

C3, serum	90-180 mg/dL	0.9-1.8 g/L
C4, serum	10-40 mg/dL	0.1-0.4 g/L
C5, serum	5.5-11.3 mg/dL	55-113 mg/L
C6, serum	17.9-23.9 mg/dL	179-239 mg/L
C7, serum	2.7-7.4 mg/dL	27-74 mg/L
C8, serum	4.9-10.6 mg/dL	49-106 mg/L
C9, serum	3.3-9.5 mg/dL	33-95 mg/L
Coombs test		
Direct	Negative	Negative
Indirect	Negative	Negative
Copper		
Serum		
Male	70-140 µg/dL	11-22 µmol/L
Female	80-155 µg/dL	13-24 µmol/L
Urine	3-35 µg/24 h	0.05-0.55 µmol/24 h
Corpuscular values of erythrocytes (values are for adults; in children values vary with age)		
Mean corpuscular hemoglobin (MCH)	27-31 pg	0.42-0.48 fmol
Mean corpuscular hemoglobin concentration (MCHC)	33-37 g/dL	330-370 g/L
Mean corpuscular volume (MCV)	Male 80-94 µ^3	80-94 fL
	Female 81-99 µ^3	81-99 fL
Cortisol, serum		
Plasma (Hep, EDTA, Ox)		
8 a.m.	5-23 4g/dL	138-635 nmol/L
4 p.m.	3-16 4g/dL	83-441 nmol/L
10 p.m.	<50% of 8 a.m. value	<0.5 of 8 a.m. value
Free, urine	<50 4g/24 h	<138 mmol/24 h
†*Creatine kinase (CK), serum		
Male	15-105 U/L (30°C)	0.26-1.79 µkat/L (30°C)
Female	10-80 U/L (30°C)	0.17-1.36 µkat/L (30°C)

Note: Strenuous exercise or intramuscular injections may cause transient elevation of CK.

*Creatine kinase MB isoenzyme, serum	0-7 ng/mL	0-7 µg/L
*Creatinine		
Serum or plasma, adult		
Male	0.7-1.3 mg/dL	62-115 µmol/L
Female	0.6-1.1 mg/dL	53-97 µmol/L
Urine		
Male	14-26 mg/kg body weight/24 h	124-230 µmol/kg body weight/24 h
Female	11-20 mg/kg body weight/24 h	97-177 µmol/kg body weight/24 h
*Creatinine clearance, serum or plasma and urine		
Male	94-140 mL/min/1.73 m2	0.91-1.35 mL/s/m2
Female	72-110 mL/min/1.73 m2	0.69-1.06 mL/s/m2

Cryoglobulins, serum	0	0
C-reactive protein, serum	<0.5 mg/dL	<5 mg/L
‡*Cyclosporine, whole blood		
Therapeutic, trough	100-200 ng/mL	83-166 nmol/L
Fibrin degradation products	<10 µg/mL	<10 mg/L
Gamma-glutamyltransferase (GGT), serum		
Male	2-30 U/L (37°C)	0.03-0.51 µkat/L (37°C)
Female	1-24 U/L (37oC)	0.02-0.41 µkat/L (37°C)
Haptoglobin, serum	30-200 mg/dL	0.3-2.0 g/L
Homogentisic acid, urine, qualitative	Negative	Negative
Immunoglobulins, serum		
IgG	700-1600 mg/dl	7-16 g/L
IgA	70-400 mg/dl	0.7-4.0 g/L
IgM	40-230 mg/dl	0.4-2.3 g/L
IgD	0-8 mg/dl	0-80 mg/L
IgE	3-423 mg/dl	3-423 kIU/L
Immunoglobulin G (IgG), CSF	0.5-6.1 mg/dL	0.5-6.1 g/L
Insulin, plasma (fasting)	2-25 µU/mL	13-174 pmol/L
*Iron, serum		
Male	65-175 µg/dL	11.6-31.3 µmol/L
Female	50-170 µg/dL	9.0-30.4 µmol/L
Iron binding capacity, serum total (TIBC)	250-425 µg/dL	44.8-71.6 µmol/L
Iron saturation, serum		
Male	20-50%	0.2-0.5
Female	15-50%	0.15-0.5
L-lactate		
Plasma (NaF)		
Venous	4.5-19.8 mg/dL	0.5-2.2 mmol/L
Arterial	4.5-14.4 mg/dL	0.5-1.6 mmol/L
Whole blood (Hep), at bedrest		
Venous	8.1-15.3 mg/dL	0.9-1.7 mmol/L
Arterial	<11.3 mg/dL	<1.3 mmol/L
Urine, 24 h	496-1982 mg/d	5.5-22 mmol/d
CSF	10-22 mg/dL	1.1-2.4 mmol/L
*Lactate dehydrogenase (LDH)		
Total (L*P), 37°C, serum		
Newborn	290-775 U/L	4.9-13.2 µkat/L
Neonate	545-2000 U/L	9.3-34 µkat/L
Infant	180-430 U/L	3.1-7.3 µkat/L
Child	110-295 U/L	1.9-5 µkat/L
Adult	100-190 U/L	1.7-3.2 µkat/L
>60 y	110-210 U/L	1.9-3.6 µkat/L

Appendix 2

*Isoenzymes, serum by agarose gel electrophoresis		
Fraction 1	14-26% of total	0.14-0.26 fraction of total
Fraction 2	29-39% of total	0.29-0.39 fraction of total
Fraction 3	20-26% of total	0.20-0.26 fraction of total
Fraction 4	8-16% of total	0.08-0.16 fraction of total
Fraction 5	6-16% of total	0.06-0.16 fraction of total
*Lactate dehydrogenase, CSF	10% of serum value	0.10 fraction of serum value
Magnesium		
Serum	1.3-2.1 mEq/L	0.65-1.07 mmol/L
	1.6-2.6 mg/dL	16-26 mg/L
Urine	6-10 mEq/24 h	3-5 mmol/24 h
Methotrexate, serum or plasma (Hep or EDTA)		
Therapeutic	Variable	Variable
Toxic		
1-2 wk after low-dose therapy post-IV infusion	≥0.02 μmol/L	≥0.02 μmol/L
24 h	≥5 μmol/L	≥5 μmol/L
48 h	≥0.5 μmol/L	≥0.5 μmol/L
72 h	≥0.05 μmol/L	≥0.05 μmol/L
Partial thromboplastin time activated (APTT)	<35 sec	<35 sec
Phenolsulfonphthalein excretion (PSP), urine	28-51% in 15 min	0.28-0.51 in 15 min
	13-24% in 30 min	0.13-0.24 in 30 min
	9-17% in 60 min	0.09-0.17 in 60 min
	3-10% in 2 h	0.03-0.10 in 2 h
	(After injection of 1 mL PSP intravenously)	(After injection of 1 mL PSP intravenously)
*Phosphatase, alkaline, total, serum	38-126 U/L (37˚C)	0.65-2.14 μkat/L
*Protein, serum		
Total	6.4-8.3 g/dL	64-83 g/L
Albumin	3.9-5.1 g/dL	39-51 g/L
Globulin		
alpha$_1$	0.2-0.4 g/dL	2-4 g/L
alpha$_2$	0.4-0.8 g/dL	4-8 g/L
beta	0.5-1.0 g/dL	5-10 g/L
gamma	0.6-1.3 g/dL	6-13 g/L
Urine		
Qualitative	Negative	Negative
Quantitative	50-80 mg/24 h (at rest)	50-80 mg/24 h (at rest)
CSF, total	8-32 mg/dL	80-320 mg/dL
*Prothrombin time (PT)	12-14 sec	12-14 sec
Sedimentation rate		
Wintrobe		
Male	0-10 mm in 1 h	0-10 mm/h

Female	0-20 mm in 1 h	0-20 mm/h
Westergren		
Male (<50 yr)	0-15 mm in 1 h	0-15 mm/h
Female (<50 yr)	0-20 mm in 1 h	0-20 mm/h
Theophylline, serum or plasma (Hep or EDTA)		
Therapeutic		
Bronchodilator	8-20 µg/mL	44-111 µmol/L
Prem. apnea	6-13 µg/mL	33-72 µmol/L
Toxic	>20 µg/mL	>110 µmol/L
Transferrin, serum		
Newborn	130-275 mg/dL	1.30-2.75 g/L
Adult	212-360 mg/dL	2.12-3.60 g/L
>60 yr	190-375 mg/dL	1.9-3.75 g/L
Urea nitrogen, serum	6-20 mg/dL	2.1-7.1 mmol urea/L
Urea nitrogen/creatinine ratio, serum	12:1 to 20:1	48-80 urea/creatinine mole ratio
*Uric acid		
Serum, enzymatic		
Male	4.5-8.0 mg/dL	0.27-0.47 mmol/L
Female	2.5-6.2 mg/dL	0.15-0.37 mmol/L
Child	2.0-5.5 mg/dL	0.12-0.32 mmol/L
Urine	250-750 mg/24 h (with normal diet)	1.48-4.43 mmol/24 h (with normal diet)

* Test values are method dependent.

† Test values are race dependent.

‡ Actual therapeutic range should be adjusted for individual patient.

§ "Fatty acids" include a mixture of different aliphatic acids of varying molecular weight; a mean molecular weight of 284 daltons has been assumed.

Common Allergens

Environmental
aerosol spray
automobile exhaust
barn dust
cigarette smoke
cottonseed
elevator grain dust mite
rain dust
gum arabic
house dust
house dust mite
jute
karaya gum
mite
mold
newsprint
nylon
orris root
parakeet feather
parrot feather
pigeon feather
perfume
pyrethrum
roundworm
silk
soybean grain dust mite
tobacco
wool

Epidermals and Animal Proteins

budgerigar droppings
budgerigar feathers
canary feathers
cat dander
cat epithelium
cattle epithelium
chicken droppings

chicken feathers
chinchilla epithelium
cockatiel feathers
cow dander
deer epithelium
dog dander
dog epithelium
duck feathers
ferret epithelium
finch feathers
fox epithelium
gerbil epithelium
goat epithelium
goose feathers
guinea pig epithelium
hamster epithelium
horse dander
mink epithelium
mouse epithelium
parrot feathers
pigeon droppings
pigeon feathers
rabbit epithelium
rat epithelium
reindeer epithelium
sheep epithelium
swine epithelium
turkey feathers

Foods of Animal and Plant Origin
abalone
almond
allspice
anchovy
anise
apple
apricot
arrowroot

artichoke
asparagus
avocado
banana
barley
basil
bay leaf
bass
beef
beet
blackberry
black mulberry
black pepper
blue mussel
blue vetch
Brazil nut
broccoli
Brussel sprouts
buckwheat
cabbage
cantaloupe
caraway
cardamon
carob
carrot
casein
cashew
cauliflower
celery
cheese
cherry
chicken
chickpea
chili pepper
chive
chub
chocolate
cinnamon
clam
clove
cocoa
coconut

codfish
coffee
common millet
coriander
corn
cornmeal
cottonseed
cow milk
cow whey
crab
cranberry
cucumber
currant
curry
date
dill
duck
eel
eggplant
egg white
egg yolk
elk
fennel
fenugreek
fig
foxtail millet
garlic
gelatin
ginger
gluten
goat milk
gooseberry
grape
grapefruit
green bean
green pepper
guava
hake
halibut
hazelnut
herring
honey

hop
Japanese millet
jujube
kale
Karaya gum
kidney bean
kiwi
lamb
leek
lemon
lentil
lettuce
lentil
licorice
lima bean
lime
linseed
lupine seed
lobster
macadamia
mackerel
maize
malt
mandarin
mango
marjoram
melon
mint
monosodium glutamate (MSG)
mushroom
mussel
mustard
mutton
navy bean
nutmeg
oat
octopus
olive
onion
orange
oregano
oyster

papaya
paprika
parsley
parsnip
passion fruit
pea
peach
peanut
pear
pecan
perch
persimmon
pineapple
pine nut
pistachio
plum
poppy
pork
potato
prune
pumpkin
rabbit
radish
raisin
raspberry
red currant
rhubarb
rice
rose hip
rye
saffron
sage
salmon
sardine
scallop
sesame
sheep milk
sheep whey
shrimp
snail
sole
soybean meal

spinach
squash
squid
strawberry
string bean
sweet chestnut
sweet potato
Swiss chard
Swiss cheese
swordfish
tarragon
tea
thyme
tomato
trout
tuna
turkey
turnip
vanilla
walnut
watermelon
wheat
whole wheat
yeast

Grass Pollens
alfalfa
annual bluegrass
Bahia
barley
Bermuda
brome
Canada bluegrass
canary
common reed
corn
crab grass
cultivated barley
cultivated corn
cultivated oat
cultivated rye
cultivated wheat

false oat-grass
Johnson
June
Kentucky blue
maize
meadow fescue
meadow foxtail
oat
orchard
perennial rye
redtop
reed canary
rye
salt
sorghum
sweet vernal
timothy
velvet
wild rye
zoysia

Insects
American cockroach
bee venom
Berlin beetle
black ant
black fly
blood worm
bumblebee
cockroach
cricket
deer fly
fire ant
flea
German cockroach
grain weevil
honeybee
horsefly
housefly
Hymenopterous vespid
louse
mayfly

mosquito
moth
nimitti midge
Oriental cockroach
paper wasp
red ant
sweat bee
wasp
white-faced hornet
yellow hornet
yellow jacket

Sporotrichum
Staphylococcus
Stemphylium
Torulopsis
Trichoderma
Trichophyton
Ulocladium
Ustilago
Verticillium
Zygomycetes

Molds and Fungi

Acremonium
Alternaria
Aspergillus
Aureobasidium
Botryomyces
Candida
Chaetomium
Cladosporium
Curvularia
Dematiaceae
Drechslera
Epicoccum
Epidermophyton
Fusarium
Gliocladium
Helminthosporium
Micropolyspora
Microsporum
Monilia
Mucor
Neurospora
Nigrospora
Paecilomyces
Penicillium
Phoma
Pityrosporum
Rhizopus
Rhodotorula
Saccharomyces

Occupational

amprolium hydrochloride
anthraquinone
benzene
carbamate
chicken feather
chromate
diisocyanate
epoxy resin
ethylenediamine
formaldehyde
gelatin
green coffee bean
hexahydrophthalic anhydride
himic anhydride
ispaghula (laxative)
latex
2-mercaptobenzothiazole
MSP (mouse serum protein)
MUP (mouse urine protein)
nickel salt
persulfate salt
phthalic anhydride
piperazine hydrochloride
platinum salt
polyvinyl difluoride
PSP (pigeon serum protein)
RSP (rat serum protein)
RUP (rat urine protein)
tetrachlorophthalic anhydride

thiuram
toluene
trichloroethylene
triethylene tetramine
tryptophan
vinyl chloride
xylene

Preservatives
formaldehyde
quaternium-15
Kathon-CG

Tree and Shrub Pollens
acacia
alder
American beech
American elm
Arizona ash
Arizona cypress
Arizona/Fremont cottonwood
aspen
Australian pine
bald cypress
bayberry
beech
Betula verrucosa
birch
black locust
black walnut
box elder
Brazilian rubber
California peppertree
cedar
chestnut
Chinese elm
common silver birch
cottonwood
cypress
date
Douglas fir
elder
elm

eucalyptus
funeral cypress
Gambel oak
grey alder
green ash
groundsel
hackberry
hazel
hickory
horn beam
horse chestnut
Italian cypress
Japanese cedar
Japanese cypress
jasmine
juniper mix
lilac
linden
live oak
loblolly pine
lodgepole pine
Lombardy poplar
Mediterranean cypress
maple
marsh elder
mesquite
Monterey cypress
mountain cedar
mountain juniper
mulberry
oak
oil palm
olive
orange blossom
Oregon ash
palm
paper mulberry
pecan
peppertree
pine
ponderosa pine
poplar
privet

queen palm
red alder
red birch
red cedar
red maple
red mulberry
redwood
river birch
rough marsh elder
Russian olive
Russian thistle
saltbush
salt cedar
saltwort
shagbark hickory
slash pine
slippery elm
spruce
sugar maple
sweetgum
sycamore
walnut
wax myrtle
weeping fig
weeping willow
Western juniper
Western red cedar
white ash
white mulberry
white oak
white pine
white poplar
willow
Virginia live oak

Venoms

bumble bee
common wasp
European hornet
paper wasp
white-faced hornet
yellow hornet

Weeds

bitter dock
burrobrush
burweed
camomile
careless
canyon ragweed
castor bean
Chenopodium
coast sage
cocklebur
dandelion
desert ragweed
dog fennel
elder
English plantain
false ragweed
firebush
fireweed
giant ragweed
goldenrod
greasewood
green amaranth
iodine bush
Japanese hop
kochia
lamb's quarter
lupin
mugwort
mustard
nettle
oxeye daisy
pigweed
plantain
poverty weed
rabbit bush
ragweed
ragwort
redroot pigweed
rough marsh elder
Russian thistle
sagebrush

saltwort
sheep sorrel
short ragweed
slender ragweed
smotherweed
spiney pigweed
sugar beet
sunflower
tall dock
tumbleweed
western ragweed
western water hemp
white burrobrush
wild tobacco
wormwood
yellow dock
yellow mustard

Appendix 4
Sample Reports

Acupuncture for Acne Rosacea

Chief Complaint
1. Acne rosacea.
2. Tendinitis, left wrist.

History of Present Illness: The patient is a 44-year-old Caucasian female who seeks traditional chinese medicine treatment for a 2-year history of acne rosacea. The acne occurs primarily on her cheeks, although she has had rare flare-ups on her nose. She has been treated in the past with tetracycline, but this works only as long as she continues taking it.

She complains of chronic left wrist tendinitis for which she takes over-the-counter ibuprofen.

Past History: The patient had a hysterectomy last year for uterine fibroid tumors. She occasionally has trouble sleeping through the night.

Social History: The patient is married and has teenage boys. She denies a history of smoking or alcohol intake. She works part-time as a legal secretary.

Diagnosis: Liver qi stagnation, which may be turning into yang rising.

Treatment: We will concentrate on the acne rosacea first, with treatment for tendinitis to follow. Needling will be done today in the following points: bi tong LI4, LI11, LV3, ST36, ST44, GB20.

Allergic Contact Dermatitis

This 27-year-old Chinese patient comes to us to report a history of back pain for which she self-medicated, using an external topical plaster that contained Chinese herbal medicine. She used 3 plasters in sequence on 3 locations, and she left each of them on her back for 24 hours. The 1st was placed on the lower lumbar spine, the 2nd on the mid lumbar spine, and the 3rd was placed on the thoracic area. Pruritic erythematous papular eruption appeared after the 2nd application.

After removing the 3rd plaster, she used supplements primarily of Western herbal medicine, which she had used for some time. She states that these were Isotonix OPC-

3 and Tension Tamer Celestial Seasonings tea. Urticaria and angioedema of the lips occurred within 10 minutes. She was treated by her family physician with prednisone for 9 days and an unknown ointment.

It was explained that the allergic reaction from the plaster was most likely caused by the myrrh that is used in the type of plaster that she used. Western herbal medicines have been reported to cause allergic reactions, including anaphylaxis, after the use of chamomile.

She was advised that patch testing would be helpful in identifying what caused her allergic reaction. She will contact her family physician to discuss allergy testing.

DIAGNOSIS: Allergic dermatitis.

CADAVERIC RENAL TRANSPLANT RECIPIENT WITH NAUSEA CONSULTATION

REASON FOR CONSULTATION: This 49-year-old female is seen at the request of her attending physician because of a renal transplant

HISTORY OF PRESENT ILLNESS: This patient, who received a 2nd cadaveric renal transplant in January of this year, had been doing very well until recently, when she underwent parathyroid surgery for secondary hyperparathyroidism. The patient was discharged the day after surgery, following which she had experienced some nausea. She also started to notice increase in her diarrhea, and she presented to the hospital with these symptoms and was admitted to the hospital for further management.

PAST MEDICAL HISTORY: The patient is known to have primary glomerular disease leading to end-stage renal failure requiring dialysis, followed by a cadaveric renal transplant several years ago. Unfortunately, after 9 years the patient completely rejected the 1st renal transplant and was back on hemodialysis. Fortunately, she received a 2nd cadaveric renal transplant in January of this year and since then has been doing well with the serum creatinine, now 0.8 mg%.

MEDICATIONS: The patient's current rejection medicines include Rapamune 4 mg every day, CellCept 500 mg b.i.d., and prednisone 7.5 mg every day.

PHYSICAL EXAMINATION: On my examination, this patient appears to be in no acute distress. Her blood pressure is 120/70 mmHg. She is afebrile at this time. Examination of her head, eyes, ears, nose and throat is unremarkable. Neck veins are not distended. Chest is symmetrical. Heart sounds are regular. There is a loud murmur heard all over the precordium. Lungs are clear. Abdominal examination reveals previous surgical scars, and there is a large incisional hernia in the left lower quadrant, which is reducible. There is no edema of the lower extremities. There is an arteriovenous fistula in the left arm with marked tortuosity of the veins. Bones and joints appear normal. Neurological examination grossly within normal limits.

LABORATORY DATA: Hemoglobin 12.3 with normal white blood count and differential. BUN is 11, creatinine 0.8. Electrolytes are normal. Calcium level is 9 mg% with a serum albumin of 3.9.

CLINICAL IMPRESSION: This is a young female who is status post 2nd cadaveric renal transplant, doing very well from a renal standpoint. She is recently status post parathyroid surgery for secondary hyperparathyroidism. We need to be cautious of postoperative hypocalcemia.

PLAN: At this time, we need to continue all her medications. If her diarrhea persists, we may have to consider temporarily decreasing the CellCept, but I would not do this without the consent of her transplant team. At the present time, we will simply treat her symptomatically with Imodium.

COMBINED LIVER AND SMALL BOWEL TRANSPLANTATION

PREOPERATIVE DIAGNOSIS: End-stage liver failure and end-stage intestinal failure.

POSTOPERATIVE DIAGNOSIS: End-stage liver failure and end-stage intestinal failure.

PROCEDURE PERFORMED: Combined liver and small bowel transplantation.

INDICATIONS FOR PROCEDURE: Impending death from end-stage liver and intestinal.

COMPLICATIONS: Intraoperative death.

DRAINS: None.

BRIEF HISTORY: The patient is a baby who was born and suffered an extreme mesenteric infarction, leaving him with extreme short bowel syndrome and total parenteral nutrition dependent. He developed severe refractory cholestasis and end-stage liver disease associated with parenteral nutrition use and was progressively deteriorating. He had significant malnutrition and was transferred for evaluation for possible combined liver and small bowel transplantation. He underwent this evaluation, was found to be an acceptable candidate for combined liver/small bowel transplant but, unfortunately, deteriorated to an extreme stage of debility and malnutrition prior to organs becoming available. During this period of time, he developed some degree of renal insufficiency and possible hepatorenal syndrome as well as severe hepatomegaly, portal hypertension, thrombocytopenia, anemia, and encephalopathy.

At the time that organs became available, he was a high-risk surgical candidate with rise in creatinine, bilirubin > 50, extremely low platelet count. However, he faced clear and impending death without transplantation. Therefore, it was elected, after discussion with the family, that although there is extremely high risk, with 100% mortality without transplant, that we would undertake attempted transplantation to possibly save his life.

DESCRIPTION OF PROCEDURE: The patient was brought to the operating room, prepped and draped in the usual sterile fashion after the induction of general endotracheal anesthesia and placement of adequate volume and monitoring lines. Thereafter, a bilateral subcostal incision with upper midline extension was made through the skin and subcutaneous tissues and the anterior rectus sheath. We divided the rectus and were able to enter the abdominal cavity.

It was immediately evident, on seeing the abdomen after opening, that there were dense adhesions and that portal hypertension was quite severe. On entering the abdominal cavity, we drained a large volume of ascites and the liver was extremely large, with severe hepatomegaly and cholestasis.

We began the dissection by using the electrocautery to identify the edge of the liver and with gentle dissection were able to remove and isolate some portion of overlying colon and duodenum from the underside of the edge of the liver. As this was being performed, some degree of coagulopathy was evident, and electrocautery was used for control. Communication with Anesthesia was made in recognition that significant transfusion would likely be required throughout the case in order accomplish successful transplantation. We continued with some adhesiolysis along the edge of the liver and placed the self-retaining retractor in order to start performing the hilar dissection.

Unexpectedly at this point, Anesthesia immediately alerted us that the patient was having atypical cardiac rhythm and suffered cardiac arrest. This was completely unexpected, and we immediately began CPR. CPR was performed for approximately 15 minutes, during which multiple anesthesiologists came to the room to assist with resuscitation, which ultimately led to reversal of cardiac arrest. However, the patient was extremely hypotensive on high-dose pressors and with an unstable rhythm. He began to develop a severe acidosis and it was clearly evident that the coagulopathy had worsened after this significant requirement for CPR.

Since he had regained a pulse, we attempted to continue with the operation, knowing that death was certain without accomplishing organ replacement. We began the dissection of the porta hepatis and were able to identify and ligate the left and right hepatic arteries, dividing these, and then identifying the common bile duct. This was then identified. This was then circumferentially surrounded, and the bile duct cleared and the anterior portal vein identified. Again, the patient seemed to suffer another cardiac arrest, and again CPR was required. Once again, we performed extensive CPR until the patient again recovered from cardiac arrest, and then at some point we were told that we could resume attempted transplantation.

Naturally, the patient's prognosis appeared grim at this juncture; however, because he again had a cardiac rhythm and death was certain without organ replacement, we attempted to perform the rapid hepatectomy and placement of new organ in the hopes that removal of the progressively ischemic, injured end-stage liver and replacement with viable liver might improve his situation.

A rapid identification of the portal vein was performed, and this was skeletonized, clamped, divided, and retrohepatic dissection of short pedicle vessels was undertaken. The inferior vena cava above and below the liver was identified, clamps were placed on the suprahepatic and infrahepatic cava, and the liver removed. Thereafter, we were able to turn attention towards identification of the infrarenal aorta by performing an extensive Kocher maneuver and retroperitoneal dissection onto the anterior wall of the aorta. A rapid exposure of the aorta allowed control of this with the Satinsky clamp.

The liver and bowel graft were taken out of the box and sutures were placed on the suprahepatic vena cava in order to begin a proximal anastomosis. Unfortunately, once again, the patient had an unstable rhythm with extreme hypotension and instability. We brought the thoracic conduit from the donor organs up to the field and in the hurried fashion used 6-0 Prolene sutures to perform an anterior aortotomy and place the thoracic inflow graft onto the aorta. Once this was accomplished, the organs were brought to the field and we began a suprahepatic caval anastomosis with 6-0 Prolene sutures.

While this was being sewn, the patient once again underwent a cardiac arrest, which was at this time irreversible, despite extensive CPR and ultimately the baby was pronounced expired in the operating room.

Thereafter, the clamps were removed and the baby's abdominal cavity was closed with running suture while the surgery team undertook extensive consultation with the family, to explain the poor outcome.

EROSIVE POLYARTICULAR RHEUMATOID ARTHRITIS FOLLOWUP NOTE

HISTORY OF PRESENT ILLNESS: The patient returned to the Rheumatology Clinic today for a routine followup visit. The patient has erosive polyarticular rheumatoid arthritis but now appears under excellent control. His current antiarthritics consist of methotrexate 10 mg once weekly, Plaquenil 400 mg daily, and prednisone 10 mg daily. He is not using a nonsteroidal antiinflammatory drug because of concerns about the Coumadin he is taking for a cardiac arrhythmia. All his medications are well tolerated, taken without side effect or toxicity, and all methotrexate-related blood monitoring is normal.

The patient appears to have had very good relief of joint pain and early morning stiffness, and only has residual problems in 2 areas, his left knee and right shoulder. He notes pain in the shoulder when he rolls over onto it at night and then a little pain through the day that is not as much of a problem. He also notes significant left knee pain, much exacerbated by walking. I understand that the patient has longstanding degenerative arthritis involving the left knee, and this probably accounts for his knee pain to a much greater extent than does any coincidental rheumatoid arthritis in that joint.

PHYSICAL EXAMINATIONS: On musculoskeletal examination, the small joints of the hands, the wrists, the elbows, the cervical spine, the lumbosacral spine, the hips, the ankles, and the feet were unremarkable. There was inability to abduct the right shoulder beyond 45 degrees and, in addition, both internal and external rotation was uncomfortable and much limited. The left shoulder was normal. On examination of the knees, the left was swollen. There did appear to be free synovial fluid within the joint; however, there was no joint margin tenderness. The knee moved fully and freely, and was stable, although there was significant coarse and fine crepitus through the full range of movement. The right knee was unaffected.

ASSESSMENT AND PLAN: After discussion with the patient, and after appropriate local antisepsis and anesthesia, I injected 80 mg of Kenalog into the left knee; I was unable to withdraw any synovial fluid preceding this injection. I hope this has the desired effect in settling down his knee pain. If not, it is possible that he may be a candidate for an arthroscopy and arthroscopic surgery, but that would be preceded by some more focused investigations of his knee anatomy. An MRI scan would probably be the most productive approach. Again, while it is possible he has some significant rheumatoid arthritis activity in the knee, I think it is much more likely that the knee pain is as a result of longstanding degenerative arthritis.

On this occasion, I did not offer to inject the patient's right shoulder, but would certainly be prepared to do this at some time in the future, and I invited him to contact me by telephone if he wished this to be performed. I asked the patient to return for the next visit in 4 months' time, or to contact me earlier by telephone if he has any intercurrent concerns.

EXCISION OF BASAL CELL CARCINOMA OF THE NOSE

PROCEDURES PERFORMED
1. Excision of lesion, right side of bony nasal pyramid.
2. Frozen section to pathology consultation showing basal cell carcinoma with clear margins.
3. V-Y closure.

COMPLICATIONS: None.

INDICATIONS
1. Coronary artery disease.
2. Congestive heart failure.
3. Ventricular tachycardia.
4. Palpitations.

DESCRIPTION OF PROCEDURE: With the patient in the supine position and after satisfactory induction of general LMA anesthesia, the patient was prepped with Betadine scrub and draped with sterile towels and drapes. The line of proposed circular excision of the lesion of the right dorsum of the bony nasal pyramid of the nose was outlined with a marking pen. It was infiltrated with local anesthetic solution, and the lesion was excised as outlined. The 12 o'clock border was marked with a marking pen and was submitted for frozen section pathology consultation, showing basal cell carcinoma with margins clear. V-Y flaps were outlined approximately 1.2 cm wide by about 2.5 cm long, one on the left side and one on the right side of the nose. These areas were infiltrated with local anesthetic solution. The flaps were elevated as outlined. Several small bleeders were controlled with electrocautery. The flaps were rotated into the defect, and the wound edges were approximated with interrupted 5-0 black nylon sutures. The patient was dressed with Steri-Strips. He tolerated the procedure very well. Total estimated blood loss was about 5 mL. He was taken to the recovery room in satisfactory condition.

EYELID FULL-THICKNESS RESECTION AND RECONSTRUCTION

PREOPERATIVE DIAGNOSIS: Left lower eyelid mass, rule out tumor.

POSTOPERATIVE DIAGNOSIS: Left lower eyelid mass, rule out tumor.

PROCEDURES PERFORMED: Left lower eyelid full-thickness resection and reconstruction.

INDICATIONS FOR PROCEDURE: The patient has had a left lower lid lesion off and on for 1 year that has not gone away. Examination revealed an elevated vascular lesion of the left lower lid. There was possible thickening of the tarsus associated with this. It was felt that this could conceivably be a sebaceous carcinoma or some other type of eyelid cancer, and therefore a full-thickness lid resection was appropriate to absolutely exclude sebaceous carcinoma. Other possibilities included a benign chronic inflammatory condition refractory to treatment.

DESCRIPTION OF PROCEDURE: Topical tetracaine was applied to each eye. The face was prepped and draped in the usual manner. A protective contact lens was placed in the left eye. Lidocaine 1% with epinephrine was injected in the central left upper lid, and a 5-0 Mersilene was placed through the skin, orbicularis, and superficial tarsus to retract the upper lid out of the way. A small pentagon was constructed, surrounding the left lower lid lesion. This measured 4 mm in horizontal dimension. Lidocaine 1% with epinephrine was injected, a 15 blade incised the skin, and Westcott scissors removed the pentagon. Cautery was used for hemostasis. The specimen was sent for permanent pathological examination. The lid margin was reconstructed with two 6-0 silk sutures; the tarsus was reconstructed with a 6-0 Vicryl suture. The skin was closed with additional 6-0 silk, and 6-0 silk sutures were tied in order to keep them out of the eye. Polysporin ointment was applied, and ice was applied. The patient tolerated the procedure well and left the operating room in good condition.

FURUNCLE TREATMENT

HISTORY OF PRESENT ILLNESS: The patient is a 23-year-old Caucasian male who presents with a painful, red, swollen bump under the skin of his left inner thigh. He says it has been present for about a week but today there is considerably more tenderness.

PHYSICAL EXAMINATION: There is an approximately 1 x 1-cm, indurated area of the inner portion of the left thigh. It is red, warm, swollen, and quite tender.

ASSESSMENT: This area represents a developing furuncle, most likely a staphylococcal abscess.

PLAN: The patient was advised to apply warm compresses to the area for 20 minutes, 3 to 4 times a day, in order to bring pus to the surface. He was advised not to attempt to squeeze it or lance it. When the pus comes to the surface, he is to return so we can take a culture from the lesion. He was given a prescription for dicloxacillin 500 mg and was instructed to take it 4 times a day.

HYPOGAMMOGLOBULINEMIA WITH NEED FOR VASCULAR ACCESS CONSULTATION

CHIEF COMPLAINT: Lack of vascular access, hypogammaglobulinemia

HISTORY OF PRESENT ILLNESS: The patient is a 61-year-old white female who previously underwent a lung transplant for emphysema and emphysema-like syndrome. She now requires a monthly infusion of gamma globulin and also has multiple blood draws. She has utilized all of her vascular access and has not been able to have blood drawn or to receive gamma globulin. She presents requesting port placement on that basis.

PAST MEDICAL HISTORY: Significant for a lung transplant in 2002, osteoporosis versus osteopenia, open cholecystectomy, hypercholesterolemia, chronic essential hypertension, total abdominal hysterectomy, prior right salpingo-oophorectomy for tubal pregnancy, bilateral cataract extraction with lens implant, non-insulin-dependent diabetes, benign colon polyps, status post colonoscopy and polypectomy, previously negative cardiac catheterization in 2000. She is gravida 2, para 1, spontaneous abortion x1.

CURRENT MEDICATIONS: Medications include CellCept 1000 mg p.o. b.i.d.; Prograf 3 mg p.o. q.a.m., 2.5 mg p.o. every night; Uro-Mag 140 mg x4 tablets p.o. q.i.d.; Deltasone 5 mg p.o. q.a.m.; Prevacid 30 mg p.o. q.a.m.; Cozaar 100 mg p.o. q.a.m.; Bactrim DS 1 p.o. every Monday, Wednesday, Friday; acyclovir 400 mg p.o. t.i.d.; Lipitor 20 mg p.o. every day, though she has not been on it for the past month; calcium and vitamin D oyster shell t.i.d.; Actonel weekly; Miacalcin nasal spray every day; multivitamins; Combivent inhaler p.r.n.; Xanax 0.25 mg p.o. every night and p.r.n.; Gammagard IV every month.

ALLERGIES: Allergies include Tricor and Lopid, which cause her hands to peel and muscle pain; codeine causes fever; and, Isovue caused urticaria.

SOCIAL HISTORY: The patient previously smoked half pack of cigarettes per day and smoked for 25 years, but has not smoked since 1999. She denies any significant history of ethanol intake. She is on disability. She previously worked doing auditing for grocery stores.

FAMILY HISTORY: Positive for hypertension, hypercholesterolemia, and prostate cancer in a paternal grandfather. Her brother had deep venous thrombosis and pulmonary embolism, but had morbid obesity. There is no family history of coronary artery disease, diabetes, or adverse anesthesia reactions.

REVIEW OF SYSTEMS: GENERAL: The patient denies any recent illnesses. HEENT: The patient has occasional headaches without recent change. Eyes: The patient wears glasses and denies any acute visual changes. Ears: The patient denies hearing loss or tinnitus. Nose: The patient denies rhinorrhea. Throat: The patient denies sore throat. NEUROLOGIC: The patient denies dizziness or a history of falls, seizures, syncope, strokes or amaurosis fugax. RESPIRATORY: The patient has exertional dyspnea, though none at rest. She denies orthopnea, cough, or a history of hemoptysis. CARDIAC: The patient denies chest pain, pressure, squeezing, heaviness, tightness, or palpitations. BREASTS: The patient denies new or changing masses, skin changes, nipple discharge or significant mastalgia. GASTROINTESTINAL: The patient denies nausea, vomiting, diarrhea, constipation, hematochezia, melena or heartburn. GENITOURINARY: The patient denies dysuria, hematuria, or nocturia. MUSCULOSKELETAL: The patient has mild diffuse muscular pain.

PHYSICAL EXAMINATION: GENERAL: Physical examination reveals a mildly obese, 61-year-old white female in no acute distress. VITAL SIGNS: Temperature 96.1, heart rate 84, respirations 16, blood pressure 148/82. HEENT: Head is normocephalic and atraumatic. Eyes: Pupils are equal, round, reactive to light. Extraocular motions are intact. Sclerae are anicteric. Nose and throat are clear. NECK: Supple, nontender, with no JVD, carotid bruit, adenopathy, thyromegaly, or thyroid nodularity. BACK: Back shows no costovertebral angle tenderness. CHEST: Symmetric other than a left posterolateral thoracotomy scar. Respirations are clear to auscultation throughout. HEART: Heart sounds S1, S2, regular rate and rhythm without rubs, gallops, or murmurs. ABDOMEN: Mildly obese, soft, and nontender with no palpable masses, hepatosplenomegaly or fluid wave. She has a large right subcostal scar and a Pfannenstiel scar. There is a tiny, soft, nontender umbilical hernia. EXTREMITIES: No edema. Pulses are palpable. Range of motion is intact. NEUROLOGIC: The patient is alert and oriented x3. Cranial nerves II-XII are grossly intact. There are no obvious focal motor or sensory deficits. INTEGUMENTARY: Warm, dry, and without focal lesions. LYMPHATICS: There is no evidence of cervical, supraclavicular, or inguinal adenopathy.

IMPRESSION
1. Lack of vascular access.
2. Hypogammaglobulinemia.

PLAN: Right subclavian subcutaneous port placement.

KINDLER SYNDROME CONSULTATION

HISTORY OF PRESENT ILLNESS: The patient is a 23-year-old male who is hospitalized for dermatologic assessment. We have been asked to see him because of swollen blisters on his hands and feet, dystrophic nails, and webbing between the fingers. These blisters have occurred since he was born and are not caused by trauma.

PHYSICAL EXAMINATION: The skin is fragile and has the appearance of wrinkled cigarette paper. The patient has had progressive changes in his skin, including dystrophic nails, atrophic spots, and webbing between his fingers. He also suffers from sensitivity to the sun that results in erythema, pruritus, and blisters. Examination of the cutis by our electronic microscope reveals flaking of the epidermis at several points. There appears to be normal keratinization and compact stratum corneum unguis and stratum spinosum epidermidis. The epidermis is very thin.

IMPRESSION: The patient appears to have Kindler syndrome, a rare congenital disorder that is characterized by blistering, photosensitivity, and progressive poikiloderma.

Thank you for referring this interesting patient. We will follow him with you.

LIVER TRANSPLANT AND BROVIAC CATHETER PLACEMENT

PREOPERATIVE DIAGNOSIS: Biliary atresia.

POSTOPERATIVE DIAGNOSIS: Biliary atresia.

PROCEDURE PERFORMED
1. Liver transplant.
2. Broviac catheter placement.

INDICATIONS FOR PROCEDURE: This child has biliary atresia. She was evaluated by our multidisciplinary transplant committee, and a liver transplant was recommended. The parents gave informed written consent to proceed.

DESCRIPTION OF PROCEDURE: The patient was brought to the operating room, and general anesthesia was induced. A urinary catheter was subsequently placed in the bladder, and anesthesiology placed monitoring devices and infusion lines. The abdomen, neck, and chest were prepped with Betadine and draped in sterile towels. An incision over the right neck was made and carried down until the external jugular vein was identified. It was divided proximally, and then a 7-French double-lumen Broviac catheter was placed in the subcutaneous tunnel exiting in the anterior chest and guided down through the external jugular vein and into the central venous system. Fluoroscopy revealed the catheter to be in satisfactory position. The wound was closed with 2 layers of absorbable suture after securing the catheter to the vein with a silk suture. The catheter was affixed to the skin at the exit site with nylon suture.

The bilateral subcostal incision was made at the site of the portoenterostomy. When the peritoneal cavity was entered, it was apparent there was a dense amount of adhesions throughout the abdomen. These were painstakingly dissected free, exposing the liver. During the course of the dissection, a colotomy occurred at the splenic flexure on the transverse colon. This was closed with a single layer of silk suture. Attention was turned to the porta, which was skeletonized. The previous Roux-en-Y limb was identified and dissected free. It was divided as close as possible to the liver. The hepatic artery was identified, and we divided the right and left hepatic arteries individually. There were numerous large lymph nodes present, which were carefully dissected free and resected. The lymphatics were ligated with silk sutures. The portal limb was identified and was noted to be extremely diminutive. This had been expected based on the MRA. It was carefully dissected free up to the bifurcation and divided. It was noted that there was very little flow in the portal vein.

The attachments of the liver to retroperitoneum were then divided medially and laterally. It was apparent that the caudate lobe encircled the vena cava, and it was not possible to remove the liver with the cava in situ. Therefore, clamps were placed on the cava above and below the liver, and the liver was resected. It was apparent that the portal vein would not be satisfactory for portal inflow, but the inferior vena cava appeared satisfactory in position and size. Therefore, the decision was made to use the vena cava as portal inflow.

The new liver was then sutured into place using a 5-0 Prolene running suture for the suprahepatic anastomosis and a 7-0 Prolene suture for the hepatic artery anastomosis, which was from an aortic patch of the donor to a branch going to the right and left hepatic arteries on the recipient. The portal vein of the donor was then anastomosed to the inferior vena cava of the recipient using running 6-0 sutures. The clamps were released, and the liver flushed nicely. Prior to releasing the clamps, the infrahepatic cava of the donor was oversewn with 4-0 Prolene suture. The liver achieved satisfactory color and texture and began to make bile. There was a strong pulse palpable in the hepatic artery, and the portal vein anastomosis appeared satisfactory. The previous Roux-en-Y limb was then used to fashion a hepaticojejunostomy using interrupted 5-0 PDS sutures. This was fashioned over a 5-French biliary stent that had been placed on the back table through the donor cystic duct and guided up the gallbladder fossa, where the peritoneum had been oversewn. Some silk sutures were used to suture the Roux-en-Y limb up to the porta and some connective tissue to relieve any tension that might occur at a later time. There was no tension on the anastomosis at this time. It was checked by infusion of the biliary catheter with saline, and there was no evidence of a leakage. The catheter was then brought out the right flank and secured with nylon suture to the skin.

The abdomen was irrigated with warm saline and, after a final check for hemostasis, was closed with running 2-0 Prolene suture in the fascia and running subcuticular stitch in the skin. The patient tolerated the procedure well.

MALIGNANT MELANOMA OF THE FOOT

HISTORY OF PRESENT ILLNESS: The patient is an 84-year-old Caucasian male who was stationed in the South Pacific during World War II. He was exposed to atomic radiation while working with survivors in Hiroshima not long after the atomic bomb was dropped.

Approximately a year ago, the patient developed an asymptomatic lesion on the plantar surface of his right foot. It did not cause him difficulty until about a month prior to seeing his primary care physician about it. It had also begun to grow and change color.

His physician performed a biopsy of the lesion. The pathology report indicated that the lesion was a malignant melanoma, so he was referred to our office for a 2nd opinion.

PHYSICAL EXAMINATION: Initial examination revealed a 2-mm diameter mass, varying in color from black to brown to pink, on the medial plantar surface of his right foot. It was firm and was not tender to palpation. It appeared to have no core, and there were no obvious bleeding papillary tips. Palpable adenopathy was absent in the popliteal fossa and in the inguinal canal. No other suspicious lesions were noted. We referred the patient to a plastic surgeon for removal of the lesion.

TREATMENT: He underwent wide excision and skin grafting. Pathology confirmed the diagnosis of Clark level IV malignant melanoma, with a tumor thickness of 4.25 mm. The surrounding skin and femoral lymph nodes were negative for metastases, as was a metastatic workup.

Following surgery, the patient was sent to a skilled nursing facility. His primary care physician is currently following him.

OPEN DONOR NEPHRECTOMY

PREOPERATIVE DIAGNOSIS: The patient is acting as a living, related kidney donor to her brother.

POSTOPERATIVE DIAGNOSIS: The patient is acting as a living, related kidney donor to her brother.

INDICATIONS FOR PROCEDURE: The patient has volunteered to be a living, related kidney donor to her brother, who suffers from end-stage renal disease. The patient was referred for evaluation as a prospective live kidney donor, and she was deemed to be a suitable candidate.

PROCEDURE PERFORMED: Open left donor nephrectomy.

DESCRIPTION OF PROCEDURE: After informed consent was obtained from the patient, she was brought to the operating room and placed supine on the operative table. After successful induction of general endotracheal anesthesia, a Foley catheter as well as an IV line were placed. An orogastric tube was also placed. The patient was then placed in the left lateral decubitus position, at which time her entire left side was placed perpendicular to the operating table. A kidney rest was then applied to an area superior to the iliac crest to make the skin by the left-sided kidney. Her left shoulder was also placed over on top of her, and so she was essentially perpendicular to the operating table. After we were content with how she was placed on the operating table, we next prepped in the usual sterile fashion for a donor nephrectomy. We identified the 12th rib, and approximately 1 fingerbreadth below the 12th rib an incision was made for an approximate length of about 18 cm. The incision ended close to the lateral border of the rectus muscle. Electrocautery was then used to cut the skin and the subcutaneous fat. The latissimus dorsi, as well as the 3 layers of the abdominal wall, was then excised in its entirety. This was done with cautery. Once this was done, we were able to gently palpate the kidney, which was superior and lateral, and using careful blunt as well as cautery dissection, we were able to find the peritoneum. We were able to reflect this medially while keeping the kidney in the retroperitoneal space.

Once this was done, a Bookwalter retractor was placed into the operative field for retraction both cephalad and caudad, and laterally and medially. Using careful dissection, we were able to open up Gerota fascia, the plane on top of the kidney. This was extended with electrocautery superiorly, and we were able to use the cautery to excise all of the attachments this had in adventitia to the superior pole of the kidney.

We next identified the adrenal gland, which was noted in its entirety. We found the adrenal vein. This was divided between silk sutures. We were able to essentially circumferentially dissect out the entire kidney, 1st at the superior pole, then extending medially and inferiorly, and then finally the inferior pole. We next found a large ovarian vein, and this was divided between silk ties. In addition, a posterior-lying lumbar vein was identified and also divided between silk sutures. We reflected the kidney, observing its inferior side, and we found the ureter. We dissected this on top of the psoas, and we left a large amount of adventitious tissue around the entire circumference of the ureter.

Once the veins were identified, we were able to manipulate the kidney and find both renal arteries. The superior pole, which was the main renal artery, had a diameter of approximately 4 to 5 mm. We dissected this with some difficulty to its entrance into the aorta. The lower pole artery, which was approximately 3 mm, was also found and dissected along its entire length to the aorta. The dissection was a little bit difficult based upon the size of the kidney, which was large, and the fact that the patient was relatively big herself and the kidney lay relatively deep. We then carefully inspected the hilum of the kidney, and it was noted to be intact.

Once this major dissection was completed, we placed a right-angle clamp quite distally on the ureter. We did not trace it on top of the iliac, and we divided it and we tied off the distal end with a 3-0 silk tie. A very minimal amount of urine was noted to emanate from the ureter. Once this was done, we had vessel loops placed around all the major vessels. We clamped off the inferior artery with a right-angle clamp right on top of the aorta; the vessel was cut. We placed a right-angle clamp on top of the main artery, which was the more superior one; this was cut. Finally, we placed a Satinsky clamp on the renal vein, and we cut on top of this. Once this was done, the kidney was removed.

On the back table, both renal arteries, the major one and the lower pole one, were irrigated with approximately 200 to 300 mL of Urecholine. We placed 200 mL through the main renal artery and approximately 100 mL through the inferior artery. The kidney was noted to blanch well, and there was good emanation of the effluent through the renal vein. The kidney was then packaged in 3 sterile bags and taken to the operating room for implantation.

We next turned our attention back to the donor. We tied off both renal arteries with double suture of 2-0 silk. Our attention was then directed towards the cut renal vein. The renal vein orifice was oversewn using a 5-0 Prolene suture, which was sutured in a double-row fashion. When we removed the Satinsky clamp, there was excellent hemostasis.

The operative field was then flooded with antibiotic saline, and hemostasis was really quite excellent. We next turned our attention to closing the wound. The wound was closed in 2 running layers of 1-0 Novafil. The transversalis muscle was closed first with a buried stitch of running Novafil, and once this was closed the external and internal oblique muscles were closed in a single layer of running Novafil. The fascia was noted to coapt together very well. Prior to closing the fascia, we brought down the kidney rest and repositioned the table. Finally, the skin was closed using a subcuticular stitch of 4-0 Monocryl. The skin was noted to coapt together very well. Once this was done, the skin was washed off of all preparatory Betadine, and Steri-Strips were placed on top of the wound. Finally, sterile gauze was placed on top of this.

OSTEOARTHRITIS CONSULTATION NOTE

HISTORY OF PRESENT ILLNESS: The patient has a history of chronic pain in the lumbosacral spine, which has progressively gotten worse over the past 2 years. She was scheduled to have an MRI but never completed it because of claustrophobia. She also has pain in the hands and both shoulders, with significant morning stiffness. She has difficulty getting up from a sitting position. She reports pain in the knees with swelling of the left knee. She has moderate swelling of both ankles, which may be related more to her history of hypertension. She has just recently had an angiogram and is currently on Coumadin.

PERTINENT PHYSICAL FINDINGS: Hands have no evidence of synovitis. There are Heberden and Bouchard nodes, with changes of osteoarthritis. Wrist movement is normally maintained. There is tenderness of both shoulders with decreased range of mobility. There is also gluteal tenderness. Hip movement is decreased. There is bilateral crepitus of the knees with decreased range of mobility. The ankles have no swelling. The feet are normal.

ASSESSMENT: Osteoarthritis of the knees.

PLAN: We will start Vioxx at 12.5 mg every day, and if no response, can be increased to 12.5 mg b.i.d. We will check for inflammation with a sedimentation rate, C-reactive protein, rheumatoid factor, ANA and uric acid levels. Physical therapy was recommended. Local injections are an option to consider in the future.

PSORIATIC ARTHRITIS FOLLOWUP NOTE

HISTORY OF PRESENT ILLNESS: I saw the patient for the first time in over 6 months. He has gotten along reasonably well with Celebrex taken to subdue arthritic pains. His psoriasis has been variably active, helped along some by topical agents you have recently prescribed and found to be useful from personal experience. He describes a gouty attack occurring in his right foot a few weeks back. He called here and was heard by the "rheumatologist on call," who tried a Medrol Dosepak to good effect.

Lately, his knees have been sore, particularly the right, which feels stiff as well.

He recently went to you for a head-to-toe physical evaluation and brought with him papers from that visit. Laboratory work included slightly raised total cholesterol of 228 with an HDL of 38, along with a uric acid of 11.4.

He recalls receiving allopurinol before and having a "reaction," but upon closer questioning, this turned out to have been exacerbation of an existing gout attack by prescribed full-strength allopurinol. This is not unexpected and does not indicate any particular sensitivity to the drug.

PHYSICAL EXAMINATION: The patient has scattered fading of plaques of psoriasis about his hands, elbows, and legs. There is restriction of motion about his hand joints. There is tenderness at the base of the thumb on the right, the hand he says he has been working with quite extensively lately. The elbows are okay except for the psoriatic changes. His right knee has a tense effusion with ulcers about the popliteal fossa. The left knee is normal by comparison. The toes are okay today. I tapped his right knee, obtaining about 45 mL of type 2 fluid. In this, I instilled triamcinolone 40 mg and some associated lidocaine to make up 10 mL.

ASSESSMENT AND PLAN: He wonders about having a different medication than Celebrex. I have provided him with some samples of Vioxx. He can take 25 mg to 50 mg a day. I also started him on a low dose of allopurinol at 50 mg a day to be increased every 2 weeks until he is on a full dose of 300 mg a day.

I think he is generally coping well with his psoriatic arthritis. I think the gout is probably contributing from time to time preemptively to his migratory arthralgias. He has been hyperuricemic for a while, but I think it is now time to begin to bring it down. I will see him back in 3 to 4 months or earlier, if needed.

PYOGENIC GRANULOMA OF SCALP, EXCISED

HISTORY: This 17-year-old female presents to our office with a growth on her scalp. She became aware of it approximately 2 months ago when it bled as a result of fixing her hair.

PHYSICAL EXAMINATION: There is a 0.8-cm nodule on the vertex that is erythematous and slightly tender. There are no other remarkable findings on cutaneous examination.

TREATMENT: The lesion was removed in the office by shave excision, followed by electrodesiccation. The specimen will be sent for pathologic evaluation to rule out a more serious lesion.

DIAGNOSIS: Pyogenic granuloma, scalp.

REPAIR OF BLEED IN INTESTINAL TRANSPLANT RECIPIENT

PREOPERATIVE DIAGNOSIS: Hemoperitoneum.

POSTOPERATIVE DIAGNOSIS: Hemoperitoneum with intact and healthy allograft intestine transplant.

PROCEDURE PERFORMED: Repair of bleed.

INDICATIONS FOR THE PROCEDURE: Postoperative bleeding.

COMPLICATIONS: None.

BRIEF HISTORY: The patient had undergone isolated small-bowel transplantation in the setting of cholestatic liver disease for potential liver salvage approximately 1 day prior. He developed some postoperative bleeding and required reexploration.

DESCRIPTION OF PROCEDURE: The patient was brought to the OR, already intubated and with lines intact from his prior transplant procedure. We opened the midline laparotomy and encountered hemoperitoneum on entering the abdominal cavity. We were able to extract approximately 2 to 3 units' worth of blood in the form of clot and fresh blood and explored the abdominal cavity. Initially on exploration, we were able to identify the superior mesenteric artery and venous anastomoses to the native blood vessels. These were intact with no evidence of bleeding. They were healthy. There was good blood flow into and out of the transplanted allograft. We explored the entirety of the abdominal cavity extensively. The finding was of some oozing from the surface of the right lobe of the liver, where it had been mobilized from the underside of the abdominal wall.

This area of the liver was very friable. The liver had a severe hepatomegaly and cholestasis and was soft, and there was a small crack in the superficial right lobe. We attempted to use argon beam electrocoagulator to accomplish perfect hemostasis of this area; however, it was unsuccessful. We also used electrocautery and attempted tacking of this area. The right lobe of the liver was extremely densely adherent to the underlying tissue and the surrounding abdominal wall, such that it could not be completely mobilized off and it appeared there was small crack in an area where attempted prior mobilization of the right lobe had taken place. Because it appeared that further attempts at aggressive mobilization of the right lobe of the liver would result in even more bleeding, we used local measures to the best that we could. We used thrombin and Gelfoam packing as well as Surgicel and extensive argon beam coagulopathy therapy to this area.

Once we had achieved what we thought was relatively good hemostasis, albeit not perfect, this was extensively packed with thrombin and Gelfoam and a 10 flat Jackson-Pratt drain was placed next to the area where the oozing had been. There was no further active bleeding at this time, and the abdominal cavity was copiously irrigated with saline and antibiotic solution. Again, the allograft and the blood vessels were checked and they were in perfect order. There was no need for further manipulation of the bowel graft, its vessels, or anything else in the abdominal cavity. Therefore, the closure was undertaken with a #1 PDS suture. Again, the closure was performed and results in no change of significance of the peak inspiratory pressure, and it was not particularly tight. The patient was left intubated, taken back to the PICU for further recovery.

RHEUMATOID ARTHRITIS CONSULTATION NOTE

HISTORY OF PRESENT ILLNESS: For several years, the patient had pain in the small joints of the hands that was localized to 1 or 2 fingers only and was of short duration without any evidence of inflammation. These episodes were infrequent. Lately, however, the patient had for the first time a very well-organized onset of joint pain and inflammation located in the PIP joints, wrists, and MCP joints. The pain was associated with morning stiffness of up to 2 hours. Regarding major joints, she has had only mild pain in the left shoulder. At some point in her disease, the patient apparently had involvement of tendons with pain in the arms and both hands. When the inflammation has been at the highest point, the patient was unable to make a fist, and it was difficult for her to perform activities of daily life and take care of herself. However, the patient could massage herself, give herself baths with warm water, and remain active and working. On 2 occasions, the patient received steroids in systemic form with very important improvement of her symptoms. For the last few months, the patient has been taking hydroxychloroquine 400 mg a day; however, her synovitis has persisted. Currently, the patient has morning stiffness of about 1 hour as well as pain and inflammation in the MCP and PIP joints.

The patient denies fever, hair loss, mouth ulcers, adenopathy, shortness of breath, chest pain, abdominal pain, or skin rashes. Before her illness, the patient used to exercise regularly, riding a bike.

PHYSICAL EXAMINATION: Musculoskeletal examination shows normal range of motion in all joints with evident synovitis localized to the 2nd, 3rd, and 4th PIP joints and over the styloid apophysis in the right hand. There is a subluxation of both 1st CMC joints bilaterally and significant tenderness to palpation in the right MCP joints. The left shoulder is minimally tender on mobilization..

PERTINENT LABORATORY FINDINGS: CBC with WBC 15.3, hemoglobin 12.3 and platelets 362,000. LFTs normal. TSH 0.33. Rheumatoid factor negative and ANA negative. X-rays of the hands show only a very mild osteopenia in the carpals; feet are normal. There are no erosions at any level.

ASSESSMENT AND PLAN: We agree with your impression that this patient has a seronegative rheumatoid arthritis. Despite the use of hydroxychloroquine for 5 months, the patient is still showing signs of active inflammation. We think that the patient may benefit with the addition of a 2nd drug, and we are recommending the initiation of methotrexate. The benefits and risks of this medication were explained to the patient, who accepted the treatment. On the other hand, given the acute inflammation, we are also recommending the initiation of prednisone 5 mg a day. We expect that after probably 1 or 2 months the patient may be able to discontinue prednisone. Regarding her treatment, there is duplication on COX-2 inhibitors, and we suggested to the patient to continue with only one of them. The patient will discontinue Vioxx. The patient will obtain an appointment with her ophthalmologist to initiate her regular checking for hydroxychloroquine. Finally, given the fact that the patient has early disease and is in to see us regarding treatment and is a very active person, we think that she may have a good prognosis. We are scheduling an appointment in 2 months.

RHEUMATOID ARTHRITIS FOLLOWUP NOTE

HISTORY OF PRESENT ILLNESS: The patient is a 38-year-old woman who has an illness of about 3 to 4 years, characterized by myalgias, arthralgias and arthritis located in the MCP joints, PIP joints, wrists, and ankles. In addition, the patient has had intermittent Raynaud syndrome, mild hair loss, and a transient rash located on the face and the neck. Other problems are sleep abnormalities and problems with equilibrium that are under evaluation by neurology. In our initial evaluation, we considered that the patient may have an undifferentiated connective tissue disease, and the possibilities were rheumatoid arthritis, lupus, or scleroderma. A trial of prednisone 15 mg was initiated. Two days after the patient started taking prednisone, she felt an impressive improvement that she describes as a miracle. The chronic sensation of fatigue was almost eliminated, and the myalgias are very mild, as well as the arthritis. The patient has not had episodes of arthritis since. The patient has been unusually active at work with energy and is able to do gardening. There is no significant change in morning stiffness, and this is still about 30 minutes.

PHYSICAL EXAMINATION: The general examination is benign. There is no hair loss. There is very mild erythema on the neck with fine telangiectasias that were mentioned before. There are no other skin lesions, and there are no mucosal lesions either. Musculoskeletal examination shows a motor power of 5/5 in all 4 extremities, range of motion is normal in all joints, and there is no evidence of synovitis at any level.

PERTINENT LABORATORY FINDINGS: CBC showed a WBC of 10,000, hemoglobin 12.9, and hematocrit 37.3. Sodium was 139, potassium 3.3, chloride 104, CO2 24, BUN 21, creatinine 0.9 and glucose 87. Liver function tests are normal. Sedimentation rate is 28, and CRP is 0.9; both of them are only slightly elevated. Normal C3 at 143, normal C4 at 25. CK 70 and aldolase 3, both normal, and immunoelectrophoresis is normal. All of her antibodies are negative, including rheumatoid arthritis. These antibodies are Scl-70, Ro, Sm, RNP, ANCA, and antiphospholipid, IgG, and IgM.

X-rays of hands show only mild osteopenia around the MCP and PIP joints. There are no erosions.

ASSESSMENT AND PLAN: The patient is a 38-year-old woman with an undifferentiated inflammatory polyarthritis. Considering the family history of a father and a brother with rheumatoid arthritis, it is possible that the patient is at the stage of an early rheumatoid arthritis, which is seronegative. Given the presence of Raynaud syndrome and fine telangiectasias, we have to keep in mind the possibility of this illness evolving to scleroderma. We do not have serologic evidence of lupus, and there is no biochemical evidence of myositis. Our plan at the moment will be to initiate high-dose chloroquine at 400 mg every day, evaluation by an ophthalmologist, and a slow reduction of prednisone to 10 mg in 1 month and then 1 mg per week. We are scheduling an appointment in 2 months and requesting a complete blood count and sedimentation rate for the next visit.

TATTOO REMOVAL

HISTORY: This is the 2nd visit for this 24-year-old Latino female. She wishes to have eyelid tattoos removed. A cosmetologist placed the tattoos at a local beauty salon. She reports that the tattoos were placed first by swabbing the eyelids with an alcohol pledget. Following this, 10 mg topical lidocaine was applied to each eyelid margin with a cotton-tipped applicator. Using a triple-pronged needle, Meicha permanent makeup was implanted along the edge of each eyelid. Saline solution was used to clean the eyelids at the conclusion of the tattooing process. The patient decided almost immediately following the procedure that she wanted the tattooing removed from the eyelids.

PLAN OF TREATMENT: We gave her 0.025% tretinoin, which she uses for acne, with instructions to apply it 4 times a day with a Q-Tip or other cotton-tipped applicator, and to apply petroleum jelly to the distal rim of the lids to protect her eyes. She was advised to expect some swelling, redness, and tenderness. She will report back to us in 1 week for followup.

TOTAL HIP ARTHOPLASTY

PREOPERATIVE DIAGNOSIS: Osteoarthritis of the right hip.

POSTOPERATIVE DIAGNOSIS: Osteoarthritis of the right hip.

PROCEDURE PERFORMED: Right total hip arthroplasty with completely cemented technique.

DESCRIPTION OF PROCEDURE: With the patient under satisfactory general anesthesia, the patient was turned in the left lateral position and placed on the Montreal frame with the pelvis and torso appropriately positioned with the towels. Prepping and draping was complete.

A direct lateral incision was placed over the right hip and carried down through the skin and subcutaneous tissue. The fascia lata was split in line with the skin incision. A relaxing incision was placed in the anterior one-third of the hip abductors, and the capsule and abductors reflected anteriorly. We opened the capsule widely and dislocated the femoral head anteriorly. The femoral head was markedly distorted with marked amount of periarticular osteophytes and periarticular osteophytes in the acetabulum. These were removed in the appropriate fashion. We then removed the femoral head.

The box chisel was used to remove the top of the femoral neck and the medial aspect of the greater trochanter. Using a T-Bar seeker, we determined the direction of the femoral canal. We then reamed the femoral canal to the appropriate transverse diameter as template revealed on the x-rays. Having then impacted the medullary broaches distally, we planed the calcar down to the throat of the broach. We then placed an absorbable wick in the medullary canal and turned our attention to the acetabulum. As mentioned, all periarticular osteophytes were removed. We then obliterated the old triradiate horseshoe in the depth of the acetabulum, having removed all synovium, and then reamed to the appropriate transverse diameter, getting good cortical cutting at the upper limits of the reamers.

Having prepared both the femur and the acetabulum, the following sizes were determined to be the appropriate fit: a 13.5 hydroxyapatite femoral stem, a 53-mm acetabulum, and a neutral femoral head of Metasul type. Having determined that these were the appropriate sizes and fits by templating and trial reduction, these were then implanted appropriately, referable to the patient's anatomic characteristics. Again, the range of motion and stability were measured and deemed to be very satisfactory.

We then rinsed copiously with saline, as we did throughout the case. The deep musculature was then closed with figure-of-8 #1 Ethibond. The gluteus medius was placed back on the greater trochanter with #1 Ethibond doubled on itself, figure-of-8 sutures, cinched down firmly. The fascia lata was closed with figure-of-eight #1 Ethibond, the subcutaneous tissue with 2-0 plain, and the skin with stainless steel staples. A sterile dressing was placed over the wound. Blood loss was approximately 400 mL. None was replaced. The patient had been given 1 g Ancef IV piggyback one-half hour prior to the surgery in the holding room.

The patient was recovered from anesthesia. The patient was carefully transferred back onto her back, the leg being held in the appropriate position of abduction and internal rotation for stability and was transferred into the hospital bed. The patient tolerated the procedure well and returned to the recovery room in satisfactory condition.

TOTAL KNEE ARTHOPLASTY

PREOPERATIVE DIAGNOSIS: Osteoarthritis of the left knee.

POSTOPERATIVE DIAGNOSIS: Osteoarthritis of the left knee.

PROCEDURE PERFORMED: Left total knee arthroplasty with completely cemented technique.

DESCRIPTION OF PROCEDURE: With the patient under satisfactory general anesthesia, the patient was placed on the operating table. The buttocks were elevated with a small sandbag, rotating the leg to the neutral position. Prepping and draping was complete. The tourniquet was applied high on the thigh and was elevated to 300 mmHg. The leg was exsanguinated with an Esmarch bandage. A long medial parapatellar incision was placed over knee, carried down through the skin and subcutaneous tissue. The vastus medialis was split obliquely, then down into the medial retinaculum to the tibial tubercle. The patella was rotated 180 degrees on itself and the knee was flexed.

The long medullary rod was placed down the medullary canal, and the end-cutting jig was placed over the end of the femur and the femur was amputated with the oscillating saw. We then turned our attention to the tibia. The tibial alignment block was fine tuned to the upper portion of the tibia, and the top of the tibia was removed and this measured a size 2. The bear claw template was affixed to the end of the femur. The bear claw indicated a size 2. We amputated the anterior and posterior condyles and beveled the corner with the chamfer block and cut the slot. We then returned to the tibia. The tibial template measured a size 2. We cut the cutting fin down top of the tibia and drilled the drill holes and cut the cutting fin appropriately. We then tried various size inserts, and the following sizes were used: The patient had a 2 tibial base plate. An 11-mm insert fit the best; 9 was too loose and 13 had a flexion contracture. The femur measured a size 2. The patella was measured a size 0-10. The patella was undercut 2 mm with the cutting drill and, having prepared all surfaces, we pulse lavaged to a dry cheesecloth appearance and then sequentially cemented the tibial base plate, snapped in the polyethylene liner. The femur was cemented, and the patella was cemented as well.

Tourniquet time was 52 minutes. We deflated the tourniquet. The circulation returned immediately. We did spot coagulation with the Bovie unit and, assuring good hemostasis and having put a cement bone plug down the medullary canal, the wound was quite dry by the time of closure. We then closed the medial retinaculum with #1 Ethibond figure-of-8 sutures, the musculature with 2-0 plain, the subcutaneous tissue with 2-0 plain, the skin with stainless steel staples. Blood loss was under 100 mL. None was replaced. The patient received 1 g Ancef IV piggyback in the holding room prior to the surgery. The patient was sterilely dressed, recovered from anesthesia, and returned to the recovery room in satisfactory condition.

VARICELLA VIRUS (CHICKENPOX VIRUS)

CHIEF COMPLAINT: Itching, blister-like rash.

HISTORY OF PRESENT ILLNESS: This 12-year-old boy comes with a 24-hour history of an itchy, blister-like rash. He also has a temperature and feeling of general malaise.

PAST HISTORY: The patient has been a healthy child, with occasional earache and stuffy nose. He has no idea where he came in contact with the varicella virus.

SOCIAL HISTORY: The patient is a vegetarian, as are the other members of his family. They do supplement their diet with vitamin and mineral supplements.

REVIEW OF SYSTEMS: Findings are insignificant, other than the rash.

PHYSICAL EXAMINATION: VITAL SIGNS: Temperature is 102 degrees Fahrenheit, blood pressure 130/70 HEENT: There are several blisters on the cheeks and forehead. Exam is otherwise normal. No blisters are seen near the eyes. NECK: There are a few blisters on each side of the neck and over the throat. CHEST: Most of the blisters appear over the torso area. This includes the back and abdomen. Heart is normal sinus rhythm. EXTREMITIES: A few blisters are up and down the extremities. NEUROLOGIC: Normal.

DIAGNOSIS: Chickenpox.

TREATMENT: The child's mother was advised that Calamine lotion helps relieve the itching. Tylenol can be given to reduce his temperature. They were advised that he should remain at home until the rash has dried up. They should also discourage visitors during this time.

Common Terms by Procedure

Acupuncture for Acne Rosacea

acne rosacea
hysterectomy
ibuprofen
liver qi stagnation
needling
tendinitis
tetracycline
traditional chinese medicine
uterine fibroid tumor

Allergic Contact Dermatitis

allergic dermatitis
allergic reaction
anaphylaxis
angioedema
chamomile
Chinese herbal medicine
external topical plaster
Isotonix OPC-3
lumbar spine
patch testing
pruritic erythematous papular eruption
Tension Tamer Celestial Seasonings tea
thoracic area
urticaria
Western herbal medicine

Cadaveric Renal Transplant Recipient with Nausea Consultation

arteriovenous fistula
blood urea nitrogen (BUN)
cadaveric renal transplant
calcium
CellCept
differential
electrolytes
end-stage renal failure

hemodialysis
hemoglobin
Imodium
incisional hernia
parathyroid surgery
postoperative hypocalcemia
precordium
prednisone
primary glomerular disease
Rapamune
renal transplant
secondary hyperparathyroidism
serum albumin
serum creatinine
tortuosity of the vein
transplant team
white blood count

Combined Liver and Small Bowel Transplantation

abdominal cavity
adhesiolysis
anemia
anterior aortotomy
anterior rectus sheath
anterior wall of the aorta
ascites
atypical cardiac rhythm
bilirubin
bowel graft
cardiac arrest
cardiopulmonary resuscitation (CPR)
caval anastomosis
cholestasis
coagulopathy
colon
combined liver and small bowel
    transplantation
common bile duct

creatinine
debility
dense adhesion
donor organ
duodenum
encephalopathy
end-stage intestinal failure
end-stage liver failure
general endotracheal anesthesia
gentle dissection
hepatectomy
hepatic artery
hepatomegaly
hepatorenal syndrome
high-dose pressor
high-risk surgical candidate
hilar dissection
hypotension and instability
impending death
inferior vena cava
infrahepatic vena cava
infrarenal aorta
intraoperative death
Kocher maneuver
liver graft
liver transplantation
low platelet count
malnutrition
mesenteric infarction
monitoring line
porta hepatis
portal hypertension
portal vein
prepped and draped
6-0 Prolene suture
proximal anastomosis
refractory cholestasis
renal insufficiency
retrohepatic dissection
retroperitoneal dissection
running suture

Satinsky clamp
self-retaining retractor
severe acidosis
short bowel syndrome
short pedicle vessel
skeletonized, clamped, and divided
skin and subcutaneous tissue
small bowel transplantation
subcostal incision
subcutaneous tissue
suprahepatic vena cava
thoracic conduit
thoracic inflow graft
thrombocytopenia
total parenteral nutrition
unstable rhythm
upper midline extension
usual sterile fashion

Erosive Polyarticular Rheumatoid Arthritis Followup Note

abduct
anesthesia
antiarthritic
antisepsis
arthroscopic surgery
arthroscopy
blood monitoring
cardiac arrhythmia
cervical spine
coarse and fine crepitus
Coumadin
degenerative arthritis
erosive polyarticular rheumatoid
    arthritis
exacerbated
external rotation
followup visit
free synovial fluid
full range of movement

internal rotation
joint margin tenderness
joint pain
Kenalog
lumbosacral spine
methotrexate
morning stiffness
magnetic resonance imaging (MRI)
MRI scan
musculoskeletal examination
nonsteroidal antiinflammatory drug
Plaquenil
polyarticular rheumatoid arthritis
prednisone
range of movement
residual problem
rheumatoid arthritis
Rheumatology Clinic
routine followup visit
side effect
small joint
toxicity

Excision of Basal Cell Carcinoma of the Nose

basal cell carcinoma
Betadine scrub
5-0 black nylon suture
bony nasal pyramid
circular excision
clear margin
controlled with electrocautery
electrocautery
estimated blood loss
flaps were rotated
frozen section pathology
general LMA anesthesia
infiltrated with local anesthetic solution
laryngeal mask airway (LMA)
local anesthetic solution
marking pen

12 o'clock border
pathology consultation
recovery room
satisfactory condition
satisfactory induction
small bleeder
Steri-Strips
sterile towel and drape
supine position
V-Y closure
wound edge

Eyelid Full-Thickness Resection and Reconstruction

benign chronic inflammatory condition
15 blade
cautery
eyelid cancer
full-thickness lid resection
hemostasis
lidocaine 1% with epinephrine
lower eyelid mass
lower lid lesion
5-0 Mersilene
pentagon
permanent pathological examination
Polysporin ointment
prepped and draped
protective contact lens
reconstruction
refractory to treatment
sebaceous carcinoma
6-0 silk suture
superficial tarsus
topical tetracaine
usual manner
vascular lesion
6-0 Vicryl suture
Westcott scissors

Furuncle Treatment
dicloxacillin
furuncle
indurated area
lance
painful, red, swollen bump
pus
staphylococcal abscess
warm compress

Hypogamma Globulinemia with Need for Vascular Access Consultation
Actonel
acyclovir
adenopathy
adverse anesthesia reaction
alert and oriented
amaurosis fugax
Bactrim DS
benign colon polyp
cardiac catheterization
carotid bruit
cataract extraction
CellCept
cervical, supraclavicular, or inguinal
    adenopathy
clear to auscultation
codeine
colonoscopy
Combivent
coronary artery disease
costovertebral angle tenderness
Cozaar
cranial nerves II-XII
deep venous thrombosis
Deltasone
diabetes
dysuria
emphysema
emphysema-like syndrome
essential hypertension
equal, round, reactive to light
exertional dyspnea
extraocular motions are intact
focal lesion
Gammagard
gamma globulin
grossly intact
hematochezia
hematuria
hemoptysis
hypercholesterolemia
hypertension
hypogammaglobulinemia
Isovue
jugular venous distention (JVD)
lens implant
Lipitor
Lopid
lung transplant
mastalgia
melena
Miacalcin
morbid obesity
motor deficit
nocturia
non-insulin-dependent diabetes
normocephalic and atraumatic
open cholecystectomy
orthopnea
osteopenia
osteoporosis
oyster shell
palpitation
polypectomy
port placement
Prevacid
Prograf
prostate cancer
pulmonary embolism
range of motion is intact
right salpingo-oophorectomy
sclerae are anicteric

sensory deficit
thoracotomy scar
thyroid nodularity
thyromegaly
tinnitus
total abdominal hysterectomy
Tricor
tubal pregnancy
Uro-Mag
urticaria
vascular access
Xanax

Kindler Syndrome Consultation

atrophic spot
congenital disorder
cutis
dystrophic nail
electronic microscope
epidermis
erythema
keratinization
Kindler syndrome
photosensitivity
progressive change
progressive poikiloderma
pruritus
stratum corneum unguis
stratum spinosum epidermidis
webbing between fingers

Liver Transplant and Broviac Catheter Placement

absorbable suture
aortic patch
biliary atresia
biliary catheter
biliary stent
Broviac catheter placement
caudate lobe
central venous system

colotomy
connective tissue
dissected free
double-lumen Broviac catheter
external jugular vein
fluoroscopy
gallbladder fossa
general anesthesia
hepatic artery
hepaticojejunostomy
informed written consent
infusion line
in situ
liver transplant
lymphatic
lymph node
monitoring device
multidisciplinary transplant committee
nylon suture
5-0 PDS sutures
peritoneum
portal inflow
portal limb
portal vein
prepped with Betadine and draped
5-0 Prolene suture
recipient
retroperitoneum
Roux-en-Y limb
running suture
satisfactory position
silk suture
skeletonized
splenic flexure
subcostal incision
subcutaneous tunnel
suprahepatic anastomosis
transverse colon
urinary catheter
vena cava

Malignant Melanoma of the Foot

asymptomatic lesion
atomic radiation
biopsy
Clark level IV malignant melanoma
femoral lymph node
inguinal canal
malignant melanoma
medial plantar surface
metastasis
metastatic workup
palpable adenopathy
papillary tip
plantar surface
popliteal fossa
skilled nursing facility
skin grafting
tender to palpation
tumor thickness
wide excision

Open Donor Nephrectomy

abdominal wall
adrenal vein
adventitia
adventitious tissue
antibiotic saline
Betadine
blunt dissection
Bookwalter retractor
buried stitch
careful dissection
caudad
cautery dissection
cephalad
circumferentially
dissect out
donor nephrectomy
double-row fashion
double suture
electrocautery

end-stage renal disease
excellent hemostasis
external oblique muscle
fingerbreadth
Foley catheter
general endotracheal anesthesia
Gerota fascia
hemostasis
hilum of the kidney
iliac crest
implantation
inferior artery
inferior pole
informed consent was obtained
internal oblique muscle
kidney rest
lateral border
laterally and medially
latissimus dorsi
left lateral decubitus position
live kidney donor
living, related kidney donor
lower pole artery
lumbar vein
major dissection
4-0 Monocryl
open left donor nephrectomy
operating room
operative field
orogastric tube
ovarian vein
oversewn
palpate the kidney
peritoneum
perpendicular to the operating table
placed supine on the operative table
prepped in the usual sterile fashion
psoas muscle
rectus muscle
renal artery
renal vein
renal vein orifice
retroperitoneal space

right-angle clamp
running Novafil
Satinsky clamp
silk suture
silk tie
sterile gauze
Steri-Strips
subcutaneous fat
subcuticular stitch
successful induction of general
  endotracheal anesthesia
suitable candidate
superior pole
Urecholine
ureter
vessel loop

Osteoarthritis Consultation Note

antinuclear antibody (ANA)
angiogram
Bouchard node
chronic pain
claustrophobia
Coumadin
C-reactive protein
crepitus of the knee
gluteal tenderness
Heberden node
local injection
lumbosacral spine
magnetic resonance imaging (MRI)
morning stiffness
osteoarthritis
range of mobility
rheumatoid factor
sedimentation rate
synovitis
uric acid
Vioxx

Psoriatic Arthritis Followup Note

allopurinol
arthritic pain
Celebrex
exacerbation
gouty attack
high-density lipoprotein (HDL)
hyperuricemic
lidocaine
Medrol Dosepak
migratory arthralgia
plaque of psoriasis
popliteal fossa
psoriasis
psoriatic change
restriction of motion
tense effusion
topical agent
total cholesterol
triamcinolone
type 2 fluid

Pyogenic Granuloma of Scalp, Excised

cutaneous examination
electrodesiccation
erythematous
pathologic evaluation
pyogenic granuloma
shave excision

Repair of Bleed in Intestinal Transplant Recipient

abdominal cavity
abdominal wall
aggressive mobilization
allograft intestine transplant
antibiotic solution
argon beam coagulopathy therapy

argon beam electrocoagulator
blood vessel
bowel graft
cholestasis
cholestatic liver disease
closure
clot and fresh blood
copiously irrigated
electrocautery
extensive argon beam coagulopathy
 therapy
10 flat Jackson-Pratt drain
friable
Gelfoam packing
hemoperitoneum
hepatomegaly
intubated
Jackson-Pratt drain
liver salvage
lobe of the liver
midline laparotomy
mobilization
mobilized
native blood vessel
#1 PDS suture
peak inspiratory pressure
pediatric intensive care unit (PICU)
perfect hemostasis
postoperative bleeding
reexploration
saline and antibiotic solution
small-bowel transplantation
superior mesenteric artery
superficial right lobe
Surgicel
thrombin
transplanted allograft
transplant procedure
underlying tissue
underside of the abdominal wall
venous anastomosis

Rheumatoid Arthritis Consultation Note

abdominal pain
active inflammation
acute inflammation
adenopathy
antinuclear antibody (ANA)
carpometacarpal (CMC)
carpals
chest pain
CMC joint
complete blood count (CBC)
COX-2 inhibitor
cyclooxygenase-2 (COX-2)
hair loss
hemoglobin
hydroxychloroquine
liver function test (LFT)
major joint
MCP joint
metacarpophalangeal (MCP)
methotrexate
morning stiffness
mouth ulcer
musculoskeletal examination
normal range of motion
osteopenia
pain and inflammation
PIP joint
platelet
prednisone
proximal interphalangeal (PIP)
range of motion
rheumatoid arthritis
rheumatoid factor
seronegative rheumatoid arthritis
shortness of breath
skin rash
small joint of the hand
steroid
styloid apophysis
subluxation

synovitis
systemic form
tenderness to palpation
thyroid-stimulating hormone (TSH)
white blood count (WBC)

Rheumatoid Arthritis Followup Note

antineutrophil cytoplasmic antibody (ANCA)
antiphospholipid antibody
arthralgia
arthritis
blood urea nitrogen (BUN)
carbon dioxide (CO2)
chloride
chloroquine
complete blood count (CBC)
connective tissue disease
creatine kinase (CK)
creatinine
C-reactive protein (CRP)
equilibrium
erythema
fine telangiectasis
GF-1 antibody
glucose
hair loss
hematocrit
IgG antibody
IgM antibody
immunoglobulin G (IgG)
immunoglobulin M (IgM)
liver function test
lupus
MCP joint
metacarpophalangeal (MCP)
musculoskeletal examination
myalgia
PIP joint
polyarthritis
potassium

prednisone
proximal interphalangeal (PIP)
range of motion is normal
Raynaud syndrome
rheumatoid arthritis
ribonucleoprotein (RNP)
RNP antibody
Ro antibody
Rose (Ro)
Scl-70 antibody
scleroderma
sedimentation rate
seronegative
sleep abnormality
Sm antibody
Smith (Sm)
sodium
synovitis
telangiectasias
thyroid-stimulating hormone (TSH)
transient rash
undifferentiated inflammatory polyarthritis
white blood count (WBC)

Tattoo Removal

alcohol pledget
cotton-tipped applicator
distal rim of the lid
eyelid tattoo
Meicha permanent makeup
petroleum jelly
saline solution
swelling, redness, and tenderness
topical lidocaine
0.025% tretinoin
triple-pronged needle

Total Hip Arthroplasty

absorbable wick
acetabulum
Ancef IV piggyback

blood loss
box chisel
calcar
cinched down
#1 Ethibond suture
fascia lata
femoral canal
femoral head
femoral neck
femoral stem
figure-of-8 suture
general anesthesia
gluteus medius
greater trochanter
hip abductor
hydroxyapatite femoral stem
intravenous (IV)
lateral incision
left lateral position
medullary broach
medullary canal
Metasul type
Montreal frame
osteoarthritis
osteophyte
periarticular osteophyte
prepping and draping
relaxing incision
satisfactory general anesthesia
stainless steel staple
sterile dressing
subcutaneous tissue
synovium
T-Bar seeker
template
templating
transverse diameter
trial reduction
triradiate horseshoe

Total Knee Arthroplasty
Ancef IV piggyback

bear claw template
beveled
blood loss
Bovie unit
cement bone plug
chamfer block
completely cemented technique
cutting drill
cutting fin
drill hole
dry cheesecloth appearance
end-cutting jig
Esmarch bandage
exsanguinated
femur
flexion contracture
general anesthesia
good hemostasis
hemostasis
holding room
intravenous (IV)
left total knee arthroplasty
medial reticulum
medullary canal
medullary rod
neutral position
oscillating saw
osteoarthritis
parapatellar incision
patella
2-0 plain suture
polyethylene liner
posterior condyle
prepping and draping
recovery room
satisfactory condition
satisfactory general anesthesia
spot coagulation
stainless steel staple
sterilely dressed
subcutaneous tissue
tibia
tibial alignment block

tibial base plate
tibial template
total knee arthroplasty
tourniquet time
vastus medialis

Varicella Virus (Chickenpox) Diagnosis

blister-like rash
Calamine lotion
chickenpox
general malaise
mineral supplement
normal sinus rhythm
Tylenol
varicella virus
vegetarian

Drugs by Indication

ACNE
Acne Product
  Acetoxyl® [Can]
  adapalene
  Akne-Mycin® [US]
  Alti-Clindamycin [Can]
  Apo®-Clindamycin [Can]
  A/T/S® [US]
  Benoxyl® [Can]
  Benzac® AC Wash [US]
  Benzac® [US]
  Benzac® W Wash [US/Can]
  Benzagel® [US]
  Benzagel® Wash [US]
  Benzamycin® [US]
  Benzashave® [US]
  benzoyl peroxide
  benzoyl peroxide and
    hydrocortisone
  Brevoxyl® Cleansing [US]
  Brevoxyl® [US]
  Brevoxyl® Wash [US]
  Cleocin HCl® [US]
  Cleocin Pediatric® [US]
  Cleocin Phosphate® [US]
  Cleocin T® [US]
  Cleocin® [US]
  Clinac™ BPO [US]
  Clindagel(TM) [US]
  ClindaMax [US]
  clindamycin
  Clindets® [US]
  Clindoxyl® Gel [Can]
  cyproterone and ethinyl estradiol
    (Canada only)
  Dalacin® C [Can]
  Dalacin® T [Can]
  Del Aqua® [US]
  Desquam-E™ [US]

Desquam-X® [US/Can]
Diane®-35 [Can]
Differin® [US/Can]
Emgel® [US]
Erycette® [US]
EryDerm® [US]
Erygel® [US]
Erythra-Derm™ [US]
erythromycin and benzoyl peroxide
erythromycin (ophthalmic/topical)
Exact® Acne Medication [US-OTC]
Fostex® 10% BPO [US-OTC]
Loroxide® [US-OTC]
Neutrogena® Acne Mask [US-OTC]
Neutrogena® On The Spot® Acne
  Treatment [US-OTC]
Novo-Clindamycin [Can]
Oxy 10® Balanced Medicated Face
  Wash [US-OTC]
Oxyderm™ [Can]
Palmer's® Skin Success Acne [US-
  OTC]
PanOxyl®-AQ [US]
PanOxyl® Bar [US-OTC]
PanOxyl® [US/Can]
ratio-Clindamycin [Can]
Romycin® [US]
Seba-Gel™ [US]
Solugel® [Can]
Staticin® [US]
Theramycin Z® [US]
Triaz® Cleanser [US]
Triaz® [US]
T-Stat® [US]
Vanoxide-HC® [US/Can]
Zapzyt® [US-OTC]

Antibiotic, Topical
  Apo®-Metronidazole [Can]
  Flagyl ER® [US]
  Flagyl® [US/Can]
  Florazole ER® [Can]
  MetroCream® [US/Can]
  MetroGel® Topical [US/Can]
  MetroLotion® [US]
  metronidazole
  Nidagel™ [Can]
  Noritate® [US/Can]
  Novo-Nidazol [Can]
  Trikacide® [Can]
Antiseborrheic Agent, Topical
  AVAR™ Cleanser [US]
  AVAR™ Green [US]
  AVAR™ [US]
  Aveeno® Cleansing Bar [US-OTC]
  Clenia™ [US]
  Fostex® [US-OTC]
  Nocosyn™ [US]
  Pernox® [US-OTC]
  Plexion SCT™ [US]
  Plexion™ TS [US]
  Plexion® [US]
  Rosanil™ [US]
  Rosula® [US]
  Sastid® Plain Therapeutic Shampoo
    and Acne Wash [US-OTC]
  Sulfacet-R® [US]
  sulfur and salicylic acid
  sulfur and sulfacetamide
  Zetacet® [US]
Estrogen and Androgen Combination
  cyproterone and ethinyl estradiol
    (Canada only)
  Diane®-35 [Can]
Keratolytic Agent
  Avage™ [US]
  Compound W® One Step Wart
    Remover [US-OTC]
  Compound W® [US-OTC]
  DHS™ Sal [US-OTC]

Dr. Scholl's® Callus Remover [US-OTC]
Dr. Scholl's® Clear Away [US-OTC]
Duoforte® 27 [Can]
Freezone® [US-OTC]
Fung-O® [US-OTC]
Gordofilm® [US-OTC]
Hydrisalic™ [US-OTC]
Ionil® Plus [US-OTC]
Ionil® [US-OTC]
Keralyt® [US-OTC]
LupiCare™ Dandruff [US-OTC]
LupiCare™ II Psoriasis [US-OTC]
LupiCare™ Psoriasis [US-OTC]
Mediplast® [US-OTC]
MG217 Sal-Acid® [US-OTC]
Mosco® Corn and Callus Remover
  [US-OTC]
NeoCeuticals™ Acne Spot
  Treatment [US-OTC]
Neutrogena® Acne Wash [US-OTC]
Neutrogena® Body Clear™ [US-OTC]
Neutrogena® Clear Pore Shine
  Control [US-OTC]
Neutrogena® Clear Pore [US-OTC]
Neutrogena® Healthy Scalp [US-OTC]
Neutrogena® Maximum Strength
  T/Sal® [US-OTC]
Neutrogena® On The Spot® Acne
  Patch [US-OTC]
Occlusal™ [Can]
Occlusal®-HP [US/Can]
Oxy® Balance Deep Pore [US-OTC]
Oxy Balance® [US-OTC]
Palmer's® Skin Success Acne
  Cleanser [US-OTC]
Pedisilk® [US-OTC]
Propa pH [US-OTC]
Sal-Acid® [US-OTC]
Salactic® [US-OTC]
SalAc® [US-OTC]
salicylic acid

Sal-Plant® [US-OTC]
Sebcur® [Can]
Soluver® [Can]
Soluver® Plus [Can]
Stri-dex® Body Focus [US-OTC]
Stri-dex® Facewipes To Go™ [US-OTC]
Stri-dex® Maximum Strength [US-OTC]
Stri-dex® [US-OTC]
tazarotene
Tazorac® [US/Can]
Tinamed® [US-OTC]
Tiseb® [US-OTC]
Trans-Ver-Sal® [US-OTC/Can]
Wart-Off® Maximum Strength [US-OTC]
Zapzyt® Acne Wash [US-OTC]
Zapzyt® Pore Treatment [US-OTC]
Retinoic Acid Derivative
Accutane® [US/Can]
Altinac™ [US]
Amnesteem™ [US]
Avita® [US]
Claravis™ [US]
isotretinoin
Isotrex® [Can]
Rejuva-A® [Can]
Renova® [US]
Retin-A® Micro [US/Can]
Retin-A® [US/Can]
Retinova® [Can]
tretinoin (topical)
Tetracycline Derivative
Alti-Minocycline [Can]
Apo®-Minocycline [Can]
Apo®-Tetra [Can]
Brodspec® [US]
Declomycin® [US/Can]
demeclocycline
Dynacin® [US]
EmTet® [US]
Gen-Minocycline [Can]

Minocin® [US/Can]
minocycline
Novo-Minocycline [Can]
Novo-Tetra [Can]
Nu-Tetra [Can]
ratio-Minocycline [Can]
Rhoxal-minocycline [Can]
Sumycin® [US]
tetracycline
Wesmycin® [US]
Topical Skin Product
azelaic acid
Azelex® [US]
BenzaClin® [US]
clindamycin and benzoyl peroxide
Duac™ [US]
Finacea™ [US]
Finevin® [US]
Topical Skin Product, Acne
BenzaClin® [US]
clindamycin and benzoyl peroxide
Duac™ [US]

ACQUIRED IMMUNODEFICIENCY SYNDROME (AIDS)
Antiretroviral Agent, Fusion Protein Inhibitor
enfuvirtide
Fuzeon™ [US/Can]
Antiretroviral Agent, Non-nucleoside Reverse Transcriptase Inhibitor (NNRTI)
Kaletra™ [US/Can]
lopinavir and ritonavir
Antiretroviral Agent, Nucleoside Reverse Transcriptase Inhibitor (NRTI)
abacavir, lamivudine, and zidovudine
Trizivir® [US/Can]

Antiretroviral Agent, Protease Inhibitor
  atazanavir
  Reyataz™ [US]
Antiretroviral Agent, Reverse
    Transcriptase Inhibitor
    (Nucleoside)
  emtricitabine
  Emtriva™ [US]
Antiretroviral Agent, Reverse
    Transcriptase Inhibitor
    (Nucleotide)
  tenofovir
  Viread(TM) [US]
Antiviral Agent
  Apo®-Zidovudine [Can]
  AZT™ [Can]
  Combivir® [US/Can]
  Crixivan® [US/Can]
  delavirdine
  didanosine
  Epivir-HBV® [US]
  Epivir® [US]
  Fortovase® [US/Can]
  Heptovir® [Can]
  Hivid® [US/Can]
  indinavir
  Invirase® [US/Can]
  lamivudine
  nelfinavir
  nevirapine
  Norvir® SEC [Can]
  Norvir® [US/Can]
  Novo-AZT [Can]
  Rescriptor® [US/Can]
  Retrovir® [US/Can]
  ritonavir
  saquinavir
  stavudine
  3TC® [Can]
  Videx® EC [US/Can]
  Videx® [US/Can]
  Viracept® [US/Can]
  Viramune® [US/Can]

  zalcitabine
  Zerit® [US/Can]
  zidovudine
  zidovudine and lamivudine
Nonnucleoside Reverse Transcriptase
    Inhibitor (NNRTI)
  efavirenz
  Sustiva® [US/Can]
Nucleoside Reverse Transcriptase
    Inhibitor (NRTI)
  abacavir
  Ziagen® [US/Can]
Protease Inhibitor
  Agenerase® [US/Can]
  amprenavir

ADDISON DISEASE

Adrenal Corticosteroid
  A-HydroCort® [US]
  Betaject™ [Can]
  betamethasone (systemic)
  Betnesol® [Can]
  Celestone® Phosphate [US]
  Celestone® Soluspan® [US/Can]
  Celestone® [US]
  Cel-U-Jec® [US]
  Cortef® Tablet [US/Can]
  cortisone acetate
  Cortone® [Can]
  hydrocortisone (systemic)
  Solu-Cortef® [US/Can]
Adrenal Corticosteroid
    (Mineralocorticoid)
  Florinef® Acetate [US/Can]
  fludrocortisone
Diagnostic Agent
  Cortrosyn® [US/Can]
  cosyntropin

ADENOSINE DEAMINASE DEFICIENCY
Enzyme
    Adagen™ [US/Can]
    pegademase (bovine)

ADRENOCORTICAL FUNCTION ABNORMALITY
Adrenal Corticosteroid
    Acthar® [US]
    A-HydroCort® [US]
    A-methapred® [US]
    Apo®-Prednisone [Can]
    Aristocort® Forte Injection [US]
    Aristocort® Intralesional Injection [US]
    Aristocort® Tablet [US/Can]
    Aristospan® Intraarticular Injection
        [US/Can]
    Aristospan® Intralesional Injection
        [US/Can]
    Betaject™ [Can]
    betamethasone (systemic)
    Betnesol® [Can]
    Celestone® Phosphate [US]
    Celestone® Soluspan® [US/Can]
    Celestone® [US]
    Cel-U-Jec® [US]
    Cortef® Tablet [US/Can]
    corticotropin
    cortisone acetate
    Cortone® [Can]
    Decadron®-LA [US]
    Decadron® [US/Can]
    Decaject-LA® [US]
    Decaject® [US]
    Deltasone® [US]
    Depo-Medrol® [US/Can]
    Depopred® [US]
    dexamethasone (systemic)
    Dexasone® L.A. [US]
    Dexasone® [US/Can]
    Dexone® LA [US]

    Dexone® [US]
    Hexadrol® [US/Can]
    H.P. Acthar® Gel [US]
    hydrocortisone (systemic)
    Kenalog® Injection [US/Can]
    Medrol® Dosepak™ [US/Can]
    Medrol® Tablet [US/Can]
    methylprednisolone
    Orapred™ [US]
    Pediapred® [US/Can]
    PMS-Dexamethasone [Can]
    Prednicot® [US]
    prednisolone (systemic)
    Prednisol® TBA [US]
    prednisone
    Prednisone Intensol™ [US]
    Prelone® [US]
    ratio-Dexamethasone [Can]
    Solu-Cortef® [US/Can]
    Solu-Medrol® [US/Can]
    Solurex L.A.® [US]
    Sterapred® DS [US]
    Sterapred® [US]
    Tac™ -3 Injection [US]
    Triam-A® Injection [US]
    triamcinolone (systemic)
    Triam Forte® Injection [US]
    Winpred™ [Can]
Adrenal Corticosteroid
        (Mineralocorticoid)
    Florinef® Acetate [US/Can]
    fludrocortisone

ALLERGIC DISORDER
Adrenal Corticosteroid
    Acthar® [US]
    Aeroseb-Dex® [US]
    A-HydroCort® [US]
    A-methapred® [US]
    Apo®-Prednisone [Can]
    Aristocort® Forte Injection [US]
    Aristocort® Intralesional Injection [US]
    Aristocort® Tablet [US/Can]

Aristospan® Intraarticular Injection [US/Can]

Aristospan® Intralesional Injection [US/Can]

Betaject™ [Can]

betamethasone (systemic)

Betnesol® [Can]

Celestone® Phosphate [US]

Celestone® Soluspan® [US/Can]

Celestone® [US]

Cel-U-Jec® [US]

Cortef® Tablet [US/Can]

corticotropin

cortisone acetate

Cortone® [Can]

Decadron®-LA [US]

Decadron® [US/Can]

Decaject-LA® [US]

Decaject® [US]

Deltasone® [US]

Depo-Medrol® [US/Can]

Depopred® [US]

dexamethasone (systemic)

dexamethasone (topical)

Dexasone® L.A. [US]

Dexasone® [US/Can]

Dexone® LA [US]

Dexone® [US]

Hexadrol® [US/Can]

H.P. Acthar® Gel [US]

hydrocortisone (systemic)

Kenalog® Injection [US/Can]

Medrol® Dosepak(TM) [US/Can]

Medrol® Tablet [US/Can]

methylprednisolone

Orapred(TM) [US]

Pediapred® [US/Can]

PMS-Dexamethasone [Can]

Prednicot® [US]

prednisolone (systemic)

Prednisol® TBA [US]

prednisone

Prednisone Intensol™ [US]

Prelone® [US]

ratio-Dexamethasone [Can]

Solu-Cortef® [US/Can]

Solu-Medrol® [US/Can]

Solurex L.A.® [US]

Sterapred® DS [US]

Sterapred® [US]

Tac(TM)-3 Injection [US]

Triam-A® Injection [US]

™ triamcinolone (systemic)

Triam Forte® Injection [US]

Winpred™ [Can]

Adrenergic Agonist Agent

Adrenalin® Chloride [US/Can]

Epifrin® [US]

epinephrine

EpiPen® Jr [US/Can]

EpiPen® [US/Can]

Primatene® Mist [US-OTC]

Vaponefrin® [Can]

Antihistamine

Alavert™ [US-OTC]

Aler-Dryl [US-OTC]

Allegra® [US/Can]

Aller-Chlor® [US-OTC]

Allerdryl® [Can]

AllerMax® [US-OTC]

Allernix [Can]

Apo®-Cetirizine [Can]

Apo®-Dimenhydrinate [Can]

Apo®-Loratadine [Can]

azatadine

Banophen® [US-OTC]

Benadryl® Dye-Free Allergy [US-OTC]

Benadryl® Gel Extra Strength [US-OTC]

Benadryl® Gel [US-OTC]

Benadryl® Injection [US]

Benadryl® [US/Can]

cetirizine

chlorpheniramine

Chlor-Trimeton® [US-OTC]

Chlor-Tripolon® [Can]
Claritin® RediTabs® [US]
Claritin® [US-OTC/Can]
clemastine
Compoz® Nighttime Sleep Aid
   [US-OTC]
cyproheptadine
dexchlorpheniramine
dimenhydrinate
Diphen® AF [US-OTC]
Diphen® Cough [US-OTC]
Diphenhist [US-OTC]
diphenhydramine
Diphen® [US-OTC]
Dramamine® Oral [US-OTC]
fexofenadine
Genahist® [US-OTC]
Gravol® [Can]
Hydramine® Cough [US-OTC]
Hydramine® [US-OTC]
Hyrexin-50® [US]
loratadine
Nolahist® [US/Can]
Novo-Dimenate [Can]
Novo-Pheniram® [Can]
Nytol™ Extra Strength [Can]
Nytol® Maximum Strength [US-OTC]
Nytol® [US/Can]
Optimine® [US/Can]
phenindamine
PMS-Diphenhydramine [Can]
Reactine™ [Can]
Siladryl® Allergy [US-OTC]
Silphen® [US-OTC]
Sleepinal® [US-OTC]
Sominex® Maximum Strength [US-
   OTC]
Sominex® [US-OTC]
Tavist®-1 [US-OTC]
Tavist® [US]
TripTone® Caplets® [US-OTC]
Tusstat® [US]
Twilite® [US-OTC]

Unisom® Maximum Strength
   SleepGels® [US-OTC]
Zyrtec® [US]
Antihistamine/Decongestant
   Combination
   Andehist NR Drops [US]
   Carbaxefed RF [US]
   carbinoxamine and pseudoephedrine
   Hydro-Tussin™-CBX [US]
   Palgic®-DS [US]
   Palgic®-D [US]
   Rondec® Drops [US]
   Rondec® Tablet [US]
   Rondec-TR® [US]
   Sildec [US]
Phenothiazine Derivative
   Anergan® [US]
   Phenergan® [US/Can]
   promethazine

ALLERGIC DISORDER (NASAL)

Corticosteroid, Topical
   Nasacort® AQ [US/Can]
   triamcinolone (inhalation, nasal)
   Trinasal® [Can]
Mast Cell Stabilizer
   Apo®-Cromolyn [Can]
   Crolom® [US]
   cromolyn sodium
   Gastrocrom® [US]
   Intal® [US/Can]
   Nalcrom® [Can]
   Nasalcrom® [US-OTC]
   Nu-Cromolyn [Can]
   Opticrom® [US/Can]

ALLERGIC DISORDER (OPHTHALMIC)

Adrenal Corticosteroid
   HMS Liquifilm® [US]
   medrysone

ALLERGIC RHINITIS

Antihistamine
  Astelin® [US/Can]
  azelastine
  Optivar™ [US]

ALOPECIA

Antiandrogen
  finasteride
  Propecia® [US/Can]
  Proscar® [US/Can]
Progestin
  hydroxyprogesterone caproate
  Hylutin® [US]
  Prodrox® [US]
Topical Skin Product
  Apo®-Gain [Can]
  Minox [Can]
  minoxidil
  Rogaine® [Can]
  Rogaine® Extra Strength for Men
    [US-OTC]
  Rogaine® for Men [US-OTC]
  Rogaine® for Women [US-OTC]

ALPHA-1-ANTITRYPSIN DEFICIENCY (CONGENITAL)

Antitrypsin Deficiency Agent
  alpha-1-proteinase inhibitor
  Aralast™ [US]
  Prolastin® [US/Can]
  Zemaira™ [US]

ANAPHYLACTIC SHOCK

Adrenergic Agonist Agent
  Adrenalin® Chloride [US/Can]
  epinephrine

ANAPHYLACTIC SHOCK (PROPHYLAXIS)

Plasma Volume Expander
  dextran 1
  Promit® [US]

ANEMIA

Anabolic Steroid
  Anadrol® [US]
  oxymetholone
Androgen
  Deca-Durabolin® [Can]
  Durabolin® [Can]
  nandrolone
Antineoplastic Agent
  cyclophosphamide
  Cytoxan® [US/Can]
  Neosar® [US]
  Procytox® [Can]
Colony-Stimulating Factor
  Aranesp™ [US/Can]
  darbepoetin alfa
  epoetin alfa
  Epogen® [US]
  Eprex® [Can]
  Procrit® [US]
Electrolyte Supplement, Oral
  Apo®-Ferrous Gluconate [Can]
  Apo®-Ferrous Sulfate [Can]
  Dexferrum® [US]
  Dexiron™ [Can]
  Fe-40® [US-OTC]
  Femiron® [US-OTC]
  Feosol® Tablet [US-OTC]
  Feostat® [US-OTC]
  Feratab® [US-OTC]
  Fer-Gen-Sol [US-OTC]
  Fergon® [US-OTC]
  Fer-In-Sol® Drops [US/Can]
  Fer-Iron® [US-OTC]
  Ferodan™ [Can]
  Feronate® [US-OTC]
  Ferro-Sequels® [US-OTC]
  ferrous fumarate
  ferrous gluconate
  ferrous sulfate
  Fe-Tinic™ 150 [US-OTC]
  Hemocyte® [US-OTC]
  Hytinic® [US-OTC]

INFeD® [US]
Infufer® [Can]
Ircon® [US-OTC]
iron dextran complex
Nephro-Fer™ [US-OTC]
Niferex® 150 [US-OTC]
Niferex® [US-OTC]
Novo-Ferrogluc [Can]
Nu-Iron® 150 [US-OTC]
Palafer® [Can]
polysaccharide-iron complex
Slow FE® [US-OTC]
Growth Factor
Aranesp™ [US/Can]
darbepoetin alfa
Immune Globulin
BayGam® [US/Can]
immune globulin (intramuscular)
Immunosuppressant Agent
Apo®-Cyclosporine [Can]
Atgam® [US/Can]
cyclosporine
Gengraf™ [US]
lymphocyte immune globulin
Neoral® [US/Can]
Restasis™ [US]
Rhoxal-cyclosporine [Can]
Sandimmune® [US/Can]
Iron Salt
iron sucrose
Venofer® [US/Can]
Recombinant Human Erythropoietin
Aranesp™ [US/Can]
darbepoetin alfa
Vitamin
Fero-Grad 500® [US-OTC]
ferrous sulfate and ascorbic acid
ferrous sulfate, ascorbic acid, and
vitamin B-complex
ferrous sulfate, ascorbic acid,
vitamin B-complex, and folic acid
Iberet-Folic-500® [US]

Iberet®-Liquid 500 [US-OTC]
Iberet®-Liquid [US-OTC]
Vitelle™ Irospan® [US-OTC]
Vitamin, Water Soluble
Apo®-Folic [Can]
Cobal® [US]
Cobolin-M® [US]
cyanocobalamin
folic acid
Nascobal® [US]
Neuroforte-R® [US]
Scheinpharm B12 [Can]
Twelve Resin-K® [US]
Vita® #12 [US]
Vitabee® 12 [US]

ANGIOEDEMA (HEREDITARY)
Anabolic Steroid
stanozolol
Winstrol® [US]
Androgen
Cyclomen® [Can]
danazol
Danocrine® [US/Can]

ANTHRAX
Penicillin
amoxicillin
Amoxicot® [US]
Amoxil® [US]
Apo®-Amoxi [Can]
Gen-Amoxicillin [Can]
Lin-Amox [Can]
Moxilin® [US]
Novamoxin® [Can]
Nu-Amoxi [Can]
penicillin G (parenteral/aqueous)
penicillin G procaine
Pfizerpen® [US/Can]
PMS-Amoxicillin [Can]
Trimox® [US]

Wycillin® [US/Can]
Quinolone
　Ciloxan® [US/Can]
　ciprofloxacin
　Cipro® [US/Can]
　Cipro® XR [US/Can]
Tetracycline Derivative
　Adoxa™) [US]
　Alti-Minocycline [Can]
　Apo®-Doxy [Can]
　Apo®-Doxy Tabs [Can]
　Apo®-Minocycline [Can]
　Apo®-Tetra [Can]
　Brodspec® [US]
　Declomycin® [US/Can]
　demeclocycline
　Doryx® [US]
　Doxy-100® [US]
　Doxycin [Can]
　doxycycline
　Dynacin® [US]
　EmTet® [US]
　Gen-Minocycline [Can]
　Minocin® [US/Can]
　minocycline
　Monodox® [US]
　Novo-Doxylin [Can]
　Novo-Minocycline [Can]
　Novo-Tetra [Can]
　Nu-Doxycycline [Can]
　Nu-Tetra [Can]
　oxytetracycline
　Periostat® [US]
　ratio-Doxycycline [Can]
　ratio-Minocycline [Can]
　Rhoxal-minocycline [Can]
　Sumycin® [US]
　Terramycin® I.M. [US/Can]
　tetracycline
　Vibramycin® [US]
　Vibra-Tabs® [US/Can]
　Wesmycin® [US]
Vaccine
　anthrax vaccine, adsorbed

BioThrax™ [US]

ARTHRITIS
Aminoquinoline (Antimalarial)
　Apo®-Hydroxyquine [Can]
　Aralen® Phosphate [US/Can]
　chloroquine phosphate
　hydroxychloroquine
　Plaquenil® [US/Can]
Analgesic, Topical
　Antiphlogistine Rub A-535
　　Capsaicin [Can]
　ArthriCare® for Women Extra
　　Moisturizing [US-OTC]
　ArthriCare® for Women Silky Dry
　　[US-OTC]
　Capsagel® [US-OTC]
　capsaicin
　Capzasin-HP® [US-OTC]
　TheraPatch® Warm [US-OTC]
　Zostrix®-HP [US/Can]
　Zostrix® [US/Can]
Antiinflammatory Agent
　Arava™ [US/Can]
　leflunomide
Antineoplastic Agent
　Apo®-Methotrexate [Can]
　cyclophosphamide
　Cytoxan® [US/Can]
　methotrexate
　Neosar® [US]
　Procytox® [Can]
　ratio-Methotrexate [Can]
　Rheumatrex® [US]
　Trexall™ [US]
Antirheumatic, Disease Modifying
　adalimumab
　anakinra
　Enbrel® [US]
　etanercept
　Humira™ [US]
　Kineret™ [US/Can]
Chelating Agent
　Cuprimine® [US/Can]

Depen® [US/Can]
penicillamine
Gold Compound
auranofin
Aurolate® [US]
aurothioglucose
gold sodium thiomalate
Myochrysine® [Can]
Ridaura® [US/Can]
Solganal® [US/Can]
Immunosuppressant Agent
Alti-Azathioprine [Can]
Apo®-Azathioprine [Can]
Apo®-Cyclosporine [Can]
azathioprine
cyclosporine
Gen-Azathioprine [Can]
Gengraf™ [US]
Imuran® [US/Can]
Neoral® [US/Can]
ratio-Azathioprine [Can]
Restasis™ [US]
Rhoxal-cyclosporine [Can]
Sandimmune® [US/Can]
Monoclonal Antibody
adalimumab
Humira™ [US]
Nonsteroidal Antiinflammatory Drug
(NSAID)
Advil® Children's [US-OTC]
Advil® Infants' Concentrated Drops
[US-OTC]
Advil® Junior [US-OTC]
Advil® Migraine [US-OTC]
Advil® [US/Can]
Albert® Tiafen [Can]
Aleve® [US-OTC]
Amigesic® [US/Can]
Anaprox® DS [US/Can]
Anaprox® [US/Can]
Ansaid® Oral [US/Can]
Apo®-Diclo [Can]

Apo®-Diclo SR [Can]
Apo®-Diflunisal [Can]
Apo®-Flurbiprofen [Can]
Apo®-Ibuprofen [Can]
Apo®-Indomethacin [Can]
Apo®-Keto [Can]
Apo®-Keto-E [Can]
Apo®-Keto SR [Can]
Apo®-Nabumetone [Can]
Apo®-Napro-Na [Can]
Apo®-Napro-Na DS [Can]
Apo®-Naproxen [Can]
Apo®-Naproxen SR [Can]
Apo®-Oxaprozin [Can]
Apo®-Sulin [Can]
Apo®-Tiaprofenic [Can]
Argesic®-SA [US]
Asaphen [Can]
Asaphen E.C. [Can]
Ascriptin® Arthritis Pain [US-OTC]
Ascriptin® Enteric [US-OTC]
Ascriptin® Extra Strength [US-OTC]
Ascriptin® [US-OTC]
Aspercin Extra [US-OTC]
Aspercin [US-OTC]
aspirin
Bayer® Aspirin Extra Strength [US-
OTC]
Bayer® Aspirin Regimen Adult
Low Strength [US-OTC]
Bayer® Aspirin Regimen Adult
Low Strength with Calcium [US-
OTC]
Bayer® Aspirin Regimen Children's
[US-OTC]
Bayer® Aspirin Regimen Regular
Strength [US-OTC]
Bayer® Aspirin [US-OTC]
Bayer® Plus Extra Strength [US-
OTC]
Bufferin® Arthritis Strength [US-
OTC]

Bufferin® Extra Strength [US-OTC]
Bufferin® [US-OTC]
Cataflam® [US/Can]
choline magnesium trisalicylate
Clinoril® [US]
Daypro™ [US/Can]
diclofenac
diflunisal
Doan's®, Original [US-OTC]
Dolobid® [US]
Easprin® [US]
EC-Naprosyn® [US]
Ecotrin® Adult Low Strength [US-OTC]
Ecotrin® Maximum Strength [US-OTC]
Ecotrin® [US-OTC]
Entrophen® [Can]
Extra Strength Doan's® [US-OTC]
Feldene® [US/Can]
fenoprofen
flurbiprofen
Froben® [Can]
Froben-SR® [Can]
Gen-Nabumetone [Can]
Gen-Naproxen EC [Can]
Gen-Piroxicam [Can]
Genpril® [US-OTC]
Halfprin® [US-OTC]
Haltran® [US-OTC]
ibuprofen
Ibu-Tab® [US]
Indocid® [Can]
Indocid® P.D.A. [Can]
Indocin® SR [US]
Indocin® [US]
Indo-Lemmon [Can]
indomethacin
I-Prin [US-OTC]
ketoprofen
Keygesic-10® [US]
magnesium salicylate
meclofenamate

Menadol® [US-OTC]
Midol® Maximum Strength Cramp Formula [US-OTC]
Momentum® [US-OTC]
Mono-Gesic® [US]
Motrin® Children's [US/Can]
Motrin® IB [US/Can]
Motrin® Infants' [US-OTC]
Motrin® Junior Strength [US-OTC]
Motrin® Migraine Pain [US-OTC]
Motrin® [US/Can]
nabumetone
Nalfon® [US/Can]
Naprelan® [US]
Naprosyn® [US/Can]
naproxen
Naxen® [Can]
Novasen [Can]
Novo-Difenac® [Can]
Novo-Difenac-K [Can]
Novo-Difenac® SR [Can]
Novo-Diflunisal [Can]
Novo-Flurprofen [Can]
Novo-Keto [Can]
Novo-Keto-EC [Can]
Novo-Methacin [Can]
Novo-Naprox [Can]
Novo-Naprox Sodium [Can]
Novo-Naprox Sodium DS [Can]
Novo-Naprox SR [Can]
Novo-Pirocam® [Can]
Novo-Profen® [Can]
Novo-Sundac [Can]
Novo-Tiaprofenic [Can]
Nu-Diclo [Can]
Nu-Diclo-SR [Can]
Nu-Diflunisal [Can]
Nu-Flurprofen [Can]
Nu-Ibuprofen [Can]
Nu-Indo [Can]
Nu-Ketoprofen [Can]
Nu-Ketoprofen-E [Can]
Nu-Naprox [Can]

Nu-Pirox [Can]
Nu-Sundac [Can]
Nu-Tiaprofenic [Can]
Ocufen® Ophthalmic [US/Can]
Orudis® KT [US-OTC]
Orudis® SR [Can]
Oruvail® [US/Can]
oxaprozin
Pennsaid® [Can]
Pexicam® [Can]
piroxicam
PMS-Diclofenac [Can]
PMS-Diclofenac SR [Can]
PMS-Tiaprofenic [Can]
ratio-Flurbiprofen [Can]
ratio-Indomethacin [Can]
Relafen® [US/Can]
Rhodacine® [Can]
Rhodis™ [Can]
Rhodis-EC™ [Can]
Rhodis SR™ [Can]
Rhoxal-nabumetone [Can]
Riva-Diclofenac [Can]
Riva-Diclofenac-K [Can]
Riva-Naproxen [Can]
Salflex® [US/Can]
salsalate
Solaraze™ [US]
St. Joseph® Pain Reliever [US-OTC]
sulindac
Sureprin 81™ [US-OTC]
Surgam® [Can]
Surgam® SR [Can]
tiaprofenic acid (Canada only)
Tolectin® DS [US]
Tolectin® [US/Can]
tolmetin
Tricosal® [US]
Trilisate® [US]
Voltaren Rapide® [Can]
Voltaren® [US/Can]
Voltaren®-XR [US]

Voltare Ophtha® [Can]
ZORprin® [US]
Nonsteroidal Antiinflammatory Drug (NSAID), COX-2 Selective
Celebrex® [US/Can]
celecoxib

ARTHRITIS (RHEUMATOID)
Nonsteroidal Antiinflammatory Drug (NSAID), COX-2 Selective
Bextra™ [US/Can]
valdecoxib

ASCARIASIS
Anthelmintic
albendazole
Albenza® [US]

ASPERGILLOSIS
A Antifungal Agent
Abelcet® [US/Can]
Amphocin® [US]
Amphotec® [US/Can]
amphotericin B cholesteryl sulfate complex
amphotericin B (conventional)
amphotericin B lipid complex
Ancobon® [US/Can]
flucytosine
Fungizone® [US/Can]
VFEND® [US]
voriconazole
Antifungal Agent, Systemic
AmBisome® [US/Can]
amphotericin B liposomal
Cancidas® [US/Can]
caspofungin

ASTHMA
Adrenal Corticosteroid
Apo®-Beclomethasone [Can]
Azmacort® [US]

beclomethasone
Beconase® AQ [US]
Decadron®-LA [US]
Decadron® [US/Can]
Decaject-LA® [US]
Decaject® [US]
dexamethasone (systemic)
Dexasone® L.A. [US]
Dexasone® [US/Can]
Dexone® LA [US]
Dexone® [US]
Flovent® HFA [Can]
Flovent® Rotadisk® [US]
Flovent® [US]
fluticasone (oral inhalation)
Gen-Beclo [Can]
Hexadrol® [US/Can]
Nu-Beclomethasone [Can]
PMS-Dexamethasone [Can]
Propaderm® [Can]
QVAR™ [US/Can]
ratio-Dexamethasone [Can]
Rivanase AQ [Can]
Solurex L.A.® [US]
triamcinolone (inhalation, oral)
Adrenergic Agonist Agent
AccuNeb™ [US]
Adrenalin® Chloride [US/Can]
Airomir [Can]
albuterol
Alti-Salbutamol [Can]
Alupent® [US]
Apo®-Salvent [Can]
Brethine® [US]
Bricanyl® [Can]
ephedrine
epinephrine
Gen-Salbutamol [Can]
isoetharine
isoproterenol
Isuprel® [US]
Levophed® [US/Can]
Maxair™ Autohaler™ [US]

Maxair™ [US]
metaproterenol
norepinephrine
pirbuterol
PMS-Salbutamol [Can]
Pretz-D® [US-OTC]
Primatene® Mist [US-OTC]
Proventil® HFA [US]
Proventil® Repetabs® [US]
Proventil® [US]
ratio-Salbutamol [Can]
Rhoxal-salbutamol [Can]
Salbu-2 [Can]
Salbu-4 [Can]
salmeterol
Serevent® [Can]
Serevent® Diskus® [US]
terbutaline
Vaponefrin® [Can]
Ventolin® HFA [US]
Ventrodisk [Can]
Volmax® [US]
VoSpire ER™ [US]
Anticholinergic Agent
Apo®-Ipravent [Can]
Atrovent® [US/Can]
Gen-Ipratropium [Can]
ipratropium
Novo-Ipramide [Can]
Nu-Ipratropium [Can]
PMS-Ipratropium [Can]
ratio-Ipratropium [Can]
Beta-2-Adrenergic Agonist Agent
Advair™ Diskus® [US/Can]
Berotec® [Can]
budesonide and formoterol (Canada only)
fenoterol (Canada only)
fluticasone and salmeterol
Foradil® Aerolizer™ [US/Can]
formoterol
Symbicort® Turbuhaler [Can]
Corticosteroid, Inhalant

Advair™ Diskus® [US/Can]
fluticasone and salmeterol
Corticosteroid, Inhalant (Oral)
budesonide and formoterol (Canada only)
Symbicort® Turbuhaler [Can]
Leukotriene Receptor Antagonist
Accolate® [US/Can]
montelukast
Singulair® [US/Can]
zafirlukast
Mast Cell Stabilizer
Apo®-Cromolyn [Can]
Crolom® [US]
cromolyn sodium
Intal® [US/Can]
Nalcrom® [Can]
Nasalcrom® [US-OTC]
nedocromil (inhalation)
Nu-Cromolyn [Can]
Opticrom® [US/Can]
Tilade® [US/Can]
Monoclonal Antibody
omalizumab
Xolair® [US]
Theophylline Derivative
aminophylline
Apo®-Theo LA [Can]
Dilor® [US/Can]
dyphylline
Elixophyllin-GG® [US]
Elixophyllin® [US]
Lufyllin® [US/Can]
Neoasma® [US]
Novo-Theophyl SR [Can]
Phyllocontin®-350 [Can]
Phyllocontin® [Can]
Quibron®-T/SR [US/Can]
Quibron®-T [US]
Quibron® [US]
Theo-24® [US]
Theochron® [US]
Theocon® [US]

Theolair™ [US/Can]
Theolate® [US]
Theomar® GG [US]
theophylline
theophylline and guaifenesin
T-Phyl® [US]
Uniphyl® [US/Can]

ASTHMA (CORTICOSTEROID-DEPENDENT)
Macrolide (Antibiotic)
Tao® [US]
troleandomycin

ASTHMA (DIAGNOSTIC)
Diagnostic Agent
methacholine
Provocholine® [US/Can]

ATOPIC DERMATITIS
Immunosuppressant Agent
Elidel® [US/Can]
pimecrolimus
Topical Skin Product
Elidel® [US/Can]
pimecrolimus

BEHÇET SYNDROME
Immunosuppressant Agent
Alti-Azathioprine [Can]
Apo®-Azathioprine [Can]
Apo®-Cyclosporine [Can]
azathioprine
cyclosporine
Gen-Azathioprine [Can]
Gengraf™ [US]
Imuran® [US/Can]
Neoral® [US/Can]
ratio-Azathioprine [Can]
Restasis™ [US]
Rhoxal-cyclosporine [Can]
Sandimmune® [US/Can]

BITE (INSECT)
Adrenergic Agonist Agent
   Adrenalin® Chloride [US/Can]
   epinephrine
   EpiPen® Jr [US/Can]
   EpiPen® [US/Can]
Analgesic, Topical
   Anestacon® [US]
   Band-Aid® Hurt-Free™ Antiseptic
      Wash [US-OTC]
   Betacaine® [Can]
   LidaMantle® [US]
   lidocaine
   Lidoderm® [US/Can]
   L-M-X™ 4 [US-OTC]
   L-M-X™ 5 [US-OTC]
   Premjact® [US-OTC]
   Topicaine® [US-OTC]
   Xylocaine® MPF [US]
   Xylocaine® [US/Can]
   Xylocaine® Viscous [US]
   Xylocard® [Can]
Antidote
   Ana-Kit® [US]
   epinephrine and chlorpheniramine
Antihistamine
   Aler-Dryl [US-OTC]
   Allerdryl® [Can]
   AllerMax® [US-OTC]
   Allernix [Can]
   Banophen® [US-OTC]
   Benadryl® Dye-Free Allergy [US-
      OTC]
   Benadryl® Gel Extra Strength [US-
      OTC]
   Benadryl® Gel [US-OTC]
   Benadryl® Injection [US]
   Benadryl® [US/Can]
   Diphenhist [US-OTC]
   diphenhydramine
   Diphen® [US-OTC]
   Genahist® [US-OTC]
   Hydramine® [US-OTC]
   Hyrexin-50® [US]
   PMS-Diphenhydramine [Can]
   Siladryl® Allergy [US-OTC]
   Silphen® [US-OTC]
Corticosteroid, Topical
   Aclovate® [US]
   Acticort® [US]
   Aeroseb-HC® [US]
   alclometasone
   amcinonide
   Amcort® [Can]
   Anusol® HC-1 [US-OTC]
   Anusol® HC-2.5% [US-OTC]
   Aquacort® [Can]
   Aristocort® A Topical [US]
   Aristocort® Topical [US]
   Bactine® Hydrocortisone [US-
      OTC]
   CaldeCORT® Anti-Itch Spray [US]
   CaldeCORT® [US-OTC]
   Capex™ [US/Can]
   Carmol-HC® [US]
   Cetacort®
   clobetasol
   Clocort® Maximum Strength [US-
      OTC]
   clocortolone
   Cloderm® [US/Can]
   Cordran® SP [US]
   Cordran® [US/Can]
   Cormax® [US]
   CortaGel® [US-OTC]
   Cortaid® Maximum Strength [US-
      OTC]
   Cortaid® with Aloe [US-OTC]
   Cort-Dome® [US]
   Cortizone®-5 [US-OTC]
   Cortizone®-10 [US-OTC]
   Cortoderm [Can]
   Cutivate™ [US]
   Cyclocort® [US/Can]
   Delcort® [US]

Dermacort® [US]
Dermarest Dricort® [US]
Derma-Smoothe/FS® [US/Can]
Dermatop® [US/Can]
Dermolate® [US-OTC]
Dermovate® [Can]
Dermtex® HC with Aloe [US-OTC]
Desocort® [Can]
desonide
DesOwen® [US]
Desoxi® [Can]
desoximetasone
diflorasone
Eldecort® [US]
Elocon® [US/Can]
Embeline™ E [US]
fluocinolone
fluocinonide
Fluoderm [Can]
flurandrenolide
fluticasone (topical)
Gen-Clobetasol [Can]
Gynecort® [US-OTC]
halcinonide
halobetasol
Halog®-E [US]
Halog® [US/Can]
Hi-Cor-1.0® [US]
Hi-Cor-2.5® [US]
Hyderm [Can]
hydrocortisone (topical)
Hydrocort® [US]
Hydro-Tex® [US-OTC]
Hytone® [US]
Kenalog® in Orabase® [US/Can]
Kenalog® Topical [US/Can]
LactiCare-HC® [US]
Lanacort® [US-OTC]
Lidemol® [Can]
Lidex-E® [US]
Lidex® [US/Can]
Locoid® [US/Can]
Lyderm® [Can]

Maxiflor® [US]
mometasone furoate
Nasonex® [US/Can]
Novo-Clobetasol [Can]
Nutracort® [US]
Olux® [US]
Orabase® HCA [US]
Oracort [Can]
Penecort® [US]
PMS-Desonide [Can]
prednicarbate
Prevex® HC [Can]
Psorcon™ E [US]
Psorcon™ [US/Can]
ratio-Clobetasol [Can]
Sarna® HC [Can]
Scalpicin® [US]
S-T Cort® [US]
Synacort® [US]
Synalar® [US/Can]
Taro-Desoximetasone [Can]
Tegrin®-HC [US-OTC]
Temovate E® [US]
Temovate® [US]
Tiamol® [Can]
Ti-U-Lac® H [Can]
Topicort®-LP [US]
Topicort® [US/Can]
Topsyn® [Can]
Triacet™ Topical [US]
Triaderm [Can]
triamcinolone (topical)
Tridesilon® [US]
U-Cort™ [US]
Ultravate™ [US/Can]
urea and hydrocortisone
Uremol® HC [Can]
Westcort® [US/Can]
Local Anesthetic
    AK-T-Caine™ [US]
    Ametop™ [Can]
    Anusol® [US-OTC]
    Cepacol Viractin® [US-OTC]

Fleet® Pain Relief [US-OTC]
Itch-X® [US-OTC]
Opticaine® [US]
Phicon® [US-OTC]
Pontocaine® [US/Can]
PrameGel® [US-OTC]
pramoxine
Prax® [US-OTC]
ProctoFoam® NS [US-OTC]
tetracaine
Tronolane® [US-OTC]
Tronothane® [US-OTC]

BITE (SNAKE)
Antivenin
antivenin (Crotalidae) polyvalent
antivenin (Micrurus fulvius)
Antivenin Polyvalent [Equine] [US]
CroFab™ [Ovine] [US]

BITE (SPIDER)
Antivenin
antivenin (Latrodectus mactans)
Electrolyte Supplement, Oral
calcium gluconate
Calfort® [US]
Cal-G® [US]
Skeletal Muscle Relaxant
methocarbamol
Robaxin® [US/Can]

BLASTOMYCOSIS
Antifungal Agent
Apo®-Ketoconazole [Can]
itraconazole
ketoconazole
Ketoderm® [Can]
Nizoral® A-D [US-OTC]
Nizoral® [US/Can]
Novo-Ketoconazole [Can]
Sporanox® [US/Can]

BLEPHARITIS
Antifungal Agent
Natacyn® [US/Can]
natamycin
urokinase

BULLOUS SKIN DISEASE
Antibacterial, Topical
Dermazin™ [Can]
Flamazine® [Can]
Silvadene® [US]
silver sulfadiazine
SSD® AF [US]
SSD® Cream [US/Can]
Thermazene® [US]
Gold Compound
Aurolate® [US]
aurothioglucose
gold sodium thiomalate
Myochrysine® [Can]
Solganal® [US/Can]
Immunosuppressant Agent
Alti-Azathioprine [Can]
Apo®-Azathioprine [Can]
azathioprine
Gen-Azathioprine [Can]
Imuran® [US/Can]
ratio-Azathioprine [Can]

BURN
Antibacterial, Topical
Dermazin™ [Can]
Flamazine® [Can]
mafenide
nitrofurazone
Silvadene® [US]
silver sulfadiazine
SSD® AF [US]
SSD® Cream [US/Can]
Sulfamylon® [US]
Thermazene® [US]
Protectant, Topical
A and D® Ointment [US-OTC]

Baza® Clear [US-OTC]
Clocream® [US-OTC]
Desitin® [US-OTC]
vitamin A and vitamin D
zinc oxide, cod liver oil, and talc

CANDIDIASIS
Antifungal Agent
Abelcet® [US/Can]
Absorbine Jr.® Antifungal [US-OTC]
Aftate® Antifungal [US-OTC]
Aloe Vesta® 2-n-1 Antifungal [US-OTC]
Amphocin® [US]
Amphotec® [US/Can]
amphotericin B cholesteryl sulfate complex
amphotericin B (conventional)
amphotericin B lipid complex
Ancobon® [US/Can]
Apo®-Fluconazole [Can]
Apo®-Ketoconazole [Can]
Baza® Antifungal [US-OTC]
Bio-Statin® [US]
Blis-To-Sol® [US-OTC]
butoconazole
Candistatin® [Can]
Canesten® Topical [Can]
Canesten® Vaginal [Can]
Carrington Antifungal [US-OTC]
ciclopirox
Clotrimaderm [Can]
clotrimazole
Cruex® [US-OTC]
1-Day™ [US-OTC]
Dermasept Antifungal [US-OTC]
Diflucan® [US/Can]
econazole
Ecostatin® [Can]
Exelderm® [US/Can]
Femizol-M™ [US-OTC]
Femstat® One [Can]

fluconazole
flucytosine
Fungi-Guard [US-OTC]
Fungizone® [US/Can]
Fungoid® Tincture [US-OTC]
Gen-Fluconazole [Can]
Gold Bond® Antifungal [US-OTC]
Gynazole-1™ [US]
Gyne-Lotrimin® 3 [US-OTC]
Gyne-Lotrimin® [US-OTC]
Gynix® [US-OTC]
itraconazole
ketoconazole
Ketoderm® [Can]
Lamisil® Cream [US]
Loprox® [US/Can]
Lotrimin® AF Athlete's Foot Cream [US-OTC]
Lotrimin® AF Athlete's Foot Solution [US-OTC]
Lotrimin® AF Jock Itch Cream [US-OTC]
Lotrimin® AF Powder/Spray [US-OTC]
Micaderm® [US-OTC]
Micatin® [US/Can]
miconazole
Micozole [Can]
Micro-Guard® [US-OTC]
Mitrazol™ [US-OTC]
Monistat® 1 Combination Pack [US-OTC]
Monistat® 3 [US-OTC]
Monistat® 7 [US-OTC]
Monistat® [Can]
Monistat-Derm® [US]
Mycelex®-3 [US-OTC]
Mycelex®-7 [US-OTC]
Mycelex® Twin Pack [US-OTC]
Mycostatin® [US/Can]
naftifine
Naftin® [US]

Nizoral® A-D [US-OTC]
Nizoral® [US/Can]
Novo-Fluconazole [Can]
Novo-Ketoconazole [Can]
Nyaderm [Can]
nystatin
Nystat-Rx® [US]
Nystop® [US]
oxiconazole
Oxistat® [US/Can]
Pedi-Dri® [US]
Penlac™ [US/Can]
Pitrex [CAN]
PMS-Nystatin [Can]
ratio-Nystatin [Can]
Spectazole™) [US/Can]
Sporanox® [US/Can]
sulconazole
Terazol® 3 [US/Can]
Terazol® 7 [US/Can]
terbinafine (topical)
terconazole
Tinactin® Antifungal Jock Itch [US-OTC]
Tinactin® Antifungal [US-OTC]
Tinaderm [US-OTC]
Ting® [US-OTC]
tioconazole
TipTapToe [US-OTC]
tolnaftate
Triple Care® Antifungal [OTC]
Trosyd™ AF [Can]
Trosyd™ J [Can]
Vagistat®-1 [US-OTC]
Zeasorb®-AF [US-OTC]
Antifungal Agent, Systemic
AmBisome® [US/Can]
amphotericin B liposomal
Antifungal/Corticosteroid
Mycolog®-II [US]
Mytrex® [US]
nystatin and triamcinolone

CANKER SORE
Antiinfective Agent, Oral
Cankaid® [US-OTC]
carbamide peroxide
Gly-Oxide® Oral [US-OTC]
Orajel® Perioseptic® [US-OTC]
Antiinflammatory Agent, Locally Applied
amlexanox
Aphthasol™ [US]
Local Anesthetic
Anbesol® Maximum Strength [US-OTC]
Anbesol® [US-OTC]
benzocaine
Benzodent® [US-OTC]
HDA® Toothache [US-OTC]
Hurricaine® [US]
Mycinettes® [US-OTC]
Orabase®-B [US-OTC]
Orajel® Maximum Strength [US-OTC]
Orajel® [US-OTC]
Orasol® [US-OTC]
Zilactin®-B [US/Can]
Protectant, Topical
gelatin, pectin, and methylcellulose
Orabase® Plain [US-OTC]

CHICKENPOX
Antiviral Agent
acyclovir
Apo®-Acyclovir [Can]
Gen-Acyclovir [Can]
Nu-Acyclovir [Can]
Zovirax® [US/Can]
Vaccine, Live Virus
varicella virus vaccine
Varivax® [US/Can]

CHROMOBLASTOMYCOSIS
Antifungal Agent
  Apo®-Ketoconazole [Can]
  ketoconazole
  Nizoral® [US/Can]
  Novo-Ketoconazole [Can]

CIRRHOSIS
Bile Acid Sequestrant
  cholestyramine resin
  Novo-Cholamine [Can]
  Novo-Cholamine Light [Can]
  PMS-Cholestyramine [Can]
  Prevalite® [US]
  Questran® Light [US/Can]
  Questran® Powder [US/Can]
Chelating Agent
  Cuprimine® [US/Can]
  Depen® [US/Can]
  penicillamine
Electrolyte Supplement, Oral
  Alcalak [US-OTC]
  Alka-Mints® [US-OTC]
  Amitone® [US-OTC]
  Apo®-Cal [Can]
  Calbon® [US]
  Calcarb 600 [US-OTC]
  Cal Carb-HD® [US-OTC]
  Calci-Chew™ [US-OTC]
  Calci-Mix™ [US-OTC]
  Calcionate® [US-OTC]
  Calciquid® [US-OTC]
  Cal-Citrate® 250 [US-OTC]
  calcium carbonate
  calcium citrate
  calcium glubionate
  calcium lactate
  Cal-Gest [US-OTC]
  Cal-Lac® [US]
  Cal-Mint [US-OTC]
  Caltrate® 600 [US/Can]
  Chooz® [US-OTC]

Citracal® [US-OTC]
Florical® [US-OTC]
Mallamint® [US-OTC]
Mylanta® Children's [US-OTC]
Nephro-Calci® [US-OTC]
Os-Cal® 500 [US/Can]
Oysco 500 [US-OTC]
Oyst-Cal 500 [US-OTC]
Oystercal® 500 [US]
Ridactate® [US]
Rolaids® Extra Strength [US-OTC]
Titralac™ Extra Strength [US-OTC]
Titralac™ [US-OTC]
Tums® 500 [US-OTC]
Tums® E-X Extra Strength Tablet
  [US-OTC]
Tums® E-X [US-OTC]
Tums® Smooth Dissolve [US-OTC]
Tums® Ultra [US-OTC]
Tums® [US-OTC]
Immunosuppressant Agent
  Alti-Azathioprine [Can]
  Apo®-Azathioprine [Can]
  azathioprine
  Gen-Azathioprine [Can]
  Imuran® [US/Can]
  ratio-Azathioprine [Can]
Vitamin D Analog
  Calciferol™ [US]
  Drisdol® [US/Can]
  ergocalciferol
  Ostoforte® [Can]
Vitamin, Fat Soluble
  AquaMEPHYTON® [US/Can]
  Aquasol A® [US]
  Mephyton® [US/Can]
  Palmitate-A® [US-OTC]
  phytonadione
  vitamin A

COCCIDIOIDOMYCOSIS
Antifungal Agent
   Apo®-Ketoconazole [Can]
   ketoconazole
   Ketoderm® [Can]
   Nizoral® A-D [US-OTC]
   Nizoral® [US/Can]
   Novo-Ketoconazole [Can]

COLD SORE
Antiviral Agent
   Denavir™ [US]
   penciclovir

COLLAGEN DISORDER
Adrenal Corticosteroid
   Acthar® [US]
   A-HydroCort® [US]
   A-methapred® [US]
   Apo®-Prednisone [Can]
   Aristocort® Forte Injection [US]
   Aristocort® Intralesional Injection
     [US]
   Aristocort® Tablet [US/Can]
   Aristospan® Intraarticular Injection
     [US/Can]
   Aristospan® Intralesional Injection
     [US/Can]
   Betaject™ [Can]
   betamethasone (systemic)
   Betnesol® [Can]
   Celestone® Phosphate [US]
   Celestone® Soluspan® [US/Can]
   Celestone® [US]
   Cel-U-Jec® [US]
   Cortef® Tablet [US/Can]
   corticotropin
   cortisone acetate
   Cortone® [Can]
   Decadron®-LA [US]
   Decadron® [US/Can]
   Decaject-LA® [US]
   Decaject® [US]
   Deltasone® [US]
   Depo-Medrol® [US/Can]
   Depopred® [US]
   dexamethasone (systemic)
   Dexasone® L.A. [US]
   Dexasone® [US/Can]
   Dexone® LA [US]
   Dexone® [US]
   Hexadrol® [US/Can]
   H.P. Acthar® Gel [US]
   hydrocortisone (systemic)
   Kenalog® Injection [US/Can]
   Medrol® Dosepak™ [US/Can]
   Medrol® Tablet [US/Can]
   methylprednisolone
   Orapred™ [US]
   Pediapred® [US/Can]
   PMS-Dexamethasone [Can]
   Prednicot® [US]
   prednisolone (systemic)
   Prednisol® TBA [US]
   prednisone
   Prednisone Intensol™ [US]
   Prelone® [US]
   ratio-Dexamethasone [Can]
   Solu-Cortef® [US/Can]
   Solu-Medrol® [US/Can]
   Solurex L.A.® [US]
   Sterapred® DS [US]
   Sterapred® [US]
   Tac™ -3 Injection [US]
   Triam-A® Injection [US]
   triamcinolone (systemic)
   Triam Forte® Injection [US]
   Winpred™ [Can]

CONDYLOMA ACUMINATUM
Antiviral Agent
   interferon alfa-2b and ribavirin
     combination pack
   Rebetron™ [US/Can]
Biological Response Modulator
   Alferon® N [US/Can]
   interferon alfa-2a

interferon alfa-2b
interferon alfa-2b and ribavirin
 combination pack
interferon alfa-n3
Intron® A [US/Can]
Rebetron™ [US/Can]
Roferon-A® [US/Can]
Immune Response Modifier
 Aldara™ [US/Can]
 imiquimod
Keratolytic Agent
 Condyline™ [Can]
 Condylox® [US]
 Podocon-25™ [US]
 Podofilm® [Can]
 podofilox
 podophyllum resin
 Wartec® [Can]

CONJUNCTIVITIS (ALLERGIC)

Adrenal Corticosteroid
 HMS Liquifilm® [US]
 medrysone
Antihistamine
 Alavert™ [US-OTC]
 Aler-Dryl [US-OTC]
 Aller-Chlor® [US-OTC]
 Allerdryl® [Can]
 AllerMax® [US-OTC]
 Allernix [Can]
 ANX® [US]
 Apo®-Dimenhydrinate [Can]
 Apo®-Hydroxyzine [Can]
 Apo®-Loratadine [Can]
 Atarax® [US/Can]
 azatadine
 Banophen® [US-OTC]
 Benadryl® Dye-Free Allergy [US-OTC]
 Benadryl® [US/Can]
 brompheniramine

chlorpheniramine
Chlor-Trimeton® [US-OTC]
Chlor-Tripolon® [Can]
Claritin® RediTabs® [US]
Claritin® [US-OTC/Can]
clemastine
cyproheptadine
dexchlorpheniramine
dimenhydrinate
Dimetane® Extentabs® [US-OTC]
Dimetapp® Allergy Children's [US-OTC]
Dimetapp® Allergy [US-OTC]
Diphen® AF [US-OTC]
Diphenhist [US-OTC]
diphenhydramine
Genahist® [US-OTC]
Gravol® [Can]
hydroxyzine
Hyrexin-50® [US]
levocabastine
Livostin® [US/Can]
Lodrane® 12 Hour [US-OTC]
loratadine
ND-Stat® Solution [US-OTC]
Nolahist® [US/Can]
Novo-Dimenate [Can]
Novo-Hydroxyzin [Can]
Novo-Pheniram® [Can]
olopatadine
Optimine® [US/Can]
Patanol® [US/Can]
phenindamine
PMS-Diphenhydramine [Can]
PMS-Hydroxyzine [Can]
Polytapp® Allergy Dye-Free
 Medication [US-OTC]
Siladryl® Allergy [US-OTC]
Silphen® [US-OTC]
Tavist®-1 [US-OTC]
Tavist® [US]
Vistacot® [US]

Vistaril® [US/Can]
Antihistamine/Decongestant
    Combination
    Andehist NR Drops [US]
    Carbaxefed RF [US]
    carbinoxamine and pseudoephedrine
    Hydro-Tussin™ -CBX [US]
    Palgic®-DS [US]
    Palgic®-D [US]
    Rondec® Drops [US]
    Rondec® Tablet [US]
    Rondec-TR® [US]
    Sildec [US]
Antihistamine, H-1 Blocker,
    Ophthalmic
    Apo®-Ketotifen [Can]
    Emadine® [US]
    emedastine
    ketotifen
    Novo-Ketotifen [Can]
    Zaditen® [Can]
    Zaditor™ [US/Can]
Antihistamine, Ophthalmic
    Astelin® [US/Can]
    azelastine
    Optivar™ [US]
Corticosteroid, Ophthalmic
    Alrex® [US/Can]
    Lotemax® [US/Can]
    loteprednol
Mast Cell Stabilizer
    Alamast™ [US/Can]
    Alocril™ [US/Can]
    nedocromil (ophthalmic)
    pemirolast
Nonsteroidal Antiinflammatory Drug
    (NSAID)
    Acular LS™ [US]
    Acular® P.F. [US]
    Acular® [US/Can]
    Apo®-Ketorolac [Can]
    ketorolac
    Novo-Ketorolac [Can]

ratio-Ketorolac [Can]
    Toradol® [US/Can]
Ophthalmic Agent, Miscellaneous
    Alamast™ [US/Can]
    pemirolast

Phenothiazine Derivative
    Anergan® [US]
    Phenergan® [US/Can]
    promethazine

CONJUNCTIVITIS (BACTERIAL)

Antibiotic, Ophthalmic
    levofloxacin
    Quixin™ Ophthalmic [US]

CONJUNCTIVITIS (VERNAL)

Adrenal Corticosteroid
    HMS Liquifilm® [US]
    medrysone
Mast Cell Stabilizer
    Alomide® [US/Can]
    lodoxamide tromethamine

CRYPTOCOCCOSIS

Antifungal Agent
    Abelcet® [US/Can]
    Amphocin® [US]
    Amphotec® [US/Can]
    amphotericin B cholesteryl sulfate
      complex
    amphotericin B (conventional)
    amphotericin B lipid complex
    Ancobon® [US/Can]
    Apo®-Fluconazole [Can]
    Diflucan® [US/Can]
    fluconazole
    flucytosine
    Fungizone® [US/Can]
    Gen-Fluconazole [Can]
    itraconazole

Novo-Fluconazole [Can]
Sporanox® [US/Can]
Antifungal Agent, Systemic
AmBisome® [US/Can]
amphotericin B liposomal

DANDRUFF
Antiseborrheic Agent, Topical
Aveeno® Cleansing Bar [US-OTC]
Balnetar® [US/Can]
Betatar® [US-OTC]
Capitrol® [US/Can]
chloroxine
coal tar
coal tar and salicylic acid
coal tar, lanolin, and mineral oil
Cutar® [US-OTC]
DHS™ Targel [US-OTC]
DHS™ Tar [US-OTC]
DHS™ Zinc [US-OTC]
Doak® Tar [US-OTC]
Estar® [US-OTC]
Exorex® [US]
Fostex® [US-OTC]
Head & Shoulders® Classic Clean 2-In-1 [US-OTC]
Head & Shoulders® Classic Clean [US-OTC]
Head & Shoulders® Dry Scalp Care [US-OTC]
Head & Shoulders® Extra Fullness [US-OTC]
Head & Shoulders® Intensive Treatment [US-OTC]
Head & Shoulders® Refresh [US-OTC]
Head & Shoulders® Smooth & Silky 2-In-1 [US-OTC]
Ionil T® Plus [US-OTC]
Ionil T® [US-OTC]
MG 217® Medicated Tar [US-OTC]
MG 217® [US-OTC]

Neutrogena® T/Gel Extra Strength [US-OTC]
Neutrogena® T/Gel [US-OTC]
Oxipor® VHC [US-OTC]
Pentrax® [US-OTC]
Pernox® [US-OTC]
Polytar® [US-OTC]
PsoriGel® [US-OTC]
pyrithione zinc
Reme-T™ [US-OTC]
Sastid® Plain Therapeutic Shampoo and Acne Wash [US-OTC]
Sebcur/T® [Can]
selenium sulfide
Selsun Blue® [US-OTC]
Selsun® [US]
sulfur and salicylic acid
Tarsum® [US-OTC]
Tegrin® [US-OTC]
Versel® [Can]
X-Seb™ T [US-OTC]
Zetar® [US-OTC]
Zincon® [USOTC]
ZNP® Bar [US-OTC]

DEBRIDEMENT OF CALLOUS TISSUE
Keratolytic Agent
trichloroacetic acid
Tri-Chlor® [US]

DEBRIDEMENT OF ESCHAR
Protectant, Topical
Granulex [US]
trypsin, balsam Peru, and castor oil

DECUBITUS ULCER
Enzyme
collagenase
Santyl® [US/Can]
Enzyme, Topical Debridement

Accuzyme™ [US]
papain and urea
Protectant, Topical
Granulex [US]
trypsin, balsam Peru, and castor oil
Topical Skin Product
Accuzyme™ [US]
papain and urea

DERMATITIS
Antiseborrheic Agent, Topical
Betatar® [US-OTC]
coal tar
Cutar® [US-OTC]
DHS™ Targel [US-OTC]
DHS™ Tar [US-OTC]
Doak® Tar [US-OTC]
Estar® [US-OTC]
Exorex® [US]
Ionil T® Plus [US-OTC]
Ionil T® [US-OTC]
MG 217® Medicated Tar [US-OTC]
MG 217® [US-OTC]
Neutrogena® T/Gel Extra Strength
[US-OTC]
Neutrogena® T/Gel [US-OTC]
Oxipor® VHC [US-OTC]
Pentrax® [US-OTC]
Polytar® [US-OTC]
PsoriGel® [US-OTC]
Reme-T™ [US-OTC]
Tegrin® [US-OTC]
Zetar® [US-OTC]
Dietary Supplement
ME-500® [US]
methionine
Pedameth® [US]
Topical Skin Product
aluminum sulfate and calcium
acetate
Apo®-Doxepin [Can]
Bluboro® [US-OTC]

Domeboro® [US-OTC]
doxepin
Novo-Doxepin [Can]
Pedi-Boro® [US-OTC]
Prudoxin™ [US]
Sinequan® [US/Can]
Zonalon® Cream [US/Can]

DERMATOLOGIC DISORDER
Adrenal Corticosteroid
Acthar® [US]
Aeroseb-Dex® [US]
A-HydroCort® [US]
A-methapred® [US]
Anusol-HC® Suppository [US]
Apo®-Prednisone [Can]
Aristocort® Forte Injection [US]
Aristocort® Intralesional Injection
[US]
Aristocort® Tablet [US/Can]
Aristospan® Intraarticular Injection
[US/Can]
Aristospan® Intralesional Injection
[US/Can]
Betaject™ [Can]
betamethasone (systemic)
Betnesol® [Can]
Celestone® Phosphate [US]
Celestone® Soluspan® [US/Can]
Celestone® [US]
Cel-U-Jec® [US]
Colocort™ [US]
Cortef® Tablet [US/Can]
corticotropin
Cortifoam® [US/Can]
cortisone acetate
Cortone® [Can]
Decadron®-LA [US]
Decadron® [US/Can]
Decaject-LA® [US]
Decaject® [US]

Deltasone® [US]
Depo-Medrol® [US/Can]
Depopred® [US]
dexamethasone (systemic)
dexamethasone (topical)
Dexasone® L.A. [US]
Dexasone® [US/Can]
Dexone® LA [US]
Dexone® [US]
Emo-Cort® [Can]
Hexadrol® [US/Can]
H.P. Acthar® Gel [US]
Hycort® [US]
hydrocortisone (rectal)
hydrocortisone (systemic)
Kenalog® Injection [US/Can]
Medrol® Dosepak™ [US/Can]
Medrol® Tablet [US/Can]
methylprednisolone
Orapred™ [US]
Pediapred® [US/Can]
PMS-Dexamethasone [Can]
Prednicot® [US]
prednisolone (systemic)
Prednisol® TBA [US]
prednisone
Prednisone Intensol™ [US]
Prelone® [US]
Proctocort™ Rectal [US]
ProctoCream ® HC Cream [US]
ratio-Dexamethasone [Can]
Solu-Cortef® [US/Can]
Solu-Medrol® [US/Can]
Solurex L.A.® [US]
Sterapred® DS [US]
Sterapred® [US]
Tac™ -3 Injection [US]
Triam-A® Injection [US]
triamcinolone (systemic)
Triam Forte® Injection [US]
Winpred™ [Can]

DERMATOMYCOSIS
Antifungal Agent
Aloe Vesta® 2-n-1 Antifungal [US-OTC]
Apo®-Ketoconazole [Can]
Baza® Antifungal [US-OTC]
Carrington Antifungal [US-OTC]
Femizol-M™ [US-OTC]
Fulvicin® P/G [US]
Fulvicin-U/F® [US/Can]
Fungoid® Tincture [US-OTC]
Grifulvin® V Suspension [US]
griseofulvin
Gris-PEG® [US]
ketoconazole
Ketoderm® [Can]
Lotrimin® AF Powder/Spray [US-OTC]
Micaderm® [US-OTC]
Micatin® [US/Can]
miconazole
Micozole [Can]
Micro-Guard® [US-OTC]
Mitrazol™ [US-OTC]
Monistat® 1 Combination Pack [US-OTC]
Monistat® 3 [US-OTC]
Monistat® 7 [US-OTC]
Monistat® [Can]
Monistat-Derm® [US]
naftifine
Naftin® [US]
Nizoral® A-D [US-OTC]
Nizoral® [US/Can]
Novo-Ketoconazole [Can]
oxiconazole
Oxistat® [US/Can]
Triple Care® Antifungal [OTC]
Zeasorb®-AF [US-OTC]

DERMATOSIS
Anesthetic/Corticosteroid
  AnaMantle® HC [US]
  Lida-Mantle® HC [US]
  lidocaine and hydrocortisone
Antibiotic, Topical
  clioquinol and flumethasone
    (Canada only)
  Locacorten® Vioform® Eardrops
    [Can]
Corticosteroid, Topical
  Aclovate® [US]
  Acticort® [US]
  Aeroseb-HC® [US]
  alclometasone
  Alphatrex® [US]
  amcinonide
  Amcort® [Can]
  Anusol® HC-1 [US-OTC]
  Anusol® HC-2.5% [US-OTC]
  Aquacort® [Can]
  Aristocort® A Topical [US]
  Aristocort® Topical [US]
  Bactine® Hydrocortisone [US-OTC]
  Betaderm® [Can]
  Betamethacot® [US]
  betamethasone (topical)
  Betatrex® [US]
  Beta-Val® [US]
  Betnovate® [Can]
  CaldeCORT® Anti-Itch Spray [US]
  CaldeCORT® [US-OTC]
  Capex™ [US/Can]
  Carmol-HC® [US]
  Celestoderm®-EV/2 [Can]
  Celestoderm®-V [Can]
  Cetacort®
  clioquinol and flumethasone
    (Canada only)
  clobetasol
  Clocort® Maximum Strength [US-OTC]

clocortolone
Cloderm® [US/Can]
Cordran® SP [US]
Cordran® [US/Can]
Cormax® [US]
CortaGel® [US-OTC]
Cortaid® Maximum Strength [US-OTC]
Cortaid® with Aloe [US-OTC]
Cort-Dome® [US]
Cortizone®-5 [US-OTC]
Cortizone®-10 [US-OTC]
Cortoderm [Can]
Cutivate™ [US]
Cyclocort® [US/Can]
Del-Beta® [US]
Delcort® [US]
Dermacort® [US]
Dermarest Dricort® [US]
Derma-Smoothe/FS® [US/Can]
Dermatop® [US/Can]
Dermolate® [US-OTC]
Dermovate® [Can]
Dermtex® HC with Aloe [US-OTC]
Desocort® [Can]
desonide
DesOwen® [US]
Desoxi® [Can]
desoximetasone
diflorasone
Diprolene® AF [US]
Diprolene® [US/Can]
Diprosone® [Can]
Eldecort® [US]
Elocon® [US/Can]
Embeline™ E [US]
fluocinolone
fluocinonide
Fluoderm [Can]
flurandrenolide
fluticasone (topical)
Gen-Clobetasol [Can]

Gynecort® [US-OTC]
halcinonide
halobetasol
Halog®-E [US]
Halog® [US/Can]
Hi-Cor-1.0® [US]
Hi-Cor-2.5® [US]
Hyderm [Can]
hydrocortisone (topical)
Hydrocort® [US]
Hydro-Tex® [US-OTC]
Hytone® [US]
Kenalog® in Orabase® [US/Can]
Kenalog® Topical [US/Can]
LactiCare-HC® [US]
Lanacort® [US-OTC]
Lidemol® [Can]
Lidex-E® [US]
Lidex® [US/Can]
Locacorten® Vioform® Eardrops
    [Can]
Locoid® [US/Can]
Luxiq™ [US]
Lyderm® [Can]
Maxiflor® [US]
Maxivate® [US]
mometasone furoate
Nasonex® [US/Can]
Novo-Clobetasol [Can]
Nutracort® [US]
Olux® [US]
Orabase® HCA [US]
Oracort [Can]
Penecort® [US]
PMS-Desonide [Can]
prednicarbate
Prevex® [Can]
Prevex® HC [Can]
Psorcon™ E [US]
Psorcon™ [US/Can]
Qualisone® [US]
ratio-Clobetasol [Can]
ratio-Ectosone [Can]

ratio-Topilene® [Can]
ratio-Topisone® [Can]
Sarna® HC [Can]
Scalpicin® [US]
S-T Cort® [US]
Synacort® [US]
Synalar® [US/Can]
Taro-Desoximetasone [Can]
Taro-Sone® [Can]
Tegrin®-HC [US-OTC]
Temovate E® [US]
Temovate® [US]
Tiamol® [Can]
Ti-U-Lac® H [Can]
Topicort®-LP [US]
Topicort® [US/Can]
Topsyn® [Can]
Triacet™ Topical [US]
Triaderm [Can]
triamcinolone (topical)
Tridesilon® [US]
U-Cort™ [US]
Ultravate™ [US/Can]
urea and hydrocortisone
Uremol® HC [Can]
Valisone® Scalp Lotion [Can]
Westcort® [US/Can]

DISCOID LUPUS ERYTHEMATOSUS (DLE)
Aminoquinoline (Antimalarial)
    Apo®-Hydroxyquine [Can]
    Aralen® Phosphate [US/Can]
    chloroquine phosphate
    hydroxychloroquine
    Plaquenil® [US/Can]
Corticosteroid, Topical
    Aclovate® [US]
    Acticort® [US]
    Aeroseb-HC® [US]
    alclometasone
    Alphatrex® [US]

amcinonide
Amcort® [Can]
Anusol® HC-1 [US-OTC]
Anusol® HC-2.5% [US-OTC]
Aquacort® [Can]
Aristocort® A Topical [US]
Aristocort® Topical [US]
Bactine® Hydrocortisone [US-OTC]
Betaderm® [Can]
Betamethacot® [US]
betamethasone (topical)
Betatrex® [US]
Beta-Val® [US]
Betnovate® [Can]
CaldeCORT® Anti-Itch Spray [US]
CaldeCORT® [US-OTC]
Capex™ [US/Can]
Carmol-HC® [US]
Celestoderm®-EV/2 [Can]
Celestoderm®-V [Can]
Cetacort®
clobetasol
Clocort® Maximum Strength [US-OTC]
clocortolone
Cloderm® [US/Can]
Cordran® SP [US]
Cordran® [US/Can]
Cormax® [US]
CortaGel® [US-OTC]
Cortaid® Maximum Strength [US-OTC]
Cortaid® with Aloe [US-OTC]
Cort-Dome® [US]
Cortizone®-5 [US-OTC]
Cortizone®-10 [US-OTC]
Cortoderm [Can]
Cutivate™ [US]
Cyclocort® [US/Can]
Del-Beta® [US]
Delcort® [US]
Dermacort® [US]
Dermarest Dricort® [US]

Derma-Smoothe/FS® [US/Can]
Dermatop® [US/Can]
Dermolate® [US-OTC]
Dermovate® [Can]
Dermtex® HC with Aloe [US-OTC]
Desocort® [Can]
desonide
DesOwen® [US]
Desoxi® [Can]
desoximetasone
diflorasone
Diprolene® AF [US]
Diprolene® [US/Can]
Diprosone® [Can]
Eldecort® [US]
Elocon® [US/Can]
Embeline™ E [US]
fluocinolone
fluocinonide
Fluoderm [Can]
flurandrenolide
fluticasone (topical)
Gen-Clobetasol [Can]
Gynecort® [US-OTC]
halcinonide
halobetasol
Halog®-E [US]
Halog® [US/Can]
Hi-Cor-1.0® [US]
Hi-Cor-2.5® [US]
Hyderm [Can]
hydrocortisone (topical)
Hydrocort® [US]
Hydro-Tex® [US-OTC]
Hytone® [US]
Kenalog® in Orabase® [US/Can]
Kenalog® Topical [US/Can]
LactiCare-HC® [US]
Lanacort® [US-OTC]
Lidemol® [Can]
Lidex-E® [US]
Lidex® [US/Can]
Locoid® [US/Can]

Luxiq™ [US]
Lyderm® [Can]
Maxiflor® [US]
Maxivate® [US]
mometasone furoate
Nasonex® [US/Can]
Novo-Clobetasol [Can]
Nutracort® [US]
Olux® [US]
Orabase® HCA [US]
Oracort [Can]
Penecort® [US]
PMS-Desonide [Can]
prednicarbate
Prevex® [Can]
Prevex® HC [Can]
Psorcon™ E [US]
Psorcon™ [US/Can]
Qualisone® [US]
ratio-Clobetasol [Can]
ratio-Ectosone [Can]
ratio-Topilene® [Can]
ratio-Topisone® [Can]
Sarna® HC [Can]
Scalpicin® [US]
S-T Cort® [US]
Synacort® [US]
Synalar® [US/Can]
Taro-Desoximetasone [Can]
Taro-Sone® [Can]
Tegrin®-HC [US-OTC]
Temovate E® [US]
Temovate® [US]
Tiamol® [Can]
Ti-U-Lac® H [Can]
Topicort®-LP [US]
Topicort® [US/Can]
Topsyn® [Can]
Triacet™ Topical [US]
Triaderm [Can]
triamcinolone (topical)
Tridesilon® [US]
U-Cort™ [US]

Ultravate™ [US/Can]
urea and hydrocortisone
Uremol® HC [Can]
Valisone® Scalp Lotion [Can]
Westcort® [US/Can]

DRACUNCULIASIS
Amebicide
Apo®-Metronidazole [Can]
Flagyl ER® [US]
Flagyl® [US/Can]
Florazole ER® [Can]
metronidazole
Noritate® [US/Can]
Novo-Nidazol [Can]
Trikacide® [Can]

DRY SKIN
Topical Skin Product
AmLactin® [US-OTC]
Aquacare® [US-OTC]
Aquaphilic® With Carbamide [US-OTC]
camphor, menthol, and phenol
Carmol® 10 [US-OTC]
Carmol® 20 [US-OTC]
Carmol® 40 [US]
Carmol® Deep Cleaning [US]
DPM™ [US-OTC]
Gormel® [US-OTC]
Lac-Hydrin® [US]
LAClotion™ [US]
lactic acid and sodium-PCA
lactic acid with ammonium hydroxide
LactiCare® [US-OTC]
Lactinol-E® [US]
Lactinol® [US]
Lanaphilic® [US-OTC]
lanolin, cetyl alcohol, glycerin, and petrolatum
Lubriderm® Fragrance Free [US-OTC]
Lubriderm® [US-OTC]

Nutraplus® [US-OTC]
Rea-Lo® [US-OTC]
Sarna® [US-OTC]
Ultra Mide® [US-OTC/Can]
urea
Ureacin® [US-OTC]
Uremol® [Can]
Urisec® [Can]
Vanamide™ [US]
Vitamin, Topical
   Amino-Opti-E® [US-OTC]
   Aquasol E® [US-OTC]
   E-Complex-600® [US-OTC]
   E-Vitamin® [US-OTC]
   vitamin E
   Vita-Plus® E Softgels® [US-OTC]
   Vitec® [US-OTC]
   Vite E® Creme [US-OTC]

ECZEMA

Antibiotic/Corticosteroid, Topical
   neomycin and hydrocortisone
Antifungal/Corticosteroid
   Ala-Quin® [US]
   clioquinol and hydrocortisone
   Dek-Quin® [US]
   Dermazene® [US]
   iodoquinol and hydrocortisone
   Vioform® Hydrocortisone [Can]
   Vytone® [US]
Corticosteroid, Topical
   Aclovate® [US]
   Acticort® [US]
   Aeroseb-HC® [US]
   alclometasone
   Alphatrex® [US]
   amcinonide
   Amcort® [Can]
   Aquacort® [Can]
   Aristocort® A Topical [US]
   Aristocort® Topical [US]
   Bactine® Hydrocortisone [US-OTC]

Betaderm® [Can]
Betamethacot® [US]
betamethasone (topical)
Betatrex® [US]
Beta-Val® [US]
Betnovate® [Can]
CaldeCORT® Anti-Itch Spray [US]
CaldeCORT® [US-OTC]
Capex™ [US/Can]
Carmol-HC® [US]
Celestoderm®-EV/2 [Can]
Celestoderm®-V [Can]
Cetacort®
clobetasol
Clocort® Maximum Strength [US-OTC]
clocortolone
Cloderm® [US/Can]
Cordran® SP [US]
Cordran® [US/Can]
Cormax® [US]
CortaGel® [US-OTC]
Cortaid® Maximum Strength [US-OTC]
Cortaid® with Aloe [US-OTC]
Cort-Dome® [US]
Cortizone®-5 [US-OTC]
Cortizone®-10 [US-OTC]
Cortoderm [Can]
Cutivate™ [US]
Cyclocort® [US/Can]
Del-Beta® [US]
Delcort® [US]
Dermacort® [US]
Dermarest Dricort® [US]
Dermatop® [US/Can]
Dermolate® [US-OTC]
Dermovate® [Can]
Dermtex® HC with Aloe [US-OTC]
Desocort® [Can]
desonide
DesOwen® [US]
Desoxi® [Can]

desoximetasone
diflorasone
Diprolene® AF [US]
Diprolene® [US/Can]
Diprosone® [Can]
Eldecort® [US]
Elocon® [US/Can]
Embeline™ E [US]
fluocinolone
fluocinonide
Fluoderm [Can]
flurandrenolide
fluticasone (topical)
Gen-Clobetasol [Can]
Gynecort® [US-OTC]
halcinonide
halobetasol
Halog®-E [US]
Halog® [US/Can]
Hi-Cor-1.0® [US]
Hi-Cor-2.5® [US]
Hyderm [Can]
hydrocortisone (topical)
Hydrocort® [US]
Hydro-Tex® [US-OTC]
Hytone® [US]
Kenalog® Topical [US/Can]
LactiCare-HC® [US]
Lanacort® [US-OTC]
Lidemol® [Can]
Lidex-E® [US]
Lidex® [US/Can]
Locoid® [US/Can]
Luxiq™ [US]
Lyderm® [Can]
Maxiflor® [US]
Maxivate® [US]
mometasone furoate
Novo-Clobetasol [Can]
Nutracort® [US]
Olux® [US]
Penecort® [US]
PMS-Desonide [Can]

prednicarbate
Prevex® [Can]
Prevex® HC [Can]
Psorcon™ E [US]
Psorcon™ [US/Can]
Qualisone® [US]
ratio-Clobetasol [Can]
ratio-Ectosone [Can]
ratio-Topilene® [Can]
ratio-Topisone® [Can]
Scalpicin® [US]
S-T Cort® [US]
Synacort® [US]
Synalar® [US/Can]
Taro-Desoximetasone [Can]
Taro-Sone® [Can]
Tegrin®-HC [US-OTC]
Temovate E® [US]
Temovate® [US]
Tiamol® [Can]
Ti-U-Lac® H [Can]
Topicort® [US/Can]
Topicort®-LP [US]
Topsyn® [Can]
Triacet™ Topical [US]
Triaderm [Can]
triamcinolone (topical)
Tridesilon® [US]
U-Cort™ [US]
Ultravate™ [US/Can]
urea and hydrocortisone
Uremol® HC [Can]
Valisone® Scalp Lotion [Can]
Westcort® [US/Can]

EPISCLERITIS
Adrenal Corticosteroid
    HMS Liquifilm® [US]
   medrysone

ERYTHROPOIETIC PROTOPORPHYRIA (EPP)
Vitamin, Fat Soluble
  A-Caro-25® [US]
  B-Caro-T™ [US]
  beta-carotene
  Lumitene™ [US]

EYELID INFECTION
Antibiotic, Ophthalmic
  mercuric oxide
  Ocu-Merox® [US]
Pharmaceutical Aid
  boric acid

FABRY DISEASE
Enzyme
  agalsidase beta
  Fabrazyme® [US]

FUNGUS (DIAGNOSTIC)
Diagnostic Agent
  Candin® [US]
  Dermatophytin® [US]
  Histolyn-CYL® [US]
  histoplasmin
  Trichophyton skin test

GENITAL HERPES
Antiviral Agent
  famciclovir
  Famvir™ [US/Can]
  valacyclovir
  Valtrex® [US/Can]

GENITAL WART
Immune Response Modifier
  Aldara™ [US/Can]
  imiquimod

GIANT PAPILLARY CONJUNCTIVITIS
Mast Cell Stabilizer
  Apo®-Cromolyn [Can]
  cromolyn sodium
  Nu-Cromolyn [Can]
  Opticrom® [US/Can]

GONOCOCCAL OPHTHALMIA NEONATORUM
Topical Skin Product
  silver nitrate

GONORRHEA
Antibiotic, Macrolide
  Rovamycine® [Can]
  spiramycin (Canada only)
Antibiotic, Miscellaneous
  spectinomycin
  Trobicin® [US]
Antibiotic, Quinolone
  gatifloxacin
  Tequin® [US/Can]
  Zymar™ [US]
Cephalosporin (Second Generation)
  Apo®-Cefuroxime [Can]
  cefoxitin
  Ceftin® [US/Can]
  cefuroxime
  Mefoxin® [US/Can]
  ratio-Cefuroxime [Can]
  Zinacef® [US/Can]
Cephalosporin (Third Generation)
  cefixime
  ceftriaxone
  Rocephin® [US/Can]
  Suprax® [Can]
Quinolone
  Apo®-Oflox [Can]
  ciprofloxacin
  Cipro® [US/Can]

Cipro® XR [US/Can]
Floxin® [US/Can]
ofloxacin
Tetracycline Derivative
Adoxa™ [US]
Apo®-Doxy [Can]
Apo®-Doxy Tabs [Can]
Apo®-Tetra [Can]
Brodspec® [US]
Doryx® [US]
Doxy-100® [US]
Doxycin [Can]
doxycycline
EmTet® [US]
Monodox® [US]
Novo-Doxylin [Can]
Novo-Tetra [Can]
Nu-Doxycycline [Can]
Nu-Tetra [Can]
ratio-Doxycycline [Can]
Sumycin® [US]
tetracycline
Vibramycin® [US]
Vibra-Tabs® [US/Can]
Wesmycin® [US]

GOUT

Antigout Agent
colchicine
colchicine and probenecid
ratio-Colchicine [Can]
Nonsteroidal Antiinflammatory Drug
(NSAID)
Advil® [US/Can]
Aleve® [US-OTC]
Anaprox® DS [US/Can]
Anaprox® [US/Can]
Apo®-Diclo [Can]
Apo®-Diclo SR [Can]
Apo®-Ibuprofen [Can]
Apo®-Indomethacin [Can]
Apo®-Napro-Na [Can]
Apo®-Napro-Na DS [Can]

Apo®-Naproxen [Can]
Apo®-Naproxen SR [Can]
Apo®-Sulin [Can]
Cataflam® [US/Can]
Clinoril® [US]
diclofenac
EC-Naprosyn® [US]
Gen-Naproxen EC [Can]
Genpril® [US-OTC]
Haltran® [US-OTC]
ibuprofen
Ibu-Tab® [US]
Indocid® [Can]
Indocid® P.D.A. [Can]
Indocin® SR [US]
Indocin® [US]
Indo-Lemmon [Can]
indomethacin
I-Prin [US-OTC]
Menadol® [US-OTC]
Motrin® IB [US/Can]
Motrin® [US/Can]
Naprelan® [US]
Naprosyn® [US/Can]
naproxen
Naxen® [Can]
Novo-Difenac® [Can]
Novo-Difenac-K [Can]
Novo-Difenac® SR [Can]
Novo-Methacin [Can]
Novo-Naprox [Can]
Novo-Naprox Sodium [Can]
Novo-Naprox Sodium DS [Can]
Novo-Naprox SR [Can]
Novo-Profen® [Can]
Novo-Sundac [Can]
Nu-Diclo [Can]
Nu-Diclo-SR [Can]
Nu-Ibuprofen [Can]
Nu-Indo [Can]
Nu-Naprox [Can]
Nu-Sundac [Can]
PMS-Diclofenac [Can]

PMS-Diclofenac SR [Can]
ratio-Indomethacin [Can]
Rhodacine® [Can]
Riva-Diclofenac [Can]
Riva-Diclofenac-K [Can]
Riva-Naproxen [Can]
sulindac
Voltaren Rapide® [Can]
Voltaren® [US/Can]
Voltaren®-XR [US]
Uricosuric Agent
Apo®-Sulfinpyrazone [Can]
Benuryl™ [Can]
Nu-Sulfinpyrazone [Can]
probenecid
sulfinpyrazone
Xanthine Oxidase Inhibitor
allopurinol
Aloprim™ [US]
Apo®-Allopurinol [Can]
Zyloprim® [US/Can]

GRAFT VERSUS HOST DISEASE
Immunosuppressant Agent
Apo®-Cyclosporine [Can]
Atgam® [US/Can]
CellCept® [US/Can]
cyclosporine
Gengraf™ [US]
lymphocyte immune globulin
muromonab-CD3
mycophenolate
Neoral® [US/Can]
Orthoclone OKT® 3 [US/Can]
Prograf® [US/Can]
Protopic® [US]
Restasis™ [US]
Rhoxal-cyclosporine [Can]
Sandimmune® [US/Can]
tacrolimus

GRAM-NEGATIVE INFECTION
Aminoglycoside (Antibiotic)
AKTob® [US]
Alcomicin® [Can]
amikacin
Amikin® [Can]
Apo®-Tobramycin [Can]
Diogent® [Can]
Garamycin® [US/Can]
Genoptic® [US]
Gentacidin® [US]
Gentak® [US]
gentamicin
kanamycin
Kantrex® [US/Can]
Nebcin® [US/Can]
PMS-Tobramycin [Can]
ratio-Gentamicin [Can]
TOBI® [US/Can]
tobramycin
Tobrex® [US/Can]
Antibiotic, Carbapenem
ertapenem
Invanz™ [US/Can]
Antibiotic, Miscellaneous
Apo®-Nitrofurantoin [Can]
Azactam® [US/Can]
aztreonam
colistimethate
Coly-Mycin® M [US/Can]
Furadantin® [US]
Macrobid® [US/Can]
Macrodantin® [US/Can]
nitrofurantoin
Novo-Furantoin [Can]
Antibiotic, Penicillin
pivampicillin (Canada only)
Pondocillin® [Can]
Antibiotic, Quinolone
gatifloxacin
Levaquin® [US/Can]

levofloxacin
Quixin™ Ophthalmic [US]
Tequin® [US/Can]
Zymar™ [US]
Carbapenem (Antibiotic)
  imipenem and cilastatin
  meropenem
  Merrem® I.V. [US/Can]
  Primaxin® [US/Can]
Cephalosporin (First Generation)
  Ancef® [US]
  Apo®-Cefadroxil [Can]
  Apo®-Cephalex [Can]
  Biocef® [US]
  cefadroxil
  cefazolin
  cephalexin
  cephalothin
  cephradine
  Ceporacin® [Can]
  Duricef® [US/Can]
  Keflex® [US]
  Keftab® [US/Can]
  Novo-Cefadroxil [Can]
  Novo-Lexin® [Can]
  Nu-Cephalex® [Can]
  Velosef® [US]
Cephalosporin (Second Generation)
  Apo®-Cefaclor [Can]
  Apo®-Cefuroxime [Can]
  Ceclor® CD [US]
  Ceclor® [US/Can]
  cefaclor
  Cefotan® [US/Can]
  cefotetan
  cefoxitin
  cefpodoxime
  cefprozil
  Ceftin® [US/Can]
  cefuroxime
  Cefzil® [US/Can]
  Mefoxin® [US/Can]
  Novo-Cefaclor [Can]

Nu-Cefaclor [Can]
PMS-Cefaclor [Can]
ratio-Cefuroxime [Can]
Vantin® [US/Can]
Zinacef® [US/Can]
Cephalosporin (Third Generation)
  Cedax® [US]
  cefixime
  Cefizox® [US/Can]
  cefotaxime
  ceftazidime
  ceftibuten
  ceftizoxime
  ceftriaxone
  Claforan® [US/Can]
  Fortaz® [US/Can]
  Rocephin® [US/Can]
  Suprax® [Can]
  Tazicef® [US]
  Tazidime® [US/Can]
Cephalosporin (Fourth Generation)
  cefepime
  Maxipime® [US/Can]
Genitourinary Irrigant
  neomycin and polymyxin B
  Neosporin® Cream [Can]
  Neosporin® G.U. Irrigant [US/Can]
Macrolide (Antibiotic)
  Apo®-Erythro Base [Can]
  Apo®-Erythro E-C [Can]
  Apo®-Erythro-ES [Can]
  Apo®-Erythro-S [Can]
  azithromycin
  Biaxin® [US/Can]
  Biaxin® XL [US/Can]
  clarithromycin
  Diomycin® [Can]
  dirithromycin
  Dynabac® [US]
  E.E.S.® [US/Can]
  Erybid™ [Can]
  Eryc® [US/Can]
  EryPed® [US]

Ery-Tab® [US]
Erythrocin® [US]
erythromycin and sulfisoxazole
erythromycin (systemic)
Eryzole® [US]
Nu-Erythromycin-S [Can]
PCE® [US/Can]
Pediazole® [US/Can]
PMS-Erythromycin [Can]
Tao® [US]
troleandomycin
Zithromax® [US/Can]
Z-PAK® [US/Can]

Penicillin
Alti-Amoxi-Clav® [Can]
amoxicillin
amoxicillin and clavulanate
   potassium
Amoxicot® [US]
Amoxil® [US]
ampicillin
ampicillin and sulbactam
Apo®-Amoxi [Can]
Apo®-Amoxi-Clav® [Can]
Apo®-Ampi [Can]
Apo®-Pen VK [Can]
Augmentin ES-600™ [US]
Augmentin® [US/Can]
Augmentin XR™ [US]
Bicillin® C-R 900/300 [US]
Bicillin® C-R [US]
Bicillin® L-A [US]
carbenicillin
Clavulin® [Can]
Gen-Amoxicillin [Can]
Geocillin® [US]
Lin-Amox [Can]
Marcillin® [US]
Moxilin® [US]
Nadopen-V® [Can]
Novamoxin® [Can]
Novo-Ampicillin [Can]
Novo-Pen-VK® [Can]

Nu-Amoxi [Can]
Nu-Ampi [Can]
Nu-Pen-VK® [Can]
penicillin G benzathine
penicillin G benzathine and
   procaine combined
penicillin G procaine
penicillin V potassium
Permapen® Isoject® [US]
piperacillin
piperacillin and tazobactam sodium
Pipracil® [Can]
PMS-Amoxicillin [Can]
Principen® [US]
PVF® K [Can]
ratio-AmoxiClav
Suspen® [US]
Tazocin® [Can]
ticarcillin
ticarcillin and clavulanate potassium
Ticar® [US]
Timentin® [US/Can]
Trimox® [US]
Truxcillin® [US]
Unasyn® [US/Can]
Veetids® [US]
Wycillin® [US/Can]
Zosyn® [US]

Quinolone
Apo®-Norflox [Can]
Apo®-Oflox [Can]
Ciloxan® [US/Can]
Cinobac® [US/Can]
cinoxacin
ciprofloxacin
Cipro® [US/Can]
Cipro® XR [US/Can]
Floxin® [US/Can]
lomefloxacin
Maxaquin® [US]
nalidixic acid
NegGram® [US/Can]
norfloxacin

Noroxin® [US/Can]
Novo-Norfloxacin [Can]
Ocuflox® [US/Can]
ofloxacin
PMS-Norfloxacin [Can]
Riva-Norfloxacin [Can]
sparfloxacin
Zagam® [US]
Sulfonamide
    Apo®-Sulfatrim [Can]
    Bactrim™ DS [US]
    Bactrim™ [US]
    erythromycin and sulfisoxazole
    Eryzole® [US]
    Gantrisin® Pediatric Suspension
      [US]
    Novo-Trimel [Can]
    Novo-Trimel D.S. [Can]
    Nu-Cotrimox® [Can]
    Pediazole® [US/Can]
    Septra® DS [US/Can]
    Septra® [US/Can]
    sulfadiazine
    sulfamethoxazole and trimethoprim
    Sulfatrim® DS [US]
    Sulfatrim® [US]
    sulfisoxazole
    sulfisoxazole and phenazopyridine
    Sulfizole® [Can]
    Truxazole® [US]
Tetracycline Derivative
    Adoxa™ [US]
    Alti-Minocycline [Can]
    Apo®-Doxy [Can]
    Apo®-Doxy Tabs [Can]
    Apo®-Minocycline [Can]
    Apo®-Tetra [Can]
    Brodspec® [US]
    Doryx® [US]
    Doxy-100® [US]
    Doxycin [Can]
    doxycycline
    Dynacin® [US]

EmTet® [US]
Gen-Minocycline [Can]
Minocin® [US/Can]
minocycline
Monodox® [US]
Novo-Doxylin [Can]
Novo-Minocycline [Can]
Novo-Tetra [Can]
Nu-Doxycycline [Can]
Nu-Tetra [Can]
oxytetracycline
Periostat® [US]
ratio-Doxycycline [Can]
ratio-Minocycline [Can]
Rhoxal-minocycline [Can]
Sumycin® [US]
Terramycin® I.M. [US/Can]
tetracycline
Vibramycin® [US]
Vibra-Tabs® [US/Can]
Wesmycin® [US]

HARTNUP DISEASE
Vitamin, Water Soluble
    niacinamide

HAY FEVER
Adrenergic Agonist Agent
    Afrin® Extra Moisturizing [US-OTC]
    Afrin® Original [US-OTC]
    Afrin® Severe Congestion [US-OTC]
    Afrin® Sinus [US-OTC]
    Afrin® [US-OTC]
    Dristan® Long Lasting Nasal [Can]
    Drixoral® Nasal [Can]
    Duramist® Plus [US-OTC]
    Duration® [US-OTC]
    Genasal [US-OTC]
    Neo-Synephrine® 12 Hour Extra
      Moisturizing [US-OTC]
    Neo-Synephrine® 12 Hour [US-
      OTC]
    Nostrilla® [US-OTC]

oxymetazoline
Twice-A-Day® [US-OTC]
Vicks Sinex® 12 Hour Ultrafine
   Mist [US-OTC]
Visine® L.R. [US-OTC]
4-Way® Long Acting [US-OTC]
Antihistamine
   Allegra® [US/Can]
   fexofenadine
Antihistamine/Decongestant
   Combination
acrivastine and pseudoephedrine
Actifed® [Can]
Actifed® Cold and Allergy [US-OTC]
Allerest® Maximum Strength [US-
   OTC]
Allerfrim® [US-OTC]
Allerphed® [US-OTC]
Aphedrid™ [US-OTC]
Aprodine® [USOTC]
A.R.M® [US-OTC]
chlorpheniramine and
   pseudoephedrine
Chlor-Trimeton® Allergy D [US-
   OTC]
C-Phed Tannate [US]
Deconamine® SR [US-OTC]
Deconamine® [US-OTC]
Genac® [US-OTC]
Genaphed Plus [US-OTC]
Hayfebrol® [US-OTC]
Histex™ [US]
Kronofed-A®-Jr [US]
Kronofed-A® [US]
PediaCare® Cold and Allergy
   [OTC]
Rhinosyn-PD® [US-OTC]
Rhinosyn® [US-OTC]
Semprex®-D [US]
Silafed® [US-OTC]
Sudafed® Cold & Allergy [US-OTC]

Triaminic® Cold and Allergy [US-
   OTC]
triprolidine and pseudoephedrine
Tri-Sudo® [US-OTC]
Uni-Fed® [US-OTC]

HERPES SIMPLEX

Antiviral Agent
   acyclovir
   Apo®-Acyclovir [Can]
   Cytovene® [US/Can]
   famciclovir
   Famvir™ [US/Can]
   foscarnet
   Foscavir® [US/Can]
   ganciclovir
   Gen-Acyclovir [Can]
   Nu-Acyclovir [Can]
   trifluridine
   Viroptic® [US/Can]
   Vitrasert® [US/Can]
   Zovirax® [US/Can]
Antiviral Agent, Topical
   Abreva™ [US-OTC]
   docosanol

HERPES ZOSTER

Analgesic, Topical
   Antiphlogistine Rub A-535
      Capsaicin [Can]
   ArthriCare® for Women Extra
      Moisturizing [US-OTC]
   ArthriCare® for Women Silky Dry
      [US-OTC]
   Capsagel® [US-OTC]
   capsaicin
   Capzasin-HP® [US-OTC]
   TheraPatch® Warm [US-OTC]
   Zostrix®-HP [US/Can]
   Zostrix® [US/Can]
Antiviral Agent
   acyclovir

Apo®-Acyclovir [Can]
famciclovir
Famvir™ [US/Can]
Gen-Acyclovir [Can]
Nu-Acyclovir [Can]
valacyclovir
Valtrex® [US/Can]
Zovirax® [US/Can]

HISTOPLASMOSIS
Antifungal Agent
Amphocin® [US]
amphotericin B (conventional)
Apo®-Ketoconazole [Can]
Fungizone® [US/Can]
itraconazole
ketoconazole
Ketoderm® [Can]
Nizoral® A-D [US-OTC]
Nizoral® [US/Can]
Novo-Ketoconazole [Can]
Sporanox® [US/Can]

HOOKWORM
Anthelmintic
albendazole
Albenza® [US]
Combantrin™ [Can]
mebendazole
Pin-X® [US-OTC]
pyrantel pamoate
Reese's® Pinworm Medicine [US-OTC]
Vermox® [US/Can]

HYPERHIDROSIS
Topical Skin Product
aluminum chloride hexahydrate
Certain Dri® [US-OTC]
Drysol™ [US]
Xerac AC™ [US]

HYPERKERATOSIS (FOLLICULARIS)
Keratolytic Agent
Compound W® One Step Wart Remover [US-OTC]
Compound W® [US-OTC]
DHS™ Sal [US-OTC]
Dr. Scholl's® Callus Remover [US-OTC]
Dr. Scholl's® Clear Away [US-OTC]
Duoforte® 27 [Can]
Freezone® [US-OTC]
Fung-O® [US-OTC]
Gordofilm® [US-OTC]
Hydrisalic™ [US-OTC]
Ionil® Plus [US-OTC]
Ionil® [US-OTC]
Keralyt® [US-OTC]
LupiCare™ Dandruff [US-OTC]
LupiCare™ II Psoriasis [US-OTC]
LupiCare™ Psoriasis [US-OTC]
Mediplast® [US-OTC]
MG217 Sal-Acid® [US-OTC]
Mosco® Corn and Callus Remover [US-OTC]
NeoCeuticals™ Acne Spot Treatment [US-OTC]
Neutrogena® Acne Wash [US-OTC]
Neutrogena® Body Clear™ [US-OTC]
Neutrogena® Clear Pore Shine Control [US-OTC]
Neutrogena® Clear Pore [US-OTC]
Neutrogena® Healthy Scalp [US-OTC]
Neutrogena® Maximum Strength T/Sal® [US-OTC]
Neutrogena® On The Spot® Acne Patch [US-OTC]
Occlusal™ [Can]
Occlusal®-HP [US/Can]
Oxy® Balance Deep Pore [US-OTC]
Oxy Balance® [US-OTC]

Palmer's® Skin Success Acne
  Cleanser [US-OTC]
Pedisilk® [US-OTC]
Propa pH [US-OTC]
Sal-Acid® [US-OTC]
Salactic® [US-OTC]
SalAc® [US-OTC]
salicylic acid
Sal-Plant® [US-OTC]
Sebcur® [Can]
Soluver® [Can]
Soluver® Plus [Can]
Stri-dex® Body Focus [US-OTC]
Stri-dex® Facewipes To Go™ [US-OTC]
Stri-dex® Maximum Strength [US-OTC]
Stri-dex® [US-OTC]
Tinamed® [US-OTC]
Tiseb® [US-OTC]
Trans-Ver-Sal® [US-OTC/Can]
Wart-Off® Maximum Strength [US-OTC]
Zapzyt® Acne Wash [US-OTC]
Zapzyt® Pore Treatment [US-OTC]

HYPERPIGMENTATION
Topical Skin Product
  Alphaquin HP [US]
  Alustra™ [US]
  Claripel™ [US]
  Eldopaque Forte® [US]
  Eldopaque® [US-OTC]
  Eldoquin® Forte® [US]
  Eldoquin® [US/Can]
  EpiQuin™ Micro [US]
  Esoterica® Facial [US-OTC]
  Esoterica® Regular [US-OTC]
  Glyquin® [US]
  hydroquinone
  Lustra-AF™ [US]
  Lustra® [US]
  Melanex® [US]

Melpaque HP® [US]
Melquin-3® [US-OTC]
Melquin HP® [US]
NeoStrata® AHA [US/Can]
Nuquin HP® Cream [US]
Palmer's® Skin Success Fade
  Cream™ [US-OTC]
Solaquin Forte® [US/Can]
Solaquin® [US/Can]
Ultraquin™ [Can]

ICHTHYOSIS
Keratolytic Agent
  Duofilm® Solution [US]
  Keralyt® Gel [US-OTC]
  salicylic acid and lactic acid
  salicylic acid and propylene glycol

IMMUNODEFICIENCY
Enzyme
  Adagen™ [US/Can]
  pegademase (bovine)
Immune Globulin
  Carimune™ [US]
  Gamimune® N [US/Can]
  Gammagard® S/D [US/Can]
  Gammar®-P I.V. [US]
  Gamunex® [Can]
  immune globulin (intravenous)
  Iveegam EN [US]
  Iveegam Immuno® [Can]
  Panglobulin® [US]
  Polygam® S/D [US]
  Venoglobulin®-S [US]

IMPETIGO
Antibiotic, Topical
  bacitracin, neomycin, and
    polymyxin B
  Bactroban® Nasal [US]
  Bactroban® [US/Can]
  mupirocin
  Mycitracin® [US-OTC]

Neosporin® Ophthalmic Ointment
[US/Can]
Neosporin® Topical [US/Can]
Triple Antibiotic® [US]
Penicillin
Apo®-Pen VK [Can]
Nadopen-V® [Can]
Novo-Pen-VK® [Can]
Nu-Pen-VK® [Can]
penicillin G procaine
penicillin V potassium
PVF® K [Can]
Suspen® [US]
Truxcillin® [US]
Veetids® [US]
Wycillin® [US/Can]

INFLAMMATION (NONRHEUMATIC)

Adrenal Corticosteroid
Acthar® [US]
A-HydroCort® [US]
A-methapred® [US]
Apo®-Prednisone [Can]
Aristocort® Forte Injection [US]
Aristocort® Intralesional Injection [US]
Aristocort® Tablet [US/Can]
Aristospan® Intraarticular Injection
[US/Can]
Aristospan® Intralesional Injection
[US/Can]
Betaject™ [Can]
betamethasone (systemic)
Betnesol® [Can]
Celestone® Phosphate [US]
Celestone® Soluspan® [US/Can]
Celestone® [US]
Cel-U-Jec® [US]
Cortef® Tablet [US/Can]
corticotropin
cortisone acetate
Cortone® [Can]

Decadron®-LA [US]
Decadron® [US/Can]
Decaject-LA® [US]
Decaject® [US]
Deltasone® [US]
Depo-Medrol® [US/Can]
Depopred® [US]
dexamethasone (systemic)
Dexasone® L.A. [US]
Dexasone® [US/Can]
Dexone® LA [US]
Dexone® [US]
Hexadrol® [US/Can]
H.P. Acthar® Gel [US]
hydrocortisone (systemic)
Kenalog® Injection [US/Can]
Medrol® Dosepak™ [US/Can]
Medrol® Tablet [US/Can]
methylprednisolone
Orapred™[US]
Pediapred® [US/Can]
PMS-Dexamethasone [Can]
Prednicot® [US]
prednisolone (systemic)
Prednisol® TBA [US]
prednisone
Prednisone Intensol™ [US]
Prelone® [US]
ratio-Dexamethasone [Can]
Solu-Cortef® [US/Can]
Solu-Medrol® [US/Can]
Solurex L.A.® [US]
Sterapred® DS [US]
Sterapred® [US]
Tac™-3 Injection [US]
Triam-A® Injection [US]
triamcinolone (systemic)
Triam Forte® Injection [US]
Winpred™ [Can]

IRON DEFICIENCY ANEMIA
Iron Salt
    ferric gluconate

KAPOSI SARCOMA
Antineoplastic Agent
    daunorubicin citrate (liposomal)
    DaunoXome® [US]
    Doxil® [US/Can]
    doxorubicin (liposomal)
    Onxol™ [US]
    paclitaxel
    Taxol® [US/Can]
    Velban® [Can]
    vinblastine
Antineoplastic Agent, Miscellaneous
    alitretinoin
    Panretin™ [US/Can]
Biological Response Modulator
    interferon alfa-2a
    interferon alfa-2b
    Intron® A [US/Can]
    Roferon-A® [US/Can]
Retinoic Acid Derivative
    alitretinoin
    Panretin™ [US/Can]

KAWASAKI DISEASE
Immune Globulin
    BayGam® [US/Can]
    Carimune™ [US]
    Gamimune® N [US/Can]
    Gammagard® S/D [US/Can]
    Gammar®-P I.V. [US]
    Gamunex® [Can]
    immune globulin (intramuscular)
    immune globulin (intravenous)
    Iveegam EN [US]
    Iveegam Immuno® [Can]
    Panglobulin® [US]
    Polygam® S/D [US]
    Venoglobulin®-S [US]

KERATITIS
Adrenal Corticosteroid
    Eflone® [US]
    Flarex® [US/Can]
    fluorometholone
    Fluor-Op® [US]
    FML® Forte [US/Can]
    FML® [US/Can]
Anticholinergic Agent
    Diotrope® [Can]
    Mydriacyl® [US/Can]
    Opticyl® [US]
    Tropicacyl® [US]
    tropicamide
Mast Cell Stabilizer
    cromolyn sodium
    Opticrom® [US/Can]

KERATITIS (EXPOSURE)
Ophthalmic Agent, Miscellaneous
    Akwa Tears® [US-OTC]
    AquaSite® [US-OTC]
    artificial tears
    Bion® Tears [US-OTC]
    HypoTears PF [US-OTC]
    HypoTears [US-OTC]
    Isopto® Tears [US/Can]
    Liquifilm® Tears [US-OTC]
    Moisture® Eyes PM [US-OTC]
    Moisture® Eyes [US-OTC]
    Murine® Tears [US-OTC]
    Murocel® [US-OTC]
    Nature's Tears® [US-OTC]
    Nu-Tears® II [US-OTC]
    Nu-Tears® [US-OTC]
    OcuCoat® PF [US-OTC]
    OcuCoat® [US/Can]
    Puralube® Tears [US-OTC]
    Refresh® Plus [US/Can]
    Refresh® Tears [US/Can]
    Refresh® [US-OTC]
    Teardrops® [Can]
    Teargen® II [US-OTC]

Teargen® [US-OTC]
Tearisol® [US-OTC]
Tears Again® [US-OTC]
Tears Naturale® Free [US-OTC]
Tears Naturale® II [US-OTC]
Tears Naturale® [US-OTC]
Tears Plus® [US-OTC]
Tears Renewed® [US-OTC]
Ultra Tears® [US-OTC]
Viva-Drops® [US-OTC]

KERATITIS (FUNGAL)
Antifungal Agent
 Natacyn® [US/Can]
 natamycin

KERATITIS (HERPES SIMPLEX)
Antiviral Agent
 trifluridine
 Viroptic® [US/Can]

KERATITIS (VERNAL)
Antiviral Agent
 trifluridine
 Viroptic® [US/Can]
Mast Cell Stabilizer
 Alomide® [US/Can]
 lodoxamide tromethamine

KERATOCONJUNCTIVITIS (VERNAL)
Mast Cell Stabilizer
 Alomide® [US/Can]
 lodoxamide tromethamine

KERATOSIS (ACTINIC)
Photosensitizing Agent, Topical
 aminolevulinic acid
 Levulan® Kerastick™ [US/Can]
Porphyrin Agent, Topical
 aminolevulinic acid
 Levulan® Kerastick™ [US/Can]

LEPROSY
Immunosuppressant Agent
 thalidomide
 Thalomid® [US/Can]
Leprostatic Agent
 clofazimine
 Lamprene® [US/Can]
Sulfone
 dapsone

LICE
Scabicides/Pediculicides
 A-200™ [US-OTC]
 Acticin® [US]
 Elimite® [US]
 End Lice® [US-OTC]
 Hexit™ [Can]
 Kwellada-P™ [Can]
 lindane
 malathion
 Nix® Dermal Cream [Can]
 Nix® [US/Can]
 Ovide™ [US]
 permethrin
 PMS-Lindane [Can]
 Pronto® [US-OTC]
 pyrethrins
 Pyrinex® Pediculicide [US-OTC]
 Pyrinyl Plus® [US-OTC]
 Pyrinyl® [US-OTC]
 R & C™ II [Can]
 R & C™ Shampoo/Conditioner [Can]
 R & C® [US-OTC]
 RID® Mousse [Can]
 Rid® Spray [US-OTC]
 Tisit® Blue Gel [US-OTC]
 Tisit® [US-OTC]

LICHEN SIMPLEX CHRONICUS
Topical Skin Product
 doxepin
 Zonalon® Cream [US/Can]

LYME DISEASE
Antibiotic, Penicillin
   pivampicillin (Canada only)
   Pondocillin® [Can]
Cephalosporin (Third Generation)
   ceftriaxone
   Rocephin® [US/Can]
Macrolide (Antibiotic)
   Apo®-Erythro Base [Can]
   Apo®-Erythro E-C [Can]
   Apo®-Erythro-ES [Can]
   Apo®-Erythro-S [Can]
   Diomycin® [Can]
   E.E.S.® [US/Can]
   Erybid™ [Can]
   Eryc® [US/Can]
   EryPed® [US]
   Ery-Tab® [US]
   Erythrocin® [US]
   erythromycin (systemic)
   Nu-Erythromycin-S [Can]
   PCE® [US/Can]
   PMS-Erythromycin [Can]
Penicillin
   amoxicillin
   Amoxicot® [US]
   Amoxil® [US]
   ampicillin
   Apo®-Amoxi [Can]
   Apo®-Ampi [Can]
   Apo®-Pen VK [Can]
   Gen-Amoxicillin [Can]
   Lin-Amox [Can]
   Marcillin® [US]
   Moxilin® [US]
   Nadopen-V® [Can]
   Novamoxin® [Can]
   Novo-Ampicillin [Can]
   Novo-Pen-VK® [Can]
   Nu-Amoxi [Can]
   Nu-Ampi [Can]
   Nu-Pen-VK® [Can]
   penicillin V potassium
   PMS-Amoxicillin [Can]
   Principen® [US]
   PVF® K [Can]
   Suspen® [US]
   Trimox® [US]
   Truxcillin® [US]
   Veetids® [US]
Tetracycline Derivative
   Adoxa™ [US]
   Apo®-Doxy [Can]
   Apo®-Doxy Tabs [Can]
   Apo®-Tetra [Can]
   Brodspec® [US]
   Doryx® [US]
   Doxy-100® [US]
   Doxycin [Can]
   doxycycline
   EmTet® [US]
   Monodox® [US]
   Novo-Doxylin [Can]
   Novo-Tetra [Can]
   Nu-Doxycycline [Can]
   Nu-Tetra [Can]
   Periostat® [US]
   ratio-Doxycycline [Can]
   Sumycin® [US]
   tetracycline
   Vibramycin® [US]
   Vibra-Tabs® [US/Can]
   Wesmycin® [US]

MASTOCYTOSIS
Histamine H-2 Antagonist
   Alti-Ranitidine [Can]
   Apo®-Cimetidine [Can]
   Apo®-Famotidine [Can]
   Apo®-Ranitidine [Can]
   cimetidine
   famotidine
   Gen-Cimetidine [Can]
   Gen-Famotidine [Can]
   Gen-Ranitidine [Can]

Novo-Cimetidine [Can]
Novo-Famotidine [Can]
Novo-Ranidine [Can]
Nu-Cimet® [Can]
Nu-Famotidine [Can]
Nu-Ranit [Can]
Pepcid® AC [US/Can]
Pepcid® [US/Can]
PMS-Cimetidine [Can]
ranitidine hydrochloride
ratio-Famotidine [Can]
ratio-Ranitidine [Can]
Rhoxal-famotidine [Can]
Tagamet® HB 200 [US/Can]
Tagamet® [US]
Zantac® 75 [US-OTC]
Zanta [Can]
Zantac® [US/Can]
Mast Cell Stabilizer
Apo®-Cromolyn [Can]
Crolom® [US]
cromolyn sodium
Gastrocrom® [US]
Intal® [US/Can]
Nalcrom® [Can]
Nasalcrom® [US-OTC]
Nu-Cromolyn [Can]
Opticrom® [US/Can]

MEASLES
Vaccine, Live Virus
Attenuvax® [US]
measles, mumps, and rubella
vaccines, combined
measles virus vaccine (live)
M-M-R® II [US/Can]
Priorix™ [Can]

MEASLES (RUBEOLA)
Immune Globulin
BayGam® [US/Can]
immune globulin (intramuscular)

MELANOMA
Antineoplastic Agent
Blenoxane® [US/Can]
bleomycin
CeeNU® [US/Can]
cisplatin
Cosmegen® [US/Can]
dacarbazine
dactinomycin
Droxia™[US]
DTIC® [Can]
DTIC-Dome® [US]
Hydrea® [US/Can]
hydroxyurea
lomustine
Mylocel™ [US]
Platinol®-AQ [US]
Platinol® [US]
teniposide
Vumon® [US/Can]
Antiviral Agent
interferon alfa-2b and ribavirin
combination pack
Rebetron™ [US/Can]
Biological Response Modulator
interferon alfa-2a
interferon alfa-2b
interferon alfa-2b and ribavirin
combination pack
Intron® A [US/Can]
Rebetron™ [US/Can]
Roferon-A® [US/Can]

MELASMA (FACIAL)
Corticosteroid, Topical
fluocinolone, hydroquinone, and
tretinoin
Tri-Luma™ [US]
Depigmenting Agent
fluocinolone, hydroquinone, and
tretinoin
Tri-Luma™ [US]

Retinoic Acid Derivative
    fluocinolone, hydroquinone, and
        tretinoin
    Tri-Luma™ [US]

MOUTH INFECTION
Antibacterial, Topical
    Dequadin® [Can]
    dequalinium (Canada only)
Antifungal Agent, Topical
    Dequadin® [Can]
    dequalinium (Canada only)

MUMPS
Vaccine, Live Virus
    measles, mumps, and rubella
        vaccines, combined
    M-M-R® II [US/Can]
    Mumpsvax® [US/Can]
    mumps virus vaccine, live,
        attenuated
    Priorix™ [Can]

MUMPS (DIAGNOSTIC)
 Diagnostic Agent
    MSTA® Mumps [US/Can]
    mumps skin test antigen

MYCOBACTERIUM AVIUM-INTRACELLULARE
Antibiotic, Aminoglycoside
    streptomycin
Antibiotic, Miscellaneous
    Mycobutin® [US/Can]
    rifabutin
    Rifadin® [US/Can]
    rifampin
    Rimactane® [US]
    Rofact™ [Can]
Antimycobacterial Agent
    ethambutol

Etibi® [Can]
    Myambutol® [US]
Antitubercular Agent
    streptomycin
Carbapenem (Antibiotic)
    imipenem and cilastatin
    meropenem
    Merrem® I.V. [US/Can]
    Primaxin® [US/Can]
Leprostatic Agent
    clofazimine
    Lamprene® [US/Can]
Macrolide (Antibiotic)
    azithromycin
    Biaxin® [US/Can]
    Biaxin® XL [US/Can]
    clarithromycin
    Zithromax® [US/Can]
    Z-PAK® [US/Can]
Quinolone
    Ciloxan® [US/Can]
    ciprofloxacin
    Cipro® [US/Can]
    Cipro® XR [US/Can]

MYCOSIS (FUNGOIDES)
Psoralen
    methoxsalen
    8-MOP® [US/Can]
    Oxsoralen® Lotion [US/Can]
    Oxsoralen-Ultra® [US/Can]
    Ultramop™ [Can]
    Uvadex® [US/Can]

NIPPLE CARE
 Topical Skin Product
    glycerin, lanolin, and peanut oil
    Massae® Breast Cream [US-OTC]

OILY SKIN
Antiseborrheic Agent, Topical
    Aveeno® Cleansing Bar [US-OTC]
    Fostex® [US-OTC]

Pernox® [US-OTC]
Sastid® Plain Therapeutic Shampoo
and Acne Wash [US-OTC]
sulfur and salicylic acid

ONYCHOMYCOSIS
Antifungal Agent
Fulvicin® P/G [US]
Fulvicin-U/F® [US/Can]
Grifulvin® V Suspension [US]
griseofulvin
Gris-PEG® [US]
Lamisil® Oral [US/Can]
terbinafine (oral)

ORAL LESION
Local Anesthetic
benzocaine, gelatin, pectin, and
sodium carboxymethylcellulose
Orabase® With Benzocaine [US-OTC]

ORGAN REJECTION
Immunosuppressant Agent
daclizumab
Zenapax® [US/Can]

ORGAN TRANSPLANT
Immunosuppressant Agent
Apo®-Cyclosporine [Can]
basiliximab
CellCept® [US/Can]
cyclosporine
Gengraf™ [US]
muromonab-CD3
mycophenolate
Neoral® [US/Can]
Orthoclone OKT® 3 [US/Can]
Prograf® [US/Can]
Protopic® [US]
Rapamune® [US/Can]
Restasis™ [US]

Rhoxal-cyclosporine [Can]
Sandimmune® [US/Can]
Simulect® [US/Can]
sirolimus
tacrolimus

OSTEOARTHRITIS
Analgesic, Nonnarcotic
Arthrotec® [US/Can]
diclofenac and misoprostol
Analgesic, Topical
Antiphlogistine Rub A-535
Capsaicin [Can]
ArthriCare® for Women Extra
Moisturizing [US-OTC]
ArthriCare® for Women Silky Dry
[US-OTC]
Capsagel® [US-OTC]
capsaicin
Capzasin-HP® [US-OTC]
TheraPatch® Warm [US-OTC]
Zostrix®-HP [US/Can]
Zostrix® [US/Can]
Miscellaneous Product
sodium hyaluronate/hylan G-F 20
Synvisc® [US/Can]
Nonsteroidal Antiinflammatory Drug
(NSAID)
Advil® Children's [US-OTC]
Advil® Infants' Concentrated Drops
[US-OTC]
Advil® Junior [US-OTC]
Advil® Migraine [US-OTC]
Advil® [US/Can]
Albert® Tiafen [Can]
Aleve® [US-OTC]
Amigesic® [US/Can]
Anaprox® DS [US/Can]
Anaprox® [US/Can]
Apo®-Diclo [Can]
Apo®-Diclo SR [Can]
Apo®-Diflunisal [Can]
Apo®-Etodolac [Can]

Apo®-Ibuprofen [Can]
Apo®-Indomethacin [Can]
Apo®-Keto [Can]
Apo®-Keto-E [Can]
Apo®-Keto SR [Can]
Apo®-Nabumetone [Can]
Apo®-Napro-Na [Can]
Apo®-Napro-Na DS [Can]
Apo®-Naproxen [Can]
Apo®-Naproxen SR [Can]
Apo®-Oxaprozin [Can]
Apo®-Sulin [Can]
Apo®-Tiaprofenic [Can]
Argesic®-SA [US]
Asaphen [Can]
Asaphen E.C. [Can]
Ascriptin® Arthritis Pain [US-OTC]
Ascriptin® Enteric [US-OTC]
Ascriptin® Extra Strength [US-OTC]
Ascriptin® [US-OTC]
Aspercin Extra [US-OTC]
Aspercin [US-OTC]
aspirin
Bayer® Aspirin Extra Strength [US-OTC]
Bayer® Aspirin Regimen Adult Low Strength [US-OTC]
Bayer® Aspirin Regimen Adult Low Strength with Calcium [US-OTC]
Bayer® Aspirin Regimen Children's [US-OTC]
Bayer® Aspirin Regimen Regular Strength [US-OTC]
Bayer® Aspirin [US-OTC]
Bayer® Plus Extra Strength [US-OTC]
Bufferin® Arthritis Strength [US-OTC]
Bufferin® Extra Strength [US-OTC]
Bufferin® [US-OTC]
Cataflam® [US/Can]
choline magnesium trisalicylate
Clinoril® [US]
Daypro™ [US/Can]

diclofenac
diflunisal
Doan's®, Original [US-OTC]
Dolobid® [US]
Easprin® [US]
EC-Naprosyn® [US]
Ecotrin® Adult Low Strength [US-OTC]
Ecotrin® Maximum Strength [US-OTC]
Ecotrin® [US-OTC]
Entrophen® [Can]
etodolac
Extra Strength Doan's® [US-OTC]
Feldene® [US/Can]
fenoprofen
Gen-Nabumetone [Can]
Gen-Naproxen EC [Can]
Gen-Piroxicam [Can]
Genpril® [US-OTC]
Halfprin® [US-OTC]
Haltran® [US-OTC]
ibuprofen
Ibu-Tab® [US]
Indocid® [Can]
Indocid® P.D.A. [Can]
Indocin® SR [US]
Indocin® [US]
Indo-Lemmon [Can]
indomethacin
I-Prin [US-OTC]
ketoprofen
Keygesic-10® [US]
Lodine® [US/Can]
Lodine® XL [US]
magnesium salicylate
meclofenamate
meloxicam
Menadol® [US-OTC]
Midol® Maximum Strength Cramp Formula [US-OTC]
Mobicox® [Can]
MOBIC® [US/Can]

Momentum® [US-OTC]
Mono-Gesic® [US]
Motrin® Children's [US/Can]
Motrin® IB [US/Can]
Motrin® Infants' [US-OTC]
Motrin® Junior Strength [US-OTC]
Motrin® Migraine Pain [US-OTC]
Motrin® [US/Can]
nabumetone
Nalfon® [US/Can]
Naprelan® [US]
Naprosyn® [US/Can]
naproxen
Naxen® [Can]
Novasen [Can]
Novo-Difenac® [Can]
Novo-Difenac-K [Can]
Novo-Difenac® SR [Can]
Novo-Diflunisal [Can]
Novo-Keto [Can]
Novo-Keto-EC [Can]
Novo-Methacin [Can]
Novo-Naprox [Can]
Novo-Naprox Sodium [Can]
Novo-Naprox Sodium DS [Can]
Novo-Naprox SR [Can]
Novo-Pirocam® [Can]
Novo-Profen® [Can]
Novo-Sundac [Can]
Novo-Tiaprofenic [Can]
Nu-Diclo [Can]
Nu-Diclo-SR [Can]
Nu-Diflunisal [Can]
Nu-Ibuprofen [Can]
Nu-Indo [Can]
Nu-Ketoprofen [Can]
Nu-Ketoprofen-E [Can]
Nu-Naprox [Can]
Nu-Pirox [Can]
Nu-Sundac [Can]
Nu-Tiaprofenic [Can]
Orudis® KT [US-OTC]
Orudis® SR [Can]

Oruvail® [US/Can]
oxaprozin
Pennsaid® [Can]
Pexicam® [Can]
piroxicam
PMS-Diclofenac [Can]
PMS-Diclofenac SR [Can]
PMS-Tiaprofenic [Can]
ratio-Indomethacin [Can]
Relafen® [US/Can]
Rhodacine® [Can]
Rhodis™ [Can]
Rhodis-EC™ [Can]
Rhodis SR™ [Can]
Rhoxal-nabumetone [Can]
Riva-Diclofenac [Can]
Riva-Diclofenac-K [Can]
Riva-Naproxen [Can]
Salflex® [US/Can]
salsalate
Solaraze™ [US]
St. Joseph® Pain Reliever [US-OTC]
sulindac
Sureprin 81™ [US-OTC]
Surgam® [Can]
Surgam® SR [Can]
tiaprofenic acid (Canada only)
Tolectin® DS [US]
Tolectin® [US/Can]
tolmetin
Tricosal® [US]
Trilisate® [US]
Utradol™ [Can]
Voltaren Rapide® [Can]
Voltaren® [US/Can]
Voltaren®-XR [US]
Voltare Ophtha® [Can]
ZORprin® [US]
Nonsteroidal Antiinflammatory Drug
(NSAID), COX-2 Selective
Celebrex® [US/Can]
celecoxib
rofecoxib

Vioxx® [US/Can]
Prostaglandin
   Arthrotec® [US/Can]
   diclofcnac and misoprostol

OSTEOPOROSIS
Bisphosphonate Derivative
   alendronate
   Aredia® [US/Can]
   Didronel® [US/Can]
   etidronate disodium
   Fosamax® [US/Can]
   Gen-Etidronate [Can]
   Novo-Alendronate [Can]
   pamidronate
Electrolyte Supplement, Oral
   Calbon® [US]
   Calcionate® [US-OTC]
   Calciquid® [US-OTC]
   calcium glubionate
   calcium lactate
   calcium phosphate (dibasic)
   Cal-Lac® [US]
   Posture® [US-OTC]
   Ridactate® [US]
Estrogen and Progestin Combination
   estrogens and medroxyprogesterone
   Premphase® [US/Can]
   Prempro™ [US/Can]
Estrogen Derivative
   Alora® [US]
   Cenestin™ [US/Can]
   Climara® [US/Can]
   Congest [Can]
   Delestrogen® [US/Can]
   Depo®-Estradiol [US/Can]
   diethylstilbestrol
   Esclim® [US]
   Estinyl® [US]
   Estrace® [US/Can]
   Estraderm® [US/Can]
   estradiol

Estring® [US/Can]
Estrogel® [Can]
estrogens (conjugated A/synthetic)
estrogens (conjugated/equine)
estrogens (esterified)
ethinyl estradiol
Femring™ [US]
Gynodiol® [US]
Honvol® [Can]
Menest® [US]
Oesclim® [Can]
Premarin® [US/Can]
Vagifem® [US/Can]
Vivelle-Dot® [US]
Vivelle® [US/Can]
Mineral, Oral
   ACT® [US-OTC]
   Fluor-A-Day® [Can]
   fluoride
   Fluorigard® [US-OTC]
   Fluorinse® [US]
   Fluotic® [Can]
   Flura-Drops® [US]
   Flura-Loz® [US]
   Gel-Kam® [US]
   Lozi-Flur™ [US]
   Luride® Lozi-Tab® [US]
   Luride® [US]
   NeutraCare® [US]
   NeutraGard® [US-OTC]
   Pediaflor® [US]
   Pharmaflur® [US]
   Phos-Flur® [US]
   PreviDent® 5000 Plus™ [US]
   PreviDent® [US]
   Stan-Gard® [US]
   Stop® [US-OTC]
   Thera-Flur-N® [US]
Polypeptide Hormone
   Calcimar® [Can]
   calcitonin
   Caltine® [Can]

Miacalcin® [US/Can]
Selective Estrogen Receptor Modulator
(SERM)
Evista® [US/Can]
raloxifene

OTITIS EXTERNA

Aminoglycoside (Antibiotic)
AKTob® [US]
Alcomicin® [Can]
amikacin
Amikin® [Can]
Apo®-Tobramycin [Can]
Diogent® [Can]
Garamycin® [US/Can]
gentamicin
kanamycin
Kantrex® [US/Can]
Myciguent [US-OTC]
Neo-Fradin™ [US]
neomycin
Neo-Rx [US]
PMS-Tobramycin [Can]
ratio-Gentamicin [Can]
tobramycin
Tobrex® [US/Can]
Antibacterial, Otic
acetic acid
VoSol® [US]
Antibiotic/Corticosteroid, Otic
Acetasol® HC [US]
acetic acid, propylene glycol
diacetate, and hydrocortisone
AntibiOtic® Ear [US]
ciprofloxacin and hydrocortisone
Cipro® HC Otic [US/Can]
Coly-Mycin® S Otic [US]
Cortimyxin® [Can]
Cortisporin® Otic [US/Can]
Cortisporin®-TC Otic [US]
neomycin, colistin, hydrocortisone,
and thonzonium

neomycin, polymyxin B, and
hydrocortisone
PediOtic® [US]
VoSol® HC [US/Can]
Antibiotic, Otic
Apo®-Oflox [Can]
chloramphenicol
Chloromycetin® Parenteral
[US/Can]
Floxin® [US/Can]
ofloxacin
Pentamycetin® [Can]
Antifungal/Corticosteroid
Dermazene® [US]
iodoquinol and hydrocortisone
Vytone® [US]
Cephalosporin (Third Generation)
ceftazidime
Fortaz® [US/Can]
Tazicef® [US]
Tazidime® [US/Can]
Corticosteroid, Topical
Aclovate® [US]
Acticort® [US]
Aeroseb-HC® [US]
alclometasone
Alphatrex® [US]
amcinonide
Aquacort® [Can]
Aristocort® A Topical [US]
Aristocort® Topical [US]
Betaderm® [Can]
Betamethacot® [US]
betamethasone (topical)
Betatrex® [US]
Beta-Val® [US]
Betnovate® [Can]
CaldeCORT® [US-OTC]
Capex™ [US/Can]
Carmol-HC® [US]
Celestoderm®-EV/2 [Can]
Celestoderm®-V [Can]

Cetacort®
clobetasol
Clocort® Maximum Strength [US-OTC]
clocortolone
Cloderm® [US/Can]
Cordran® SP [US]
Cordran® [US/Can]
Cormax® [US]
CortaGel® [US-OTC]
Cortaid® Maximum Strength [US-OTC]
Cortaid® with Aloe [US-OTC]
Cort-Dome® [US]
Cortizone®-5 [US-OTC]
Cortizone®-10 [US-OTC]
Cortoderm [Can]
Cutivate™ [US]
Cyclocort® [US/Can]
Del-Beta® [US]
Delcort® [US]
Dermacort® [US]
Dermarest Dricort® [US]
Derma-Smoothe/FS® [US/Can]
Dermatop® [US/Can]
Dermolate® [US-OTC]
Dermovate® [Can]
Dermtex® HC with Aloe [US-OTC]
Desocort® [Can]
desonide
DesOwen® [US]
Desoxi® [Can]
desoximetasone
diflorasone
Diprolene® AF [US]
Diprolene® [US/Can]
Diprosone® [Can]
Eldecort® [US]
Elocon® [US/Can]
Embeline™ E [US]
fluocinolone
fluocinonide
Fluoderm [Can]

flurandrenolide
fluticasone (topical)
Gen-Clobetasol [Can]
Gynecort® [US-OTC]
halcinonide
halobetasol
Halog®-E [US]
Halog® [US/Can]
Hi-Cor-1.0® [US]
Hi-Cor-2.5® [US]
Hyderm [Can]
hydrocortisone (topical)
Hydrocort® [US]
Hydro-Tex® [US-OTC]
Hytone® [US]
Kenalog® Topical [US/Can]
LactiCare-HC® [US]
Lanacort® [US-OTC]
Lidemol® [Can]
Lidex-E® [US]
Lidex® [US/Can]
Locoid® [US/Can]
Luxiq™ [US]
Lyderm® [Can]
Maxiflor® [US]
Maxivate® [US]
mometasone furoate
Novo-Clobetasol [Can]
Nutracort® [US]
Olux® [US]
Orabase® HCA [US]
Oracort [Can]
Penecort® [US]
PMS-Desonide [Can]
prednicarbate
Prevex® [Can]
Prevex® HC [Can]
Psorcon™ E [US]
Psorcon™ [US/Can]
Qualisone® [US]
ratio-Clobetasol [Can]
ratio-Ectosone [Can]
ratio-Topilene® [Can]

ratio-Topisone® [Can]
Sarna® HC [Can]
Scalpicin® [US]
S-T Cort® [US]
Synacort® [US]
Synalar® [US/Can]
Taro-Desoximetasone [Can]
Taro-Sone® [Can]
Tegrin®-HC [US-OTC]
Temovate E® [US]
Temovate® [US]
Tiamol® [Can]
Ti-U-Lac® H [Can]
Topicort®-LP [US]
Topicort® [US/Can]
Topsyn® [Can]
Triacet™ Topical [US]
Triaderm [Can]
triamcinolone (topical)
Tridesilon® [US]
U-Cort™ [US]
Ultravate™ [US/Can]
urea and hydrocortisone
Uremol® HC [Can]
Westcort® [US/Can]
Otic Agent, Analgesic
A/B® Otic [US]
Allergan® Ear Drops [US]
antipyrine and benzocaine
Auralgan® [US/Can]
Aurodex® [US]
Auroto® [US]
Benzotic® [US]
Dec-Agesic® A.B. [US]
Dolotic® [US]
Rx-Otic® Drops [US]
Otic Agent, Antiinfective
Cresylate® [US]
m-cresyl acetate
Quinolone
ciprofloxacin
Cipro® [US/Can]
Cipro® XR [US/Can]

lomefloxacin
Maxaquin® [US]
nalidixic acid
NegGram® [US/Can]

PAIN

Analgesic, Miscellaneous
acetaminophen and tramadol
Ultracet™ [US]
Analgesic, Narcotic
acetaminophen and codeine
Actiq® [US/Can]
alfentanil
Alfenta® [US/Can]
Anexsia® [US]
Apo®-Butorphanol [Can]
aspirin and codeine
Astramorph/PF™ [US]
Avinza™ [US]
Bancap HC® [US]
belladonna and opium
B&O Supprettes® [US]
Buprenex® [US/Can]
buprenorphine
butalbital compound and codeine
butorphanol
Capital® and Codeine [US]
Ceta-Plus® [US]
codeine
Codeine Contin® [Can]
Co-Gesic® [US]
Coryphen® Codeine [Can]
Damason-P® [US]
Darvocet-N® 50 [US/Can]
Darvocet-N® 100 [US/Can]
Darvon® Compound-65 [US]
Darvon-N® Tablet [US/Can]
Darvon® [US]
Demerol® [US/Can]
dihydrocodeine compound
Dilaudid-5® [US]
Dilaudid-HP-Plus® [Can]
Dilaudid-HP® [US/Can]

Dilaudid® [US/Can]
Dilaudid-XP® [Can]
Dolacet® [US]
Dolophine® [US/Can]
Duragesic® [US/Can]
Duramorph® [US]
Empirin® With Codeine [US]
Endocet® [US/Can]
Endodan® [US/Can]
fentanyl
Fiorinal®-C 1/2 [Can]
Fiorinal®-C 1/4 [Can]
Fiorinal® With Codeine [US]
Hydrocet® [US]
hydrocodone and acetaminophen
hydrocodone and aspirin
hydrocodone and ibuprofen
Hydromorph Contin® [Can]
hydromorphone
Infumorph® [US]
Kadian® [US/Can]
Levo-Dromoran® [US]
levorphanol
Lorcet® 10/650 [US]
Lorcet®-HD [US]
Lorcet® Plus [US]
Lortab® [US]
Margesic® H [US]
Maxidone™ [US]
Mepergan® [US]
meperidine
meperidine and promethazine
Meperitab® [US]
M-Eslon® [Can]
Metadol™ [Can]
methadone
Methadone Intensol™ [US]
Methadose® [US/Can]
Morphine HP® [Can]
morphine sulfate
M.O.S.-Sulfate® [Can]
MS Contin® [US/Can]
MSIR® [US/Can]

nalbuphine
Norco® [US]
Nubain® [US/Can]
Numorphan® [US/Can]
opium tincture
Oramorph SR® [US]
oxycodone
oxycodone and acetaminophen
oxycodone and aspirin
OxyContin® [US/Can]
Oxydose™ [US]
OxyFast® [US]
OxyIR® [US/Can]
oxymorphone
paregoric
PC-Cap® [US]
pentazocine
pentazocine compound
Percocet® [US]
Percodan® [US/Can]
Phenaphen® With Codeine [US]
PMS-Butorphanol [Can]
PMS-Hydromorphone [Can]
PMS-Morphine Sulfate SR [Can]
PMS-Oxycodone-Acetaminophen [Can]
Pronap-100® [US]
propoxyphene
propoxyphene and acetaminophen
propoxyphene and aspirin
ratio-Codeine [Can]
ratio-Emtec-30 [Can]
ratio-Lenoltec [Can]
ratio-Morphine [Can]
ratio-Morphine SR [Can]
ratio-Oxycocet [Can]
ratio-Oxycodan® [Can]
ratio-Tecnal C 1/2 [Can]
ratio-Tecnal C 1/4 [Can]
remifentanil
RMS® [US]
Roxanol 100® [US]
Roxanol®-T [US]
Roxanol® [US]

Roxicet® 5/500 [US]
Roxicet™ [US]
Roxicodone™ Intensol™ [US]
Roxicodone™ [US]
Stadol® NS [US/Can]
Stadol® [US]
Stagesic® [US]
Statex® [Can]
Sublimaze® [US]
Subutex® [US]
sufentanil
Sufenta® [US/Can]
Supeudol® [Can]
Synalgos®-DC [US]
642® Tablet [Can]
Talacen® [US]
Talwin® NX [US]
Talwin® [US/Can]
T-Gesic® [US]
Triatec-8 [Can]
Triatec-30 [Can]
Triatec-Strong [Can]
Tylenol® with Codeine [US/Can]
Tylox® [US]
Ultiva™ [US/Can]
Vicodin® ES [US]
Vicodin® HP [US]
Vicodin® [US]
Vicoprofen® [US/Can]
Zydone® [US]
Analgesic, Nonnarcotic
Abenol® [Can]
Acephen® [US-OTC]
acetaminophen
acetaminophen and
   diphenhydramine
acetaminophen and
   phenyltoloxamine
acetaminophen and tramadol
acetaminophen, aspirin, and caffeine
Acular LS™ [US]
Acular® P.F. [US]
Acular® [US/Can]

Advil® Children's [US-OTC]
Advil® Infants' Concentrated Drops
   [US-OTC]
Advil® Junior [US-OTC]
Advil® Migraine [US-OTC]
Advil® [US/Can]
Aleve® [US-OTC]
Amigesic® [US/Can]
Anaprox® DS [US/Can]
Anaprox® [US/Can]
Ansaid® Oral [US/Can]
Apo®-Acetaminophen [Can]
Apo®-Diclo [Can]
Apo®-Diclo SR [Can]
Apo®-Diflunisal [Can]
Apo®-Etodolac [Can]
Apo®-Flurbiprofen [Can]
Apo®-Ibuprofen [Can]
Apo®-Indomethacin [Can]
Apo®-Keto [Can]
Apo®-Keto-E [Can]
Apo®-Ketorolac [Can]
Apo®-Keto SR [Can]
Apo®-Mefenamic [Can]
Apo®-Nabumetone [Can]
Apo®-Napro-Na [Can]
Apo®-Napro-Na DS [Can]
Apo®-Naproxen [Can]
Apo®-Naproxen SR [Can]
Apo®-Oxaprozin [Can]
Apo®-Sulin [Can]
Argesic®-SA [US]
Asaphen [Can]
Asaphen E.C. [Can]
Ascriptin® Arthritis Pain [US-OTC]
Ascriptin® Enteric [US-OTC]
Ascriptin® Extra Strength [US-OTC]
Ascriptin® [US-OTC]
Aspercin Extra [US-OTC]
Aspercin [US-OTC]
aspirin
Atasol® [Can]

Bayer® Aspirin Extra Strength [US-OTC]

Bayer® Aspirin Regimen Adult Low Strength [US-OTC]

Bayer® Aspirin Regimen Adult Low Strength with Calcium [US-OTC]

Bayer® Aspirin Regimen Children's [US-OTC]

Bayer® Aspirin Regimen Regular Strength [US-OTC]

Bayer® Aspirin [US-OTC]

Bayer® Plus Extra Strength [US-OTC]

Brexidol® 20 [Can]

Bufferin® Arthritis Strength [US-OTC]

Bufferin® Extra Strength [US-OTC]

Bufferin® [US-OTC]

Cataflam® [US/Can]

Cetafen Extra® [US-OTC]

Cetafen® [US-OTC]

choline magnesium trisalicylate

Clinoril® [US]

Daypro™ [US/Can]

diclofenac

diflunisal

Dolobid® [US]

Easprin® [US]

EC-Naprosyn® [US]

Ecotrin® Adult Low Strength [US-OTC]

Ecotrin® Maximum Strength [US-OTC]

Ecotrin® [US-OTC]

Entrophen® [Can]

etodolac

Excedrin® Extra Strength [US-OTC]

Excedrin® Migraine [US-OTC]

Excedrin® P.M. [US-OTC]

Feldene® [US/Can]

fenoprofen

Feverall® [US-OTC]

flurbiprofen

Froben® [Can]

Froben-SR® [Can]

Genaced [US-OTC]

Genapap® Children [US-OTC]

Genapap® Extra Strength [US-OTC]

Genapap® Infant [US-OTC]

Genapap® [US-OTC]

Genebs® Extra Strength [US-OTC]

Genebs® [US-OTC]

Genesec® [US-OTC]

Gen-Nabumetone [Can]

Gen-Naproxen EC [Can]

Gen-Piroxicam [Can]

Genpril® [US-OTC]

Goody's® Extra Strength Headache Powder [US-OTC]

Goody's PM® Powder [US-OTC]

Halfprin® [US-OTC]

Haltran® [US-OTC]

ibuprofen

Ibu-Tab® [US]

Indocid® [Can]

Indocid® P.D.A. [Can]

Indocin® SR [US]

Indocin® [US]

Indo-Lemmon [Can]

indomethacin

Infantaire [US-OTC]

I-Prin [US-OTC]

ketoprofen

ketorolac

Legatrin PM® [US-OTC]

Liquiprin® for Children [US-OTC]

Lodine® [US/Can]

Lodine® XL [US]

Mapap® Children's [US-OTC]

Mapap® Extra Strength [US-OTC]

Mapap® Infants [US-OTC]

Mapap® [US-OTC]

meclofenamate

mefenamic acid

Menadol® [US-OTC]

Midol® Maximum Strength Cramp
   Formula [US-OTC]
Mono-Gesic® [US]
Motrin® Children's [US/Can]
Motrin® IB [US/Can]
Motrin® Infants' [US-OTC]
Motrin® Junior Strength [US-OTC]
Motrin® Migraine Pain [US-OTC]
Motrin® [US/Can]
nabumetone
Nalfon® [US/Can]
Naprelan® [US]
Naprosyn® [US/Can]
naproxen
Naxen® [Can]
Norgesic™ Forte [US/Can]
Norgesic™ [US/Can]
Novasen [Can]
Novo-Difenac® [Can]
Novo-Difenac-K [Can]
Novo-Difenac® SR [Can]
Novo-Diflunisal [Can]
Novo-Flurprofen [Can]
Novo-Keto [Can]
Novo-Keto-EC [Can]
Novo-Ketorolac [Can]
Novo-Methacin [Can]
Novo-Naprox [Can]
Novo-Naprox Sodium [Can]
Novo-Naprox Sodium DS [Can]
Novo-Naprox SR [Can]
Novo-Pirocam® [Can]
Novo-Profen® [Can]
Novo-Sundac [Can]
Nu-Diclo [Can]
Nu-Diclo-SR [Can]
Nu-Diflunisal [Can]
Nu-Flurprofen [Can]
Nu-Ibuprofen [Can]
Nu-Indo [Can]
Nu-Ketoprofen [Can]
Nu-Ketoprofen-E [Can]
Nu-Mefenamic [Can]

Nu-Naprox [Can]
Nu-Pirox [Can]
Nu-Sundac [Can]
Ocufen® Ophthalmic [US/Can]
orphenadrine, aspirin, and caffeine
Orphengesic Forte [US]
Orphengesic [US]
Orudis® KT [US-OTC]
Orudis® SR [Can]
Oruvail® [US/Can]
oxaprozin
Pediatrix [Can]
Pennsaid® [Can]
Percogesic® Extra Strength [US-OTC]
Percogesic® [US-OTC]
Pexicam® [Can]
Phenylgesic® [US-OTC]
piroxicam
piroxicam and cyclodextrin (Canada
   only)
PMS-Diclofenac [Can]
PMS-Diclofenac SR [Can]
PMS-Mefenamic Acid [Can]
Ponstan® [Can]
Ponstel® [US/Can]
ratio-Flurbiprofen [Can]
ratio-Indomethacin [Can]
ratio-Ketorolac [Can]
Redutemp® [US-OTC]
Relafen® [US/Can]
Rhodacine® [Can]
Rhodis™ [Can]
Rhodis-EC™ [Can]
Rhodis SR™ [Can]
Rhoxal-nabumetone [Can]
Riva-Diclofenac [Can]
Riva-Diclofenac-K [Can]
Riva-Naproxen [Can]
Salflex® [US/Can]
salsalate
Silapap® Children's [US-OTC]
Silapap® Infants [US-OTC]
sodium salicylate

Solaraze™ [US]
St. Joseph® Pain Reliever [US-OTC]
sulindac
Sureprin 81™[US-OTC]
Tempra® [Can]
Tolectin® DS [US]
Tolectin® [US/Can]
tolmetin
Toradol® [US/Can]
tramadol
Tricosal® [US]
Trilisate® [US]
Tylenol® Arthritis Pain [US-OTC]
Tylenol® Children's [US-OTC]
Tylenol® Extra Strength [US-OTC]
Tylenol® Infants [US-OTC]
Tylenol® Junior Strength [US-OTC]
Tylenol® PM Extra Strength [US-OTC]
Tylenol® Severe Allergy [US-OTC]
Tylenol® Sore Throat [US-OTC]
Tylenol® [US/Can]
Ultracet™ [US]
Ultram® [US/Can]
Utradol™ [Can]
Valorin Extra [US-OTC]
Valorin [US-OTC]
Vanquish® Extra Strength Pain Reliever [US-OTC]
Voltaren Rapide® [Can]
Voltaren® [US/Can]
Voltaren®-XR [US]
Voltare Ophtha® [Can]
ZORprin® [US]
Decongestant/Analgesic
Advil® Cold, Children's [US-OTC]
Advil® Cold & Sinus [US/Can]
Dristan® Sinus Caplets [US]
Dristan® Sinus Tablet [US/Can]
Motrin® Cold and Sinus [US-OTC]
Motrin® Cold, Children's [US-OTC]
pseudoephedrine and ibuprofen

Local Anesthetic
Alcaine® [US/Can]
Diocaine® [Can]
ethyl chloride
ethyl chloride and dichlorotetrafluoroethane
Fluro-Ethyl® Aerosol [US]
Ophthetic® [US]
Parcaine® [US]
proparacaine
Neuroleptic Agent
Apo®-Methoprazine [Can]
methotrimeprazine (Canada only)
Novo-Meprazine [Can]
Nozinan® [Can]
Nonsteroidal Antiinflammatory Drug (NSAID)
Doan's®, Original [US-OTC]
Extra Strength Doan's® [US-OTC]
Keygesic-10® [US]
magnesium salicylate
Momentum® [US-OTC]
Nonsteroidal Antiinflammatory Drug (NSAID), COX-2 Selective
rofecoxib
Vioxx® [US/Can]
Nonsteroidal Antiinflammatory Drug (NSAID), Oral
Apo®-Floctafenine [Can]
floctafenine (Canada only)
Idarac® [Can]

PAIN (ANOGENITAL)
Anesthetic/Corticosteroid
Analpram-HC® [US]
Enzone® [US]
Epifoam® [US]
Pramosone® [US]
Pramox® HC [Can]
pramoxine and hydrocortisone
ProctoFoam®-HC [US/Can]
Zone-A Forte® [US]
Zone-A® [US]

Local Anesthetic
  benzocaine
  dibucaine
  dyclonine
  Fleet® Pain Relief [US-OTC]
  Foille® [US-OTC]
  Hurricaine® [US]
  Mycinettes® [US-OTC]
  Nupercainal® [US-OTC]
  Pontocaine® [US/Can]
  pramoxine
  Prax® [US-OTC]
  ProctoFoam® NS [US-OTC]
  tetracaine
  Trocaine® [US-OTC]
  Tronolane® [US-OTC]
  Tronothane® [US-OTC]

PAIN (SKIN GRAFT HARVESTING)
Analgesic, Topical
  EMLA® [US/Can]
  lidocaine and prilocaine

PARACOCCIDIOIDOMYCOSIS
Antifungal Agent
  Apo®-Ketoconazole [Can]
  ketoconazole
  Ketoderm® [Can]
  Nizoral® [US/Can]
  Novo-Ketoconazole [Can]

PEMPHIGUS
Aminoquinoline (Antimalarial)
  Aralen® Phosphate [US/Can]
  chloroquine phosphate

PERIANAL WART
Immune Response Modifier
  Aldara™ [US/Can]
  imiquimod

PINWORM
Anthelmintic

Combantrin™ [Can]
mebendazole
Pin-X® [US-OTC]
pyrantel pamoate
Reese's® Pinworm Medicine [US-OTC]
Vermox® [US/Can]

PITYRIASIS (ROSEA)
Corticosteroid, Topical
  Aclovate® [US]
  Acticort® [US]
  Aeroseb-HC® [US]
  alclometasone
  Alphatrex® [US]
  amcinonide
  Amcort® [Can]
  Anusol® HC-1 [US-OTC]
  Anusol® HC-2.5% [US-OTC]
  Aquacort® [Can]
  Aristocort® A Topical [US]
  Aristocort® Topical [US]
  Bactine® Hydrocortisone [US-OTC]
  Betaderm® [Can]
  Betamethacot® [US]
  betamethasone (topical)
  Betatrex® [US]
  Beta-Val® [US]
  Betnovate® [Can]
  CaldeCORT® Anti-Itch Spray [US]
  CaldeCORT® [US-OTC]
  Capex™ [US/Can]
  Carmol-HC® [US]
  Celestoderm®-EV/2 [Can]
  Celestoderm®-V [Can]
  Cetacort®
  clobetasol
  Clocort® Maximum Strength [US-OTC]
  clocortolone
  Cloderm® [US/Can]
  Cordran® SP [US]
  Cordran® [US/Can]

Cormax® [US]
CortaGel® [US-OTC]
Cortaid® Maximum Strength [US-OTC]
Cortaid® with Aloe [US-OTC]
Cort-Dome® [US]
Cortizone®-5 [US-OTC]
Cortizone®-10 [US-OTC]
Cortoderm [Can]
Cutivate™ [US]
Cyclocort® [US/Can]
Del-Beta® [US]
Delcort® [US]
Dermacort® [US]
Dermarest Dricort® [US]
Derma-Smoothe/FS® [US/Can]
Dermatop® [US/Can]
Dermolate® [US-OTC]
Dermovate® [Can]
Dermtex® HC with Aloe [US-OTC]
Desocort® [Can]
desonide
DesOwen® [US]
Desoxi® [Can]
desoximetasone
diflorasone
Diprolene® AF [US]
Diprolene® [US/Can]
Diprosone® [Can]
Eldecort® [US]
Elocon® [US/Can]
Embeline™ E [US]
fluocinolone
fluocinonide
Fluoderm [Can]
flurandrenolide
fluticasone (topical)
Gen-Clobetasol [Can]
Gynecort® [US-OTC]
halcinonide
halobetasol
Halog®-E [US]
Halog® [US/Can]

Hi-Cor-1.0® [US]
Hi-Cor-2.5® [US]
Hyderm [Can]
hydrocortisone (topical)
Hydrocort® [US]
Hydro-Tex® [US-OTC]
Hytone® [US]
Kenalog® in Orabase® [US/Can]
Kenalog® Topical [US/Can]
LactiCare-HC® [US]
Lanacort® [US-OTC]
Lidemol® [Can]
Lidex-E® [US]
Lidex® [US/Can]
Locoid® [US/Can]
Luxiq™ [US]
Lyderm® [Can]
Maxiflor® [US]
Maxivate® [US]
mometasone furoate
Nasonex® [US/Can]
Novo-Clobetasol [Can]
Nutracort® [US]
Olux® [US]
Orabase® HCA [US]
Oracort [Can]
Penecort® [US]
PMS-Desonide [Can]
prednicarbate
Prevex® [Can]
Prevex® HC [Can]
Psorcon™ E [US]
Psorcon™ [US/Can]
Qualisone® [US]
ratio-Clobetasol [Can]
ratio-Ectosone [Can]
ratio-Topilene® [Can]
ratio-Topisone® [Can]
Sarna® HC [Can]
Scalpicin® [US]
S-T Cort® [US]
Synacort® [US]
Synalar® [US/Can]

Taro-Desoximetasone [Can]
Taro-Sone® [Can]
Tegrin®-HC [US-OTC]
Temovate E® [US]
Temovate® [US]
Tiamol® [Can]
Ti-U-Lac® H [Can]
Topicort®-LP [US]
Topicort® [US/Can]
Topsyn® [Can]
Triacet™ Topical [US]
Triaderm [Can]
triamcinolone (topical)
Tridesilon® [US]
U-Cort™ [US]
Ultravate™ [US/Can]
urea and hydrocortisone
Uremol® HC [Can]
Valisone® Scalp Lotion [Can]
Westcort® [US/Can]

PLANTARIS
Keratolytic Agent
Duofilm® Solution [US]
Keralyt® Gel [US-OTC]
salicylic acid and lactic acid
salicylic acid and propylene glycol

PLANTAR WART
Keratolytic Agent
Duofilm® Solution [US]
salicylic acid and lactic acid
Topical Skin Product
silver nitrate

POISON IVY
Protectant, Topical
bentoquatam
IvyBlock® [US-OTC]

POISON OAK
Protectant, Topical
bentoquatam
IvyBlock® [US-OTC]

POISON SUMAC
Protectant, Topical
bentoquatam
IvyBlock® [US-OTC]

POLYCYTHEMIA VERA
Antineoplastic Agent
busulfan
Busulfex® [US/Can]
mechlorethamine
Mustargen® [US/Can]
Myleran® [US/Can]

POLYP, NASAL
Adrenal Corticosteroid
Acthar® [US]
AeroBid®-M [US]
AeroBid® [US]
A-methapred® [US]
Apo®-Beclomethasone [Can]
Apo®-Flunisolide [Can]
Apo®-Prednisone [Can]
Aristocort® Forte Injection [US]
Aristocort® Intralesional Injection
   [US]
Aristocort® Tablet [US/Can]
Aristospan® Intraarticular Injection
   [US/Can]
Aristospan® Intralesional Injection
   [US/Can]
beclomethasone
Beconase® AQ [US]
Betaject™ [Can]
betamethasone (systemic)
Betnesol® [Can]
Celestone® Phosphate [US]
Celestone® Soluspan® [US/Can]
Celestone® [US]
Cel-U-Jec® [US]
corticotropin
cortisone acetate
Cortone® [Can]
Deltasone® [US]

Depo-Medrol® [US/Can]
Depopred® [US]
Dexacort® Phosphate Turbinaire® [US]
dexamethasone (nasal)
flunisolide
Gen-Beclo [Can]
H.P. Acthar® Gel [US]
Kenalog® Injection [US/Can]
Medrol® Dosepak™ [US/Can]
Medrol® Tablet [US/Can]
methylprednisolone
Nasalide® [US/Can]
Nasarel® [US]
Nu-Beclomethasone [Can]
Orapred™ [US]
Pediapred® [US/Can]
Prednicot® [US]
prednisolone (systemic)
Prednisol® TBA [US]
prednisone
Prednisone Intensol™ [US]
Prelone® [US]
Propaderm® [Can]
QVAR™ [US/Can]
ratio-Flunisolide [Can]
Rhinalar® [Can]
Rivanase AQ [Can]
Solu-Medrol® [US/Can]
Sterapred® DS [US]
Sterapred® [US]
Tac™-3 Injection [US]
Triam-A® Injection [US]
triamcinolone (systemic)
Triam Forte® Injection [US]
Winpred™ [Can]
Corticosteroid, Topical
Nasacort® AQ [US/Can]
triamcinolone (inhalation, nasal)
Trinasal® [Can]

PROTOZOAL INFECTION
Antiprotozoal
Apo®-Metronidazole [Can]
Flagyl ER® [US]
Flagyl® [US/Can]
Florazole ER® [Can]
metronidazole
NebuPent® [US]
Noritate® [US/Can]
Novo-Nidazol [Can]
Pentacarinat® [Can]
Pentam-300® [US]
pentamidine
Trikacide® [Can]

PRURITUS
Antihistamine
Alavert™ [US-OTC]
Aler-Dryl [US-OTC]
Aller-Chlor® [US-OTC]
Allerdryl® [Can]
AllerMax® [US-OTC]
Allernix [Can]
ANX® [US]
Apo®-Hydroxyzine [Can]
Apo®-Loratadine [Can]
Atarax® [US/Can]
azatadine
Banophen® [US-OTC]
Benadryl® Dye-Free Allergy [US-OTC]
Benadryl® Gel Extra Strength [US-OTC]
Benadryl® Gel [US-OTC]
Benadryl® Injection [US]
Benadryl® [US/Can]
brompheniramine
chlorpheniramine
Chlor-Trimeton® [US-OTC]
Chlor-Tripolon® [Can]
Claritin® RediTabs® [US]
Claritin® [US-OTC/Can]
clemastine

A151

Colhist® Solution [US-OTC]
cyproheptadine
dexchlorpheniramine
Dimetane® Extentabs® [US-OTC]
Dimetapp® Allergy Children's [US-OTC]
Dimetapp® Allergy [US-OTC]
Diphen® AF [US-OTC]
Diphenhist [US-OTC]
diphenhydramine
Diphen® [US-OTC]
Genahist® [US-OTC]
Hydramine® [US-OTC]
hydroxyzine
Hyrexin-50® [US]
Lodrane® 12 Hour [US-OTC]
loratadine
ND-Stat® Solution [US-OTC]
Nolahist® [US/Can]
Novo-Hydroxyzin [Can]
Novo-Pheniram® [Can]
Optimine® [US/Can]
Panectyl® [Can]
phenindamine
PMS-Diphenhydramine [Can]
PMS-Hydroxyzine [Can]
Polytapp® Allergy Dye-Free
   Medication [US-OTC]
Siladryl® Allergy [US-OTC]
Silphen® [US-OTC]
Tavist®-1 [US-OTC]
Tavist® [US]
trimeprazine (Canada only)
Vistacot® [US]
Vistaril® [US/Can]
Phenothiazine Derivative
   Anergan® [US]
   Phenergan® [US/Can]
   promethazine

PSEUDOGOUT
Antigout Agent
   colchicine

ratio-Colchicine [Can]
Nonsteroidal Antiinflammatory Drug
   (NSAID)
   Apo®-Indomethacin [Can]
   Indocid® [Can]
   Indocid® P.D.A. [Can]
   Indocin® SR [US]
   Indocin® [US]
   Indo-Lemmon [Can]
   indomethacin
   Novo-Methacin [Can]
   Nu-Indo [Can]
   ratio-Indomethacin [Can]
   Rhodacine® [Can]

PSORIASIS
Antibiotic/Corticosteroid, Topical
   neomycin and hydrocortisone
Antineoplastic Agent
   Apo®-Methotrexate [Can]
   methotrexate
   ratio-Methotrexate [Can]
   Rheumatrex® [US]
   Trexall™ [US]
Antipsoriatic Agent
   Balnetar® [US/Can]
   Betatar® [US-OTC]
   calcipotriene
   coal tar
   coal tar and salicylic acid
   coal tar, lanolin, and mineral oil
   Cutar® [US-OTC]
   DHS™ Targel [US-OTC]
   DHS™ Tar [US-OTC]
   Doak® Tar [US-OTC]
   Dovonex® [US]
   Estar® [US-OTC]
   Exorex® [US]
   Ionil T® Plus [US-OTC]
   Ionil T® [US-OTC]
   MG 217® Medicated Tar [US-OTC]
   MG 217® [US-OTC]

Neutrogena® T/Gel Extra Strength [US-OTC]
Neutrogena® T/Gel [US-OTC]
Oxipor® VHC [US-OTC]
Pentrax® [US-OTC]
Polytar® [US-OTC]
PsoriGel® [US-OTC]
Reme-T™ [US-OTC]
Sebcur/T® [Can]
Tarsum® [US-OTC]
Tegrin® [US-OTC]
X-Seb™ T [US-OTC]
Zetar® [US-OTC]
Corticosteroid, Topical
Aclovate® [US]
Acticort® [US]
Aeroseb-HC® [US]
alclometasone
Alphatrex® [US]
amcinonide
Amcort® [Can]
Anusol® HC-1 [US-OTC]
Anusol® HC-2.5% [US-OTC]
Aquacort® [Can]
Aristocort® A Topical [US]
Aristocort® Topical [US]
Bactine® Hydrocortisone [US-OTC]
Betaderm® [Can]
Betamethacot® [US]
betamethasone and calcipotriol
    (Canada only)
betamethasone (topical)
Betatrex® [US]
Beta-Val® [US]
Betnovate® [Can]
CaldeCORT® Anti-Itch Spray [US]
CaldeCORT® [US-OTC]
Capex™ [US/Can]
Carmol-HC® [US]
Celestoderm®-EV/2 [Can]
Celestoderm®-V [Can]
Cetacort®
clobetasol

Clocort® Maximum Strength [US-OTC]
clocortolone
Cloderm® [US/Can]
Cordran® SP [US]
Cordran® [US/Can]
Cormax® [US]
CortaGel® [US-OTC]
Cortaid® Maximum Strength [US-OTC]
Cortaid® with Aloe [US-OTC]
Cort-Dome® [US]
Cortizone®-5 [US-OTC]
Cortizone®-10 [US-OTC]
Cortoderm [Can]
Cutivate™ [US]
Cyclocort® [US/Can]
Del-Beta® [US]
Delcort® [US]
Dermacort® [US]
Dermarest Dricort® [US]
Derma-Smoothe/FS® [US/Can]
Dermatop® [US/Can]
Dermolate® [US-OTC]
Dermovate® [Can]
Dermtex® HC with Aloe [US-OTC]
Desocort® [Can]
desonide
DesOwen® [US]
Desoxi® [Can]
desoximetasone
diflorasone
Diprolene® AF [US]
Diprolene® [US/Can]
Diprosone® [Can]
Dovobet® [Can]
Eldecort® [US]
Elocon® [US/Can]
Embeline™ E [US]
fluocinolone
fluocinonide
Fluoderm [Can]
flurandrenolide

fluticasone (topical)
Gen-Clobetasol [Can]
Gynecort® [US-OTC]
halcinonide
halobetasol
Halog®-E [US]
Halog® [US/Can]
Hi-Cor-1.0® [US]
Hi-Cor-2.5® [US]
Hyderm [Can]
hydrocortisone (topical)
Hydrocort® [US]
Hydro-Tex® [US-OTC]
Hytone® [US]
Kenalog® in Orabase® [US/Can]
Kenalog® Topical [US/Can]
LactiCare-HC® [US]
Lanacort® [US-OTC]
Lidemol® [Can]
Lidex-E® [US]
Lidex® [US/Can]
Locoid® [US/Can]
Luxiq™ [US]
Lyderm® [Can]
Maxiflor® [US]
Maxivate® [US]
mometasone furoate
Nasonex® [US/Can]
Novo-Clobetasol [Can]
Nutracort® [US]
Olux® [US]
Orabase® HCA [US]
Oracort [Can]
Penecort® [US]
PMS-Desonide [Can]
prednicarbate
Prevex® [Can]
Prevex® HC [Can]
Psorcon™ E [US]
Psorcon™ [US/Can]
Qualisone® [US]
ratio-Clobetasol [Can]
ratio-Ectosone [Can]

ratio-Topilene® [Can]
ratio-Topisone® [Can]
Sarna® HC [Can]
Scalpicin® [US]
S-T Cort® [US]
Synacort® [US]
Synalar® [US/Can]
Taro-Desoximetasone [Can]
Taro-Sone® [Can]
Tegrin®-HC [US-OTC]
Temovate E® [US]
Temovate® [US]
Tiamol® [Can]
Ti-U-Lac® H [Can]
Topicort®-LP [US]
Topicort® [US/Can]
Topsyn® [Can]
Triacet™ Topical [US]
Triaderm [Can]
triamcinolone (topical)
Tridesilon® [US]
U-Cort™ [US]
Ultravate™ [US/Can]
urea and hydrocortisone
Uremol® HC [Can]
Valisone® Scalp Lotion [Can]
Westcort® [US/Can]
Keratolytic Agent
Anthraforte® [Can]
anthralin
Anthranol® [Can]
Anthrascalp® [Can]
Avage™ [US]
Compound W® One Step Wart
  Remover [US-OTC]
Compound W® [US-OTC]
DHS™ Sal [US-OTC]
Drithocreme® [US]
Dr. Scholl's® Callus Remover [US-
  OTC]
Dr. Scholl's® Clear Away [US-OTC]
Duoforte® 27 [Can]
Freezone® [US-OTC]

Fung-O® [US-OTC]
Gordofilm® [US-OTC]
Hydrisalic™ [US-OTC]
Ionil® Plus [US-OTC]
Ionil® [US-OTC]
Keralyt® Gel [US-OTC]
Keralyt® [US-OTC]
LupiCare™ Dandruff [US-OTC]
LupiCare™ II Psoriasis [US-OTC]
LupiCare™ Psoriasis [US-OTC]
Mediplast® [US-OTC]
MG217 Sal-Acid® [US-OTC]
Micanol® [US/Can]
Mosco® Corn and Callus Remover [US-OTC]
NeoCeuticals™ Acne Spot Treatment [US-OTC]
Neutrogena® Acne Wash [US-OTC]
Neutrogena® Body Clear™ [US-OTC]
Neutrogena® Clear Pore Shine Control [US-OTC]
Neutrogena® Clear Pore [US-OTC]
Neutrogena® Healthy Scalp [US-OTC]
Neutrogena® Maximum Strength T/Sal® [US-OTC]
Neutrogena® On The Spot® Acne Patch [US-OTC]
Occlusal™ [Can]
Occlusal®-HP [US/Can]
Oxy® Balance Deep Pore [US-OTC]
Oxy Balance® [US-OTC]
Palmer's® Skin Success Acne Cleanser [US-OTC]
Pedisilk® [US-OTC]
Propa pH [US-OTC]
Sal-Acid® [US-OTC]
Salactic® [US-OTC]
SalAc® [US-OTC]
salicylic acid
salicylic acid and propylene glycol
Sal-Plant® [US-OTC]

Sebcur® [Can]
Soluver® [Can]
Soluver® Plus [Can]
Stri-dex® Body Focus [US-OTC]
Stri-dex® Facewipes To Go™ [US-OTC]
Stri-dex® Maximum Strength [US-OTC]
Stri-dex® [US-OTC]
tazarotene
Tazorac® [US/Can]
Tinamed® [US-OTC]
Tiseb® [US-OTC]
Trans-Ver-Sal® [US-OTC/Can]
Wart-Off® Maximum Strength [US-OTC]
Zapzyt® Acne Wash [US-OTC]
Zapzyt® Pore Treatment [US-OTC]
Monoclonal Antibody
 alefacept
 Amevive® [US]
Psoralen
 methoxsalen
 8-MOP® [US/Can]
 Oxsoralen® Lotion [US/Can]
 Oxsoralen-Ultra® [US/Can]
 Ultramop™ [Can]
 Uvadex® [US/Can]
Retinoid-like Compound
 acitretin
 Soriatane® [US/Can]
Vitamin D Analog
 betamethasone and calcipotriol (Canada only)
 Dovobet® [Can]

PURPURA
Immune Globulin
 Carimune™ [US]
 Gamimune® N [US/Can]
 Gammagard® S/D [US/Can]
 Gammar®-P I.V. [US]
 Gamunex® [Can]

immune globulin (intravenous)
Iveegam EN [US]
Iveegam Immuno® [Can]
Panglobulin® [US]
Polygam® S/D [US]
Venoglobulin®-S [US]
Immunosuppressant Agent
Alti-Azathioprine [Can]
Apo®-Azathioprine [Can]
azathioprine
Gen-Azathioprine [Can]
Imuran® [US/Can]
ratio-Azathioprine [Can]

PURPURA (THROMBOCYTOPENIC)
Antineoplastic Agent
Oncovin® [Can]
Vincasar® PFS® [US/Can]
vincristine

RATTLESNAKE BITE
Antivenin
antivenin (Crotalidae) polyvalent
Antivenin Polyvalent [Equine] [US]
CroFab™ [Ovine] [US]

RENAL ALLOGRAFT REJECTION
Immunosuppressant Agent
antithymocyte globulin (rabbit)
Thymoglobulin® [US]

RHEUMATIC DISORDER
Adrenal Corticosteroid
Acthar® [US]
A-HydroCort® [US]
A-methapred® [US]
Apo®-Prednisone [Can]
Aristocort® Forte Injection [US]
Aristocort® Intralesional Injection [US]
Aristocort® Tablet [US/Can]

Aristospan® Intraarticular Injection [US/Can]
Aristospan® Intralesional Injection [US/Can]
Betaject™ [Can]
betamethasone (systemic)
Betnesol® [Can]
Celestone® Phosphate [US]
Celestone® Soluspan® [US/Can]
Celestone® [US]
Cel-U-Jec® [US]
Cortef® Tablet [US/Can]
corticotropin
cortisone acetate
Cortone® [Can]
Decadron®-LA [US]
Decadron® [US/Can]
Decaject-LA® [US]
Decaject® [US]
Deltasone® [US]
Depo-Medrol® [US/Can]
Depopred® [US]
dexamethasone (systemic)
Dexasone® L.A. [US]
Dexasone® [US/Can]
Dexone® LA [US]
Dexone® [US]
Hexadrol® [US/Can]
H.P. Acthar® Gel [US]
hydrocortisone (systemic)
Kenalog® Injection [US/Can]
Medrol® Dosepak™ [US/Can]
Medrol® Tablet [US/Can]
methylprednisolone
Orapred™ [US]
Pediapred® [US/Can]
PMS-Dexamethasone [Can]
Prednicot® [US]
prednisolone (systemic)
Prednisol® TBA [US]
prednisone
Prednisone Intensol™ [US]
Prelone® [US]

ratio-Dexamethasone [Can]
Solu-Cortef® [US/Can]
Solu-Medrol® [US/Can]
Solurex L.A.® [US]
Sterapred® DS [US]
Sterapred® [US]
Tac™-3 Injection [US]
Triam-A® Injection [US]
triamcinolone (systemic)
Triam Forte® Injection [US]
Winpred™ [Can]

RHEUMATIC FEVER
Nonsteroidal Antiinflammatory Drug
    (NSAID)
Amigesic® [US/Can]
Argesic®-SA [US]
choline magnesium trisalicylate
Doan's®, Original [US-OTC]
Extra Strength Doan's® [US-OTC]
Keygesic-10® [US]
magnesium salicylate
Momentum® [US-OTC]
Mono-Gesic® [US]
Salflex® [US/Can]
salsalate
Tricosal® [US]
Trilisate® [US]
Penicillin
Bicillin® C-R 900/300 [US]
Bicillin® C-R [US]
penicillin G benzathine and
    procaine combined

RHEUMATOID ARTHRITIS
Analgesic, Nonnarcotic
Arthrotec® [US/Can]
diclofenac and misoprostol
Prostaglandin
Arthrotec® [US/Can]
diclofenac and misoprostol

RHINITIS
Adrenal Corticosteroid
AeroBid®-M [US]
AeroBid® [US]
Apo®-Beclomethasone [Can]
Apo®-Flunisolide [Can]
beclomethasone
Beconase® AQ [US]
budesonide
Decadron®-LA [US]
Decadron® [US/Can]
Decaject-LA® [US]
Decaject® [US]
Dexacort® Phosphate Turbinaire®
    [US]
dexamethasone (nasal)
dexamethasone (systemic)
Dexasone® L.A. [US]
Dexasone® [US/Can]
Dexone® LA [US]
Dexone® [US]
Entocort™ EC [US/Can]
Flonase® [US]
flunisolide
fluticasone (nasal)
Gen-Beclo [Can]
Gen-Budesonide AQ [Can]
Hexadrol® [US/Can]
Nasalide® [US/Can]
Nasarel® [US]
Nu-Beclomethasone [Can]
PMS-Dexamethasone [Can]
Propaderm® [Can]
Pulmicort® Nebuamp®
Pulmicort Respules® [US]
Pulmicort Turbuhaler® [US/Can]
QVAR™ [US/Can]
ratio-Dexamethasone [Can]
ratio-Flunisolide [Can]
Rhinalar® [Can]
Rhinocort® Aqua™ [US/Can]
Rivanase AQ [Can]
Solurex L.A.® [US]

Adrenergic Agonist Agent
  Afrin® Extra Moisturizing [US-OTC]
  Afrin® Original [US-OTC]
  Afrin® Severe Congestion [US-OTC]
  Afrin® Sinus [US-OTC]
  Afrin® [US-OTC]
  Balminil® Decongestant [Can]
  Balminil® Nasal Decongestant [Can]
  Biofed [US-OTC]
  Decofed® [US-OTC]
  Decongest [Can]
  Dimetapp® 12-Hour Non-Drowsy
    Extentabs® [US-OTC]
  Dimetapp® Decongestant [US-OTC]
  Dristan® Long Lasting Nasal [Can]
  Drixoral® Nasal [Can]
  Duramist® Plus [US-OTC]
  Duration® [US-OTC]
  Eltor® [Can]
  ephedrine
  Genaphed® [US-OTC]
  Genasal [US-OTC]
  Kidkare Decongestant [US-OTC]
  Kodet SE [US-OTC]
  Neo-Synephrine® 12 Hour Extra
    Moisturizing [US-OTC]
  Neo-Synephrine® 12 Hour [US-OTC]
  Nostrilla® [US-OTC]
  Optigene® 3 [US-OTC]
  Oranyl [US-OTC]
  oxymetazoline
  PediaCare® Decongestant Infants
    [US-OTC]
  PMS-Pseudoephedrine [Can]
  Pretz-D® [US-OTC]
  pseudoephedrine
  Pseudofrin [Can]
  Robidrine® [Can]
  Silfedrine Children's [US-OTC]
  Sudafed® 12 Hour [US-OTC]
  Sudafed® 24 Hour [US-OTC]
  Sudafed® Children's [US-OTC]
  Sudafed® [US-OTC]

  Sudodrin [US-OTC]
  tetrahydrozoline
  Triaminic® Allergy Congestion
    [US-OTC]
  Triaminic® Infant Decongestant [Can]
  Twice-A-Day® [US-OTC]
  Tyzine® Pediatric [US]
  Tyzine® [US]
  Vicks Sinex® 12 Hour Ultrafine
    Mist [US-OTC]
  4-Way® Long Acting [US-OTC]
  xylometazoline
Antihistamine
  Alavert™ [US-OTC]
  Allegra® [US/Can]
  Aller-Chlor® [US-OTC]
  Apo®-Cetirizine [Can]
  Apo®-Loratadine [Can]
  azatadine
  brompheniramine
  cetirizine
  chlorpheniramine
  Chlor-Trimeton® [US-OTC]
  Chlor-Tripolon® [Can]
  Claritin® RediTabs® [US]
  Claritin® [US-OTC/Can]
  clemastine
  Colhist® Solution [US-OTC]
  cyproheptadine
  dexchlorpheniramine
  Dimetane® Extentabs® [US-OTC]
  Dimetapp® Allergy Children's [US-
    OTC]
  Dimetapp® Allergy [US-OTC]
  fexofenadine
  Lodrane® 12 Hour [US-OTC]
  loratadine
  ND-Stat® Solution [US-OTC]
  Nolahist® [US/Can]
  Novo-Pheniram® [Can]
  Optimine® [US/Can]
  phenindamine

Polytapp® Allergy Dye-Free
  Medication [US-OTC]
Reactine™ [Can]
Tavist®-1 [US-OTC]
Tavist® [US]
Zyrtec® [US]
Antihistamine/Decongestant/Antitussive
  Cerose-DM® [US-OTC]
  chlorpheniramine, phenylephrine,
    and codeine
  chlorpheniramine, phenylephrine,
    and dextromethorphan
  Pediacof® [US]
Antihistamine/Decongestant
  Combination
  Allegra-D® [US/Can]
  Andehist NR Syrup [US]
  Benadryl® Allergy and Sinus
    Fastmelt™ [US-OTC]
  Benadryl® Allergy/Decongestant
    [US-OTC]
  Benadryl® Children's Allergy and
    Cold Fastmelt™ [US-OTC]
  Benadryl® Children's Allergy and
    Sinus [US-OTC]
  Brofed® [US]
  Bromanate® [US-OTC]
  Bromfed-PD® [US-OTC]
  Bromfed® [US-OTC]
  Bromfenex® PD [US]
  Bromfenex® [US]
  brompheniramine and
    pseudoephedrine
  Children's Dimetapp® Elixir Cold
    & Allergy [US-OTC]
  chlorpheniramine, phenylephrine,
    and phenyltoloxamine
  Chlor-Tripolon ND® [Can]
  Claritin-D® 12-Hour [US]
  Claritin-D® 24-Hour [US]
  Claritin® Extra [Can]
  Comhist® [US]

diphenhydramine and
  pseudoephedrine
fexofenadine and pseudoephedrine
loratadine and pseudoephedrine
Nalex®-A [US]
Rondec® Syrup [US]
Touro™ Allergy [US]
Antihistamine, Nonsedating
  Aerius® [Can]
  Clarinex® [US]
  desloratadine
Corticosteroid, Intranasal
  Elocon® [US/Can]
  mometasone furoate
  Nasonex® [US/Can]
Corticosteroid, Topical
  Nasacort® AQ [US/Can]
  triamcinolone (inhalation, nasal)
  Trinasal® [Can]
Decongestant/Analgesic
  Advil® Cold, Children's [US-OTC]
  Advil® Cold & Sinus [US/Can]
  Dristan® Sinus Caplets [US]
  Dristan® Sinus Tablet [US/Can]
  Motrin® Cold and Sinus [US-OTC]
  Motrin® Cold, Children's [US-OTC]
  pseudoephedrine and ibuprofen
Mast Cell Stabilizer
  Apo®-Cromolyn [Can]
  Crolom® [US]
  cromolyn sodium
  Gastrocrom® [US]
  Intal® [US/Can]
  Nalcrom® [Can]
  Nasalcrom® [US-OTC]
  Nu-Cromolyn [Can]
  Opticrom® [US/Can]
Phenothiazine Derivative
  Anergan® [US]
  Phenergan® [US/Can]
  promethazine

RHINITIS (ALLERGIC)

Antihistamine/Decongestant
    Combination
    cetirizine and pseudoephedrine
    Reactine® Allergy and Sinus [Can]
    Zyrtec-D 12 Hour™ [US]
Corticosteroid, Intranasal
    Elocon® [US/Can]
    mometasone furoate
    Nasonex® [US/Can]

RHINORRHEA

Anticholinergic Agent
    Apo®-Ipravent [Can]
    Atrovent® [US/Can]
    Gen-Ipratropium [Can]
    ipratropium
    Novo-Ipramide [Can]
    Nu-Ipratropium [Can]
    PMS-Ipratropium [Can]
    ratio-Ipratropium [Can]

ROENTGENOGRAPHY (LIVER)

Diagnostic Agent
    IC-Green® [US]
    indocyanine green

ROUNDWORM

Anthelmintic
    Combantrin™ [Can]
    mebendazole
    Pin-X® [US-OTC]
    pyrantel pamoate
    Reese's® Pinworm Medicine [US-OTC]
    Vermox® [US/Can]

RUBELLA

Vaccine, Live Virus
    measles, mumps, and rubella
        vaccines, combined
    Meruvax® II [US]
    M-M-R® II [US/Can]
    Priorix™ [Can]
    rubella virus vaccine (live)

SARCOIDOSIS

Corticosteroid, Topical
    Aclovate® [US]
    Acticort® [US]
    Aeroseb-HC® [US]
    alclometasone
    Alphatrex® [US]
    amcinonide
    Amcort® [Can]
    Anusol® HC-1 [US-OTC]
    Anusol® HC-2.5% [US-OTC]
    Aquacort® [Can]
    Aristocort® A Topical [US]
    Aristocort® Topical [US]
    Bactine® Hydrocortisone [US-OTC]
    Betaderm® [Can]
    Betamethacot® [US]
    betamethasone (topical)
    Betatrex® [US]
    Beta-Val® [US]
    Betnovate® [Can]
    CaldeCORT® Anti-Itch Spray [US]
    CaldeCORT® [US-OTC]
    Capex™ [US/Can]
    Carmol-HC® [US]
    Celestoderm®-EV/2 [Can]
    Celestoderm®-V [Can]
    Cetacort®
    clobetasol
    Clocort® Maximum Strength [US-OTC]
    clocortolone
    Cloderm® [US/Can]
    Cordran® SP [US]
    Cordran® [US/Can]
    Cormax® [US]
    CortaGel® [US-OTC]
    Cortaid® Maximum Strength [US-OTC]

Cortaid® with Aloe [US-OTC]
Cort-Dome® [US]
Cortizone®-5 [US-OTC]
Cortizone®-10 [US-OTC]
Cortoderm [Can]
Cutivate™ [US]
Cyclocort® [US/Can]
Del-Beta® [US]
Delcort® [US]
Dermacort® [US]
Dermarest Dricort® [US]
Derma-Smoothe/FS® [US/Can]
Dermatop® [US/Can]
Dermolate® [US-OTC]
Dermovate® [Can]
Dermtex® HC with Aloe [US-OTC]
Desocort® [Can]
desonide
DesOwen® [US]
Desoxi® [Can]
desoximetasone
diflorasone
Diprolene® AF [US]
Diprolene® [US/Can]
Diprosone® [Can]
Eldecort® [US]
Elocon® [US/Can]
Embeline™ E [US]
fluocinolone
fluocinonide
Fluoderm [Can]
flurandrenolide
fluticasone (topical)
Gen-Clobetasol [Can]
Gynecort® [US-OTC]
halcinonide
halobetasol
Halog®-E [US]
Halog® [US/Can]
Hi-Cor-1.0® [US]
Hi-Cor-2.5® [US]
Hyderm [Can]
hydrocortisone (topical)

Hydrocort® [US]
Hydro-Tex® [US-OTC]
Hytone® [US]
Kenalog® in Orabase® [US/Can]
Kenalog® Topical [US/Can]
LactiCare-HC® [US]
Lanacort® [US-OTC]
Lidemol® [Can]
Lidex-E® [US]
Lidex® [US/Can]
Locoid® [US/Can]
Luxiq™ [US]
Lyderm® [Can]
Maxiflor® [US]
Maxivate® [US]
mometasone furoate
Nasonex® [US/Can]
Novo-Clobetasol [Can]
Nutracort® [US]
Olux® [US]
Orabase® HCA [US]
Oracort [Can]
Penecort® [US]
PMS-Desonide [Can]
prednicarbate
Prevex® [Can]
Prevex® HC [Can]
Psorcon™ E [US]
Psorcon™ [US/Can]
Qualisone® [US]
ratio-Clobetasol [Can]
ratio-Ectosone [Can]
ratio-Topilene® [Can]
ratio-Topisone® [Can]
Sarna® HC [Can]
Scalpicin® [US]
S-T Cort® [US]
Synacort® [US]
Synalar® [US/Can]
Taro-Desoximetasone [Can]
Taro-Sone® [Can]
Tegrin®-HC [US-OTC]
Temovate E® [US]

Temovate® [US]
Tiamol® [Can]
Ti-U-Lac® H [Can]
Topicort®-LP [US]
Topicort® [US/Can]
Topsyn® [Can]
Triacet™ Topical [US]
Triaderm [Can]
triamcinolone (topical)
Tridesilon® [US]
U-Cort™ [US]
Ultravate™ [US/Can]
urea and hydrocortisone
Uremol® HC [Can]
Valisone® Scalp Lotion [Can]
Westcort® [US/Can]

SARCOMA
Antineoplastic Agent
Adriamycin® [Can]
Adriamycin PFS® [US]
Adriamycin RDF® [US]
Apo®-Methotrexate [Can]
Blenoxane® [US/Can]
bleomycin
Caelyx® [Can]
cisplatin
Cosmegen® [US/Can]
dacarbazine
dactinomycin
doxorubicin
DTIC® [Can]
DTIC-Dome® [US]
Ifex® [US/Can]
ifosfamide
methotrexate
Myocet® [Can]
Oncovin® [Can]
Platinol®-AQ [US]
Platinol® [US]
ratio-Methotrexate [Can]
Rheumatrex® [US]
Rubex® [US]

Trexall™ [US]
Velban® [Can]
vinblastine
Vincasar® PFS® [US/Can]
vincristine

SCABIES
Scabicides/Pediculicides
A-200™ [US-OTC]
Acticin® [US]
crotamiton
Elimite® [US]
End Lice® [US-OTC]
Eurax® Topical [US]
Hexit™ [Can]
Kwellada-P™ [Can]
lindane
Nix® Dermal Cream [Can]
Nix® [US/Can]
permethrin
PMS-Lindane [Can]
Pronto® [US-OTC]
pyrethrins
Pyrinex® Pediculicide [US-OTC]
Pyrinyl Plus® [US-OTC]
Pyrinyl® [US-OTC]
R & C™ II [Can]
R & C™ Shampoo/Conditioner
  [Can]
R & C® [US-OTC]
RID® Mousse [Can]
Rid® Spray [US-OTC]
Tisit® Blue Gel [US-OTC]
Tisit® [US-OTC]

SCLERODERMA
Aminoquinoline (Antimalarial)
Aralen® Phosphate [US/Can]
chloroquine phosphate
Chelating Agent
Cuprimine® [US/Can]
Depen® [US/Can]
penicillamine

SCURVY
Vitamin, Water Soluble
Apo®-C [Can]
ascorbic acid
C-500-GR™ [US-OTC]
Cecon® [US-OTC]
Cenolate® [US]
Cevi-Bid® [US-OTC]
C-Gram [US-OTC]
Dull-C® [US-OTC]
Proflavanol C™ [Can]
Revitalose C-1000® [Can]
sodium ascorbate
Vita-C® [US-OTC]

SEBORRHEIC DERMATITIS
Antiseborrheic Agent, Topical
AVAR™ Cleanser [US]
AVAR™ Green [US]
AVAR™ [US]
Aveeno® Cleansing Bar [US-OTC]
Balnetar® [US/Can]
Betatar® [US-OTC]
Capitrol® [US/Can]
chloroxine
Clenia™ [US]
coal tar
coal tar and salicylic acid
coal tar, lanolin, and mineral oil
Cutar® [US-OTC]
DHS™ Targel [US-OTC]
DHS™ Tar [US-OTC]
DHS™ Zinc [US-OTC]
Doak® Tar [US-OTC]
Estar® [US-OTC]
Exorex® [US]
Fostex® [US-OTC]
Head & Shoulders® Classic Clean 2-In-1 [US-OTC]
Head & Shoulders® Classic Clean [US-OTC]
Head & Shoulders® Dry Scalp Care [US-OTC]
Head & Shoulders® Extra Fullness [US-OTC]
Head & Shoulders® Intensive Treatment [US-OTC]
Head & Shoulders® Refresh [US-OTC]
Head & Shoulders® Smooth & Silky 2-In-1 [US-OTC]
Ionil T® Plus [US-OTC]
Ionil T® [US-OTC]
MG 217® Medicated Tar [US-OTC]
MG 217® [US-OTC]
Neutrogena® T/Gel Extra Strength [US-OTC]
Neutrogena® T/Gel [US-OTC]
Nocosyn™ [US]
Oxipor® VHC [US-OTC]
Pentrax® [US-OTC]
Pernox® [US-OTC]
Plexion SCT™ [US]
Plexion™ TS [US]
Plexion® [US]
Polytar® [US-OTC]
PsoriGel® [US-OTC]
pyrithione zinc
Reme-T™ [US-OTC]
Rosanil™ [US]
Rosula® [US]
Sastid® Plain Therapeutic Shampoo and Acne Wash [US-OTC]
Sebcur/T® [Can]
selenium sulfide
Selsun Blue® [US-OTC]
Selsun® [US]
Sulfacet-R® [US]
sulfur and salicylic acid
sulfur and sulfacetamide
Tarsum® [US-OTC]
Tegrin® [US-OTC]
Versel® [Can]
X-Seb™ T [US-OTC]
Zetacet® [US]
Zetar® [US-OTC]

Zincon® [USOTC]
ZNP® Bar [US-OTC]
Keratolytic Agent
  Compound W® One Step Wart
    Remover [US-OTC]
  Compound W® [US-OTC]
  DHS™ Sal [US-OTC]
  Dr. Scholl's® Callus Remover [US-
    OTC]
  Dr. Scholl's® Clear Away [US-OTC]
  Duoforte® 27 [Can]
  Freezone® [US-OTC]
  Fung-O® [US-OTC]
  Gordofilm® [US-OTC]
  Hydrisalic™[US-OTC]
  Ionil® Plus [US-OTC]
  Ionil® [US-OTC]
  Keralyt® [US-OTC]
  LupiCare™ Dandruff [US-OTC]
  LupiCare™ II Psoriasis [US-OTC]
  LupiCare™ Psoriasis [US-OTC]
  Mediplast® [US-OTC]
  MG217 Sal-Acid® [US-OTC]
  Mosco® Corn and Callus Remover
    [US-OTC]
  NeoCeuticals™ Acne Spot
    Treatment [US-OTC]
  Neutrogena® Acne Wash [US-OTC]
  Neutrogena® Body Clear™ [US-
    OTC]
  Neutrogena® Clear Pore Shine
    Control [US-OTC]
  Neutrogena® Clear Pore [US-OTC]
  Neutrogena® Healthy Scalp [US-
    OTC]
  Neutrogena® Maximum Strength
    T/Sal® [US-OTC]
  Neutrogena® On The Spot® Acne
    Patch [US-OTC]
  Occlusal™ [Can]
  Occlusal®-HP [US/Can]
  Oxy® Balance Deep Pore [US-OTC]
  Oxy Balance® [US-OTC]

  Palmer's® Skin Success Acne
    Cleanser [US-OTC]
  Pedisilk® [US-OTC]
  Propa pH [US-OTC]
  Sal-Acid® [US-OTC]
  Salactic® [US-OTC]
  SalAc® [US-OTC]
  salicylic acid
  Sal-Plant® [US-OTC]
  Sebcur® [Can]
  Soluver® [Can]
  Soluver® Plus [Can]
  Stri-dex® Body Focus [US-OTC]
  Stri-dex® Facewipes To Go™ [US-
    OTC]
  Stri-dex® Maximum Strength [US-
    OTC]
  Stri-dex® [US-OTC]
  Tinamed® [US-OTC]
  Tiseb® [US-OTC]
  Trans-Ver-Sal® [US-OTC/Can]
  Wart-Off® Maximum Strength [US-
    OTC]
  Zapzyt® Acne Wash [US-OTC]
  Zapzyt® Pore Treatment [US-OTC]

SINUSITIS

Adrenergic Agonist Agent
  Balminil® Decongestant [Can]
  Biofed [US-OTC]
  Decofed® [US-OTC]
  Dimetapp® 12-Hour Non-Drowsy
    Extentabs® [US-OTC]
  Dimetapp® Decongestant [US-
    OTC]
  Eltor® [Can]
  Genaphed® [US-OTC]
  Kidkare Decongestant [US-OTC]
  Kodet SE [US-OTC]
  Oranyl [US-OTC]
  PediaCare® Decongestant Infants
    [US-OTC]
  PMS-Pseudoephedrine [Can]

pseudoephedrine
Pseudofrin [Can]
Robidrine® [Can]
Silfedrine Children's [US-OTC]
Sudafed® 12 Hour [US-OTC]
Sudafed® 24 Hour [US-OTC]
Sudafed® Children's [US-OTC]
Sudafed® [US-OTC]
Sudodrin [US-OTC]
Triaminic® Allergy Congestion
  [US-OTC]
Triaminic® Infant Decongestant
  [Can]
Aminoglycoside (Antibiotic)
Alcomicin® [Can]
Diogent® [Can]
Garamycin® [US/Can]
Genoptic® [US]
Gentacidin® [US]
Gentak® [US]
gentamicin
ratio-Gentamicin [Can]
Antibiotic, Miscellaneous
Alti-Clindamycin [Can]
Apo®-Clindamycin [Can]
Cleocin HCl® [US]
Cleocin Pediatric® [US]
Cleocin Phosphate® [US]
Cleocin T® [US]
Cleocin® [US]
Clindagel™ [US]
ClindaMax [US]
clindamycin
Clindets® [US]
Clindoxyl® Gel [Can]
Dalacin® C [Can]
Dalacin® T [Can]
Novo-Clindamycin [Can]
ratio-Clindamycin [Can]
Antibiotic, Penicillin
pivampicillin (Canada only)
Pondocillin® [Can]

Antibiotic, Quinolone
ABC Pack™ (Avelox®) [US]
Avelox® [US/Can]
gatifloxacin
Levaquin® [US/Can]
levofloxacin
moxifloxacin
Quixin™ Ophthalmic [US]
Tequin® [US/Can]
Vigamox™ [US]
Zymar™ [US]
Antihistamine/Decongestant
  Combination
Benadryl® Allergy and Sinus
  Fastmelt™ [US-OTC]
Benadryl® Allergy/Decongestant
  [US-OTC]
Benadryl® Children's Allergy and
  Cold Fastmelt™ [US-OTC]
Benadryl® Children's Allergy and
  Sinus [US-OTC]
diphenhydramine and
  pseudoephedrine
Cephalosporin (First Generation)
Apo®-Cefadroxil [Can]
Apo®-Cephalex [Can]
Biocef® [US]
cefadroxil
cephalexin
cephradine
Duricef® [US/Can]
Keflex® [US]
Keftab® [US/Can]
Novo-Cefadroxil [Can]
Novo-Lexin® [Can]
Nu-Cephalex® [Can]
Velosef® [US]
Cephalosporin (Second Generation)
Apo®-Cefaclor [Can]
Apo®-Cefuroxime [Can]
Ceclor® CD [US]
Ceclor® [US/Can]
cefaclor

cefpodoxime
cefprozil
Ceftin® [US/Can]
cefuroxime
Cefzil® [US/Can]
Novo-Cefaclor [Can]
Nu-Cefaclor [Can]
PMS-Cefaclor [Can]
ratio-Cefuroxime [Can]
Vantin® [US/Can]
Zinacef® [US/Can]
Cephalosporin (Third Generation)
Cedax® [US]
cefdinir
cefixime
ceftibuten
Omnicef® [US/Can]
Suprax® [Can]
Cold Preparation
Aquatab® C [US]
Balminil DM + Decongestant +
Expectorant [Can]
Benylin® DM-D-E [Can]
Endal® [US]
Entex® LA [US]
guaifenesin and phenylephrine
guaifenesin, pseudoephedrine, and
dextromethorphan
Guiatuss™ CF [US]
Koffex DM + Decongestant +
Expectorant [Can]
Liquibid-D [US]
Maxifed® DM [US]
Novahistex® DM Decongestant
Expectorant [Can]
Novahistine® DM Decongestant
Expectorant [Can]
PanMist®-DM [US]
Prolex-D [US]
Protuss®-DM [US]
Pseudovent™ DM [US]
Robitussin® Cold and Congestion
[US-OTC]

Robitussin® Cough and Cold Infant
[US-OTC]
Touro™ CC [US]
Tri-Vent™ DM [US]
Decongestant/Analgesic
Advil® Cold, Children's [US-OTC]
Advil® Cold & Sinus [US/Can]
Dristan® Sinus Caplets [US]
Dristan® Sinus Tablet [US/Can]
Motrin® Cold and Sinus [US-OTC]
Motrin® Cold, Children's [US-OTC]
pseudoephedrine and ibuprofen
Expectorant/Decongestant
Ami-Tex PSE [US]
Anatuss LA [US]
Aquatab® D Dose Pack [US]
Aquatab® D [US]
Aquatab® [US]
Congestac® [US]
Deconsal® II [US]
Defen-LA® [US]
Duratuss™ GP [US]
Duratuss™ [US]
Entex® PSE [US]
Eudal®-SR [US]
G-Phed-PD [US]
G-Phed [US]
Guaifed-PD® [US]
Guaifed® [US-OTC]
guaifenesin and pseudoephedrine
Guaifenex® GP [US]
Guaifenex® PSE [US]
Guaifen PSE [US]
Guai-Vent™/PSE [US]
Maxifed-G® [US]
Maxifed® [US]
Miraphen PSE [US]
Novahistex® Expectorant With
Decongestant [Can]
PanMist® Jr. [US]
PanMist® LA [US]
PanMist® S [US]
Profen® II [US-OTC]

Pseudo GG TR [US]
Pseudovent™-Ped [US]
Pseudovent™ [US]
Respa-1st® [US]
Respaire®-60 SR [US]
Respaire®-120 SR [US]
Robitussin-PE® [US-OTC]
Robitussin® Severe Congestion
  [US-OTC]
Touro LA® [US]
V-Dec-M® [US]
Versacaps® [US]
Zephrex LA® [US]
Zephrex® [US]

Macrolide (Antibiotic)
Apo®-Erythro Base [Can]
Apo®-Erythro E-C [Can]
Apo®-Erythro-ES [Can]
Apo®-Erythro-S [Can]
Biaxin® [US/Can]
Biaxin® XL [US/Can]
clarithromycin
Diomycin® [Can]
dirithromycin
Dynabac® [US]
E.E.S.® [US/Can]
Erybid™ [Can]
Eryc® [US/Can]
EryPed® [US]
Ery-Tab® [US]
Erythrocin® [US]
erythromycin (systemic)
Nu-Erythromycin-S [Can]
PCE® [US/Can]
PMS-Erythromycin [Can]

Penicillin
Alti-Amoxi-Clav® [Can]
amoxicillin
amoxicillin and clavulanate
  potassium
Amoxicot® [US]
Amoxil® [US]
ampicillin

Apo®-Amoxi [Can]
Apo®-Amoxi-Clav® [Can]
Apo®-Ampi [Can]
Apo®-Cloxi [Can]
Augmentin ES-600™[US]
Augmentin® [US/Can]
Augmentin XR™ [US]
Clavulin® [Can]
cloxacillin
Gen-Amoxicillin [Can]
Lin-Amox [Can]
Marcillin® [US]
Moxilin® [US]
nafcillin
Novamoxin® [Can]
Novo-Ampicillin [Can]
Novo-Cloxin [Can]
Nu-Amoxi [Can]
Nu-Ampi [Can]
Nu-Cloxi® [Can]
oxacillin
PMS-Amoxicillin [Can]
Principen® [US]
ratio-AmoxiClav
Trimox® [US]

Quinolone
Apo®-Oflox [Can]
Ciloxan® [US/Can]
ciprofloxacin
Cipro® [US/Can]
Cipro® XR [US/Can]
Floxin® [US/Can]
lomefloxacin
Maxaquin® [US]
Ocuflox® [US/Can]
ofloxacin
sparfloxacin
Zagam® [US]

Sulfonamide
Apo®-Sulfatrim [Can]
Bactrim™ DS [US]
Bactrim™ [US]
Novo-Trimel [Can]

Novo-Trimel D.S. [Can]
Nu-Cotrimox® [Can]
Septra® DS [US/Can]
Septra® [US/Can]
sulfamethoxazole and trimethoprim
Sulfatrim® DS [US]
Sulfatrim® [US]
Tetracycline Derivative
Adoxa™ [US]
Alti-Minocycline [Can]
Apo®-Doxy [Can]
Apo®-Doxy Tabs [Can]
Apo®-Minocycline [Can]
Apo®-Tetra [Can]
Brodspec® [US]
Doryx® [US]
Doxy-100® [US]
Doxycin [Can]
doxycycline
Dynacin® [US]
EmTet® [US]
Gen-Minocycline [Can]
Minocin® [US/Can]
minocycline
Monodox® [US]
Novo-Doxylin [Can]
Novo-Minocycline [Can]
Novo-Tetra [Can]
Nu-Doxycycline [Can]
Nu-Tetra [Can]
oxytetracycline
Periostat® [US]
ratio-Doxycycline [Can]
ratio-Minocycline [Can]
Rhoxal-minocycline [Can]
Sumycin® [US]
Terramycin® I.M. [US/Can]
tetracycline
Vibramycin® [US]
Vibra-Tabs® [US/Can]
Wesmycin® [US]

SJÖGREN SYNDROME
Cholinergic Agent
cevimeline
Evoxac™ [US/Can]

SKIN INFECTION (TOPICAL THERAPY)
Antibacterial, Topical
ACU-dyne® [US-OTC]
Betadine® Ophthalmic [US]
Betadine® [US/Can]
hexachlorophene
Mersol® [US-OTC]
Merthiolate® [US-OTC]
Minidyne® [US-OTC]
Operand® [US-OTC]
pHisoHex® [US/Can]
povidone-iodine
Proviodine [Can]
Summer's Eve® Medicated Douche [US-OTC]
thimerosal
Vagi-Gard® [US-OTC]
Antibiotic/Corticosteroid, Topical
AntibiOtic® Ear [US]
bacitracin, neomycin, polymyxin B, and hydrocortisone
Cortimyxin® [Can]
Cortisporin® Cream [US]
Cortisporin® Ointment [US/Can]
Cortisporin® Ophthalmic [US/Can]
Cortisporin® Otic [US/Can]
NeoDecadron® Ocumeter® [US]
neomycin and dexamethasone
neomycin and hydrocortisone
neomycin, polymyxin B, and hydrocortisone
PediOtic® [US]
Antibiotic, Topical
Akne-Mycin® [US]
AK-Poly-Bac® [US]
AK-Tracin® [US]
Alcomicin® [Can]

Apo®-Metronidazole [Can]
Apo®-Tetra [Can]
A/T/S® [US]
Avagard™ [US-OTC]
Baciguent® [US/Can]
Baci-IM® [US]
bacitracin
bacitracin and polymyxin B
bacitracin, neomycin, and
  polymyxin B
bacitracin, neomycin, polymyxin B,
  and lidocaine
BactoShield® CHG [US-OTC]
Bactroban® Nasal [US]
Bactroban® [US/Can]
Betadine® First Aid Antibiotics +
  Moisturizer [US-OTC]
Betasept® [US-OTC]
Brodspec® [US]
ChloraPrep® [US-OTC]
chlorhexidine gluconate
Chlorostat® [US-OTC]
Clorpactin® WCS-90 [US-OTC]
Diogent® [Can]
Dyna-Hex® [US-OTC]
Emgel® [US]
EmTet® [US]
Erycette® [US]
EryDerm® [US]
Erygel® [US]
Erythra-Derm™ [US]
erythromycin (ophthalmic/topical)
Flagyl ER® [US]
Flagyl® [US/Can]
Florazole ER® [Can]
framycetin (Canada only)
Garamycin® [US/Can]
Genoptic® [US]
Gentacidin® [US]
Gentak® [US]
gentamicin
Hibiclens® [US-OTC]
LID-Pack® [Can]

MetroCream® [US/Can]
MetroGel® Topical [US/Can]
MetroGel-Vaginal® [US]
MetroLotion® [US]
metronidazole
mupirocin
Myciguent [US-OTC]
Mycitracin® [US-OTC]
Neo-Fradin™ [US]
neomycin
neomycin and polymyxin B
Neo-Rx [US]
Neosporin® Cream [Can]
Neosporin® G.U. Irrigant [US/Can]
Neosporin® Ophthalmic Ointment
  [US/Can]
Neosporin® Topical [US/Can]
Nidagel™ [Can]
Noritate® [US/Can]
Novo-Nidazol [Can]
Novo-Tetra [Can]
Nu-Tetra [Can]
Operand® Chlorhexidine Gluconate
  [US-OTC]
Optimyxin® Ophthalmic [Can]
oxychlorosene
Peridex® [US]
Periochip® [US]
PerioGard® [US]
Polysporin® Ophthalmic [US]
Polysporin® Topical [US-OTC]
ratio-Gentamicin [Can]
Romycin® [US]
Sofra-Tulle® [Can]
Spectrocin Plus® [US-OTC]
Staticin® [US]
Sumycin® [US]
tetracycline
Theramycin Z® [US]
Trikacide® [Can]
Triple Antibiotic® [US]
T-Stat® [US]
Wesmycin® [US]

Intravenous Nutritional Therapy
  alcohol (ethyl)
  Biobase™ [Can]
  Dilusol® [Can]
  Duonalc® [Can]
  Duonalc-E® Mild [Can]
  Lavacol® [US-OTC]
Topical Skin Product
  Campho-Phenique® [US-OTC]
  camphor and phenol
  Iodex [US-OTC]
  iodine
  Iodoflex™ [US]
  Iodosorb® [US]
  merbromin
  Mercurochrome® [US]

SKIN PROTECTANT
Pharmaceutical Aid
  benzoin
  TinBen® [US-OTC]

SKIN ULCER
Enzyme
  collagenase
  Santyl® [US/Can]

SOFT TISSUE INFECTION
Aminoglycoside (Antibiotic)
  Alcomicin® [Can]
  amikacin
  Amikin® [Can]
  Apo®-Tobramycin [Can]
  Diogent® [Can]
  Garamycin® [US/Can]
  Gentak® [US]
  gentamicin
  tobramycin
  Tobrex® [US/Can]
Antibiotic, Carbacephem
  Lorabid™ [US/Can]
  loracarbef
Antibiotic, Carbapenem

ertapenem
Invanz™ [US/Can]
Antibiotic, Miscellaneous
  Alti-Clindamycin [Can]
  Apo®-Clindamycin [Can]
  Cleocin HCl® [US]
  Cleocin Pediatric® [US]
  Cleocin Phosphate® [US]
  Cleocin T® [US]
  Cleocin® [US]
  Clindagel™ [US]
  ClindaMax [US]
  clindamycin
  Clindets® [US]
  Clindoxyl® Gel [Can]
  Dalacin® C [Can]
  Dalacin® T [Can]
  Novo-Clindamycin [Can]
  ratio-Clindamycin [Can]
  Vancocin® [US/Can]
  Vancoled® [US]
  vancomycin
Antibiotic, Penicillin
  pivampicillin (Canada only)
  Pondocillin® [Can]
Antibiotic, Quinolone
  Levaquin® [US/Can]
  levofloxacin
  Quixin™ Ophthalmic [US]
Antifungal Agent, Systemic
  Fucidin® [Can]
  Fucithalmic® [Can]
  fusidic acid (Canada only)
Cephalosporin (First Generation)
  Ancef® [US]
  Apo®-Cefadroxil [Can]
  Apo®-Cephalex [Can]
  Biocef® [US]
  cefadroxil
  cefazolin
  cephalexin
  cephalothin
  cephradine

Ceporacin® [Can]
Duricef® [US/Can]
Keflex® [US]
Keftab® [US/Can]
Novo-Cefadroxil [Can]
Novo-Lexin® [Can]
Nu-Cephalex® [Can]
Velosef® [US]
Cephalosporin (Second Generation)
   Apo®-Cefaclor [Can]
   Apo®-Cefuroxime [Can]
   Ceclor® CD [US]
   Ceclor® [US/Can]
   cefaclor
   Cefotan® [US/Can]
   cefotetan
   cefoxitin
   cefpodoxime
   cefprozil
   Ceftin® [US/Can]
   cefuroxime
   Cefzil® [US/Can]
   Mefoxin® [US/Can]
   Novo-Cefaclor [Can]
   Nu-Cefaclor [Can]
   PMS-Cefaclor [Can]
   ratio-Cefuroxime [Can]
   Vantin® [US/Can]
   Zinacef® [US/Can]
Cephalosporin (Third Generation)
   Cedax® [US]
   cefixime
   Cefizox® [US/Can]
   cefotaxime
   ceftazidime
   ceftibuten
   ceftizoxime
   ceftriaxone
   Claforan® [US/Can]
   Fortaz® [US/Can]
   Rocephin® [US/Can]
   Suprax® [Can]
   Tazicef® [US]

Tazidime® [US/Can]
Cephalosporin (Fourth Generation)
   cefepime
   Maxipime® [US/Can]
Macrolide (Antibiotic)
   azithromycin
   dirithromycin
   Dynabac® [US]
   Zithromax® [US/Can]
   Z-PAK® [US/Can]
Penicillin
   Alti-Amoxi-Clav® [Can]
   amoxicillin
   amoxicillin and clavulanate
     potassium
   Amoxicot® [US]
   Amoxil® [US]
   ampicillin
   ampicillin and sulbactam
   Apo®-Amoxi [Can]
   Apo®-Amoxi-Clav® [Can]
   Apo®-Ampi [Can]
   Apo®-Cloxi [Can]
   Apo®-Pen VK [Can]
   Augmentin ES-600™ [US]
   Augmentin® [US/Can]
   Augmentin XR™ [US]
   Bicillin® C-R 900/300 [US]
   Bicillin® C-R [US]
   Bicillin® L-A [US]
   carbenicillin
   Clavulin® [Can]
   cloxacillin
   dicloxacillin
   Gen-Amoxicillin [Can]
   Geocillin® [US]
   Lin-Amox [Can]
   Marcillin® [US]
   Moxilin® [US]
   Nadopen-V® [Can]
   nafcillin
   Novamoxin® [Can]
   Novo-Ampicillin [Can]

Novo-Cloxin [Can]
Novo-Pen-VK® [Can]
Nu-Amoxi [Can]
Nu-Ampi [Can]
Nu-Cloxi® [Can]
Nu-Pen-VK® [Can]
oxacillin
penicillin G benzathine
penicillin G benzathine and
   procaine combined
penicillin G (parenteral/aqueous)
penicillin G procaine
penicillin V potassium
Permapen® Isoject® [US]
Pfizerpen® [US/Can]
piperacillin
piperacillin and tazobactam sodium
Pipracil® [Can]
PMS-Amoxicillin [Can]
Principen® [US]
PVF® K [Can]
ratio-AmoxiClav
Suspen® [US]
Tazocin® [Can]
ticarcillin
ticarcillin and clavulanate potassium
Ticar® [US]
Timentin® [US/Can]
Trimox® [US]
Truxcillin® [US]
Unasyn® [US/Can]
Veetids® [US]
Wycillin® [US/Can]
Zosyn® [US]
Quinolone
   Apo®-Oflox [Can]
   Ciloxan® [US/Can]
   ciprofloxacin
   Cipro® [US/Can]
   Cipro® XR [US/Can]
   Floxin® [US/Can]
   lomefloxacin
   Maxaquin® [US]

   Ocuflox® [US/Can]
   ofloxacin

SOFT TISSUE SARCOMA
Antineoplastic Agent
   Adriamycin® [Can]
   Adriamycin PFS® [US]
   Adriamycin RDF® [US]
   Caelyx® [Can]
   Cosmegen® [US/Can]
   dactinomycin
   doxorubicin
   Myocet® [Can]
   Rubex® [US]

SOLAR LENTIGO
Retinoic Acid Derivative
   mequinol and tretinoin
   Solagae™ [US/Can]
Vitamin A Derivative
   mequinol and tretinoin
   Solagae™ [US/Can]
Vitamin, Topical
   mequinol and tretinoin
   Solagae™ [US/Can]

STOMATITIS
Local Anesthetic
   Cepacol® Maximum Strength [US-OTC]
   dyclonine
   Sucrets® [US-OTC]

SUNBURN
Nonsteroidal Antiinflammatory Drug
   (NSAID)
   Feldene® [US/Can]
   Gen-Piroxicam [Can]
   Novo-Pirocam® [Can]
   Nu-Pirox [Can]
   Pexicam® [Can]
   piroxicam

SUN OVEREXPOSURE
Sunscreen
    methoxycinnamate and oxybenzone
    PreSun® 29 [US-OTC]
    Ti-Screen® [US-OTC]

SURFACE ANTISEPTIC
Antibacterial, Topical
    benzalkonium chloride
    Benza® [US-OTC]
    3M™ Cavilon™ Skin Cleanser
      [US-OTC]
    Ony-Clear [US-OTC]
    Zephiran® [US-OTC]

SWEATING
Alpha-Adrenergic Blocking Agent
    Dibenzyline® [US/Can]
    phenoxybenzamine

SYPHILIS
Antibiotic, Miscellaneous
    chloramphenicol
    Chloromycetin® Parenteral
      [US/Can]
    Diochloram® [Can]
    Pentamycetin® [Can]
Penicillin
    Bicillin® L-A [US]
    penicillin G benzathine
    penicillin G (parenteral/aqueous)
    penicillin G procaine
    Permapen® Isoject® [US]
    Pfizerpen® [US/Can]
    Wycillin® [US/Can]
Tetracycline Derivative
    Adoxa™ [US]
    Apo®-Doxy [Can]
    Apo®-Doxy Tabs [Can]
    Apo®-Tetra [Can]
    Brodspec® [US]
    Doryx® [US]
    Doxy-100® [US]

Doxycin [Can]
doxycycline
EmTet® [US]
Monodox® [US]
Novo-Doxylin [Can]
Novo-Tetra [Can]
Nu-Doxycycline [Can]
Nu-Tetra [Can]
Periostat® [US]
ratio-Doxycycline [Can]
Sumycin® [US]
tetracycline
Vibramycin® [US]
Vibra-Tabs® [US/Can]
Wesmycin® [US]

SYSTEMIC LUPUS ERYTHEMATOSUS (SLE)
Aminoquinoline (Antimalarial)
    Apo®-Hydroxyquine [Can]
    hydroxychloroquine
    Plaquenil® [US/Can]
Antineoplastic Agent
    cyclophosphamide
    Cytoxan® [US/Can]
    Neosar® [US]
    Procytox® [Can]

TINEA
Antifungal Agent
    Absorbine Jr.® Antifungal [US-OTC]
    Aftate® Antifungal [US-OTC]
    Aloe Vesta® 2-n-1 Antifungal [US-OTC]
    Apo®-Ketoconazole [Can]
    Baza® Antifungal [US-OTC]
    Blis-To-Sol® [US-OTC]
    butenafine
    Canesten® Topical [Can]
    Canesten® Vaginal [Can]
    carbol-fuchsin solution
    Carrington Antifungal [US-OTC]
    ciclopirox

Clotrimaderm [Can]
clotrimazole
Cruex® [US-OTC]
Dermasept Antifungal [US-OTC]
econazole
Ecostatin® [Can]
Exelderm® [US/Can]
Femizol-M™ [US-OTC]
Fulvicin® P/G [US]
Fulvicin-U/F® [US/Can]
Fungi-Guard [US-OTC]
Fungi-Nail® [US-OTC]
Fungoid® Tincture [US-OTC]
Gold Bond® Antifungal [US-OTC]
Grifulvin® V Suspension [US]
griseofulvin
Gris-PEG® [US]
Gyne-Lotrimin® 3 [US-OTC]
Gyne-Lotrimin® [US-OTC]
Gynix® [US-OTC]
ketoconazole
Ketoderm® [Can]
Lamisil® Cream [US]
Loprox® [US/Can]
Lotrimin® AF Athlete's Foot Cream [US-OTC]
Lotrimin® AF Athlete's Foot Solution [US-OTC]
Lotrimin® AF Jock Itch Cream [US-OTC]
Lotrimin® AF Powder/Spray [US-OTC]
Lotrimin® Ultra™ [US-OTC]
Mentax® [US]
Micaderm® [US-OTC]
Micatin® [US/Can]
miconazole
Micozole [Can]
Micro-Guard® [US-OTC]
Mitrazol™ [US-OTC]
Monistat® 1 Combination Pack [US-OTC]
Monistat® 3 [US-OTC]
Monistat® 7 [US-OTC]
Monistat® [Can]
Monistat-Derm® [US]
Mycelex®-7 [US-OTC]
Mycelex® Twin Pack [US-OTC]
Myco-Nail [US-OTC]
naftifine
Naftin® [US]
Nizoral® A-D [US-OTC]
Nizoral® [US/Can]
Novo-Ketoconazole [Can]
oxiconazole
Oxistat® [US/Can]
Penlac™ [US/Can]
Pitrex [CAN]
sodium thiosulfate
Spectazole™ [US/Can]
sulconazole
terbinafine (topical)
Tinactin® Antifungal Jock Itch [US-OTC]
Tinactin® Antifungal [US-OTC]
Tinaderm [US-OTC]
Ting® [US-OTC]
TipTapToe [US-OTC]
tolnaftate
triacetin
Triple Care® Antifungal [OTC]
undecylenic acid and derivatives
Versiclear™ [US]
Zeasorb®-AF [US-OTC]
Antifungal/Corticosteroid
   betamethasone and clotrimazole
   Lotriderm® [Can]
   Lotrisone® [US/Can]
Antiseborrheic Agent, Topical
   Head & Shoulders® Intensive Treatment [US-OTC]
   selenium sulfide
   Selsun Blue® [US-OTC]
   Selsun® [US]
   Versel® [Can]
Disinfectant
   sodium hypochlorite solution

TISSUE GRAFT
Immunosuppressant Agent
  Apo®-Cyclosporine [Can]
  CellCept® [US/Can]
  cyclosporine
  Gengraf™ [US]
  muromonab-CD3
  mycophenolate
  Neoral® [US/Can]
  Orthoclone OKT® 3 [US/Can]
  Prograf® [US/Can]
  Protopic® [US]
  Restasis™ [US]
  Rhoxal-cyclosporine [Can]
  Sandimmune® [US/Can]
  tacrolimus

TRANSFUSION REACTION
Antihistamine
  Alavert™ [US-OTC]
  Aller-Chlor® [US-OTC]
  Allerdryl® [Can]
  AllerMax® [US-OTC]
  Allernix [Can]
  ANX® [US]
  Apo®-Hydroxyzine [Can]
  Apo®-Loratadine [Can]
  Atarax® [US/Can]
  azatadine
  Banophen® [US-OTC]
  Benadryl® Dye-Free Allergy [US-OTC]
  Benadryl® Injection [US]
  Benadryl® [US/Can]
  brompheniramine
  chlorpheniramine
  Chlor-Trimeton® [US-OTC]
  Chlor-Tripolon® [Can]
  Claritin® RediTabs® [US]
  Claritin® [US-OTC/Can]
  clemastine
  Colhist® Solution [US-OTC]
  cyproheptadine
  dexchlorpheniramine
  Dimetane® Extentabs® [US-OTC]
  Dimetapp® Allergy Children's [US-OTC]
  Dimetapp® Allergy [US-OTC]
  Diphen® AF [US-OTC]
  Diphenhist [US-OTC]
  diphenhydramine
  Diphen® [US-OTC]
  Genahist® [US-OTC]
  Hydramine® [US-OTC]
  hydroxyzine
  Hyrexin-50® [US]
  Lodrane® 12 Hour [US-OTC]
  loratadine
  ND-Stat® Solution [US-OTC]
  Nolahist® [US/Can]
  Novo-Hydroxyzin [Can]
  Novo-Pheniram® [Can]
  Optimine® [US/Can]
  phenindamine
  PMS-Diphenhydramine [Can]
  PMS-Hydroxyzine [Can]
  Polytapp® Allergy Dye-Free Medication [US-OTC]
  Siladryl® Allergy [US-OTC]
  Silphen® [US-OTC]
  Tavist®-1 [US-OTC]
  Tavist® [US]
  Vistaril® [US/Can]
Phenothiazine Derivative
  Anergan® [US]
  Phenergan® [US/Can]
  promethazine

ULCER, DIABETIC FOOT OR LEG
Topical Skin Product
  becaplermin
  Regranex® [US/Can]

URTICARIA

Antihistamine
Alavert™ [US-OTC]
Allegra® [US/Can]
Aller-Chlor® [US-OTC]
Apo®-Cetirizine [Can]
Apo®-Loratadine [Can]
azatadine
brompheniramine
cetirizine
chlorpheniramine
Chlor-Trimeton® [US-OTC]
Chlor-Tripolon® [Can]
Claritin® RediTabs® [US]
Claritin® [US-OTC/Can]
clemastine
Colhist® Solution [US-OTC]
cyproheptadine
Dimetane® Extentabs® [US-OTC]
Dimetapp® Allergy Children's [US-OTC]
Dimetapp® Allergy [US-OTC]
fexofenadine
Lodrane® 12 Hour [US-OTC]
loratadine
ND-Stat® Solution [US-OTC]
Nolahist® [US/Can]
Novo-Pheniram® [Can]
Optimine® [US/Can]
Panectyl® [Can]
phenindamine
Polytapp® Allergy Dye-Free
Medication [US-OTC]
Reactine™ [Can]
Tavist®-1 [US-OTC]
Tavist® [US]
trimeprazine (Canada only)
Zyrtec® [US]
Phenothiazine Derivative
Anergan® [US]
Phenergan® [US/Can]
promethazine

VAGINAL ATROPHY

Estrogen and Progestin Combination
Activella™ [US]
CombiPatch® [US]
estradiol and norethindrone

VAGINITIS

Antibiotic, Vaginal
sulfabenzamide, sulfacetamide, and
sulfathiazole
V.V.S.® [US]
Estrogen and Progestin Combination
estrogens and medroxyprogesterone
Premphase® [US/Can]
Prempro™ [US/Can]
Estrogen Derivative
Alora® [US]
Cenestin™ [US/Can]
Climara® [US/Can]
Congest [Can]
Delestrogen® [US/Can]
Depo®-Estradiol [US/Can]
diethylstilbestrol
Esclim® [US]
Estinyl® [US]
Estrace® [US/Can]
Estraderm® [US/Can]
estradiol
Estring® [US/Can]
Estrogel® [Can]
estrogens (conjugated A/synthetic)
estrogens (conjugated/equine)
estrone
ethinyl estradiol
Femring™ [US]
Gynodiol® [US]
Honvol® [Can]
Kestrone® [US/Can]
Oesclim® [Can]
Oestrilin [Can]
Premarin® [US/Can]
Vagifem® [US/Can]
Vivelle-Dot® [US]
Vivelle® [US/Can]

VARICELLA
Antiviral Agent
  acyclovir
  Apo®-Acyclovir [Can]
  foscarnet
  Foscavir® [US/Can]
  Gen-Acyclovir [Can]
  Nu-Acyclovir [Can]
  Zovirax® [US/Can]
Immune Globulin
  BayGam® [US/Can]
  immune globulin (intramuscular)
  varicella-zoster immune globulin
    (human)

VARICELLA-ZOSTER
Vaccine, Live Virus
  varicella virus vaccine
  Varivax® [US/Can]

VARICOSE ULCER
Protectant, Topical
  Granulex [US]
  trypsin, balsam Peru, and castor oil

VENEREAL WART
Biological Response Modulator
  Alferon® N [US/Can]
  interferon alfa-n3

VITILIGO
Psoralen
  methoxsalen
  8-MOP® [US/Can]
  Oxsoralen® Lotion [US/Can]
  Oxsoralen-Ultra® [US/Can]
  Ultramop™ [Can]
  Uvadex® [US/Can]
Topical Skin Product
  Benoquin® [US]
  monobenzone

WILSON DISEASE

Chelating Agent
  Syprine® [US/Can]
  trientine

WORMS
Anthelmintic
  Mintezol® [US]
  thiabendazole

XEROSTOMIA
Cholinergic Agent
  pilocarpine
  Salagen® [US/Can]

Appendix 7
Transplant Organizations

ORGAN PROCUREMENT ORGANIZATIONS

ALABAMA
Alabama Organ Center
500 22nd St. S, Ste. 102
Birmingham, AL 35233
Phone: (800) 252-3677
Fax: (205) 731-9250
Web: www.uab.edu/aoc

ALASKA
LifeCenter Northwest
1407 116th Ave NE Ste. E-210
Bellevue, WA 98004
Phone: (877) 275.5269
Web: www.lcnw.org

ARIZONA
Donor Network of Arizona
201 W. Coolidge
Phoenix, AZ 85013
Phone: (602) 222-2200, (800) 94-DONOR
Fax: (602) 222-2202
Web: www.dnaz.org

Donor Network of Arizona
1239 E. Prince
Tucson, AZ 85719
Phone: (520) 747-5500
Fax: (520) 747-5599
Web: www.dnaz.org

ARKANSAS
Arkansas Regional Organ Recovery Agency
1100 N. University Ave., Ste. 200
Little Rock, AR 72207
Phone: (501) 907-9150
Web: www.arora.org

Mid-America Transplant Services
c/o St. Bernard's Emergency Department
224 East Matthews
Jonesboro, AR 72401

Phone: (870) 972-4306
Fax: (870) 802-5138
Web: www.mts.stl.org

Mid-South Transplant Foundation
910 Madison Ave., Ste. 1002
Memphis, TN 38103
Phone: (901) 328-4438, (877) 228-LIFE
Web: www.midsouthtransplant.org

Southwest Transplant Alliance
3710 Rawlins, Ste. 1100
Dallas, TX 75219
Phone: (214) 522-0255, (800) 788-8058
Web: www.organ.org

CALIFORNIA
California Transplant Donor Network
1611 Telegraph Ave., Ste. 600
Oakland, CA 94612-2149
Phone: (510) 444-8500, (800) 570-9400
Fax: (510) 444-8501
24-hour Donor Referral: (800) 55-DONOR
Web: www.ctdn.org

Golden State Donor Service
1760 Creekside Oaks Dr., Ste. 160
Sacramento, CA 95833
Phone: (916) 567-1600
Web: www.gsds.org

Life Sharing Community Organ and Tissue
  Donation
3465 Camino Del Rio South, Ste. 410
San Diego, CA 92108
Phone: (619) 521-1983
Fax: (619) 521-2833
Web: www.lifesharing.org

One Legacy
S. Mark Taper Transplant Center
2200 W. 3rd St., Ste. 400
Los Angeles, CA 90057
Phone: (213) 413-6219
Fax: (213) 413-5373
24-hour Donor Referral: (800)338-6112
Web: www.onelegacy.org

COLORADO
Donor Alliance, Inc.
3773 Cherry Creek North Dr., Ste. 601
Denver, CO 80209
Phone: (303) 329-4747, (888) 686-4747
Fax: (303) 321-0366
Web: www.donoralliance.org

CONNECTICUT
LifeChoice Donor Services
Hartford Hospital
8 Griffin Rd. N.
Windsor, CT 06095
Phone: (800) 874-5215
Web: www.harthosp.org

New England Organ Bank
One Gateway Center
Newton, MA 02458-2803
Phone: (800) 446-NEOB
Web: www.neob.org

DELAWARE
Gift of Life Donor Program
2000 Hamilton St., Ste. 201
Philadelphia, PA 19130-3813
Phone: (800) 366-6771
Web: www.donors1.org

DISTRICT OF COLUMBIA
Washington Regional Transplant
  Consortium
8110 Gatehouse Rd., Ste. 101 West
Falls Church, VA 22042
Phone: (703) 641-0100, (866) 232-3666
Fax: (703) 641-0211
Web: www.wrtc.org

FLORIDA
LifeLink of Florida
409 Bayshore Blvd.
Tampa, FL 33606
Phone: (800) 262-5775
Web: www.lifelinkfound.org

LifeLink of Southwest Florida
12655 New Brittany Blvd., Bldg. 13
Ft. Myers, FL 33907
Phone: (800) 262-5775
Web: www.lifelinkfound.org

LifeQuest Organ Recovery Services
720 SW 2nd Ave., North Tower, Ste. 570
Gainesville, FL 32601
Phone: (352) 338-7133, (800) 535-GIVE
Fax: (352) 338-7135
Web: www.lifequestfla.org

LifeQuest Organ Recovery Services
580 W. 8th St., Tower II Ste. 8001
Jacksonville, FL 32209
Phone: (904) 244-9880, (800) 535-GIVE
Fax: (904) 244-9881
Web: www.lifequestfla.org

LifeQuest Organ Recovery Services
345 S. Magnolia Dr., Ste. A-11
Tallahassee, FL 32301
Phone: (352) 338-7133, (800) 535-GIVE
Fax: (850) 877-1150
Web: www.lifequestfla.org

LifeQuest Organ Recovery Services
5150 Bayou Blvd., Ste. 2K
Pensacola, FL 32503
Phone: (352) 338-7133, (800) 535-GIVE
Fax: (850) 478-8829
Web: www.lifequestfla.org

TransLife Organ/Tissue/Transplant Services
2501 N. Orange Ave., Ste. 514
Orlando, FL 32804
Phone: (407) 303-2474, (800) 443.6667
Fax: (407) 303-2473
Web: www.translife.org

GEORGIA
Alabama Organ Center
500 22nd St. S, Ste. 102
Birmingham, AL 35233
Phone: (800) 252-3677
Web: www.uab.edu/aoc

LifeLink of Georgia
2875 Northside Pkwy.
Norcross, GA 30071
Phone: (770) 225-5465
Web: www.lifelinkfound.org/georgia/ga.asp

LifeLink of Georgia
14 Chatham Center Dr., Suite B
Savannah, GA 31405
Web: www.lifelinkfound.org/georgia/ga.asp

LifeLink of Georgia
2743 Perimeter Pkwy., Bldg. 100, Ste. 120
Augusta, GA 30909
Web: www.lifelinkfound.org/georgia/ga.asp

HAWAII
Organ Donor Center of Hawaii
900 Fort Street Mall, Ste. 1140
Honolulu, HI 96813
Phone: (808) 599-7630
Fax: (808) 599-7631
Web: www.organdonorhawaii.com

IDAHO
Intermountain Donor Services
230 S. 500 E, Ste. 290
Salt Lake City, UT 84102
Phone: (801) 521-1755, (800) 833-6667
Fax: (801)364-8815
Web: www.idslife.org

LifeCenter Northwest
1407 116th Ave NE, Ste. E-210
Bellevue, WA 98004
Phone: (877) 275.5269
Web: www.lcnw.org

Pacific Northwest Transplant Bank
2611 SW 3rd Ave., Ste. 320
Portland, OR 97201-4952
Phone: (503) 494-5560
24-hour Donor Referral: (800)344-8916
Web: www.pntb.org

ILLINOIS
Mid-America Transplant Services
1139 Olivette Executive Pkwy.
St. Louis, MO 63132
Phone: (314) 991-1661
Fax: (314) 991-2805
Web: www.mts-stl.org

Mid-America Transplant Services
P.O. Box 190
Galatia, IL 62935
Phone: (618) 268-6025
Fax: (618) 268-6625
Web: www.mts-stl.org

Gift of Hope Organ and Tissue Donor
 Network
600 N. Industrial Dr.
Elmhurst, IL 60126
Phone: (630) 758-2600
Web: www.giftofhope.org

INDIANA
Indiana Organ Procurement Organization,
 Inc.
429 N. Pennsylvania St., Ste. 201
Indianapolis, IN 46204
Phone: (888) 275-4676
Web: www.iopo.org

Kentucky Organ Donor Affiliates
106 E. Broadway
Louisville, KY 40202
Phone: (502) 581-9511, (800) 525-3456
Web: www.kyorgandonor.org

LifeCenter Fund
2925 Vernon Pl., Ste. 300
Cincinnati, OH 45219
Phone: (800) 981-5433
Web: www.lifecnt.org

Gift of Hope Organ and Tissue Donor
  Network
600 N. Industrial Dr.
Elmhurst, IL 60126
Phone: (630) 758-2600
Web: www.giftofhope.org

IOWA
Iowa Donor Network
550 Madison Ave.
North Liberty, IA 52317
Phone: (319) 665-3787, (800) 831-4131
Fax: (319) 665-3788
Web: www.iadn.org

Iowa Donor Network
8191 Birchwood Court, Suite J
Johnston, IA 50131
Phone: (515) 727-7897, (800) 831-4131
Fax: (515) 727-7911
Web: www.iadn.org

Iowa Donor Network
4240 Hickory Ln, Suite D
Sioux City, IA 51106
Phone: (712) 274-8821, (800) 831-4131
Fax: (712) 274-8829
Web: www.iadn.org

Nebraska Organ Retrieval System
5725 F St.
Omaha, NE 68117
Phone: (402) 733-4000
Fax: (402) 733-9312
Web: www.NEdonation.org

KANSAS
Midwest Transplant Network
1900 W. 47th Pl., Ste. 400
Westwood, KS 66205
Phone: (913) 262-1668
Donor referral: (800) 366-6791
Fax: (913) 262-5130
Web: www.mwtn.org

KENTUCKY
Kentucky Organ Donor Affiliates
106 E. Broadway
Louisville, KY 40202
Phone: (502) 581-9511, (800) 525-3456
Web: www.kyorgandonor.org

LifeCenter Fund
2925 Vernon Pl., Ste. 300
Cincinnati, OH 45219
Phone: (800) 981-5433
Web: www.lifecnt.org

LOUISIANA
Louisiana Organ Procurement Agency
3501 N. Causeway Blvd., Ste. 940
Metarie, LA 70002-3626
Phone: (504) 837-3355, (800) 521-4483
Fax: (504) 837-3587
Web: www.lopa.org

MAINE
New England Organ Bank
One Gateway Center
Newton, MA 02458
Phone: 800-446-NEOB
Web: www.neob.org

MARYLAND
Transplant Resource Center of Maryland
1540 Caton Center Dr., Ste. R
Baltimore, MD 21227
Phone: (410) 242-7000, (800) 641-HERO
Fax: (410) 242-1871
Web: www.mdtransplant.org

Washington Regional Transplant
  Consortium
8110 Gatehouse Rd., Ste. 101 W
Falls Church, VA 22042
Phone: (703) 641-0100
Web: www.wrtc.org

MASSACHUSETTS
New England Organ Bank
One Gateway Center
Newton, MA 02458
Phone: 800-446-NEOB
Web: www.neob.org

LifeChoice Donor Services
Hartford Hospital
8 Griffin Rd. N
Windsor, CT 06095
Phone: (800) 874-5215
Web: www.harthosp.org

MICHIGAN
Gift of Life Michigan
2203 Platt Rd.
Ann Arbor, MI 48104
Phone: (800) 482-4881
Web: www.tsm-giftoflife.org

University of Wisconsin Hospital and
  Clinics Organ Procurement Organization
600 Highland Ave.
Madison, WI 53792
Phone: (608)263-0356
Web: www.uwhealth.org

MINNESOTA
LifeSource, Upper Midwest Organ
  Procurement Organization, Inc.
2550 University Ave. W, Ste. 315 S
St. Paul, MN 55114-1904
Phone: (651) 603-7833, (888) 5DONATE
Fax: (651) 603-7801
Web: www.life-source.org

MISSISSIPPI
Mississippi Organ Recovery Agency
12 River Bend Pl.
Jackson, MS 39232
Phone: (601) 933-1000, (800) 690-8878
Fax: (601) 933-1006
Web: www.msora.org

Mid-South Transplant Foundation
910 Madison Ave., Ste. 1002
Memphis, TN 38103
Phone: (901) 328-4438, (877) 228-LIFE
Web: www.midsouthtransplant.org

MISSOURI
Mid-America Transplant Services
1139 Olivette Executive Pkwy.
St. Louis, MO 63132
Phone: (314) 991-1661
Fax: (314) 991-2805
Web: www.mts-stl.org

Mid-America Transplant Services
121 Broadview, Ste. 1
Cape Girardeau, MO 63703
Phone: (573) 332-0070
Fax: (573) 332-0080
Web: www.mts-stl.org

Mid-America Transplant Services
3854 South Ave.
Springfield, MO 65807
Phone: (417) 886-2500
Fax: (417) 886-2515
Web: www.mts-stl.org

Midwest Transplant Network
1900 W. 47th Pl., Ste. 400
Westwood, KS 66205
Phone: (913) 262-1668
Fax: (913) 262-5130
Web: www.mwob.org

MONTANA
LifeCenter Northwest
1407 116th Ave. NE Suite E-210
Bellevue, WA 98004
1.877.275.5269
Web: www.lcnw.org

NEBRASKA
Nebraska Organ Retrieval System
5725 F St.
Omaha, NE 68117
Phone: (402) 733-1800, (877) 633-1800
Web: www.nedonation.org

Iowa Donor Network
550 Madison Ave.
North Liberty, IA 52317
Phone: (319) 665-3787
Fax: (319) 665-3788
Web: www.iadn.org

NEVADA
Nevada Donor Network, Inc.
2085 E. Sahara
Las Vegas, NV 89104
Phone: (702) 796-9600
Web: www.nvdonor.org

California Transplant Donor Network
1611 Telegraph Ave., Ste. 600
Oakland, CA 94612-2149
Phone: (510) 444-8500, (888) 570-9400
Fax: (510) 444-8501
Web: www.ctdn.org

NEW HAMPSHIRE
New England Organ Bank
One Gateway Center
Newton, MA 02458-2803
Phone: (800) 446-NEOB
Web: www.neob.org

NEW JERSEY
New Jersey Organ and Tissue Donation
  Services
841 Mountain Ave.
Springfield, NJ 07081
Phone: (973) 379-4535
Web: www.sharenj.org

Gift of Life Donor Program
2000 Hamilton St., Ste. 201
Philadelphia, PA 19130-3813
Phone: (215) 557-8090, (800) 366-6771
Web: www.donors1.org

NEW MEXICO
New Mexico Donor Services
2715 Broadbent Pkwy., Ste. J
Albuquerque, NM 87107
Phone: (800) 843-7672
Web: www.dcids.org

NEW YORK
Center for Donation and Transplant
218 Great Oaks Blvd.
Albany, NY 12203
Phone: (518) 262-5606, (800) 256-7811
Web: www.cdtny.org

Center for Organ Recovery & Education
204 Sigma Dr.
RIDC Park
Pittsburgh, PA 15238
Phone: (800) 366-6777
Fax: (412) 963-3564
Web: www.core.org

New York Organ Donor Network, Inc.
475 Riverside Dr., Ste. 1244
New York, NY 10115-1244
Phone: (212) 870-2240
24-Hour Referral Line: (800) GIFT-4-NY
Fax: (212) 870-3299
Web: www.nyodn.org

Upstate New York Transplant Services, Inc.
165 Genesee St.
Buffalo, NY 14203
Phone: (716) 853-6667, (800) 227-4771
Fax: (716) 853-6674
Web: www.unyts.org

Finger Lakes Donor Recovery Network
Corporate Woods of Brighton
Building 30, Ste. 220
Rochester, NY 14623
Phone: (800) 810-5494
Fax: (585) 272-4956
Web: www.donorrecovery.org

NORTH CAROLINA
Carolina Donor Services
3622 Lyckan Pkwy., Ste. 6002
Durham, NC 27707
Phone: (919) 489-8404
Web: www.carolinadonorservices.org

LifeShare of the Carolinas
5000-D Airport Center Pkwy.
Charlotte, NC 28208
Phone: (704) 697-3303
Fax: (704) 697-3056
Web: www.lifesharecarolinas.org

LifeNet
5809 Ward Ct.
Virginia Beach, VA 23455
Phone: (757) 464-4761, (800) 847-7831
Fax: (757) 464-5721
Web: www.lifenet.org

OHIO
LifeBanc
20600 Chagrin Blvd., Ste. 350
Cleveland, OH 44122-5343
Phone: (216) 752-5433, (888) 558-5433
Fax: (216) 751-4204
Web: www.lifebanc.org

Life Connection of Ohio
1545 Holland Rd., Ste. C
Maumee, OH 43537-1694
Phone: (419) 893-4891, (800) 262-5443
Fax: (419) 893-1827
Web: www.lifeconnectionofohio.org

Lifeline of Ohio Organ Procurement Agency
770 Kinnear Rd., Ste. 200
Columbus, OH 43212
Phone: (800) 525-5667
Fax: (614) 291-0660
Web: www.lifelineofohio.org

LifeCenter Fund
2925 Vernon Pl., Ste. 300
Cincinnati, OH 45219
Phone: (800) 981-5433
Web: www.lifecnt.org

Kentucky Organ Donor Affiliates
106 E. Broadway
Louisville, KY 40202
Phone: (502) 581-9511, (800) 525-3456
Web: www.kyorgandonor.org

OKLAHOMA
LifeShare Transplant Donor Services of
  Oklahoma, Inc.
5801 N. Broadway, Ste. 300
Oklahoma City, OK 73118
Phone: (888) 580-5680
Fax: (405) 840-9748
Web: www.oosn.org

OREGON
Pacific Northwest Transplant Bank
2611 SW 3rd Ave., Ste. 320
Portland, OR 97201-4952
Phone: (503) 494-5560
Fax: (503) 494-4725
24-hour donor referral: (800) 344-8916
Web: www.pntb.org

PENNSYLVANIA
Center for Organ Recovery & Education
204 Sigma Dr.
RIDC Park
Pittsburgh, PA 15238
Phone: (800) 366-6777
Fax: (412) 963-3564
Web: www.core.org

Gift of Life Donor Program
2000 Hamilton St., Ste. 201
Philadelphia, PA 19130-3813
Phone: (800) 366-6771
Web: www.donors1.org

New York Organ Donor Network, Inc.
475 Riverside Dr., Ste. 1244
New York, NY 10115-1244
Phone: (212) 870-2240
24-Hour Referral Line: (800) GIFT-4-NY
Fax: (212) 870-3299
Web: www.nyodn.org

PUERTO RICO
LifeLink of Puerto
Daimler-Chrysler Building, Suite 100
Calle 1 #1, Metro Office Park
Guaynabo, Puerto Rico 00968
Phone: (787) 277-0900, (800)558-0977
www.lifelinkfound.org

RHODE ISLAND
New England Organ Bank
One Gateway Center
Newton, MA 02458-2803
Phone: (800) 446-NEOB
Web: www.neob.org

SOUTH CAROLINA
LifePoint Inc. Organ & Eye Tissue Services
  for South Carolina
1064 Gardner Rd., Ste. 105
Charleston, SC 29407-5711
Phone: (800) 462-0755
Web: www.lifepoint-sc.org

LifeLink of Georgia
2875 Northside Pkwy.
Norcross, GA 30071
Phone: (770) 225-5465
Web: www.lifelinkfound.org/georgia/ga.asp

SOUTII DAKOTA
LifeSource, Upper Midwest Organ
  Procurement Organization, Inc.
2550 University Ave. W, Ste. 315 South
St. Paul, MN 55114-1904
Phone: (651) 603-7833, (888) 5DONATE
Fax: (651) 603-7801
Web: www.life-source.org

TENNESSEE
Mid-South Transplant Foundation
910 Madison Ave., Ste. 1002
Memphis, TN 38103
Phone: (901) 328-4438, (877) 228-LIFE
Web: www.midsouthtransplant.org

Tennessee Donor Services
651 E. 4th St., Ste. 402
University Tower
Chattanooga, TN 37403
Phone: (423) 756-5736
Web: www.dcids.org

Tennessee Donor Services
7015 Middlebrook Pike
Knoxville, TN 37909
Phone: (865) 588-1031
Web: www.dcids.org

Tennessee Donor Services
1600 Hayes St., Ste. 300
Nashville, TN
Phone: (615) 234-5251, (888) 234-4440
Web: www.dcids.org

TEXAS
LifeGift Organ Donation Center
5615 Kirby Dr., Ste. 900
Houston, TX 77005
Phone: (713) 523-4438, (800) 633-6562
Fax: (713) 737-8100
Web: www.lifegift.org

Texas Organ Sharing Alliance
8122 Datapoint
San Antonio, TX 78229
Phone: (210) 614-7030
Web: www.txorgansharing.org

Southwest Transplant Alliance
3710 Rawlins, Ste. 1100
Dallas, TX 75219
Phone: (214) 522-0255, (800) 788-8058
Web: www.organ.org

UTAH
Intermountain Donor Services
230 S. 500 E, Ste. 290
Salt Lake City, UT 84102
Phone: (801) 521-1755, (800) 833-6667
Fax: (801)364-8815
Web: www.idslife.org

VERMONT
Center for Donation and Transplant
218 Great Oaks Blvd.
Albany, NY 12203
Phone: (518) 262-5606, (800) 256-7811
Web: www.cdtny.org

New England Organ Bank
One Gateway Center
Newton, MA 02458-2803
Phone: (800) 446-NEOB
Web: www.neob.org

VIRGINIA
LifeNet
5809 Ward Ct.
Virginia Beach, VA 23455
Phone: (757) 464-4761, (800) 847-7831
Fax: (757) 464-5721
Web: www.lifenet.org

Washington Regional Transplant
  Consortium
8110 Gatehouse Rd., Ste. 101 W
Falls Church, VA 22042
Phone: (703) 641-0100
Web: www.wrtc.org

Carolina Donor Services
205 Plaza Dr., Suite D
Greenville, NC 27858
Phone: (252) 757-0090
Fax: (252) 757-0708
Web: www.carolinadonorservices.org

WASHINGTON
LifeCenter Northwest
1407 116th Ave. NE Suite E-210
Bellevue, WA 98004
1.877.275.5269
Web: www.lcnw.org

Pacific Northwest Transplant Bank
2611 SW 3rd Ave., Ste. 320
Portland, OR 97201-4952
Phone: (503) 494-5560
24-hour Donor Referral: (800)344-8916
Web: www.pntb.org

WEST VIRGINIA
Center for Organ Recovery & Education
204 Sigma Dr.
RIDC Park
Pittsburgh, PA 15238
Phone: (800) 366-6777
Fax: (412) 963-3564
Web: www.core.org

Kentucky Organ Donor Affiliates
106 E. Broadway
Louisville, KY 40202
Phone: (502) 581-9511, (800) 525-3456
Web: www.kyorgandonor.org

Lifeline of Ohio Organ Procurement Agency
770 Kinnear Rd., Ste. 200
Columbus, OH 43212
Phone: (800) 525-5667
Fax: (614) 291-0660
Web: www.lifelineofohio.org

LifeNet
5809 Ward Ct.
Virginia Beach, VA 23455
Phone: (757) 464-4761, (800) 847-7831
Fax: (757) 464-5721
Web: www.lifenet.org

WISCONSIN
Wisconsin Donor Network
9200 W. Wisconsin
Milwaukee, WI 53226
Phone: (414) 805-2024, (800) 432-5406
Web: www.wisdonornetwork.org

University of Wisconsin Hospital and
  Clinics Organ Procurement Organization
600 Highland Ave.
Madison, WI 53792
Phone: (608)263-0356
Web: www.uwhealth.org

WYOMING
Intermountain Donor Services
230 S. 500 E, Ste. 290
Salt Lake City, UT 84102
Phone: (801) 521-1755, (800) 833-6667
Fax: (801)364-8815
Web: www.idslife.org

Donor Alliance, Inc.
3773 Cherry Creek N Dr., Ste. 601
Denver, CO 80209
Phone: (303) 329-4747, (888) 868-4747
Fax: (303) 321-0366
Web: www.donoralliance.org

ORGAN AND TISSUE ORGANIZATIONS

AMERICAN ASSOCIATION OF TISSUE BANKS
1320 Old Chain Bridge Rd., Ste. 450
McLean, VA 22101
Phone: (703) 827-9582
Fax: (703) 356-2198
Web: www.aatb.org

AMERICAN RED CROSS NATIONAL TISSUE SERVICES
c/o American Red Cross National
  Headquarters
2025 E Street, NW
Washington, DC 20006
Phone: (202) 303-4498, (800) 4-TISSUE
Web: www.redcross.org

COALITION ON DONATION
700 N. 4th Ave.
Richmond, VA 23219
Phone: (804) 782-4920
Fax: (804) 782-4643

Web: www.shareyourlife.org

EYE BANK ASSOCIATION OF AMERICA
1015 18th St. NW, Ste. 1010
Washington, DC 20036
Phone: (202) 775-4999
Fax: (202) 429-6036
Web: www.restoresight.org

LIFENET
5809 Ward Ct.
Virginia Beach, VA 23455
Phone: (757) 464-4761, (800) 847-7831
Fax: (757) 464-5721
Web: www.lifenet.org

JAMES REDFORD INSTITUTE FOR TRANSPLANT AWARENESS PRESIDENT AND FOUNDER
Annie Aft, Executive Director
10573 W. Pico Blvd., Ste. 214
Los Angeles, CA 90064-2348
Phone: (310) 559-6325
Fax: (310) 559-6370
Web: www.jrifilms.org

MINORITY ORGAN TISSUE TRANSPLANT EDUCATION PROGRAM
2041 Georgia Ave., NW
Ambulatory Care Center, Ste. 3100
Washington, DC 20060
Phone: (202) 865-4888, (800) 393-2839
Fax: (202) 865-4880
Web: www.nationalmottep.org

MUSCULOSKELETAL TRANSPLANT FOUNDATION
125 May St.
Edison, NJ 08837
Phone: (732) 661-0202
Fax: (732) 661-2298
Web: www.mtf.org

NATIONAL DONOR FAMILY COUNCIL
c/o National Kidney Foundation
30 E. 33rd St.
New York, NY 10016
Phone: (212) 889-2210, (800) 622-9010
Fax: (212) 689-9261
Web: www.kidney.org

NATIONAL MINORITY ORGAN AND TISSUE TRANSPLANT EDUCATION PROGRAM
2041 Georgia Ave., NW
Ambulatory Care Center, Ste. 3100
Washington, DC 20060
Phone: (202) 856-4888, (800) 393-2839
Fax: (202) 865-4880
Web: www.nationalmottep.org

NATIONAL TRANSPLANT ACTION COMMITTEE
Craig Irwin, President
Box 5357
Aloha, OR 97006
Phone: (503) 690-8265
Fax: (503) 629-8199

TISSUE BANKS INTERNATIONAL
815 Park Ave.
Baltimore, MD 21201
Phone: (410) 752-3800
Fax: (410) 783-0183
Web: www.tbionline.org

TRANSPLANT RECIPIENTS INTERNATIONAL ORGANIZATION, INC.
2117 L St. NW, Ste. 353
Washington, DC 20037
Phone: (202) 293-0980, (800) TRIO-386
Web: www.trioweb.org

Wendy Marx Foundation
Jeffrey Marx
Wendy Marx Foundation for Organ Donor
  Awareness
322 South Carolina Ave. SE, Ste. 201
Washington, DC 20003
Phone: (202) 546-7270
Web: www.transplantbook.com